Manual of Hospital Planning and Designing

Ajay Garg • Anil Dewan

Manual of Hospital Planning and Designing

For Medical Administrators, Architects and Planners

Springer

Ajay Garg
Hospital Administration
Teerthanker Mahaveer University
Moradabad, India

Anil Dewan
School of Planning
and Architecture Delhi
New Delhi, India

ISBN 978-981-16-8455-5 ISBN 978-981-16-8456-2 (eBook)
https://doi.org/10.1007/978-981-16-8456-2

This Springer imprint is published by the registered company Springer Nature Singapore Pte Ltd.
The registered company address is: 152 Beach Road, #21-01/04 Gateway East, Singapore 189721, Singapore

First and foremost, we would like to thank God. We could never have done this without the faith we have in God, the Almighty.

My late father Dr. R.N. Gupta for his blessings and my mother Mrs. Santosh Gupta for inspiring me to write this book.

My wife, Mohini Garg

who was the main person by my corner, pushing me to share my experience by writing this book. You are my love and inspiration! Thanks for not just believing but knowing that I could do this! I Love You Always and Forever!

To my children, Dr. Megha Garg and Parth Garg

The hard work that you put into this book and all the suggestions and improvements that you made to it have not just made this book better but have also strengthened our bond. I wish you both all the happiness and success in this world.

—Ajay Garg

My late father Dewan Hargopal for nurturing me, My Mother Shanta Rani for having faith in me, My wife, Poonam

for being my steady anchor and moral support.

My son, Gandharv

for constant encouragement and belief in me.

My students—past, present, and future—and teachers who always inspired me for academic excellence.

—Prof. Dr. Anil Dewan

Preface

As compared to any other commercial buildings, the hospital buildings are one of the most complex buildings/projects to plan, design, build, and operate. There is a direct relation between the design of hospitals and satisfaction experienced by patients, staff, and family members of the patient. The better the planning and designing, the greater will be the impact on the performance of the hospital.

Once the hospital building is planned and executed, the redesigning of hospital or modifications in the building are generally difficult and not feasible. As hospital projects involve huge investment and once constructed, it is usually not feasible to change the design and plan again and again.

Furthermore, it is also equally true that the good planning and designing of the hospital services contributes a lot to reduce errors, decrease the rate of infection and cross infection and accidents due to falls of the patients, protect staff from injury, increase patient's recovery rate from disease and sufferings, and also increase staff satisfaction.

Over a period of time, after visiting many hospitals, right from small nursing homes to the large corporate hospitals, we had noticed that there were a lot of designing faults, e.g., the beds were not laid down properly and adequate working spaces were not provided; the nursing station was not at the desired location; the required electrical points were not provided or if provided were not properly located; no proper barriers were provided for separation of different zones for infection control; the sizes of the rooms were not proper (either they were too small or they were too large); the room temperature or humidity was not controlled as required; and others like security, safety, and hygiene were not addressed to.

After seeing such a state of affairs of hospitals in respect of the poor quality of designing and planning, we were really upset. The promoters generally feel comfortable by planning and designing the hospital building based on their own experience or otherwise take the help of inexperienced friends, architects, or other persons to plan and design the hospital building. This results in inappropriate designing of the building.

We being in the healthcare industry for about 40 years, wherein we were deeply involved in the planning, designing, operations, and management of the hospital, share our experiences of planning, designing, and setting up a hospital. Therefore, this book has been written.

In this book, we have tried to detail out all the phases and steps involved in planning and designing. We have also tried to detail out the room, areas, or zones required in the hospital. After that we have elaborated the important department of the hospital along with the MEP services in detail.

We have tried to share our experiences in depth such as the location and number of electrical and communication points, the environmental details of the rooms, and the size and location of different rooms and areas.

Please note the details given in this book are based purely on the practicality of the working conditions as per our personal experience. Though we have tried to highlight the norms of various accreditation agencies like JCI and NABH, but still the promoters are advised to go through the norms of the agencies/government, applicable in their respective countries. If you feel that any of the details given in this book are not correct, it may be true for you or your country and may not be true for other countries. The requirement of the spaces and facilities varies from user to user or from country to country. Hence you may consider those issues which you may feel to be beneficial to you, and rest of the issues may be ignored.

We have tried to write this book in very easily understandable English. This book may be of great help to the students and small and large hospital promoters, planners, and designers.

Moradabad, India Ajay Garg
New Delhi, India Anil Dewan

Acknowledgments

We are thankful to Mr. Suresh Jain the Chancellor and Mr. Manish Jain the Group Vice-Chairman of Teerthanker Mahaveer University, Moradabad, and Director Prof. Dr. PSN Rao, Dean Academics, Prof. Dr. Ashok Kumar and Dean Research Prof. Dr. Sanjay Gupta of the School of Planning and Architecture, New Delhi, for providing us the platform for learning and gaining experiences in the field of health care. Without your support and inputs, it would have been difficult to write this book and share our experiences. Here, we would also like to thank Mr. Abhisekh Kapoor for providing us all his help in writing this book.

Extending our gratitude toward Dr. Rohit Varshney, we would like to thank him for his constant support toward our vision, regular discussions, and brainstorming sessions during the compilation of this book and his guidance on many small questions and tasks. We would also like to thank him for helping us in compiling and sharing his experiences in a few chapters of this book.

We would also like to extend thanks to Ar. Sandal Kapoor and his office Sandal Kapoor Associates for sharing project details which are adapted for this book and Ar. Arif Ali for helping us with the illustrations.

Lastly, we would like to thank each one who believed in our vision and supported us throughout this amazing journey. We hope this book helps everyone in some way and collectively we can make the medical society achieve great heights.

Thank You!

Ajay Garg
Prof. Dr. Anil Dewan

Introduction

As compared to any other commercial buildings, the hospital buildings are one of the most complex buildings/projects to plan, design, build, and operate. A well-planned and designed hospital contributes a lot to reduce errors, decrease or control infection rate, protect patients and staff from injury, increase patient's recovery rate, and increase staff satisfaction.

It is noticed that the promoters or the designers usually make a lot of mistakes in designing the hospital setup. Some of them may be small but have a lot of impact on the efficient working of the hospital. Once the hospital is functional, it becomes very difficult to make changes and alterations.

In this book, we have tried to address all such issues and detailed out all the phases and steps involved in planning and designing and the room, areas, or zones required in the hospital. Elaborated details of all the important department/units of the hospital along with the MEP services have been provided. Also, in-depth details of the services like the location and number of electrical and communication points, the environment of rooms, and the size and location of rooms have been mentioned. This book also describes about the furniture required in the hospital.

The book has been written keeping in mind the easy and effective movement of men, material, and patients. Special consideration has been given to infection control. The book has been written keeping in mind the norms of the accreditation agencies like JCI/NABH.

This book will be helpful to the designers and promoters in understanding the requirements well in advance. As the book is in very easily understandable English, it may be of great help to the students of hospital management, paramedical sciences, and architecture and small and large hospital promoters, planners, and designers.

Ajay Garg
Prof. Dr. Anil Dewan

Contents

Part VI Equipment Planning

About the Authors

Ajay Garg, FCA, DHA, SAP(FI) has been in the field of healthcare planning, designing, and administration for the last three decades. He has worked for about 28 years with various hospitals like Narinder Mohan Hospital & Heart Centre, Ghaziabad; Jeevan Rekha Hospital, Kashipur; and Teerthanker Mahaveer Medical College, Moradabad.

He has also completed various hospital projects like Krishna Hospital (Kashipur), Narayan Hospital (Rudrapur), Le Crest Hospital (Vasundhara, Ghaziabad), and TSM Medical College & Hospital (Lucknow) as a hospital consultant.

Anil Dewan has experience in teaching hospital programming, planning, designing, and construction and project management for healthcare facilities for more than 40 years.

He has been adviser to institutions like the World Bank, World Health Organization, and Bureau of Indian Standards. Presently, he is a professor of architecture at the School of Planning and Architecture. He is also a hospital consultant to the Institute of Medicine, Tribhuvan Teaching University, Kathmandu, Nepal.

Part I

Hospital Planning

1 Phases of Planning and Designing

A hospital or so-called Health Care Facility is one of the most complex buildings/projects to plan, design, build and operate. The quality of planning and designing has a long-term impact on the performance of the hospital. Once planned and executed, the redesigning of hospital carries its own difficulties and shortcomings. As hospital projects involve huge investment and once constructed, it is usually not feasible to change the designs and plans again and again.

It is evident that there is a direct relation between the design of hospitals and satisfaction experienced by patients, staff and family members of the patient. Furthermore, this is also equally true that the good planning and designing of the hospital services contributes a lot to reduce errors, decrease rates of infection and cross infection and accidents due to falls of the patients, protect staff from injury, increase patient's recovery rate from disease and sufferings and also increase staff satisfaction. Further, a well-designed hospital cannot only prevent harm and injury but also provide mental, physical and psychological support to the patient in the process of healing.

The following are the different phases for setting up a hospital project:

1.1 Hospital Planning

This phase includes the "wishlist" of the promoters giving considerations on master planning, predesigning issues and working on the feasibility reports along with the DPR.

1.2 Schematic Design

This phase involves drawing the initial and rough outline of the hospital project, including conceptual designing, preliminary allocation of the spaces, room layouts, structural designing along with other initial details and preliminary drawings.

1.3 Construction Documents

This phase includes converting all the aspects of the detailed drawing into a document for estimating costs and planning construction activities.

A. Garg, A. Dewan, *Manual of Hospital Planning and Designing*,
https://doi.org/10.1007/978-981-16-8456-2_1

1.4 Design and Development

This phase includes drawing of various units of the hospital and adding details of infrastructure, designing, including electrical fixtures, furniture location and decor.

1.5 MEP Planning

This phase includes the planning of the MEP services of the hospital like electricity, plumbing, MGPS, CCD Cameras, Audio-visual networking and IT networking.

1.6 Construction

This is the phase in which the hospital building is actually being built up step by step.

1.7 Equipment Planning

In this phase, the requirement of equipment is worked out, the configuration and the technical specifications are finalized, quotations are invited, the order of the equipment is placed, installation is completed and the commissioning of equipment is done.

1.8 Man Power Planning

This phase includes assessing the requirement of man power, finalizing the Standard Operating Procedures (SOPs), inviting resumes, interviews, appointments and joining of the employees.

1.9 Finalizing the Standard Operating Procedures of Hospital

In this phase, the SOP's Rules and Regulations, Rate List etc. are finalized based on which the operations of the hospital shall be carried out.

1.10 Commissioning

This phase is for testing the services, ensuring specifications, operationalizing the equipment, training the staff and disinfecting the hospital before kick-starting the hospital.

Therefore, planning, designing and building hospitals without thorough planning, thinking can ultimately lead to troubles and the purpose of the hospital services may be lost. As hospitals provide a wide range of services that are made up or supported by many other functional units of the hospital, they are one of the most complex types of building as compared to any other commercial building.

Hospitals generally render the diagnostic and therapeutic functions and each of the functionality has different requirements of infrastructure so that the concerned functionality can provide excellent results and quality.

Indeed, hospital design may also be influenced by many restraints and opportunities like the climate of the area, surrounding facilities, budget allocation and presently available technology. But the best design will be the one where the designer can overcome these hurdles to the extent possible or adopt alternate measures to tackle these hurdles.

Can anyone predict what will be the requirement of the hospital after 10, 20, 30, or say 40 years from now? The answer is "No, not at all." As the world has undergone the experience of changing health care technology so fast in a few years, the same is going to change further, maybe faster than in the past. Under those circumstances, the hospital has to accept the changing technology and adopt it at the earliest. This will only be possible if the infrastructure of the hospital allows for such adoption. If not, the hospital will lag behind in the race. Therefore, hospital designs shall be planned to look years ahead and should have the flexibility to adopt changes.

Further, due to the inevitable demographic changes, technology development, changing norms and codes of various agencies, changing political policy etc., there can be a lot of pressure on the hospitals to adopt these changes as time progresses.

It has been experienced that mostly there is a tendency to design hospital facilities thinking that the problem can be solved as and when the problem is faced. It means the immediate need is identified and within the existing resources, a design response is provided as a solution. Like an extension of ICUs, more Operating rooms, more private beds etc. This methodology can be true and feasible to a certain extent, but how many such solutions can be provided and adopted. Over a period of time, one or the other day, the designer has to say NO to these changes.

Since the last few years and till today, the planning and designing of the hospital building have undergone significant developments and changes. Therefore, it is emphasized that the initial planning and designing has to be strategic and integrating with a long-term vision considering a few factors such as the adoption of the would-be technology in future, thinking beyond the problem-based solutions, thinking the design solutions that will fit into the future changes, providing the spaces for future expansions, adopting modular technology and easing out the movement of the men and material.

It is true that to treat the patients, hospitals need to have a team of experienced and professional doctors and other paramedical staff, still the infrastructure of the hospital plays an important role in achieving the objective of the hospitals. As a huge amount of funds are being invested in infrastructure, it is not feasible to renovate the hospital frequently. Therefore, infrastructure must be designed in such a way that it looks attractive, is functional and is safe for the patients and the health workers.

The future vision of the hospital project starts the day when the idea of building a hospital is conceived by the owners. The detailed feasibility report has to be worked out, the selection of land is then another crucial factor. The most important factor is designing the individual units of the hospital like Emergency, Intensive care units and Operating complex and Indoor patient wards. Similarly, there are other few things that the designers or promoters need to carefully consider as they plan the hospital.

Further Reading

Hospital | WBDG - Whole Building Design Guide [Internet]. [cited 2021 Jun 7]. Available from: https://www.wbdg.org/building-types/health-care-facilities/hospital

Joint Commission Resources, Inc, editor. Planning, design, and construction of health care facilities. 2nd ed. Oakbrook Terrace, Ill: Joint Commission Resources; 2009. 156 p.

Political, Economic, Technological and Cultural Influences that Will Shape Service Delivery in the Next Decade [Internet]. World Meteorological Organization. 2015 [cited 2021 Jun 7]. Available from: https://public.wmo.int/en/bulletin/political-economic-technological-and-cultural-influences-will-shape-service-delivery-next

Project Management for Construction: The Design and Construction Process [Internet]. [cited 2021 Jun 7]. Available from: https://www.cmu.edu/cee/projects/PMbook/03_The_Design_And_Construction_Process.html

Walrath BJ. A Project Planning Guide for Healthcare Facility Owners [Internet] [Thesis]. Georgia Institute of Technology; 2007 [cited 2021 Jun 7]. Available from: https://smartech.gatech.edu/handle/1853/14557

2 Inception of the Idea

The Planning of the hospital starts as soon as the idea of setting up the hospital is conceived by the promoter. What comes to mind as the first thought is 'Where to set up a hospital?' The answer to this depends on personal factors and understandings of the promoter. He/she may opt for a particular place because that can be the place where he/she resides, where he/she works, the environment, the assumptions that a particular place has more patients, assumption that the number of hospitals are fewer in that particular area etc. But should we depend on such factors which are not supported by any evidence or documents of assessment? The promoter shall ask himself one question 'what is the purpose of building up a hospital, why at this place and not at other places'. The promoter shall answer these questions him/herself. The questions to which the promoter shall put answers to are:

- Why did I think of making the hospital?
- What is the purpose of this hospital?
- What is the philosophy of the hospital? Is it to serve the community or to make it a business venture?
- What is my profession? Am I a medico or non-medico? If non-medico, what are my plans to manage the hospital?
- What about hospital after my death? Are my children interested to continue the hospital project?
- Do I want to do charity in the hospital?
- If Yes, what type of charity do I want to do? Do I want to treat free of cost or at concessional cost?
- If I want to do charity, up to what extent am I planning to do so?

Once these questions are answered and the promoter is sure and affirmative for setting up the hospital, he/she shall proceed further. The next issue which he/she should answer is 'What will be the Status of the Hospital?' Will it be a trust-owned charitable hospital, community hospital, or a corporate hospital?

The next step after answering these questions and finalizing the place/city is the preparation of the Feasibility Report. This report indicates the feasibility of the success of the hospital at that place based on the surveys conducted in the nearby area of the proposed hospital location. There are different agencies that can do this job for the promoter. Some of the factors that are included and surveyed by the agency are:

- What shall be the coverage area, the residents of which shall avail the services of the hospital?
- To how many cities or villages can the hospital provide services?
- What is the approximate population that is expected to avail the services of the hospital?
- Details of the other hospitals in the vicinity and the bed strength of these hospitals along

A. Garg, A. Dewan, *Manual of Hospital Planning and Designing*,
https://doi.org/10.1007/978-981-16-8456-2_2

with the details of services being provided by them.

- Details of nursing homes and individual practitioners' clinics in the vicinity.

Answers to these questions based on the actual survey, supported by documentary evidence, can make it easy for the promoters to understand the expected business from that particular location and which in turn can help to make decisions about the location.

Once the promoters make up their mind about the location, the Geographical details are collected by the agency. Some of the factors can be like:

- The exact location of the hospital with address.
- On which road the hospital shall be located.
- The distance of the hospital from the railway Station.
- The distance of the hospital from the bus station.
- The distance of the hospital from the airport.
- What is the local mode of transport to the hospital?
- Police station jurisdiction.
- The distance of the hospital from the nearest police station.
- The distance of the hospital from the nearest fire Station.
- The main occupation of the public.
- Per capita income of the public.
- The living standard of the people.
- Paying capacity of the individuals.
- Main industries in the area.
- How many Central Govt. /State Govt. Offices/ Employees reside in that area?
- What is the awareness of Health Insurance to the population residing in that area?

Once these answers are received and the promoters are satisfied, the final decision can be taken about the location of the hospital.

3 Factors Assessing Feasibility of the Hospital

Consideration of the actual facts is an essential requirement for developing appropriate hospital facilities. There must be deep efforts of pre-programming, research surveys, and discussion to work out the most appropriate programming, planning, and designing of the hospital setup. Hospitals and facilities in the hospital shall be designed to prevent illness, detect diseases as early as possible, treat disease and then rehabilitate the patient.

3.1 Demographics

The Population trends in the area along with the life expectancy of population to be served have to be determined. The total population shall be determined according to age and gender. Also, the growth of the population in that particular area has to be determined. In some regions, there can be an accelerating growth rate of population, while others may have a significant aged population or there can be areas with fewer births etc.

3.2 Understanding the Type of Diseases

In different regions, there can be different types of diseases causing illness and death. These could range from waterborne diseases like Typhoid, Malaria and/or other chronic diseases like Tuberculosis and COPD. Each and every cause of disease or illness and death requires a well-defined approach for prevention and treatment of such illness, disease and death. For appropriate planning of the proposed hospital, this analysis shall help a lot while planning the services to be provided, spaces and equipment required and of course, the manpower needed. Also, the Non-communicable ailments such as Cardiac disease, Paraplegic Stroke, Renal Failure, Diabetes and Hypertension that are becoming more prevalent these days have to be determined. More importantly, a careful assessment is required for the infectious diseases, which in turn shall help in designing the isolation areas of the hospital.

3.3 Community

While designing a hospital, the assessment shall be done for the people in the community relating to the knowledge, awareness, and initiatives to keep their family and other individuals healthy. Also, there is a need to assess and consider the climate, culture, religion, traditions, financial wellness, education level of the population particularly the health education, and the difference between needs and wants of the population. It is very important to assess the main occupation of the population, per capita income of the popula-

A. Garg, A. Dewan, *Manual of Hospital Planning and Designing*,
https://doi.org/10.1007/978-981-16-8456-2_3

tion, living standard of the population, and of course the paying capacity of the population of that particular area where the hospital is being planned.

3.4 Healthcare Systems and Hospitals Network

Because of the increasing demand for hospitals and acceleration and sophistication of technology and communications, there has been a growth in setting up of new hospitals to cope up with the population. Health setups range from clinics and nursing homes to hospitals. The size of hospitals varies from small, medium, and large. For better planning, a deep analysis is required to assess the number and types of such healthcare facilities already available in the area. This assessment shall help to judge the requirement of services to be provided, patient load in the hospital, and also the spaces to be allotted. The assessment shall also be done for the prevailing charges of hospital services in the nearby areas. These assessments shall also help in estimating the revenue that can be generated from the proposed hospital.

3.5 Innovations in Facility Planning and Management

Before planning and designing, the designers shall be well aware about the latest innovations and developments relating to the planning, design and construction of the hospital. The designer shall also consider the innovation in the operations and maintenance of the hospital.

3.6 The Requirement of the Specialty Facilities and/or Departments

The assessment shall also be done for determining the specialty facility and/or departments to be provided. Like, on the expected number of patients—the number of OPD's shall be planned, Diseases prevalent in the area—department to be provided, Critical Care requirement in the area—the Intensive Care Units shall be planned and on the expected attendance in Emergency—Size of the Emergency shall be planned.

3.7 Medical Tourism

An assessment shall be done for the expected medical tourism. Medical tourism means travelling from different countries to other countries for health assessment, diagnosis of disease, treatment, or interventional procedures, only because of the less cost of treatment and/or good quality of the medical treatment as compared to their own country. There are countries in the world where medical care has become so expensive that people do not hesitate to fly from one country to another country to receive medical care at substantially reduced costs.

3.8 Health Insurance and Empanelment

This is an important factor to be assessed while planning the hospital as it is going to impose a significant effect on the expected number of patients and revenue earnings of the proposed hospital. It has to be seen that on average what percentage of people are insured for health care. Also, to determine how many people on average are employed in the Govt., Semi Govt., and private institutions who provide free medical facilities to their employees.

3.9 Catchment Area

While planning, consideration has to be given to the catchment area from where the patients are expected to avail the facility of the proposed hospital. For better determination, the assessment of these areas also has to be done on issues like any existing hospital, distances, conveyance, approach, referring physicians and other doctors in that area. The bigger the catchment area and more the referring physicians, better shall be the space and facility planning, and better shall be the revenue collection.

Further Reading

Ar Z. Modern Principles and Practice in Planning and Designing of Healthcare Services (An Overview: Latest Trends of Design in Indian Hospitals). J Archit Eng Technol [Internet]. 2019 [cited 2021 Jun 8];07(02). Available from: https://www.omicsonline.org/open-access/modern-principles-and-practice-in-planning-and-designing-of-healthcare-services-an-overview-latest-trends-of-design-in-indian-hosp-2168-9717-1000222-107203.html

Century I of M (US) C on A the H of the P in the 21st. Understanding Population Health and Its Determinants [Internet]. The Future of the Public's Health in the 21st Century. National Academies Press (US); 2002 [cited 2021 Jun 8]. Available from: https://www.ncbi.nlm.nih.gov/books/NBK221225/

Griffin CH, Joint Commission, Joint Commission Resources, Inc., Joint Commission International, AIA Academy of Architecture for Health, editors. Planning, design, and construction of health care facilities: addressing Joint Commission and JCI standards and other considerations--from planning to commissioning. Third edition. Oak Brook, IL: Joint Commission Resources; 2015. 138 p.

Hernandez LM, Blazer DG, Institute of Medicine (US) Committee on Assessing Interactions Among Social B. The Impact of Social and Cultural Environment on Health [Internet]. Genes, Behavior, and the Social Environment: Moving Beyond the Nature/Nurture Debate. National Academies Press (US); 2006 [cited 2021 Jun 8]. Available from: https://www.ncbi.nlm.nih.gov/books/NBK19924/

Hospital of Tomorrow The design perspective - Facilities & Operations [Internet]. [cited 2021 Jun 8]. Available from: https://www.asianhhm.com/facilities-operations/hospital-design

Naghipour M, Langarizadeh M, Razzazi M. Identification of the requirements for designing medical tourism information system of Iran. J Educ Health Promot [Internet]. 2019 Jun 27 [cited 2021 Jun 8];8. Available from: https://www.ncbi.nlm.nih.gov/pmc/articles/PMC6615129/

World Health Organization, World Bank Group, OECD. Delivering Quality Health Services: A Global Imperative for Universal Health Coverage [Internet]. Geneva: World Health Organization; 2018 [cited 2021 Jun 8]. Available from: http://hdl.handle.net/10986/29970

4 Preparation of Detailed Project Report (DPR) and Techno-Commercial Feasibility Report (TCFR)

Detailed Project Reports (DPRs) are bankable sets of documents that show the results and outputs of working and projections while planning and designing a project. DPR is detailed and elaborated projections and plans for the project indicating overall calculations, programme, financials, roles and responsibilities, time planning for project, details of required activities and resources required for completion of the project.

During the planning stage, a blueprint is prepared on paper which gives a detailed study and analysis of what has to be done to convert the investment into a feasible and profitable venture. In this set of document, top management's policies and guidelines, its impact on the project span, appraisal of financial viability is estimated and dealt with in-depth. The DPR mainly covers the issues like contract drawings, detailed technical feasibility studies, financial feasibility calculations, execution of the project from the practical point of view, the time period for completion of the project and staff planning. DPR also highlights the type and nature of inherited risks in the project and other foreseeable external risks that can influence the outcome of the hospital project. The DPR should address and provide measures for risk management and risk mitigation.

The DPR is a document that guides the management about the progress of the project on real-time basis. It also provides the tools for comparison of actual vs. projected figures in terms of costs, time period, milestone achievements etc. This actual vs. projections are measured based on:

1. Whether the project was completed on time as compared to the estimated period?
2. Whether the actual cost of the project was within reasonable limits of cost escalation?
3. Whether after completion of the project, was it able to deliver the desired results relating to the quality and quantity and whether the patient's satisfaction is achieved at a profitable cost?
4. Whether the project gestation period was within the planned duration as estimated?

4.1 Information to Be Generally Provided in DPR

To start preparing the DPR, some of the following information shall be generally provided in the DPR:

1. General Information about the hospital project.
2. Background and the experience of the project promoters in the hospital industry.
3. Details of the Bed in hospital; ward wise (Table 4.1).
4. Details of the departments and services to be given.
5. Details of the proposed project like:
   (a) Number of OPDs.

A. Garg, A. Dewan, *Manual of Hospital Planning and Designing*,
https://doi.org/10.1007/978-981-16-8456-2_4

(b) The number of Private Rooms, Semi-private Room, General Wards etc.
(c) Number of critical Units (ICU) and the number of beds in each ICU.

Table 4.1 Break up of type and number of beds

General Beds
Semi-private Beds
Private Beds
Deluxe Room
Suites
ICCU
CTVS ICU
HDU
MICU
Day Care
SICU
NICU
PICU
Pre and post-op. Gynae
Endo. Recovery
Emergency
Others
Total Number of Beds

(d) Number of Operating Rooms.
(e) Support services to be provided.
(f) Equipment to be installed.
(g) Management teams for the project.
(h) Details of land, buildings and equipment.
(i) Details of infrastructural facilities (power, water supply, transport facilities etc.).
(j) Effluents produced by the project and treatment procedures adopted.
(k) Manpower requirement and availability.

6. Schedule of implementation period of the project.
7. Detailed Project cost (Table 4.2).
8. Details of Department Wise Breakup of Required Items (Table 4.3).
9. Depreciation Statement (Table 4.4).
10. Details of Salary and Allowances (Table 4.5).
11. Staff requirement Planning (Table 4.6).
12. Resources and Means of finances for the project.

Table 4.2 List of capital items required

S. No.	Item	Unit	Quantity required	Approximate cost Rate (in USD)	Amount (in USD)	Group total (in USD)	Supplier
1	***Land***	Sq. Mtr.					
1A	Purchase of Extra FAR						
2	***Building***						
2A	**RCC Structure**	Sq. Ft.					
2B	**RCC bunkers**	Lumpsum					
2C	**Civil Construction Part of the Building Including**	Sq. Ft.					
	Cement and Steel						
	Steel						
4	***Equipment***						
4A	***ICU/ICCU/CTVS/Stepdown***						
	Bedside Monitors	Nos.					
	Bipep ventilator	Nos.					
	I.A.B.P.	Nos.					
	Pulse Oximeter	Nos.					
	Syringe Pumps	Nos.					
	Test Lungs	Nos.					
	Ventilator	Nos.					
4B	***Cath lab and cardiac OT***						
	A.C.T. Machine	Nos.					
	Total Capital Expenditure						

Likewise the details will be worked out for all the capital items, add contingency and at the end the total projected capital expenditure on the project will be calculated

Table 4.3 Department wise breakup of the required items

Name of Item	Gen. Ward	Emerg.	OPD'S	O.T	Investigation	Misc.	Total
No. of Bed							
Intensive care unit							
ICU/ICCU/CTVS/Step Down							
Bedside Monitors							
Bipep Ventilator							
I.A.B.P.							
Pulse Oximeter							
Syringe Pumps							
Test Lungs							
Ventilator							
Cath Lab and Cardiac OT							
A.C.T. Machine							
Cath Lab							

This table will be filled out for all the items ward wise to calculate the exact quantity of items required for the project

Table 4.4 Calculation of the schedule of depreciation

	Land	Building	Equipment	Furniture	Total
First Year					
W.D.V as on Start of year					
Add Allocation of Contingency					
Add Allocation of IDC					
Additions					
Total					
Less Depreciation					
W.D.V as on End of Year					

In a similar fashion, the depreciation will be calculated year by year

Table 4.5 Details of salary and allowances

Department	No. of persons	Salary/month per employee (in USD)	Salary per employee per year (in USD)	Total salary per month (In USD)	Total salary per year (In USD)
Patient care					
Nursing Care					
Nursing Superintendent					
Asst. Nursing Suptd.					
Sister in-charge					
Nurses					
Ward Boys					
Doctors					
Senior Residents					
Junior Residents					
Total					

This table shall be filled out for all the projected employees and at the end the total expenditure to be calculated

Table 4.6 Calculation of requirement of staff

Staff	Beds	Morning	Evening	Night	Reliever	Total
Nurses						
General Ward						
Semi-private Ward						
Private Ward						
Deluxe Ward						
Suites						
ICCU						
Step Down						
CTVS ICU						
ICU						
NICU						

To calculate the required number of staff members, this table shall be filled up, shift wise, mainly for Nursing Staff, Ward Assistants and Housekeeping workers etc.

Table 4.7 Proposed requirement of working capital

S. no.	Particulars	Total projected consumption during the year	Number of days/months	Amount (USD in millions)
1	Stock of medicines			
2	Stock of OT Consumables			
5	Stock of Ward Consumables			
6	Stock of Linen Consumables			
7	Stock of instruments/minor equipment (Consumable in a Year)			
8	Advance Salary to Doctors and Staff to initiate them to join Hospital			
9	Total Debts outstanding from Panels like Govt. Dept., empanelled organizations and Industries			
	Total			
	Our Margin			
	WC from Bank			
	Total			

13. Working capital requirements and arrangements thereof (Table 4.7).
14. The assumed rate of hospital services (Table 4.8).
15. Assumed Operational Expenses (Table 4.9).
16. Interest calculation on the loans (Table 4.10).
17. Assumed number of patients and procedures that can be performed (Table 4.11).
18. Statement of Bed days occupancy per year (Table 4.12).
19. Revenue earning projections (Table 4.13).
20. Revenue expenses projections (Table 4.14).
21. Profit and loss statement for the next 10 years (Table 4.15).
22. Cash Flow statement for the next 10 years (Table 4.16).
23. The financial ratio for the bank loans.
24. Projected Balance Sheets for the next 10 years.
25. Marketing and selling arrangements made.
26. Mode and means of repayment of term loans and cash credit loans.
27. Government approvals required for the project. Local authority's consents and statutory permissions required for the project.
28. Details of collateral security that can be offered to the financial institutions.

Table 4.8 Statement of schedule of charges for services

Head of income	Unit	Rate (in USD)
Admission Charges	Per admitted patient	
General bed income	Per day including nursing care	
Semi-private beds income	Per day including nursing care	
Private beds income	Per day including nursing care	
Deluxe bed income	Per day including nursing care	
Suite bed income	Per day including nursing care	
ICCU bed income	Per day including nursing care	
ICU bed income	Per day including nursing care	
CTVS bed income	Per day including nursing care	
Step down bed income	Per day including nursing care	
NICU charges	Per day including nursing care	
SICU bed income	Per day including nursing care	
PICU bed income	Per day including nursing care	
Burn ICU bed income	Per day including nursing care	
Pre and post-angio bed income	Per day including nursing care	
Recovery bed charges	Per surgery	
Emergency bed charges	Per day including nursing care	
Doctors visit charges		
General wards	Per day	
Semi-private ward	Per day	
Private ward	Per day	
Income from O.P.D specialist	Per card	
Income from O.P.D super-specialist	Per card	
TMT	Per test	
Echocardiography	Per test	
ECG's	Per ECG	
Holter	Per Holter	

This statement of schedule of charges for services shall be prepared for all the services to be provided in the Hospital

Table 4.9 Statement of assumed expenses of hospital

Head of expense	Unit	Rate/ percentage	Remarks
Fixed expenses			
Salary and allowances	Increased 10% every year		Separate working of the staff required is attached with this report
Annual maintenance contract	About 5% of the cost of equipment		In the first year, the AMC will be done by the owners and from the second year onward the AMC will be ours
Insurance	1.25% of the cost of project		
Building Maintenance	Approx. Per Month		It is assumed that the repair cost will increase in subsequent years
Provident Fund	12% of Salaries		This includes the PF and the allied expenses of the Provident Fund Department for half of the employees
Semi-variable Expenses			
Electricity	Approx. Per Month		Assumed to be fixed amount
Advertisement	Approx. Per Month		Assumed to be fixed amount
Diet charges	Per Diet		Total bed occupancy (* Rate per diet

(continued)

Table 4.9 (continued)

Head of expense	Unit	Rate/ percentage	Remarks
Variable Expenses			
Consultation Fees			
Doctors Share Visits General Ward	Percentage of Receipts		Fixed Percentage of the Receipt of Income Statement
Doctors Share Visits Deluxe Room	Percentage of Receipts		Fixed Percentage of the Receipt of Income Statement
Doctors Share Visits Suites	Percentage of Receipts		Fixed Percentage of the Receipt of Income Statement
Consumables			
O.T Drugs	Percentage of Receipts		Fixed Percentage of the Receipt of Income Statement
Cost of Medicines	Percentage of Receipts		Fixed Percentage of the Receipt of Income Statement
Other Variable Expenses			
Concession and Discount	Percentage of Receipts		Fixed Percentage of the Total Receipt of Income Statement
Other Non-Planned Expenses	Fixed		Assumed

This statement of Projected Expenses shall be prepared for all the expenditure in the Hospital

Table 4.10 Calculation of the interest payable for loan

Year/ month	Amount due	Interest	Group total	or Say
Interest rate		Interest rate in percentage		
I st Year				
1				
2				
3				
4				
5				
6				
7				
8				
9				
10				
11				
12				
IInd year				
1				

In a similar fashion, the Interest payable shall be calculated for all the years till the Loans are paid out

4.2 Documents DPR Shall Contain

As the DPR is a complete set of planning and assessment documents, it shall contain the following documents:

1. Location Profile and Geo-technical Site Characterization:
   (a) General
   (b) Climate and Rainfall
   (c) Map
   (d) Physical Characteristics
   (e) Economy and Industries
   (f) Transportation and Communications
2. Synopsis and Project at a Glance
3. Executive Summary
4. Organization Details
   (a) Name of Organization/Company with Contact Details

Table 4.11 Statement of projected number of patients

Number of patients	Unit	No. of beds	Basis of calculation	1st year	–	10th year
Bed Occupancy	Per Day		Percentage of Total Paid Beds			
OPD Specialists	Per Day		Assumption			
OPD Super Specialists	Per Day		Assumption			
TMT	Per Day		Assumption			
Echocardiography	Per Day		Assumption			
ECG's	Per Day		Assumption			
Surgeries General	Per Day		Assumption (Including Neuro, Paediatric, Plastic, Urology, Gynae, Ortho, ENT, Eye etc.)			

The projected number of patients shall be calculated for each and every service to be provided in the hospital. These numbers will be used to calculate the projected income of the hospital

Table 4.12 Statement of projected bed occupancy per year

Number of patients	Unit	No. of beds	Basis of calculation	1st year	–	10th year
General Ward	Per Day		Total Number of Beds * Percentage of Occupancy * 365 Days			
Semi-private Beds	Per Day		Total Number of Beds * Percentage of Occupancy * 365 Days			
Private Beds	Per Day		Total Number of Beds * Percentage of Occupancy * 365 Days			
Deluxe Room	Per Day		Total Number of Beds * Percentage of Occupancy * 365 Days			

This table shall be filled for all the Indoor beds in the hospital to calculate the total bed days occupied in the year

Table 4.13 Statement of projected income

						(In million)	
Head of income	Unit	Rate (in Rs.)	Basis of calculation	1st year	–	10th year	Total
General Bed Income	Per Day Including Nursing Care		Bed Occupancy Per Year * Rate Per Bed				

(continued)

Table 4.13 (continued)

						(In million)	
Head of income	Unit	Rate (in Rs.)	Basis of calculation	1st year	–	10th year	Total
Doctors visit charges							
General Wards	2 Visits per day		Bed occupancy per year * Rate of doctors visit				
Private Ward	2 Visits Per Day		Bed Occupancy Per Year * Rate of Doctors Visit				
Income from OPD	Per Card		Number of OPD Patients Per Day * 300 Days * Rate of OPD Card				
Echocardiography	Per Test		Number of Echo Per Day * 365 Days * Average Rate of Echo				
ECG's	Per ECG		Number of ECG's Per Day * 365 Days * Average Rate of ECG				
Total							

This table shall be filled for each and every service head from where the income of the hospital is expected, and at the end, the total projected income is worked out

Table 4.14 Statement of projected expenses

						Expenses (in million)	
Head of expense	Unit	Rate (in Rs.)	Basis of calculation	1st year	–	10th year	Total
Fixed expenses							
Salary and Allowances	Increased 10% Every Year		Separate Working of the Staff Required is Attached with this Report				
Building Maintenance	Approx. Per Month		Assumed to be Fixed Amount				
Total fixed expenses (A)							
Semi-variable expenses							
Electricity	Approx. Per Month		Assumed to be fixed amount				
Diet Charges	Per Diet		Total bed occupancy * Rate per diet				

Table 4.14 (continued)

						Expenses (in million)	
Head of expense	Unit	Rate (in Rs.)	Basis of calculation	1st year	–	10th year	Total
Total semi-Variable Expenses (B)							
Variable expenses							
Doctors share							
Private ward	Percentage of receipts		Fixed percentage of the receipt of income statement				
Income from OPD	Percentage of receipts		Fixed percentage of the receipt of income statement				
Echocardiography	Percentage of receipts		Fixed percentage of The receipt of income statement				
Angiography	Percentage of receipts		Fixed percentage of the receipt of income statement				
Surgeries	Percentage of receipts		Fixed Percentage of The Receipt of Income Statement				
Anaesthesia Charges	Percentage of Receipts		Fixed Percentage of The Receipt of Income Statement				
Total other variable expenses (C 1)						**2501.77**	**34621.48**
Consumables							
O.T Drugs	Percentage of Receipts	50%	Fixed Percentage of The Receipt of Income Statement				
Cost of Medicines	Percentage of Receipts	75%	Fixed Percentage of The Receipt of Income Statement				
Linen Consumables	Lumpsum	25,000	Assumed to be Fixed Amount				
Other Ward Consumables	Approx. Per Month	50,000	Assumed to be Fixed Amount				
Total Consumables (C 2)							
Other variable expenses							
Concession and Discount	Percentage of Receipts		Fixed Percentage of The Total Receipt of Income Statement				
Other Non-Planned Expenses	Fixed		Assumed				
Total other variable expenses (C 3)							
Total variable expenses (D = C1 + C2 + C3)							
Total expenses (fixed, semi-Variable, Variable) (E = A + B + D)							

(continued)

Table 4.14 (continued)

						Expenses (in million)	
Head of expense	Unit	Rate (in Rs.)	Basis of calculation	1st year	–	10th year	Total
Interest on bank loan	On loan amount @ 12.5% P.A At reducing rate		Separate working of the interest calculation attached with this report				
Interest on working capital	On working capital amount @ 13.5% PA		Amount of CC * rate of interest				
Total interest on term loans (F)							
Depreciation	**(G)**		As per schedule of calculation attached				
Total expenses (including depreciation and interest) (H = E + F + G)							

All the projected expenditures shall be filled up in this table to calculate the total expenditure of the hospital

Table 4.15 Statement of projected surplus/deficit

			(USD in million)	
	1st year	–	10th year	Total
Total income (as per income statement enclosed)				
Less operating expenses (as per the expenses statement enclosed)				
Operating surplus/(deficit)				
LessBank interest				
Operating surplus/(deficit) After interest but before depreciation				
LessDepreciation				
Net surplus/Deficit after interest and depreciation				
Cumulative Surplus/(Deficit)				

   (b) Status of the Organization
   (c) Name of Director(S)/Management
   (d) Name of Hospital
   (e) The capacity of the Hospital (Bed)
   (f) Location of the Hospital
5. Industry Analysis
   (a) Overview of the Healthcare Industry
      (i) Introduction
      (ii) Healthcare Industry Structure of the country
   (b) Structure and Segmentation of Hospital Industry
      (i) Classification of Hospitals Based on Objective
      (ii) Classification of Hospitals Based on Ownership
      (iii) Classification of Hospitals Based on the System of Medicine
   (c) Market Size of the healthcare and Growth

Table 4.16 Projected cash flow statement

			(USD in million)	
	1st year	–	10th year	Total
Opening balance of cash				
Inflow from receipts				
Less expenses with interest but without depreciation				
Operating surplus				
Induction of cash credit limit				
Total inflow of cash during the year				
Less repayment of instalment of bank				
Net cash surplus/ deficit after expenses and repayment of instalment				
Less blockage in debtors				
Less increase in current assets and stores				
Less investment in assets				
Total outflow of cash				
Net cash surplus/ deficit after expenses and repayment of instalment and additions to the fixed assets				

(i) Present Market Size of the healthcare facilities
(ii) Public Healthcare Expenditure by the Governments
(iii) Healthcare Infrastructure in the country

(d) Growth
(i) Growth drivers
(ii) Medical Tourism and improving health insurance penetration
(iii) Medical Information and Telemedicine
(iv) Trend of Outsourcing Diagnostic Services in the area
(v) Govt. Plans to enhance in Expenditure in public health
(vi) Increment in the Health Awareness amongst population
(vii) Awareness of the public for Medical Insurance

6. Hospital Management Issues
(a) Management and Commercial Plans
(i) Brief Introduction of the Hospital Management
(ii) Outpatient Services
(iii) Inpatient Services
(iv) Diagnostic Services
(v) Interventional Services
(vi) Material Management
(b) Steps that shall be involved in Setting up a Hospital project
7. Planning the Hospital
(a) Brief Description of Major Disorders
(b) Permissions and Clearances Required from the Govt. Local bodies

   (c) Advertising, Marketing and Promotional planning
   (d) Mobilisation of the Bank Loans
   (e) Critical Success Factor
   (f) Planning to get Hospital Accreditations
   (g) Tentative Project Implementation Plan
8. Planning of Hospital Building
   (a) Site Selection
   (b) Draft Site Plan
   (c) Key Flow Chart of a Hospital
   (d) Flow Chart of Various Departments
   (e) Flow Chart of Outpatient Department
   (f) Flow Chart of Inpatient Department
   (g) Vendors and Suppliers of Building materials
   (h) Contractors for construction and finishing of Building
   (i) The contractor for Air Conditioning and Refrigeration Units
9. Financials (Projections are given for the next 10 years)
   (a) Projections of the number of patients likely to avail services department wise and service wise.
   (b) Calculation of Projected Revenue/Income/Realisation from Hospital like:
      (i) From OPD
      (ii) From IPD
      (iii) From Sales of Medicine
      (iv) From Diagnostic Services
      (v) From Interventions/Operating Rooms
      (vi) From Interest
      (vii) From Rent
      (viii) Any Other Expected Revenue
   (c) Calculation of Projected Expenses/Cost of Products/Services/Items for Hospital like:
      (i) Salary and Wages
      (ii) Semi-Variable/Semi-fixed Expenses
      (iii) Variable Cost and Expenses
      (iv) Overheads
      (v) Royalty and Other Charges
      (vi) Marketing Expenses
      (vii) Consumables, Store etc.
      (viii) Employees Expenses
      (ix) Fuel Expenses
      (x) Power/Electricity Expenses
      (xi) Royalty and Other Charges
      (xii) Repairs and Maintenance Expenses
      (xiii) Administration Expenses
      (xiv) Depreciation at WDV
      (xv) Interest and Repayment—Term Loans
      (xvi) Any Other Expected Revenue
   (d) Projected Surplus/Deficit or Profit/Loss Statement
   (e) Projected Gross Profit/Loss
   (f) Financial Charges
   (g) Tax on Profits
   (h) Net Profit After Taxes
   (i) Profits and Appropriations
   (j) Projected Cash Flow
   (k) Net Cash In-Flow and Out-Flow from Operating Activities
   (l) Net Cash Accruals
   (m) Projected Balance Sheets for 10 years
      (i) Total Liabilities
      (ii) Total Assets
      (iii) Assets
      (iv) Share Capital including Equity and Preference Share Capital
      (v) Current Assets
      (vi) Gross Working Capital
      (vii) Current Liabilities
      (viii) Net Working Capital
      (ix) Calculation of Work in process
   (n) Profitability Ratios
      (i) ROI (Average of Fixed Assets)
      (ii) RONW (Average of Share Capital)
      (iii) ROI (Average of Total Assets)
      (iv) D.S.C.R
      (v) Earnings Per Share (EPS)
      (vi) Debt Equity Ratio
      (vii) Cost as % of revenue collected
      (viii) Forex Transaction
      (ix) Growth in Assets and Liabilities
      (x) Growth in Income and Expenditure
      (xi) Liquidity Ratios
      (xii) Profitability Ratio

(xiii) Return Ratios
(xiv) Structure of Assets and Liabilities (%)
(xv) Working Capital and Turnover Ratios

(o) Break-even Analysis
(i) Profit Volume Ratio (PVR)
(ii) Fixed Expenses/Cost
(iii) B.E.P.

(p) Sensitivity Analysis-Price/Volume
(i) Resultant N.P.B.T
(ii) Resultant D.S.C.R
(iii) Resultant PV Ratio
(iv) Resultant DER
(v) Resultant ROI
(vi) Resultant BEP

(q) Projected Pay-Back Period and IRR

10. Project Cost of Building

The total cost of the hospital building has to be calculated. The main heads of expenses towards building are:

(a) Land
(b) Architect Fees
(c) Consultants Fees
(d) RCC Structure
(e) RCC Bunkers
(f) Civil Construction Part of the Building Including
(g) Electrification Works Including Fittings and lights
(h) Sanitary Works Including the Fittings
(i) Site Development and External Works
(j) WTP, ETP and STP
(k) External Electric Works
(l) Central Air Conditioning
(m) Central Pipe Medical Gas Supply Line System
(n) Fire Fitting Eq.
(o) Generators
(p) Nurse Call System
(q) Civil Furniture
(r) Audio Visual System
(s) Hot Water and Solar Heating System
(t) Bed Elevators
(u) PTS
(v) Curtains/Blinds/Scrub/Wall Guards/ Corner Guards
(w) IT and EPABX
(x) Signage System
(y) Special Items
(z) Expenses During Construction Period
(aa) Any other Expenses

11. Projected Cost of Hospital Equipment/ Consumables/Disposables

(a) Brief Description of Some Common Hospital Equipment
(b) Brief Description of Major Machinery
(c) Department Wise Requirement of Medical Equipment in Quantity
(d) Cost and Vendors of:
(i) Medical/Hospital Equipment
(ii) Hospital Laundry
(iii) Misc. Small Instruments
(iv) Misc. Disposable Items
(v) Linen
(vi) Consumables
(vii) Backup Services like Ambulance, Autoclaves, Computers with Printers and UPS
(viii) Fridges, Hospital Operating Software, Televisions, Water Coolers, Oxygen Cylinders etc.
(ix) Patient Furniture
(x) Library Books
(xi) Skill Development
(xii) Simulation Lab
(xiii) Any other Item required

(e) Preoperative and Preliminary Expenses
(f) Technical Knowhow
(g) Provision of Contingencies

12. Means of Funds for Project or Sources and Disposition of Funds:

(a) Promoters Contribution
(b) Equity Share Capital
(c) Term Loan from Banks/Financial Institutions
(d) Unsecured Loans
(e) Donation/Grants
(f) Any Other Means of Funds

13. Challenges in the Hospital Industry
14. Hospital Equipment and Facilities Photograph
15. Conclusion

4.3 General Contents in DPR

Apart from the contents given above in Sect. 4.2, the DPR shall also contain information about the Guidelines, Information, Procedures and Policies that will form part of the planning and designing, based on which the work will be executed. Usually, the following are provided:

1. General guidelines and conditions that shall govern all types of contractual agreements that are likely to be entered with various agencies during the project implementation period.
2. General guidelines for resolution of any dispute that may arise in future and arbitration procedures to be indicated, specifying the nature of the issue that may be referred for arbitration or for solving the dispute, powers for solving the disputes, choice of the arbitrator by both the parties and the place where such proceedings should be held.
3. Guidelines related to supply, erection, installation, commissioning and guarantee/warranty issues of the various equipment required for the project.
4. Guidelines for choosing the vendors. Will it be a tendering process or direct quotation method? If tendering, whether to follow a single- or two-stage tendering. It may also contain model documents and formats related to an invitation to tenders, specifications etc.
5. Guidelines for vendor short-listing and terms for contracting. Some points related to vendor detailing that are highlighted in the DPR are as cited below:
   (a) Commitment concerning delivery period of the activity and penalty conditions, in case of failure to fulfil such commitment.
   (b) General terms of payment including running/progress payment.
   (c) Inspection and testing procedure and points where the customer can hold payments.
   (d) Guarantee test, schedule of testing, procedure of testing, criteria for success and failure and accompanying bank guarantee.
   (e) Responsibility for goods damaged while in transit or during erection and/or commissioning.
   (f) Condition of admissibility of any increase in the price/rates of the contract.
   (g) Contract variations and the manner of handling them.
   (h) Mobilization advance to be paid initially along with the terms and conditions so that the advance is fully secured.
   (i) Responsibility to supply the equipment and necessary accessories and spare parts.
6. DPR shall provide an estimate of the phase-wise requirement of capital funds. This plan shall be the basis of a strategic planning for raising the funds from external sources like banks and financial institutions, and/or through public issues.
7. Include a schedule for ensuring adequate flow of funds for the timely completion of the project with adequate provision for normal contingencies.
8. Include the project phase: A recommended system of monitoring and control of the financial expenses on the project, as compared to the physical progress of the project.
9. The PERT chart clearly depicting the time period required for completion of a particular activity or the project as a whole. Also, the plan of starting and ending dates of the dependent work (where one work is only possible to start after completion of some earlier ones). What shall be the remedy to cope up with the time lost due to delay in any particular activity?

4.4 Evaluation of DPR

As the final onus of the project vests with the owners, the owner must have an appropriate mechanism and methods to evaluate DPR. The owners must pose the following questions:

1. What are the sources of critical data and information that have been taken in the DPR like demand, capital cost and input cost?

2. The extent to which the strategic plan of top management has been reflected in the design or the alterations?
3. What were the various alternatives considered, and the methodology followed for choosing one among them?
4. The extent to which the plan and design fulfils the applicable statutory requirements and regulations as defined by the authorities, both currently in force and those that can be foreseen?
5. Identification of potential problems, hurdles, bottlenecks, shortcomings and/or major risks involved in the project.
6. Degree and depth of detailing.
7. Influence of complementary/completing projects.
8. Scope for future expansion/modification/adaptation of new technologies that may come in the future and so on.

The above list is a sample of the types of questions that the owners might pose during the process of selection, appraisal of the first draft and before approval.

4.5 Sample Formats of DPR

Some of the sample formats as are provided below, will make it easy to understand and prepare DPR.

Further Reading

Chopra H. Project Report on Health care Hospital Service Industry. [cited 2021 Jun 8]; Available from: https://www.academia.edu/19162092/Project_Report_on_Health_care_Hospital_Service_Industry

Detailed Project Report (DPR) I Project Management [Internet]. Your Article Library. 2016 [cited 2021 Jun 8]. Available from: https://www.yourarticlelibrary.com/project-reports/detailed-project-report-dpr-project-management/94668

Project Report on hospital (100 beds), Feasibility Report, How Much Investment, Know How, Formulations, Profitable Business, How to Start, small scale industry [Internet]. [cited 2021 Jun 8]. Available from: https://www.eiriindia.org/project-report-handbook-hospital-beds-with-formulation-technology-1335

Services NPC. Project Reports & Profiles » Hospital, Specialized (Super Speciality) Hospitals, Healthcare, Nursing Home, Diagnostic Center, Trauma Center, Children [Internet]. NIIR Project Consultancy Services. [cited 2021 Jun 8]. Available from: https://www.niir.org/profile-project-reports/profiles/hospital-specialized-super-speciality-hospitals-healthcare-nursing-home-diagnostic-center-trauma-center-children-s-hospital-mental-hospital-sanatorium-medicare-healthcare-business-ideas-in-medical-sector/z,,74,0,a/index.html

5 Site Selection

Selection of a site for construction of the hospital is an important issue. Lots of factors have to be kept in mind while selecting the site. If a wrong site is selected, it can be very harmful to the overall project. While selecting the site, the below thoughts shall be kept in mind.

5.1 Size of the Land Required for Hospital

As compared to any other commercial building, the hospital normally requires large spaces because of the varied services to be provided in the hospital. In hospitals, normally space is required for OPD, IPD, Diagnostic, Interventions, Stores, Administrative area, Waiting rooms, etc. Hence, very careful consideration has to be given as to how much space shall be needed as of now, as well as the space that may be required for expansion in future.

Provision for future expansion is very critical while planning. One shall look ahead for at least 20 years from now. Expansion can be on account of increase in the population size around the hospital resulting in a more patient load of the hospital, the addition of more disciplines, offer more specialists, addition in diagnostic or new and advanced machinery. To accommodate all these, the hospital may need extra spaces in the future. If the future expansion plans are not considered today it cannot be done in future.

5.2 Assessment of the Covered Area Required for Hospital

Before finalizing the size of the land, a detailed assessment has to be done regarding the covered area required for the hospital building. For calculating the covered area, first of all, a detailed list of the services to be provided in the hospital has to be prepared. Thereafter the rooms required for these services are worked out. Once the room list is finalized, sizes of the rooms have to be decided. Multiplying the sizes of the room with the number of rooms, the total area is calculated. Add provision of future expansion to these spaces. Total out the required area. Then add a particular percentage to this figure towards the movement spaces like corridors, staircases and elevators spaces (say 35%) and calculate the total area required for the hospital.

Now that the total required covered area has been calculated, we need to work out the land space required to accommodate a building that can accommodate the calculated covered area. Generally, it is seen that there are various norms specified by the Development authorities or the

A. Garg, A. Dewan, *Manual of Hospital Planning and Designing*,
https://doi.org/10.1007/978-981-16-8456-2_5

Govt. agencies for constructing a commercial building. Some of them are:

5.3 Total FAR Allowed

FAR means the Floor Area Ratio. FAR can be different for different cities. Based on the allowed FAR, the area of land has to be calculated.

5.4 Set Back Area

Generally, for all commercial buildings, norms have been prescribed by the authorities fixing the required Set Back areas to be kept around the building. Generally, the Set Back area has to be left on all four sides of the hospital building.

5.5 Maximum Permissible Land Coverage

Authorities also lay down the norms of allowed land coverage out of the total land area of the site. It may vary from 25 to 50%, depending on the city, town etc.

5.6 Maximum Permissible Height of the Building

Authorities also lay down the norms of allowed building height. There can be various factors affecting the maximum height like distance from the airport, the zone of the earthquake and average wind pressure.

Considering all these norms of the authorities along with the required calculated area, the required land space is calculated.

Other Factors
Some of the other factors to be considered while finalizing the land are:

5.7 Approach to the Site

The approach to the site of a hospital shall be convenient both to the community and to the service vehicles, including firefighting vehicles.

5.8 Location of the Land

The access to the exact location of the land shall be considered in terms of distance from the main road etc. The nearer the land from the main road, easier shall be the approach to the hospital. The frontage of the land is also considered. Wider the frontage, better shall be the design of the building.

5.9 Availability of Transportation

A good public transport facility shall be available in the area for easy access to the hospital. The transport can be like Taxis, Local Trains, Local Busses, Rikshaw and Auto.

5.10 Security

The area around the hospital shall have sufficient security measures to safeguard patients, families, personnel and the public.

5.11 Availability of Utilities

Facilities shall be available nearby to provide adequate and reliable utilities like water, gas, sewer and electricity. The water supply shall be sufficient to cater to the normal usage plus firefighting requirements. The electricity supply line shall be near to the hospital and shall have a stable voltage and frequency. The sewerage line shall be very near to the hospital building.

5.12 Road Network in the Area

There shall be proper and adequate roads for an easy approach to the hospital. The roads shall be wide enough for quick and easy traffic movement.

5.13 Environmental Pollution

One must try to choose the site having the least environmental pollution.

5.14 Wind and Earthquake

Before finalizing the land, the care shall be given to the history of the wind pressure and the earthquake in the area.

5.15 Flood Protection

If the planned area is prone to the occasional flood, care has to be taken to choose the area where the flood situation can be handled easily.

Further Reading

8 Important Things to Consider when Choosing a Location for the Hospital – Hospital Planning [Internet]. World's Largest Collection of Essays! Published by Experts. 2013 [cited 2021 Jun 8]. Available from: https://www.shareyouressays.com/knowledge/8-important-things-to-consider-when-choosing-a-location-for-the-hospital-hospital-planning/115957

Four criteria for selecting health care sites [Internet]. [cited 2021 Jun 8]. Available from: https://www.hfmmagazine.com/articles/3116-four-criteria-for-selecting-health-care-sites

Gul M, Guneri AF. Hospital Location Selection: A Systematic Literature Review on Methodologies and Applications. Math Probl Eng. 2021 Feb 13;2021:e6682958.

Jamali F, Sadrmousavi MS, Eshlaghi M. An introduction to hospital sites selection and design. J Hosp. 2012 Aug 10;11(2):87–98.

Moradian MJ, Ardalan A, Nejati A, Boloorani AD, Akbarisari A, Rastegarfar B. Risk Criteria in Hospital Site Selection: A Systematic Review. PLoS Curr [Internet]. 2017 May 1 [cited 2021 Jun 8];9. Available from: https://www.ncbi.nlm.nih.gov/pmc/articles/PMC5419719/

Varnakovida P, Messina JP. Hospital Site Selection Analysis. :16.

6 General Issues to Be Considered While Designing Hospital Building

6.1 Importance of Hospital Planning and Designing

A hospital is a place where patients are handled specially in the case of emergency and are provided medical treatments or surgeries. So, it is important to design the hospital building in such a way that the spaces look spacious and could store all the required equipment/instruments for the treatment. Also, it is very important for easy and quick movement of men and material.

As designing of the hospital, building is a complex procedure and as everybody cannot be an expert in all the fields, it is recommended that more and more professional experts from different disciplines are inducted and a team be formed for better designing. This professional team shall consist of Doctors from various disciplines, Hospital Administrators, Management representatives, Facility Planners, Architects, Electrical Engineers, Air Conditioning Engineers, Structure Engineer, Interior Designer, Civil Engineers, Biomedical Engineers, Medical planners, Landscape designer etc.

A good architectural firm considers several factors as they design the building. Some of these factors are location, patient's movement, staff movement and workflow, treatment options to be provided and the community's needs for health services. Modern hospitals are becoming more and more public-driven and provision to provide a greater number of specialized services to patients.

The design of the hospital shall be designed and created so that it is structured and maintained to provide quality health care. As patients and their families are becoming more involved in the course of treatment, hospitals need to respond to the changing requirements for treatment and accommodations. The design shall ensure the dignity of the patient by providing privacy and confidentiality.

As there are various standards of hospital design requirements and also overriding challenges for commissioners and regulators, the design of the hospital shall be such which reconciles with all these requirements and standards of various authorities. In India, the standards are like NABH and internationally the standards of JCI shall be followed. Apart from this, the industry standards must be followed while planning hospital building towards bed space, operation theatres, consultation and investigation rooms.

Well-designed, supportive hospital environment cannot only prevent harm and injury but also provide mental and physical support and help in the healing process. It has now become imperative to rethink hospital design as a critical element in bringing about change in the way health care is provided and experienced in hospitals.

A. Garg, A. Dewan, *Manual of Hospital Planning and Designing*,
https://doi.org/10.1007/978-981-16-8456-2_6

Before starting the designing of the hospital that designer shall always be clear on some of the issues like:

1. Assess the site location with the direction of sun/daylight positioning, air pathways etc.
2. Size, shape and dimensions of the land.
3. Regulations of Setback areas, Land Coverage and FSI/FAR and thus total buildable area allowed.
4. Height restrictions in the area, if any.
5. Efficient master planning.
6. Proper working on the rooms and area requirement.
7. Services to be offered in the hospital/departments to be operational in the hospital.
8. Future plans of the hospital related to the expansion of the services/departments.
9. Medical equipment/devices and their specific requirements in terms of area, utilities, weight, heat load and power load.
10. Which diagnostic facilities are to be provided?
11. Staffing numbers in each department and their specific needs.
12. Waiting area requirements (number of people expected in the waiting area).
13. Workflows of men and material.
14. Patient footfalls.
15. Patient needs.
16. Bed types and numbers in each category.
17. Operating room numbers, types based on surgery types.
18. Horizontal and vertical movements and flows.

Now various general issues relating to the hospital designing.

6.2 Flexibility and Expandability

Advancement in medical sciences is continuously happening and will happen in the future also. The needs and modes of treatment are changing day by day and will continue to change in future. New equipment, services, and diagnostic facilities will be added in the future. Therefore, the design shall be such which could easily accommodate all such advancement, without involving much alterations or modifications. The designer shall always think of at least 20 years ahead and shall provide sufficient extra spaces for future expansion. A successful hospital design and building project require careful designing and planning. It is also recommended that hospitals should follow more of the modular concepts of space planning and layout, wherever possible though considering the cost factors also. Similarly, it is also recommended to use generic room sizes, use modular, easily accessed and easily modifiable mechanical and electrical systems.

6.3 Design for the Patient Experience

What is the ultimate object of the hospital? It is basically the diagnosis and treatment of the patients. Additionally, the other goals of the hospital can be health education or prevention of the diseases, but the main objective is diagnosis and treatment. A designer must create an environment that promotes the well-being of patients because the design of a space is a part of the therapeutic process. The design shall be more of a Patient-focused design such as providing spaces to store patient's belongings, working places to have proper mobile charging stations, comfortable and pleasant waiting areas and designated spaces for private discussions with the physicians.

6.4 Design for Employee Productivity

Though patients are certainly the most important party in a hospital, as they are the people who utilize the services and assess the quality and readiness of the services provided to them. The feedback and satisfaction of the patients and the attendants of the patient are very important for the growth of the hospital.

But on the other hand, it is also true that the physicians and employees of the hospital are the ones who have to provide a quality service. It is these people who have to actually work and deliver the result. Then why should not the designer consider taking the views of these employees and physicians who have to actually work? Physicians and employees shall give their design and space requirements under which they can work efficiently and allow them to do their jobs flawlessly to best serve patients and their families.

6.5 Accessibility to the Patient

What is accessibility in terms of the hospital? As a hospital provides varied services in a large and different area of the hospital building, it is important how soon and by which means the patient and attendant can reach that area. This is accessibility. As everyone cannot walk in right away in the hospital and the special facilities may have to be provided to make it accessible for them to enter hospital like an ambulance or a helicopter may need access to your facility, therefore the Helipad and the Ambulance docking may have to be provided. Likewise, patients may need to be transferred to hospital who is already on a bed, or on a wheelchair or on crutches. So, the design must ensure fast and easy access to the facility. Therefore, the means like hospital corridors, staircases, and ramps shall be quite wide and sufficient. Similarly, there shall be elevators wide enough (like Bed Elevators) and fast. Likewise, sufficient spaces shall be provided for ambulance bays and a proper helipad should be built (if planned and needed).

6.6 Security and Safety of Men and Material

As the Hospitals are public places, a lot of people of different class and status visit the regularly. Therefore, there are several security concerns such as protection of hospital property, assets, public, patients and staff, consumables and drugs etc. Also, vulnerability to terrorism or mob attack because of high visibility cannot be ruled out. While designing a hospital, security and safety features must be built into the design keeping these issues in mind.

One of the greatest issues in healthcare design and operation is the safety of the patient. Therefore, a great concern is required for the safety of patients and attendants while designing a hospital. Some concerned events can be fall, jump, suicide or theft etc. To reduce such events, the designer shall include non-slippery surfaces including a ramp, double colour staircase of easy identification of steps, providing proper wall guards and handrails, unobstructed pathways, handicapped toilets, sealed windows or windows with grills etc.

Another important concern of patient safety is inpatient suicides. The two most common methods of suicide in hospitals are jumping and hanging. In a room there can be many things that the patients can use to hang themselves, such as bathroom curtain rods, showerheads, fans, hook if any etc. Thus, alternate methods shall be used and such fittings and fixtures should be avoided. To minimize jumping, provide windows that cannot be opened and are doubled-paned, making them much harder to breakthrough. Still, if open windows are to be provided, proper provision for the windows grills shall be present.

6.7 Sustainability of Resources

A hospital building is one of the highest consumers of resources like energy and water. Hospitals being a large public building, usually have a significant impact on the environment and economy of the surrounding community. Therefore, a sustainable design has to be worked out for reducing the consumption of these natural resources and reducing a hospital's costs on these resources. There are two issues, one is to minimize the wastage and the other is the alternate sources of these resources. Let us take the example of energy like Electricity. To minimize wastage, sensor technology can be used, which turns on and off depending on the entry or exit from the room, through sensors. Similarly, at places, one can use time-based switching on/off the lights. For alternate energy sources, one can plan for solar energy etc. Similarly, for water, we can consider mist showers instead of running water etc. Rainwater harvesting can be a good source of water. For petroleum conservation, design can be planned for battery vehicles etc. The Concepts of smart cities can be applied to the extent possible.

6.8 Efficiency and Cost-Effectiveness

While designing any project, particularly a hospital, the first thing to be kept in mind is efficiency and for that efficiency how much extra cost is needed. One shall not compromise with the efficiency in the hospital design whatsoever. Even though some extra cost has to shed out towards efficiency, it should be considered. What is efficiency in the hospital layout? It is like minimizing the distance of necessary travel between frequently used spaces; rushing to the patient in case of emergency; allow supervision of patients visually; efficient logistics system for supplies of consumable, medicines and food and of course removal of waste; keep spaces out of infection and cross infection; make efficient use of multi-purpose spaces and consolidate spaces to a smaller space where ever possible.

6.9 Adaptation of Technological Advancements

In the twenty-first century, everybody has seen the advancement in technology, particularly the advancement in electronics. Another major revolution has been noticed in Web Technology and the usage of Smartphones. Today most of the equipment in the hospitals is electronic-based and as there is continuous advancement in the electronic, the designs of the medical equipment are changing. Apart from this a lot of new medical equipment is being invented, resulting in more advanced medical care and diagnostic facilities. The cloud and web technologies have changed the world and so have medical services in terms of data storage, research, and clinical trials. Also with the changing technology and infectious diseases like COVID-19 have pushed the world towards the adaptation of more and more Telemedicine.

Considering this fact of continuous advancement in the technologies, the designer while designing the hospital has to keep in mind that in the coming future, these advancements have to be adopted by the hospital. Therefore, the designer shall plan and provide spaces for easy adaptation of these advancements. Also, keep in mind the required modifications that need to be done in future to adapt to the changing technology.

In order to provide timely, accurate diagnosis, treatment and interventions, physicians need to have complete and real-time information about the patient, symptoms, investigations, care required and different treatment options. Technologies such as the Internet, electronic medical records and clinical decision-support systems can help a lot in achieving the assignment.

6.10 Stress and Fear of Patients and Visitors

Stress and Fear of the patients and attendants is one of the major concerns during the course of a patient's treatment and care. People usually feel stressed and fear for their relative or friend who is suffering from the disease. Therefore, while designing the hospital, the designer shall create a design that can reduce the stress and fear of the patient. The environment of the hospital shall give a positive feeling to the people present in the hospital. While designing, the designer shall plan to give spaces for some worship area in the premises. Also, the designer can keep the provision of wall hangings having positive quotes and religious photographs. Apart from this, a provision for continuous counselling of the people in the hospital can be provided.

6.11 Quality Care of Patients

In a hospital, the quality and quick care of the patients matters a lot. The designer has to ensure that in his/her design quality care is provided without wastage of time, e.g. the provision for a separate ambulance bay has to be provided for emergency and the provision of stretcher trolley and the wheelchair is provided at the entrance of the door for quick movement of the patient. Similarly, immediately on arrival of the patient, high level of quality and competent care, availability of qualified physicians and allied health professionals leave a positive impact on the quality of service. To achieve this, the designer can plan a Medical Officer room just at the entrance of the emergency department. Likewise, so many other factors can be considered while designing the building.

6.12 Therapeutic Environment

Patients and visitors should perceive a hospital as an advanced, equipped, comfortable, safe, unthreatening, and stress-free area capable of maintaining privacy. While designing, apart from the designer, an interior designer also plays an important role in designing to create an excellent healthcare environment. For example, this can be achieved by considering ample natural lights, fresh air, using cheerful and varied colours and textures, providing outside views from the patient bed, and by providing effective signage systems. Designers should provide an environment in which the overall design of the building contributes to the process of healing and reduces the fear, noise, infection rate and that are safe and private.

6.13 Cleanliness and Sanitation

As hospitals are dealing with sick and infectious patients, an important factor to consider when building a hospital is cleanliness and sanitation. Hospitals need to be kept extremely clean to prevent the spread of diseases and infections. Therefore, the design shall be such that it provides quick and efficient cleaning, sanitizing and disinfecting. People come to the hospital with germs and bacteria, so the need is to ensure that the materials you select do not hold these items in. Very careful selection of the material is the crux to this. While choosing the material the designer has to keep in mind how easy they are to care for, how much footfall they can sustain, which methods can be used to clean them, and if they can be cleaned and/or sterilized. In addition to the other requirements, floors in hospitals must be puncture and impact-, abrasion- and stain-resistant.

6.14 Noise Reduction

In a hospital setup, noise interferes with comforts of the patients, affects communication, decreases concentration, distracts, affects cognitive performance and also increases stress and fatigue. Noise can also adversely impact healing, disturb sleep and reduce overall patient satisfaction levels. The causes of noise can be due to movement of a lot of men and materials at a particular point of time, screaming due to pain and fear, back-to-back patient beds on the same wall, vibration noise on the floor, noise of the mechanical/electrical/plumbing systems, improper flooring, outside traffic horn and unwanted announcements and music at high volume. Also, the unwanted mobile rings and loud talking create nuisance and disturbance to others.

Therefore, while designing the hospital the designer has to keep in mind all these issues and provide measures to curb the noise in the hospital building. Some of the measures can be like beds shall be placed on the opposite walls instead of common walls, flooring can be noiseless like rubber or PVC, triple glazed windows can be planned, usage of nurse call systems with a minimal tone having vibration features, proper vibration pads for electrical/mechanical machines, proper insulation of walls can be an option, special ceiling tiles that can absorb noise shall be opted and mobile phones shall be kept on vibrating mode.

6.15 Minimizing the Operative, Postoperative and Hospital-Acquired Infections

Due to the huge footfall of varied people, the chances of infection are tremendous in the hospital setup. As a lot of infected patients from various diseases land in the hospital, it is believed that the atmosphere inside the hospital building contains various types of infections. There are all the chances that a healthy patient may acquire the infection from the hospital, which is generally called Nosocomial infection. Still further, the infection acquired during the intervention or surgeries can be worse for the patient.

Therefore, while designing the hospital building, the designer has to ensure that the chances of infection are minimized. Some of the factors that can reduce the infection rate are: One-way movement in the operating complex, proper zoning of the areas wherein for the infectious patients a separate zone is provided; proper barricading of the infectious areas; internal window blinds to be provided to reduce the accumulation of dust; providing proper air filtration system including HEPA filters; ultraviolet lights clinical areas; airflow systems in which clean air passes the patient and is recycled and filtered again; cross ventilation to be provided; radiant heat panel eliminates condensation; reduction of the waiting area in the patient treatment areas etc.

6.16 Automation Where Possible

The design of the building should be in a manner that can easily adapt automation. Adaptation of automation and technology like electronic medical records, bar-coding, physician order entry, a pneumatic tube system, computers in room, sophisticated nurse call system and interfacing the diagnostic equipment with the software. The adoption of automation is definitely a necessary component for improving patient care more efficiently and relying less on manual systems.

6.17 Environmental Pollution Control

The design, construction, renovation, expansion and operation of hospitals are all subject to provisions of several environmental pollution control laws and guidelines and its associated regulatory regulations. The regulations are like air quality, handling and disposal of biomedical waste, noise pollution, underground storage tanks, hazardous materials and wastes storage and medical waste storage and disposal. While designing the hospital it has to be ensured that all the statutory regulations of environment pollution control are addressed and complied with.

Hospitals generally produce a lot of waste, including biomedical waste, which is hazardous. A properly designed system is required to handle such wastes.

Hospitals also use a large amount of energy. Hence, it is very important to adopt other means to save energy. Adoption of solar panels or using environmentally safe building products, rainwater harvesting, adding electric vehicles etc. can be a great effort to lessen the environmental impact the hospital building is going to create in the surrounding areas.

6.18 Internal Road

Roads inside the hospital property shall be either paved or cemented roads for access to all entrances and to patient landing areas and for delivery of material to the hospital. Hospitals having emergency services shall have separate emergency access, well-demarcated and marked to facilitate entry from the public roads or streets.

6.19 Parking

Adequate vehicular parking shall be made available for staff, patients, families, personnel and the public with a clear entrance to and exit from the parking area. Sufficient security for the vehicles shall be ensured.

6.20 Wind, Earthquake-Resistant and Flood Protection

Hospital buildings shall be designed in such a fashion that can address the issues relating to earthquakes, tornadoes, flooding, hurricanes and other regional disasters. Planning and design shall consider the need to protect the life and ensure the safety of all hospital workers, occupants and visitors to the hospital. Also, the design shall have the means and way-outs which shall permit for continuity of services following such a disaster.

6.21 Nature Plus Artwork

The patients and/or attendants coming to the hospital are normally in pain and are mentally disturbed. Further, if the hospital's look and ambience are not good, or the colours are not soothing (like Red is not preferred in hospitals, being the colour of blood), or there is a lot of noise and disturbance, the patients and attendants do not feel comfortable. Therefore, the hospitals shall try to include nature and artwork to the extent possible while designing the building and the colours shall be attractive etc. The windows shall be provided for better natural views. Providing all these facilities while designing, will give more positive feelings to the patient and attendants. Both nature and artwork shall contribute to patients having a greater sense of well-being.

6.22 Colours to Be Used

Colours give a different sense of place in hospitals. Also, colour has been known to be associated with mood. Colour can even help patients to have a sense of orientation. Therefore, while designing the designer must stress the choice of colours. As the choice of colour varies from person to person and the promoter may insist on the colour of his/her choice, but the designer shall insist on the colours that will fit in the use and give a soothing effect. Also, the colour shall allow easy identification of the spaces. Using different colour choices for patient private rooms, corridors, waiting areas, examination rooms, procedure rooms etc. can have a definite effect on patient motivation, stress levels and satisfaction.

6.23 Choice of Building Materials

For a hospital building, the choice of materials is a skill that the designer puts in. Right from the start of construction, the factor of choice of material comes in. Like for RCC work the choice can be pre-mix concrete, Hollow block instead of bricks can be used and flooring can have tiles instead of marble stone. It is also true that materials play an important role in the overall look and feel. When designing a hospital specifically, materials must be considered for both safety and aesthetic looks and must stand up to the steady movement of men and material. Flooring, furniture, wall coverings, lighting and even handrails and other fixtures should be conducive to infection control measures and should be glare and slip-resistant were necessary to maximize safety. Moreover, after the COVID-19 period, preference is given to a material that can be easily disinfected and sanitized.

6.24 Flooring

For a hospital, the appropriate flooring choice must live up to rigorous standards. The Flooring must meet strict health codes as provided by various standards. When choosing flooring systems for hospitals, there are several considerations to take into account and many different requirements must be met. In hospitals, different spaces may require different floorings. Like the flooring of the ramps has to be slip-resistant, similarly, the flooring of reception may differ from the flooring of patient rooms and corridors etc. Flooring shall promote safety, maintain hygiene and infection control protocols, should be easily cleanable and disinfectable, contribute to a positive patient experience and with proven durability with minimal maintenance costs. Flooring shall also look aesthetic, give a clean appearance and shall provide a positive and welcoming atmosphere for patients, attendants and healthcare workers.

Further Reading

10 Elements of the Perfect Hospital Design - Architizer Journal [Internet]. Journal. 2019 [cited 2021 Jun 1]. Available from: https://architizer.com/blog/practice/details/perfect-hospital-design/

Groeneveld B, Dekkers T, Boon B, D'Olivo P. Challenges for design researchers in healthcare. Des Health. 2018 Jul 3;2(2):305–26.

Hospital design challenges: now and into the future [Internet]. [cited 2021 Jun 10]. Available from: , http://hospitalhealth.com.au/content/design-in-health/article/hospital-design-challenges-now-and-into-the-future-1050121645

How to Ensure Patient Safety in a Healthcare Setting [Internet]. Regis College Online. 2018 [cited 2021 Jun 10]. Available from: https://online.regiscollege.edu/blog/7-tips-ensuring-patient-safety-healthcare-settings/

Indmedica - Journal of the Academy of Hospital Administration [Internet]. [cited 2021 Jun 10]. Available from: https://www.indmedica.com/journals.php?journalid=6&issueid=25&articleid=238&action=article

Lateef F. Hospital design for better infection control. J Emerg Trauma Shock. 2009;2(3):175–9.

Major Issues and Trends Impacting Health and Hospital Planning, Design, Construction, Operation and Maintenance [Internet]. [cited 2021 Jun 10]. Available from: https://www.asianhhm.com/facilities-operations/issues-trends-hospital-planning-design

Nusem E. Design in Healthcare: Challenges and Opportunities. In 2018.

Reiling J, Hughes RG, Murphy MR. The Impact of Facility Design on Patient Safety. In: Hughes RG, editor. Patient Safety and Quality: An Evidence-Based Handbook for Nurses [Internet]. Rockville (MD): Agency for Healthcare Research and Quality (US); 2008 [cited 2021 Jun 10]. (Advances in Patient Safety). Available from: http://www.ncbi.nlm.nih.gov/books/NBK2633/

Theodore D. Better design, better hospitals. CMAJ Can Med Assoc J. 2016 Sep 6;188(12):902–3.

7 Area Requirement and Planning

Now that after the preparation of the DPR and acceptance of the feasibility studies is done and final approval of the promoter is received, the designer has to proceed with the further planning part of the building. The next step is working and calculating the area requirement.

Hospitals are one of the most complexes of building types. Hospitals provide a wide range of services and functional units through its various departments and support services. These include, but are not limited to, diagnostic and therapeutic functions, such as operating rooms; emergency; imaging; clinical laboratories; support functions, such as housekeeping; food services and fundamental inpatient care or bed-related activities. Each of these functionalities of a hospital including complicated electrical, mechanical, information technology and telecommunications systems, needs specialized knowledge and expertise. Furthermore, due to various regulations, norms and code of various agencies which govern the hospital design, planning and designing of hospital becomes much more complicated.

The design process incorporates the suggestions and input from the owner and from key hospital staff who has to actually work and deliver results. The designer also has to understand the requirements of the patients, visitors, support staff, volunteers and suppliers who do not generally have direct input towards the design.

What does the area mean? The area is the space required for the particular service, functionality or department and is termed as the carpet area. The difference between the carpet area and the total area is that the carpet area is the actual functional area and if the wall spaces and the movement spaces like corridors, ramps, staircases and lifts are added to it, it is called the total area.

7.1 Functional Areas

Calculation of the area or space requirement is the foremost task the designer has to undertake, and based on these requirements only the designer can begin the work of architectural drawings. Basically, if we see the functionality of the hospital, the following are the functional areas:

1. **Emergency Services**: Is for providing the service to the patient after the OPD timing or the patient who are critically sick or injured accidentally and trauma cases.
2. **Entrance Area**: The area in which the patients or visitors land into before going to any other department or before availing any other services of the hospital.
3. **OPD Services**: The area where the outdoor consultation is provided to patients who are not critical or follow-up patients.
4. **Diagnostic Services**: The area where different types of diagnostic investigation are performed to support the physicians for the

A. Garg, A. Dewan, *Manual of Hospital Planning and Designing*,
https://doi.org/10.1007/978-981-16-8456-2_7

actual diagnosis of the disease and further management and treatment of the patient. It can be Imaging, Clinical Laboratories, Cath Lab etc.

5. **Other Treatments**: These are the areas where support para-medical treatment like dialysis or physiotherapy are provided.
6. **Intensive Care Services**: The area where the critical patients are kept under strict supervision and monitoring and the treatment is provided.
7. **Therapeutic Services**: This is the area where the interventions and surgeries are performed like Operating Room and Labour Room.
8. **Intermediate Care Area**: This is the area where the patients are actually admitted in the indoor for further management and treatment. It can be General Wards, Semi-private Rooms, Private Rooms, Deluxe Room, VIP Suites, Isolation rooms etc.
9. **Administrative/Ancillary Services**: The area from where the administration of the hospital is taken care of. This includes areas like Directors' office, MS office, NS office, IT Department and Personnel/Purchase/Marketing/Accounts office.
10. **Hospital Services**: The services which indirectly help in the management and treatment of the patients. This can be like CSSD, Kitchen, Laundry, Stores and Mortuary.
11. **Engineering Services**: The support department keeps the systems of the hospital alive so that all other services and departments work smoothly. These are like Electrical, Mechanical, Public Health, Fire Protection, Communication, Medical Gases, HVAC and various Workshops.
12. **Other Services**: All other services like Security, Transport, Housekeeping, Conference and Medical Record.

7.2 Room/Space Requirement

Once the functional areas are finalized, the next step is to prepare the list and details of the rooms that will be required for each function. There are a lot of factors and issues based on which the number of rooms required shall be worked out. Below are some of them, but are not limited to:

1. Do the promoters desire to follow the norms of agencies like NABH or JCI which provide the minimum standards for hospitals?
2. What are the projections on the numbers of patients expected to utilize the services of the hospital?
3. How much footfall is expected in the entrance lobby?
4. How many service counters and how many shops are planned in the entrance hall?
5. How big the pharmacy shall be? How many patients are expected to take medicine from the pharmacy? What will be the quantum of stock in the pharmacy?
6. How many specialities and super speciality departments are to be made operational initially and in future?
7. What will be the system of conducting OPD? Will a single OPD chamber be allotted to one speciality or otherwise there will be a chamber sharing system based on time slot?
8. For which departments do the OPD's have to be designed specifically?
9. What all procedures and diagnostic services will be provided in the OPD? For example, in Ophthalmology will the service be given for laser, A-Scan, B-Scan etc. and for Cardiology which investigations will be carried out like ECG, Echocardiography, Holter, Tilt Test, TMT, ABP, Thallium Test, Nuclear Heart Scan, ElectroPhysiology studies and Dobutamine Stress Echocardiography?
10. What services will be provided in Radiology initially and in future like X-Rays, Ultrasound, Mammography, CT Scan, MRI, PET CT, PET MRI and Gamma Scan?
11. Which investigations will be carried out in clinical laboratories in-house, and which will be sent to outside labs?
12. Which investigations are planned to be provided in future?
13. Will the blood bank deal only with whole blood or the components as well and whether the apheresis is planned today or in future?

14. Will the high-end procedures be done in the hospital like Cath Lab?
15. Will the department of Oncology be provided? If yes will Radiotherapy be provided?
16. How many and what type of patients are expected to land in emergency and triage?
17. Is a major operating room required in an emergency or is a minor OT enough?
18. What all paramedical treatment facilities to be provided like Physiotherapy, Orthotics, Speech Therapy and Occupational Therapy?
19. Will the facility of Dialysis be provided? If yes, how many patients are expected per day?
20. How many ICUs are to be planned along with the future expansion plans, e.g. MICU, SICU, RICU, NICU, Neuro ICU, ICCU, Gynae ICU, Paedia ICU, Ortho ICU and Pulmonary ICU?
21. How many beds are to be provided in each ICU?
22. Is the HDU/Step Down ICU required?
23. How many Operating Rooms are to be planned? Will there be any dedicated operating rooms for specialized surgeries like Organ Transplants?
24. How many delivery rooms are to be planned? Out of which, how many are expected to be infectious?
25. What shall be the bed capacity in each ward/function? For example, the number of beds planned for Triage, Emergency ward, General Wards etc.?
26. How many Private, Semi-Private, Deluxe and VIP Suits are planned?
27. How many administrative staff are planned to be seated at a time?
28. Will the services of Laundry and Kitchen be in-house or outsourced?
29. Whether the Oxygen supply is made through a cylinder manifold or liquid oxygen plant has to be installed?

Before working out the actual room requirement initially and keeping provision for the future, the answers to these types of questions have to be provided. To answer such questions, it is felt that a team of experts be formed, including the physicians and statisticians, to collect details either from the other such hospitals or by their own experience. The feasibility studies already done in this regard earlier shall be of great help to answer most of such questions.

Once the answers to such questions are provided, the actual work of room requirements is started. For preparing the list of rooms, it has to be assessed how many rooms shall be required for every functionality and each service of that functionality.

Another important issue comes out regarding the ancillary rooms required attached to or along with the main service room. For example, the Surgery OPD may require the dressing room, Eye OPD may require a refraction room, laser room, dark room, procedure room etc. Hence, the detailed work about the ancillary rooms has to be done for each and every service room.

Based on the experience and practical uses, we have worked out a list of such ancillary rooms required along with the main service room, which has been given in Table 7.1.

Based on the above example, the final list of rooms required has to be finalized.

Table 7.1 Rooms required for various zones/units/departments

Zone	Function/room
Entrance area	
Entrance lobby	Trolley park
	General waiting
	Public utilities
Reception	Enquiry counter
	Registration counter
	Queuing tracks
	Records
	Admission counter
	Discharge counter
	Cash counter
	Health insurance counter
	Empanelled patients counter

(continued)

Table 7.1 (continued)

Zone	Function/room
Pharmacy	Storage and disbursing hall
	Bulk storage
	Cold room
	Expiry medicine room
	Costly medicine room
	Cut strip sorting room
	Pharmacist office
	Public utility for staff
Arcade	Temple
	Snack counter
	Book shop
	Gift shop
	Other shop—1
	Other shop—2
	ATM
Control rooms for	Security
	Housekeeping
	Fire safety
	Water supply
	Electrical safety
	Ambulance
Service/staff entrance	**Staff utilities**
	Lockers
	Change rooms
	Time keeping
OPD services	
Specialities	
Medicine block	Examination room with exam. cubicles
	Rooms for special clinics
	Clinical demonstration room
	Extra rooms for future expansion
	Reception inquiry
	Registration
	Record room
	Store
	Public utility for faculty
	Public utility for patients and attendants
	Sub waiting
Surgery block	Examination room with exam. cubicles
	Rooms for special clinics
	Clinical demonstration room
	Extra rooms for future expansion
	Reception and enquiry
	Registration
	Record room
	Dressing room—Male
	Dressing room—Female
	Endoscopy room
	Change room
	Store
	Reporting room
	Minor operation theatre
	Change room for OT
	Sluice room
	Store
	Store
	Public utility for faculty
	Public utility for patients and attendants
	Sub waiting
Ophthalmology block	Examination room with examination cubicles
	Rooms for special clinics
	Clinical demonstration room
	Extra rooms for future expansion
	Reception and enquiry
	Registration
	Record room
	Refraction
	Orthopty
	Treatment
	Dark room
	Dressing room
	Store
	Public utility for faculty
	Public utility for patients and attendants
	Sub waiting

Table 7.1 (continued)

Zone	Function/room
ENT block	Examination room with exam. cubicles
	Rooms for special clinics
	Clinical demonstration room
	Extra rooms for future expansion
	Reception and enquiry
	Registration
	Record room
	Audiometry
	ENG Lab
	Speech Therapy room
	Store
	Public utility for faculty
	Public utility for patients and attendants
	Sub waiting
Dental block	Examination room with Dental Chairs
	Rooms for special clinics
	Clinical demonstration room
	Extra rooms for future expansion
	Reception and enquiry
	Registration
	Record room
	Dental laboratory
	Dental X-ray
	Dental surgery
	Prosthetic dentistry
	Store
	Public utility for faculty
	Public utility for patients and attendants
	Sub waiting

Table 7.1 (continued)

Zone	Function/room
Obs. and Gynae. block	Examination room with exam. cubicles
	Rooms for special clinics
	Clinical demonstration room
	Extra rooms for future expansion
	Reception and enquiry
	Registration
	Record room
	D & C room
	IVF clinic
	Antenatal clinic
	Family welfare clinic
	Sterility clinic
	Cancer detection Clinic
	Ultrasound room
	Colposcopy room
	Store
	Public utility for faculty
	Public utility for patients and attendants
	Sub waiting
Paediatric block	Examination room with exam. cubicles
	Rooms for special clinics
	Clinical demonstration room
	Extra rooms for future expansion
	Reception and enquiry
	Registration
	Record room
	Play area
	Child welfare including immunization clinic
	Child guidance clinic
	Child rehabilitation clinic including facilities for speech therapy and occupational therapy
	Counselling
	Store
	Public utility for faculty
	Public utility for patients and attendants
	Sub waiting

(continued)

Table 7.1 (continued)

Zone	Function/room
Orthopaedics block	Examination room with exam. cubicles
	Rooms for special clinics
	Clinical demonstration room
	Extra rooms for future expansion
	Reception and enquiry
	Registration
	Record room
	Plaster room
	Plaster-cutting room
	Splint store
	Store
	Public utility for faculty
	Public utility for patients and attendants
	Sub waiting
Dermatology/VD block	Examination room with exam. cubicles
	Rooms for special clinics
	Clinical demonstration room
	Extra rooms for future expansion
	Reception and enquiry
	Registration
	Record room
	Skin lab
	Treatment Room
	Store
	Public utility for faculty
	Public utility for patients and attendants
	Sub waiting
Psychiatry block	Examination room with exam. cubicles
	Rooms for special clinics
	Clinical demonstration room
	Extra rooms for future expansion
	Reception and enquiry
	Registration
	Record room
	Counselling
	ECT/Recovery
	EEG room
	NCV/EMG room
	Store
	Public utility for faculty
	Public utility for patients and attendants
	Sub waiting

Table 7.1 (continued)

Zone	Function/room
TB and chest block	Examination room with exam. cubicles
	Rooms for special clinics
	Clinical demonstration room
	Extra rooms for future expansion
	Reception and enquiry
	Registration
	Record room
	ICTC centre
	DOT centre
	PFT room
	Store
	Public utility for faculty
	Public utility for patients and attendants
	Sub waiting
Dietary	Examination room with exam. cubicles
	Extra rooms for future expansion
	Reception and enquiry
	Registration
	Record room
	Store
	Public utility for faculty
	Public utility for patients and attendants
	Sub waiting
Super specialities	
Cardiology	Exam/Consultation
	Sub waiting
Cardiac surgery	Exam/Consultation
	Sub waiting
Burns and plastic surgery	Exam/Consultation
	Sub waiting
Diabetes and endocrinology	Exam/Consultation
	Sub waiting
Geriatric medicine	Exam/Consultation
	Sub waiting
Gastroenterology medicine	Exam/Consultation
	Sub waiting
Gastroenterology surgery	Exam/Consultation
	Sub waiting
Pulmonology	Exam/Consultation
	Procedure room
	Sub waiting
Nephrology	Exam/Consultation
	Sub waiting
Neurology	Exam/Consultation
	Sub waiting

Table 7.1 (continued)

Zone	Function/room
Neurosurgery	Exam/Consultation
	Sub waiting
Oncology medicine	Exam/Consultation
	Sub waiting
Oncology surgery	Exam/Consultation
	Sub waiting
Oncology radiation therapy	Exam/Consultation
	Sub waiting
Paediatric surgery	Exam/Consultation
	Sub waiting
Urology	Exam/Consultation
	UroDynamics study room
	Uro flow meter room
	Sub waiting
Diagnostic services	
Imaging	
Utility area	Reception and enquiry
	Registration
	Record room
	Store for unused films and related material
	Store for used films
	Public utility for faculty
	Public utility for patients and attendants
	Report delivery room
	Sub waiting
	Extra rooms for future expansion
X-ray	Radiography rooms for DR or X-ray machine
	Radiography Room IITV system and fluoroscopy
	Room for 60 mA mobile X-ray system
	Change rooms
	Sub waiting
	Barium preparation
	CR room
Ultrasound	Ultrasound
	Change room
	Toilets
	Sub waiting
CT Scan	Examination room
	Control room
	UPS room
	Change room
	Store
	Sub waiting

Table 7.1 (continued)

Zone	Function/room
MRI	Examination room
	Control room
	UPS room
	Machine room
	Change room
	Store
	Sub waiting
Mammography	Examination room
	Change room
	Store
	Sub waiting
PET scan	Examination room
	Control room
	UPS room
	Machine room
	Holding cubicles
	Medicine storage
	Medicine preparation room
	Medicine infusion room
	Change room
	Toilet with settlement tank
	Store
	Sub waiting
Other new investigations	Examination room
	Control room
	UPS room
	Machine room
	Change room
	Store
	Sub-waiting
Support	Electric panel room
	Reporting room
	Seminar cum library
Staff accommodation	HOD with toilet
	PA to HOD
	Doctors rooms
	Senior resident room
Clinical laboratories	
Utility area	Sample collection room
	Sample receipt/preparation
	Reception and enquiry
	Registration
	Record room
	Store for unused reagents, kits and related materials
	Public utility for faculty
	Public utility for patients and attendants
	Report delivery room
	Sub waiting
	Extra rooms for future expansion

(continued)

Table 7.1 (continued)

Zone	Function/room
Clinical laboratories	Biochemistry
	Microbiology
	Pathology
	Histopathology
	Histology
	Cytology
Support	Washing and disinfection
	Media preparation
	Clinical demonstration room
	Seminar cum library
Blood bank	Reception waiting
	Bleeding
	Apheresis' room
	Refreshment/Rest room
	Blood testing room
	Record
	Blood lab/Storage
	Doctors rest room
Other investigations	
Cardiac investigations	ECG room
	TMT room
	Echocardiography
	Holter rooms
	ABP Rooms
	Ultrasound rooms
	Tilt test room
	Thallium scan
	Nuclear heart scan camera (gamma camera)
	Electrophysiology lab
	Dobutamine Stress Echocardiography (DSE)
	Reception and enquiry
	Registration
	Record room
	Store
	Public utility for faculty
	Public utility for patients and attendants
	Report delivery room
	Sub waiting
	Extra rooms for future expansion

Table 7.1 (continued)

Zone	Function/room
Cath lab	Reception and enquiry
	Registration
	Record room
	Report delivery room
	Sub waiting
	Extra rooms for future expansion
	Examination
	Control
	UPS
	Panel
	Doctors change
	Staff change
	Scrub
	Cath wash
	Toilet
	CD store
	Store
Pulmonology investigations	**Sleep clinic**
	Spirometer rooms
	Body box diffusion
	Seno room
	6 min walk test room
	Diffusion room for DLCO
	ET/CT room
	Pulmonary rehabilitation
	Endoscopic room
	TBNA room
Neurology investigations	Transcranial Doppler
	Neuro physiotherapy room
	Speech and swallowing clinic
	EEG lab
	NVC/EMG
	EEG lab
Department of radiotherapy	
Utility area	Reception and enquiry
	Registration
	Record room
	Store
	Public utility for faculty
	Public utility for patients and attendants
	Report delivery room
	Sub waiting
	Extra rooms for future expansion

Table 7.1 (continued)

Zone	Function/room
Treatment area	Teletherapy unit
	Intracavitary treatment room
	Interstitial, endocavitary, surface mould therapy room
	Planning room
	Metalling treatment planning equipment, mould room
	Medical Physics Laboratory
	Chemotherapy/Radiotherapy procedures etc.
	Control room
	Doctors change
	Staff change
	Scrub
	Toilet
	Store
Radiotherapy ward	Patient beds
	Nurses duty room
	Store
	Dirty utility/Sluice room
	Clean supply room
	Examination and treatment room
	Ward pantry
	Resident doctors and student duty room
	Extra rooms for future expansion
	Public utility for staff
	Public utility for patients and attendants
Emergency services	
Entrance lobby	Trolley park
	General waiting
	Public utilities
Reception	Enquiry counter
	Registration counter
	Queuing tracks
	Records
	Admission counter
	Cash counter
Attached rooms	Procedure rooms
	Plaster room
	Clean utility
	ECG room
	Medico-legal specimen and record
	Dirty linen
	Store
	Portable X-ray room
	Disaster storage room

Table 7.1 (continued)

Zone	Function/room
Triage	Examination resuscitation
	Waiting
	Examination cubicles
	EMO duty room
	Public utility for faculty
	Public utility for patients and attendants
Minor operating suite	Minor OT
	Scrub/Gowning
	Dirty utility
Staff accommodation	Nurse duty
	Doctors duty
	Ambulance driver/Nursing assistant
Emergency operation theatre complex	Operation theatre
	Pre-operative room
	Post-operative recovery
	Sterilization
	Clean storage
	Toilet
	Sluice room
	Instrument/Linen wash
	Store
	Change room doctors—Male
	Change room doctors—Female
	Change room staff—Male
	Change room staff—Female
Emergency ward	Ward
	Store
	Examination and treatment room
	Nurses duty room
	Ward pantry
	Resident doctors and student duty room
	Night duty room for junior residents
	Public utility for faculty
	Public utility for patients and attendants

(continued)

Table 7.1 (continued)

Zone	Function/room
Other treatments	
Physiotherapy	Examination room with exam. cubicles
	Clinical demonstration room
	Extra rooms for future expansion
	Reception and enquiry
	Registration
	Record room
	Electrotherapy
	Thermotherapy
	Massage therapy
	Traction
	Gymnasium
	Store
	Public utility for faculty
	Public utility for patients and attendants
	Sub waiting
Dialysis	Procedure room
	Procedure room for positive patients
	Dialyser wash
	Toilet cum change room
	Media preparation room
	Store
	RO plant room
	Sub waiting
Intensive care area	
MICU, CCU, RICU, SICU, CTVS, PICU, Burn ICU etc.	Patient beds
	Intensive care beds
	Clean utility
	Equipment park/store
	Dirty utility/Sluice room
	Examination and treatment room
	Formula Room
	Public utility for staff
	Public utility for patients and attendants
	Sub waiting area
Staff accommodation	Change room—Male
	Change room—Female
	Resident doctors and student duty room
	Nurses night duty room
	Night duty room for junior residents

Table 7.1 (continued)

Zone	Function/room
Step down ICU/ HDU	Patient beds
	Intensive care beds
	Clean utility
	Equipment park/store
	Dirty utility/sluice room
	Examination and treatment room
	Ward pantry
	Public utility for staff
	Public utility for patients and attendants
	Sub waiting area
Staff accommodation	Change room—Male
	Change room—Female
	Resident doctors and student duty room
	Nurses night duty room
	Night duty room for junior residents
Neonatal ICU	Patient beds
	Clean baby room
	Infected baby room
	Ventilator room
	Clean utility
	Equipment park/store
	Dirty utility/sluice room
	Examination and treatment room
	Mothers feeding room
	Cloth wash area
	Formula Room
	Public utility for staff
	Public utility for patients and attendants
	Sub waiting area
Staff accommodation	Change room—Male
	Change room—Female
	Resident doctors and student duty room
	Nurses night duty room
	Night duty room for junior residents
Therapeutic services	
Operation theatre suite	
Unsterile zone	Waiting area for attendants
	Public utility for patients and attendants

Table 7.1 (continued)

Zone	Function/room
Protective zone	Staff changing technicians with toilet—Males
	Staff changing technicians with toilet—Females
	Staff changing Class IV with toilet—Males
	Staff changing Class IV with toilet—Females
	Students changing with toilet—Males
	Students changing with toilet—Females
	Doctors change room with toilet—Male
	Doctors change room with toilet—Female
	Lockers
	Unsterile store
	Office
	Restroom for staff—Males
	Restroom for staff—Females
	Pantry
	Surgeons restroom
	Observation gallery for students
	Soiled linen pre-wash room
	Soiled instruments wash room
Clean zone	Dirty utility
	Pre-operative room
	Preparation room
	Post-operative recovery
	Public utility for patients
Sterile zone	Main operating theatres
	Septic operation theatre
	Endoscopy room
	Scrub/Gowning
	Instrument trolley layup
	Clean supply room
	Sterilization room
	Clean store

Table 7.1 (continued)

Zone	Function/room
Delivery suite	
Protective zone	Nursing station
	Trolley park
	Pre-labour patient beds
	Eclampsia beds
	Exam/Prep
	Post-natal recovery
	Public utilities for patients
	Staff changing technicians with toilet—Males
	Staff changing technicians with toilet—Females
	Staff changing Class IV with toilet—Males
	Staff changing Class IV with toilet—Females
	Students changing with toilet—Males
	Students changing with toilet—Females
	Doctors change room with toilet—Male
	Doctors change room with toilet—Female
	Lockers
	Unsterile store
	Office
	Duty room for students—Males
	Duty room for students—Females
	Pantry
	Surgeons restroom
	Observation gallery for students
	Soiled linen pre-wash room
	Soiled instruments wash room
Delivery area	Labour room
	Scrub/Gowning
	Clean utility
	Nursery baby bath
	Dirty utility
	Store

(continued)

Table 7.1 (continued)

Zone	Function/room
Intermediate care area	
General ward	Patient beds
	Nurses duty room
	Store
	Dirty utility/sluice room
	Clean supply room
	Examination and treatment room
	Ward pantry
	Resident doctors and student duty room
	Extra rooms for future expansion
	Public utility for staff
	Public utility for patients and attendants
	Visitors bay
Semi-private ward	Patient beds (twin sharing) with toilet
	Nurse desk
	Store
	Dirty utility/Sluice room
	Clean supply room
	Examination and treatment room
	Ward pantry
	Resident doctors and student duty room
	Nurses duty room
	Extra rooms for future expansion
	Public utility for Staff
	Visitors bay
Private ward	Patient beds (single bed) with toilet
	Nurse desk
	Store
	Dirty utility/Sluice room
	Clean supply room
	Examination and treatment room
	Ward pantry
	Resident doctors and student duty room
	Nurses duty room
	Extra rooms for future expansion
	Public utility for staff
	Visitors bay

Table 7.1 (continued)

Zone	Function/room
Deluxe ward	Patient beds (single bed) with toilet
	Nurse desk
	Store
	Dirty utility/Sluice room
	Clean supply room
	Examination and treatment room
	Ward pantry
	Resident doctors and student duty room
	Nurses duty room
	Extra rooms for future expansion
	Public utility for staff
	Visitors bay
Family suites	Patient beds (single bed) with toilet
	Family room
	Nurse desk
	Store
	Dirty utility/Sluice room
	Clean supply room
	Examination and treatment room
	Ward pantry
	Resident doctors and student duty room
	Nurses duty room
	Extra rooms for future expansion
	Public utility for staff
	Visitors bay
Administrative/Ancillary services	
Hospital administration	
Directors office	Office
	Toilet
	Directors P.A. room
	Secretarial staff
	Waiting area for visitors
Medical superintendent office	Office
	Toilet
	P.A. room
	Secretarial staff
	Waiting area for visitors
Dy. medical superintendent office	Office
	Toilet
	P.A. room
	Secretarial staff
	Waiting area for visitors

Table 7.1 (continued)

Zone	Function/room
Nursing administration	
Nursing superintendent office	Office
	Toilet
	P.A. room
	Secretarial staff
	Waiting area for visitors
Dy. nursing superintendent office	Office
	Toilet
General administration	
Personnel office	Personnel manager
	Training and skill development manager
	Attendance management
	Leaves record
	Clerks
	Toilet
Account office	Finance manager
	Chief cashier
	Officers
	Clerks
	Stores
	Sub waiting
	Public utility for staff
Marketing office	Marketing manager
	Marketing staff
	Design room
	Meeting room
	Stores
	Sub waiting
	Public utility for staff
Purchase office	**Purchase manager**
	Purchase officer
	Stores
	Sub waiting
	Public utility for staff
Hospital information	IT Manager
	IT control room
	Server room
	Public utility for staff

Table 7.1 (continued)

Zone	Function/room
Hospital services	
Hospital kitchen	Entry of staff
	Airlock entry
	Change rooms cum hand wash
	Receipt area for supplies
	Bulk storage for tableware, linen, crockery and utensils
	Fruit/Vegetable storage
	Refrigerator/s, cool rooms and freezers
	Storage areas for dry ration/goods
	Pre-preparation
	Cooking/Baking
	Reheating facilities
	Packing/Plating areas
	Trolley parking area
	Loading/Distribution
	Trolley/cart washing area
	Pot wash
	Dishwashing
	Waste disposal area
	Manifold room and cylinder storage
	Staff accommodation
	Kitchen manager
	Dietician
	Dietetics staff
	Public utility for staff
Central sterile supply	Staff change
	Dirty receipt
	Washing/Disinfection
	Assembly/Packing
	Sterilization
	Sterile storage
	Delivery room
	ETO room
	CSSD supervisor
	Staff room
	Public utility for staff
Hospital laundry	Dirty receipt
	Mending and tailoring
	Sorting/Weighing
	Washing
	Ironing
	Clean storage
	Public utility for staff

(continued)

Table 7.1 (continued)

Zone	Function/room
Medical and general stores	**Medical and general stores**
	Surgical and dressing
	Linen and livery
	Stationery and printing
	Chemicals and glassware
	Sanitation and misc.
	Furniture
	Awaiting condemnation
	Staff accommodation
	Stores officer
	Public utility for staff
Mortuary	Body store
	Body wash
Engineering services	
Electrical	Substation
	Standby generator
	Workshop
	Switch room
	Office
	Public utility for staff
Mechanical	Lifts
	Air conditioning plant
	Air handling unit
Public health	Health officer
	Staff
	Public utility for staff
	Water supply
	Sewage disposal
	Biomedical waste storage
	ETP/STP tank
Fire protection	Fire detection
	Fire fitting (water storage)
	Fire Extinguishers
Communication	Telephone exchange
Medical gases and vacuum	Liquid oxygen tank area
	Landing bay
	Manifold
	Compressor
	Vacuum
	Medical gases control room
	Public utility for staff

Table 7.1 (continued)

Zone	Function/room
Workshop	Electromechanical workshop
	Biomedical workshop
	Civil maintenance workshop
	Aluminium Works Workshop
	Painting workshop
	Steel workshop
	Air conditioning workshop
	Wooden works workshop
	Medical gases workshop
	Maintenance control manager
	Office staff for maintenance
	Public utility for staff
Other services	
Security	Supervisor
	CCTV control room
	Public utility for staff
Mobile transport	Supervisor
	Ambulance parking
	Public utility for staff
Housekeeping	Supervisor
	Material storage
Hospital and staff committee (Conference) room	Conference room
	Central lecture theatre gallery type
	Library
Medical records	Receipt
	Compilation desk
	Indexing/Coding
	Statistical analysis
	Computer lab
	Storage files/Register
	Binding room
	Staff accommodation
	Medical record officer
	Secretarial staff
	Public utility for staff

7.3 Sizes of the Rooms

Once the list of the required rooms is finalized, then comes a question: WHAT SHALL BE THE SIZES OF THESE ROOMS. To answer this question, firstly the practical experience of the physicians, secondly the norms and codes of the regulating agencies, thirdly the load of patients availing such services and lastly the space availability for such rooms out of the total area available, shall be calculated.

It is recommended that while deciding the room sizes, it shall be borne in mind that the rooms shall be of reasonable size and not to be too big resulting in the wastage of space, neither too small which may hamper working in that room.

For deciding the final size of the room, one has to plan the internal layout of the room, i.e. how the equipment/machinery shall be placed in the room, how the bed/couch shall be placed, what all furniture shall be required in the room, how many people shall be present at a particular point of time and how much working and movement space is required in the room.

Based on this layout, the length and breadth of the room are decided. Based on these dimensions, the area of the room shall be worked out. It is better if such a list is prepared in a spreadsheet. In the first column, the room name is mentioned, the second column is for the number of such rooms required, third is for length, fourth is for breadth, the fifth is for area per room and sixth is for the total area of all such rooms. After this exercise, the total area required for services and functionalities has been finalized. Let us call it a **Functional Area**.

The format of such a spreadsheet can be as shown in Table 7.2.

Once the functional area of the rooms has been worked out, then comes the addition of movement spaces like corridors, staircases, staircase lobbies, lift wells, lift lobbies and ramps to the functional area. These areas are not directly related to any service or functionality but are common to all.

The best way to provide provision for these movement spaces is to add a percentage area to the functional area actually worked out for each service and functionalities. Again a question that arises is: What Percentage to add for Movement Areas. The percentage shall again depend on the norms and codes of regulating agencies or otherwise be based on the practical experience of users.

Normally, it is believed that somewhere between 35 and 40% of the total functional area should be added towards the movement areas.

After adding the movement area to the functional area, the total area required for the building shall be finalized. It is this sheet on which the designer will start the work of placing the departments, functionalities and services in the architectural drawings.

7.4 Zoning

The next step after the calculation of the area requirement is to divide the entire building into different zones. What is Zoning? It is grouping different areas of a hospital according to functionality and accessibility to the patient. Normally the hospitals have the following zones:

1. **Outer Zone—Fast movement Zone**: These are the areas that are mostly visited by the patients/attendants. This zone shall be open for all and immediately accessible to the public. These areas are like emergency service, outpatient service, cafeteria, entrance hall and administrative service.
2. **Second Zone—Semi-movement zone**: These are the areas that receive and serve the patients but patients are generally not in direct contact with the workers of this zone neither the patients nor the attendants are required to visit this zone. But truly speaking some of the services of this zone requires the physical attendance of the patients like radiology. The department like laboratory, pharmacy and radiology fall in this zone.
3. **Inner Zone—Limited movement zone**: In this zone mostly the indoor wards are covered. Here the services of nursing care and management of patients are provided. This zone includes Intermediate Care Areas like General Wards, Semi-Private Rooms, Private Rooms, Deluxe Rooms and VIP suites. Generally, the patients/attendants and guests of the patients are allowed in this zone.
4. **Deep Zone—Banned Zone**: This zone includes the critical units and the operating theatre complex. As this needs to be highly sterilized and free from any types of infection,

Table 7.2 Sample of working out the room requirement and area calculation for hospital building

Zone	Function/room	No. of rooms	Size		Covered area per unit	Total covered area in sq. ft.	Total covered area in sq. mt.
			Length	Breadth			
OPD services							
Specialities	**Medicine block**						
	Examination room with exam. cubicles	4	12	15	180.00	720.00	66.89
	Rooms for special clinics	4	12	15	180.00	720.00	66.89
	Clinical demonstration room	1	25	15	375.00	375.00	34.84
	Extra rooms for future expansion	2	12	15	180.00	360.00	33.45
	Reception and enquiry	1	8	8	64.00	64.00	5.95
	Registration	1	8	8	64.00	64.00	5.95
	Record room	1	12	12	144.00	144.00	13.38
	Store	1	8	8	64.00	64.00	5.95
	Public utility for faculty	1	8	8	64.00	64.00	5.95
	Public utility for patients and attendants	1	12	15	180.00	180.00	16.72
	Sub waiting	1	30	30	900.00	900.00	83.61
	Total					3655.00	339.58
	Add movement area	35%				1279.25	118.85
	Total required area					4934.25	458.43

the movement in this zone is banned. This zone is totally segregated from the other public zones like outer, second and inner zones. This zone includes functionalities like all ICUs, operation theatres, surgical service, delivery service and NICU.

5. **Isolation Zone—Restricted Zone**: This zone is reserved for the infected patient, who can easily transmit the disease to other patients or healthy people. The patients suffering from infections like COVID-19 are kept in this zone. All the services required for such patients like isolation ICU, wards and rooms are located in this zone. The movement to this zone shall be careful and with all the necessary precautions.
6. **Service Zone**—This zone is for all other services department that provides support services to the functionality of the hospital. This zone includes areas like dietary service, housekeeping service, laundry, MGPS, Workshops and Medical Records.

7.5 Placement of Zones in the Building

Now the time has come to allot the floors and spaces to different zones in the hospital building. The designer shall keep in mind the distances to be travelled and the movement of men and material from one zone to another. Moreover, two different zones providing support to each other shall not be far off but in the vicinity to each other (Fig. 7.1).

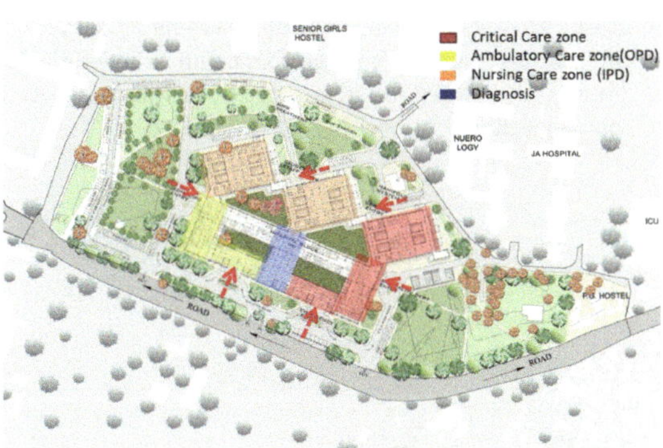

Fig. 7.1 Sample drawing of zoning of the hospital buildings

Let us take an example of a building having 12 stories with a breakup of:

1. Second basement
2. First basement
3. Ground floor
4. First floor
5. Second floor
6. Service floor
7. Third floor
8. Fourth floor
9. Fifth floor
10. Sixth floor
11. Seventh floor
12. Eighth floor

If we want to allot spaces to different zones in this building, it can be done as follows:

1. Second basement: The Services Zone can be placed in this basement. Some of the services that can be placed are like Medical Records, Hospital and Staff Committee (Conference) Room, Housekeeping, Mobile Transport, Security Control, Workshops, MGPS, Communication, Fire Protection Control, Mechanicals like AC plant, Electrical Panel and UPS room, Medical and General Stores, Hospital Information Control including Server room, Purchase Officer, Marketing Officer, Account Office and Personnel Office. Please avoid the services requiring heavy water consumption or the services which drain heavy amounts of water, because it is a very cumbersome job to drain water from the basements. Placement of Bunkers for Radiotherapy is a good option to be done in this basement.
2. First Basement: We can place the administrative department and diagnostic department along with some of the OPD's in this basement. The departments and services are like Radiology, Clinical Laboratories, Blood Bank, Physiotherapy, Directors Office, Medical Superintendent Office, Dy. Medical Superintendent Office, Nursing Superintendent Office, Dy. Nursing Superintendent Office, Central Sterile Supply, Hospital Kitchen and Mortuary.

3. Ground Floor: As the approach to this floor is accessible easily, so the departments and services most often used by the public are placed on this floor. The departments and services that can be placed at this floor can be like Emergency Department along with Emergency Operation theatre complex, Entrance Lobby, Reception, Billing and Registration, Help Desk, Pharmacy, Waiting areas, Cardiac Investigations, Pulmonology Investigations, Neurology Investigations, Other Investigations and Sample Collection room.
4. First Floor: The leftover OPD's and investigations can be taken on this floor along with the waiting areas.
5. Second Floor: This floor can be used for the Intensive Care Unit and the Operation Theatre complex. The departments and the functionality that can be placed here are Operation Theatre Suite, Cath Lab, CCU, SICU and CTVS ICU, MICU, RICU, PICU, Burn ICU etc. Also, the Delivery Suite along with OBS OT can be placed here. If the Delivery suite is placed here then Neonatal ICU also has to be placed near to that only.
6. Service Floor: This floor is mainly used for the services like BioMedical Workshops, other workshops and the placing of the AHU's of HVAC.
7. Third Floor: This floor can be used for Semi-intensive Care Floor and the functionalities like Step Down ICU/HDU and Dialysis can be placed here.
8. Fourth Floor to Seventh Floor: These floors can be used for placement of all the General Wards, Semi-private Ward, Private Ward, Deluxe Ward and Family Suites.
9. Eighth Floor: This Floor can be dedicated to Isolation and only infected patients shall be admitted here. The set up shall include all types of wards, ICU's and diagnostic facilities like mobile radiology.

Further Reading

A new method for calculating health care spaces [Internet]. [cited 2021 Jun 10]. Available from: https://www.hfmmagazine.com/articles/3244-calculating-health-care-spaces

Academy of architecture for health. Guidelines for design and construction of hospital and health care facilities: 2001 edition. Washington, D.C.: AIA; 2002.

Almansi K. DEVELOPING A TECHNIQUE TO CALCULATE THE HOSPITAL SERVICE AREA AND MEASURE THE ACCESSIBILITY LEVELS TO TERTIARY HOSPITALS USING GIS. Int J Sci Knowl. 2015 Aug 31;6:9.

Benitez GB, Da Silveira GJC, Fogliatto FS. Layout Planning in Healthcare Facilities: A Systematic Review. HERD Health Environ Res Des J. 2019 Jul 1;12(3):31–44.

Gibson I. An approach to hospital planning and design using discrete event simulation. In 2007. p. 1501–9.

Griffin CH, Joint Commission, Joint Commission Resources, Inc, Joint Commission International, AIA Academy of Architecture for Health, editors. Planning, design, and construction of health care facilities: addressing Joint Commission and JCI standards and other considerations--from planning to commissioning. Third edition. Oak Brook, IL: Joint Commission Resources; 2015. 138 p.

Jiang S, Verderber S. On the Planning and Design of Hospital Circulation Zones: A Review of the Evidence-Based Literature. HERD Health Environ Res Des J. 2016 Oct 14;10.

Lavy S, Hamilton DK, Jiang Y, Kircher A, Dixit MK, Lee J-T. Hospital Building and Departmental Area Calculation: Comparison of 36 Recent North American Projects. HERD Health Environ Res Des J. 2019 Oct 1;12(4):174–85.

Staff CC. Hospital Space Planners: Planning Hospitals of the Future [Internet]. [cited 2021 Jun 10]. Available from: https://blog.cmecorp.com/hospital-space-planners-planning-hospitals-of-the-future

Part II

Schematic Design of Hospital

Schematic Design 8

Once the designer is out of the planning phase, he/she starts working on the Second Phase, i.e. Schematic Design.

8.1 What Is the Schematic Design?

It is an exercise to produce the complete design of a project on papers, in the shape of drawings, as planned in phase 1. The schematic design phase aims to develop a plan of action relating to the building that how the building will look based on the planning and designing and also based on the client's budget.

While preparing the designs, the designer needs to consider the relationship between different functionalities of the hospital. It includes the complete description of building systems such as structural design, mechanical works, HVAC system, firefighting system, CCTV, plumbing and electrical systems. The designer also designs the rough interior and exterior finishes. Schematic Design also includes descriptions of all engineering considerations that are to be used during the construction and operation of the hospital, materials, equipment, systems and spaces to be included in the project. These designs also include the floor plans, site plans and building elevations produced.

The designer starts with preparing rough plans, or schematics, showing a general model of the location of rooms, placement of doors and windows and the overall structure of the building. The outlines of spaces for different functionalities planned during phase 1 are produced as a design. Once these are defined, the designer shall produce several different hospital designs utilizing these spaces in several unique ways.

The hospital promoters thereafter review and refine the designs, keeping in mind the issues related to the functionality and usability of the spaces. Also to see that the issues like required adjacencies, safety, security, code compliance and aesthetics have been taken care of. The promoter and other planning team members then carefully scrutinize these schematic drawings for any errors or omissions. The owners choose one design that best aligns with their vision for the finished hospital project. Once a schematic design is settled on, the scale at which the project will move forward is defined.

Further Reading

Code C and. Understanding the Architects Design Phases: Schematic Design; Design Development; Construction Documents [Internet]. [cited 2021 Jun 10]. Available from: http://canadiantimberframes.com/understanding-the-architects-design-phases-schematic-design-design-development-construction-documents

Fig. 1.Design schematic from a hospital construction project [Internet]. ResearchGate. [cited 2021 Jun 10]. Available from: https://www.researchgate.net/figure/

A. Garg, A. Dewan, *Manual of Hospital Planning and Designing*,
https://doi.org/10.1007/978-981-16-8456-2_8

Design-schematic-from-a-hospital-construction-project_fig1_266323773
Gibson IW, Lease BL. An approach to hospital planning and design using discrete event simulation. In: 2007 Winter Simulation Conference [Internet]. Washington, DC, USA: IEEE; 2007 [cited 2021 Jun 10]. p. 1501–9. Available from: http://ieeexplore.ieee.org/document/4419763/
Project Design Phases | UCOP [Internet]. [cited 2021 Jun 10]. Available from: https://www.ucop.edu/construction-services/facilities-manual/volume-3/vol-3-chapter-1.html
Schematic Design Phase [Internet]. Western Michigan University. 2015 [cited 2021 Jun 10]. Available from: https://wmich.edu/facilities/planning/schematicdesign
What Are Schematic Designs? [Internet]. Home Guides | SF Gate. [cited 2021 Jun 10]. Available from: https://homeguides.sfgate.com/what-are-schematic-designs-13401027.html

9 Effects of COVID-19 on the Design of the Hospital

After a schematic design is finalized, the next step is to prepare the final working drawings. However, the recent COVID-19 pandemic has defined that the world will have to live with such viruses indefinitely. Hospitals being healthcare providers, are affected by such pandemics due to a variety of reasons. This chapter will highlight some potential issues that arise in a hospital during a pandemic and provide possible solutions to them which can be practised during the designing phase.

Nobody can deny that pandemics are not new, but it is this time that the world has known about the major threat that such pandemics can deliver if not handled properly, efficiently and in time. Globally, the leaders of hospitals are dealing with unprecedented levels of demand for healthcare in their hospitals and struggling about the solution to provide optimal medical care to all the needed patients and the public as a whole. If living with diseases is what we eventually will end up with, there should be certain long-term measures that shall become a part of our lives. Out of all these, Hospital Architecture, Design and Planning are the most important.

During the recent COVID-19 pandemic, hospitals faced a large number of problems such as shortage of space to handle the patient surge, infection spread, scarcity of hospital beds, advanced equipment, doctors and paramedical staff, and poor awareness of health care, insurance and prevention of the disease among the general public.

In almost all countries, the experience of COVID-19 has demonstrated the potential for fundamental shifts, changes or alterations in the hospitals. This includes the design and construction of hospitals, training of healthcare workers, maintenance of hygiene in the healthcare facility, curbing the rate of cross-infection and nosocomial infection, procurement and management of critical care equipment along with the personal protective equipment (PPE) etc.

9.1 What Will Be the Design of Future Hospitals

What will be the design of future healthcare institutions capable enough to handle pandemics?

In the past, designers have always concentrated on the patient and healthcare workers' safety while designing hospitals. However, experts predict that post-COVID-19, there are more areas to focus on leading to the changes to be incorporated in a healthcare facility. Strategies need to be developed for handling such diseases beyond the current scope and capacities. At the same time, a careful balance needs to be maintained to ensure that we do not build such facilities that lay under or unutilized, leading to wastage of critical resources like trained staff, medical equipment and money. To do this, we

A. Garg, A. Dewan, *Manual of Hospital Planning and Designing*,
https://doi.org/10.1007/978-981-16-8456-2_9

need an advanced and extensive network of accessible, available and affordable hospital-like facilities.

For example, locally available healthcare facility centres can be redeveloped to serve as healthcare provider centres that can address the rising needs of beds in hospitals and act as an extension of larger hospitals or neighbourhood clinics. Coupled with similar screening and treatment infrastructure protocols, these facilities can prove to be an asset to the communities. Also, as the virus spread rapidly, a new approach is known as 'isolation and containment zones' is essential in the hospital building, design and architecture. If existing healthcare institutions cannot redesign their facilities, they shall modify them to a possible extent.

9.2 Issues to Be Addressed While Planning and Designing a Hospital in Post-COVID-19 Era

While designing a new healthcare facility, the following issues must be simultaneously addressed to a hospital design:

1. **Changes in the design of building, location, spaces and sizes of the rooms of the healthcare facility**.
2. **Changes in the layout and facilities of various departments such as emergency rooms, operating rooms, intensive care area, diagnostic facilities, waiting lobbies, staff zones and administrative zones**.
3. **Acceptance of the new and improved building materials which seems to be more appropriate as per the new building designs or which can ease out the concept of a new and better-designed building**.
4. **Temporary conversion of spaces in the hospital to treatment units, emergency suites, ICU's and isolation units to handle the patient surge**.
5. **Modification and adoption of improved working systems and SOPs that are in consensus with the new or modified design of the healthcare facility**.

Let us discuss the above issues in a few more details:

9.3 Changes in the Design of Building, Location, Spaces and Sizes of the Rooms in the Healthcare Facility

One has to consider that COVID-19 will force experts to think about the transformation of both design and material to be used in all spaces of the hospital. It has made the world aware of the threat from large-scale infectious diseases, the crippling effect they can have on human lives and this should lead to a better design in places we live, work and entertain. Thus, we suggest the following architectural changes that can be implemented while designing a new hospital facility or redesigning an existing one.

9.3.1 Hybrid Design of Building

For more cross ventilation, natural air and light, it is recommended that during the post-COVID era, hospitals must design the buildings which are more climate and natural light-sensitive, and friendly. Therefore, designers have to shift from a box-type monolithic design to a hybrid building design, which offers more courtyards, building offsets and outdoor interactions. Another advantage is, the more natural light and air, the more energy consumption and savings because it reduces dependence on electricity and air conditioning. In simple terms, the concept of 'Green Building' has to be adopted.

9.3.2 Improving Infection Prevention

The Hospitals' design should stress more and more on improving the infection control, be it cross-infection or nosocomial infection. To achieve this, the following factors shall be considered:

9.3.2.1 Zoning

Proper zoning of the hospitals shall have to be designed. For this, we recommend a **Green Zone** which should be a clean zone where one can be sure that nobody in this zone is infected, **Blue Zone** is a space where COVID-infected patients are placed and treated, and an **Amber Zone** where the state of the patient is yet not yet known whether he/she is infected.

9.3.2.2 Ultraviolet and Chemical Disinfection

The hospitals shall be designed to withstand cleaning using harsh chemicals, UV-C light, or sterilizing mists without compromising on the finishing of the surfaces.

9.3.2.3 Defined Protocol for Flow

The most challenging aspect is to create a proper and well-defined protocol for the flow of patients, staff and material within hospitals. This helps to ensure absolute sterility, infection prevention and operational efficiency.

9.3.2.4 Segregation of Patients

Hospitals need to devise strategies and protocols for segregating infectious and non-infectious patients. We recommend developing two separate infrastructures within a hospital with separate entries to the building, separate diagnostic services like radiology, laboratory, operating rooms and in-patient services, including Critical Care Units. Of course, this is the best solution, but not always practically feasible and cost-efficient. Therefore, it is advised to create virtual barriers and segregate patients by zoning.

9.3.2.5 Separate Entries

For better control of the infection, separate entries for OPD, emergency and diagnostic facilities are recommended. This will not only control the infection but also reduce the rush of patients and attendants at a single point, thereby allowing social distancing.

9.3.2.6 Personal Protective Care

Several steps need to be taken to keep the healthcare workers safe and ensure that they have access to personal protective equipment such as gloves and masks. We have to plan where to make the donning and doffing rooms, where to stock the PPE kits and other items like masks, gloves and shoe covers. Similarly, several spaces have to be made in the hospitals for hand sanitization. Sanitization stations can be planned at places like a hallway, entrances, toilets, waiting lobbies and reception. The idea is to place them closer to the point of care, which could improve staff hand hygiene.

9.3.2.7 Lesser Horizontal Surfaces

Reducing the number of horizontal surfaces like reception counters, Wash Basins, tables and ledges and working counters can help reduce the spread of infection. The lesser the horizontal surfaces, the lesser will be the area and chances for particles to land up. This will also minimize the nicks and corners where usually the debris can collect making it easier to clean and sterilize/ sanitize them.

9.3.2.8 Facilities for Staff

Some healthcare workers in a hospital can be on long shift duties and they may come from far-off places. For such staff, extended staff amenities such as dining spaces, restrooms, recreation rooms and sleeping spaces/pods shall be provided. These spaces should adhere to social distancing protocols and should be small in size but more in number to avoid the rush at a single place.

9.3.2.9 Barriers and Vestibules

For segregating different zones in a hospital, barriers such as air curtains shall be installed. Also, vestibules shall be created by providing double doors so that the air mixing of two zones can be avoided.

9.3.2.10 Isolation Areas/Units/Rooms

It is recommended that negative pressure isolation rooms shall not be distributed throughout the hospital but shall be concentrated in a particular zone. Segregation of patients can easily be achieved in such a design and the entry of outsiders can also be restricted to avoid the spread of infection.

9.3.2.11 HVAC and Air Handling System

HVAC systems play a very important role in hospitals, not only by maintaining comfortable climatic conditions for patients and employees but also by maintaining a clean and germ-free environment to contribute to the wellness of the patients and to prevent further spread of disease. Also, medical equipment in hospitals is very sensitive to temperature and humidity levels and requires perfect air control for them to function accurately and uninterrupted. These important factors for air control means the design of air conditioning systems for the hospitals must consider the characteristics that need special attention in this sector. Details of the HVAC system have been provided in another chapter of this book under the section 'Air-Conditioning'.

9.4 Changes in the Layout, Facilities of Various Departments, Emergency Rooms, Operating Rooms, Intensive Care Area, Diagnostic Facilities, Waiting Lobbies, Staff Zones, the Administrative Zones etc.

Hospitals have various departments like Out Patient Department, Indoor Patient Department, Emergency Department, Intensive Care Suits, Operating Rooms, Waiting lobbies and Diagnostic departments like Radiology and Laboratory. In the post-COVID era, the design of these departments needs to be altered (redesigned) to avoid the spread of infection. If a new hospital is to be set up, changes must be planned and implemented during the designing phase while keeping in mind the effect of current pandemic and more infections to come in the future.

For an existing hospital, the following alterations must be performed to a possible extent:

9.4.1 Entrance Lobbies

The entrance lobbies are the first place where the patients, workers and visitors land into. This is the place from where onwards the segregation, distancing, and infection control begins. Normally, services like Reception, Inquiry desk, Help desk, Registration, Admission and Discharge desk and Cash Counter are provided in the entrance lobby. Following are some of the technological advancements that help reduce the spread of infection in the entrance lobbies:

9.4.1.1 Reduction of People Landing in the Entrance Lobby

It is recommended that the entrance, waiting, gathering and sitting areas in the entrance lobby should be reduced to a possible extent. The arrangement should be made to provide such services through using online registrations, admissions and discharges over the phone etc. There shall be no sitting provision in the lobby (if essential very few can be allowed with proper social distancing, used majorly for disabled people, pregnant ladies or sick patients).

9.4.1.2 Portal Technology

As the patients are increasingly becoming more and more technology savvy, the portal helps them do most of the hospital-related bits of help and tasks. Portals can ease the registration, collection of reports, inquiry and bookings etc. without visiting a hospital.

9.4.1.3 Self-service Kiosks

Similar to portals, self-service kiosks can help to expedite processes like registration in hospital, enquiry and healthcare information. Patients can increasingly do the work that could have been done at counters without having to come in contact with anyone. This can help with staff savings while increasing patient comfort. Automated kiosks can assist patients with paying charges of hospital, checking identification numbers, signing consents and paperwork and other registration requirements of the hospital.

9.4.1.4 Screening Areas

It is recommended to provide a screening area at the hospital entrance and any other main public entry to perform screening through questionnaires, and measurements of body temperature and basic vitals. For this, isolated screening cabins can be used. The screening chamber is a closed chamber with a provision of negative pressure and UV sterilization with a glass partition on the front side. There are two holes in the glass to fix the long elbow gloves. A healthcare worker sitting in the cabin can examine the patient standing on the other side of the glass through the gloves. This allows hospital staff to identify the highly contagious patients and isolate them or restrict their access to the hospital right from the entry point.

9.4.1.5 Handwash/Sanitizer Stations

Hospitals should place handwash stations or hand sanitizer dispensers at the doors, entrances and inside patient treatment rooms and near-patient beds, and encourage staff, patients and visitors to use them on a more frequent basis. Before placing these stations, analysis of the building layout for other accessible locations should be done.

9.4.1.6 Face Masks/Shoe Covers Dispensers

Hospitals should also make arrangements for placing the face mask/shoe cover dispensers at the doors and entrances of the hospital. Any staff, patients and visitors entering the hospital shall be encouraged to use them on a more frequent basis. As in the case of handwash and sanitizer stations, before placing these dispensers, an analysis of the building layout for other accessible locations should be done.

9.4.1.7 Acrylic or Glass Partitions

It is believed that despite automation, some patients/visitors will be using the counters and service desks. Under such circumstances, there are all the chances of the staff getting infected. To overcome this, it is advised to make a proper 1829 mm high acrylic or glass partition at the top of the staff counter or desk and ensure that the staff is always on the other side of the partition (Fig. 9.1).

9.4.2 Waiting Lobbies

These are the areas created to allow patients or visitors to wait for their turn while using the services of a hospital. They can also be used as a waiting area for the patient's attendants. During the pre-COVID era, more and more waiting lobbies with a capacity to allow a large number of people

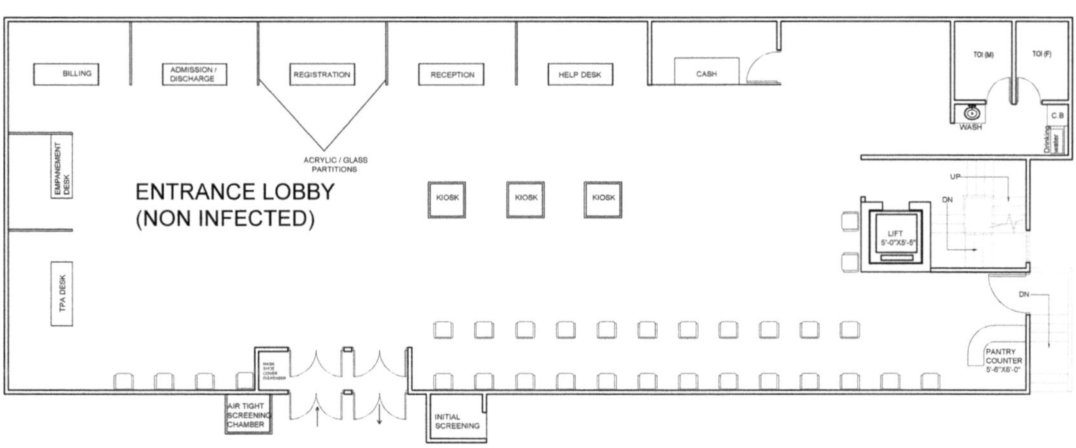

Fig. 9.1 Suggested layout of an entrance lobby

to sit were preferred. But now, post-COVID-19, all public spaces, like waiting areas, lobbies and dining halls, will have to be carefully planned and designed to create a greater physical separation between people by introducing an efficient queuing system. Following are the few suggestions to redesign waiting rooms and public spaces:

9.4.2.1 Individual Seats

The foremost principle to be followed is that individual seats shall be provided to aid social distancing.

9.4.2.2 Sub-waiting Lobbies

It is recommended that instead of large waiting lobbies, hospitals shall design small and sub-waiting lobbies. For example, instead of providing a large lobby with a seating capacity of 200 in the OPD block, a separate sub-waiting lobby of around 30 seats serving one or two OPD rooms shall be created. However, such measures may not be practical in all situations, especially for small hospitals, nursing homes and clinics. The number of people who can be allowed to wait in hospital lobbies shall be limited to a certain maximum number with a specific minimum spacing between their seats. So, future waiting lobbies could be smaller but in scattered clusters.

9.4.2.3 Minimize Interaction with Others

The concept of a smaller enclave waiting space that separates the sick from other patients or visitors will be preferred. The seating has to be in the clusters of small numbers of chairs, say 2–3 chairs per cluster. Further, each cluster shall be portioned from the other with at least 5 ft. acrylic or glass partition to reduce exposure with other patients/visitors.

9.4.2.4 Outside Waiting

Patients and families shall be encouraged and advised to wait outside or in their car instead of waiting in the lobby.

9.4.2.5 Adopting a Token System

To reduce the crowd in waiting lobbies, a token system shall be introduced, where the patient or visitor is issued a token at the time of registration so that they are well aware of their turn. They need not be in the waiting lobby or near the service room but can wait somewhere else. For information about the status of the token, LCDs can be provided at various places in the hospital. We can even use advanced technology, where an SMS will be sent to the mobile number of the token holder as and when his/her turn arrives.

9.4.3 Outpatient Department

9.4.3.1 Design of OPD to Be Modified

In the future, the design of an OPD has to be modified to maintain social distancing and avoid direct contact with patients. For this, some type of acrylic or glass partitions will have to be used, wherein on one side of the partition is a staff member, and on the other side is the patient. For communication between the two, a two-way audio system shall be preferred. Also, doctors can use the telemedicine approach to see the patient remotely on video, and conduct examinations remotely using IoT-enabled devices.

9.4.3.2 Use of Touch-Free Medical Devices

To avoid direct and close contact with the patient, it is advised to replace current medical devices such as BP apparatus, Stethoscope, Pulse Oximeter and Thermometer with their wireless and touch-free counterparts.

9.4.3.3 OPD Consultation Rooms with Videoconferencing Solutions

It is evident that in the near future, patients would avoid going to hospitals until and unless it is really necessary. This would result in patients adopting more and more video consultations rather than OPD visits, thereby allowing OPDs to be less crowded. This would completely change the layout and design of the OPD consultation rooms, which would now need to incorporate more elements for videoconferencing solutions.

9.4.3.4 Creating Virtual OPD

We recommend to adopt and introduce the concept of Virtual OPD, wherein IT infrastructure shall play a major role in designing. The patient to doctor communication interface and doctor-to-staff communication will be carried out through AV controls. In today's world, the widely available technologies such as video chat and virtual reality headsets will have to be incorporated to help patients stay connected to friends and family.

9.4.3.5 Sterilization and Pressure

A provision shall be made to protect the OPD by UV-C light disinfection and sanitization from time to time. Also, the OPD should be positively pressurized.

9.4.3.6 Telemedicine Impact on the Facility

Telemedicine has boomed during this crisis of COVID-19 era, thus forcing healthcare workers to perform routine check-ups and treat patients without putting either doctor, staff or patient at risk. The technology of telemedicine is relatively cheap and enables physicians to see more patients in less time, and virtually requires no space. Increased use of telemedicine could possibly increase the number of patients. Also, it may give chances to increase the medical tourism for international patients because it will be easy for the patients sitting at far off places to connect to the doctors. Initial consultations can be done over videoconferences and test reports can be shared likewise. Only the patients requiring procedural intervention could come down to the hospital. All tests are done in the hospital within 15 min using Point of Care diagnostics and medicines are dispensed automatically using a combination of machines.

9.4.3.7 Mobile Health

Mobile health is becoming more and more popular these days as the elimination of wires and cords and enabling physicians and patients to check healthcare processes online. Smartphones and tablets allow healthcare providers to freely access and send information to the desired. Physicians and service providers can use Mobile Health tools for orders, documentation or simply search for more patient information.

9.4.4 Emergency Department

The emergency care area that was originally designed for patient resuscitation and attendant waiting will now need to be redesigned to prevent the spread of the virus and cross infection.

9.4.4.1 Entrance to Emergency

First of all, emergency shall have a separate entrance. There shall be a design to route all the patients, attendants, visitors and others through a channel where the thermal screening cameras are fixed and the sanitization facility is provided. At the entrance, a provision of vestibule and air curtain shall be provided. Preferably in the vestibule, a provision shall be made for sanitizer, face masks and shoe cover dispensers. Also, a suitable place shall be allotted for the hand wash station.

9.4.4.2 Medical Officer Cabin

The room of the medical officer shall be the first room after entering the emergency. This cabin shall be properly air-tightened with glass partitions and shall be under negative pressure.

9.4.4.3 Triage

Triage is the area where all the patients land. Triage shall have the provision for normal beds and few beds for infected patients called Isolation cabins. The isolation shall be properly air-tightened and negatively pressurized. These isolation cabins shall not be mixed with other beds in the same hall but shall be a separate zone with a barrier in between. Separate staff shall take care of the patients in isolation cabins.

9.4.4.4 Attendant Waiting Lobby

The waiting lobby shall not be large in size and the chairs shall be placed keeping in mind social distancing protocols. Attendants shall be discouraged to enter the emergency lobby and shall be asked to stay out as much as possible. This can help a lot in controlling infection spread keeping the patients and attendants safer.

9.4.4.5 Connecting Emergency with the In-Patient Department

For entering the in-patient department from emergency, doors/barriers shall be provided. The door shall be fixed in the corridor and be guarded, and this shall not be a thorough passage.

9.4.5 In-Patient Department

9.4.5.1 Zoning of the Indoor Patient Areas

One important factor is to dedicate specific areas (preferably within hospital) where infectious patients can be managed. If such an area is not available in the hospital premises, any other dedicated non-infectious spaces can be dedicated where such care may be delivered. Post-COVID-19 designs shall be such where the zoning of the indoor patient area shall be a necessity. The first zone shall be for the non-infected patients and the second shall be for the critical patients like those requiring ICUs and HDUs. The third zone shall be for infected patients. Normally, hospitals have different categories of indoor units like General ward, Semi-private rooms, Private rooms, Deluxe rooms and Suites. It is recommended that all the categories of indoor units of a particular zone shall be in a cluster (maybe on the same floor/block/building or adjoining floors/blocks/buildings).

9.4.5.2 Separation of Zones

Zones shall be separated from each other with proper barriers so that the patient/visitors of one zone are restricted to enter another unless allowed.

9.4.5.3 Intensive Care Units

Normally, the intensive care units are designed to be in a single zone, which helps to provide intensive care to critical patients. If that is the case, then the infective and non-infective ICUs have to be in a separate Unit or room/hall. There shall be proper barriers to restrict the movement between them.

9.4.5.4 Isolation Unit

For infected patients, there shall be Isolation rooms (preferably hosting a single patient) and the unit shall be under negative pressure with 100% fresh air. The exhausted air has to be treated and then pushed back to the atmosphere. If it is an isolation ICU with more than one bed, each bed shall preferably have a separate air handling system so that anyone bed can be converted to a negatively pressurized bed if needed.

9.4.5.5 Single Bed Rooms

Multiple occupancy rooms are on their way out. Most hospitals now shall prefer a single bed unit concept, as it creates isolation and helps a lot to control the spread of infection.

9.4.5.6 Multiple Bed Indoor Wards

If it is necessary to have a multiple bed ward, it is recommended that the entire ward shall be divided into cubicles with glass partitions and each cubicle shall not have more than four beds. Also, more inter-bed space shall be provided. In such a case, each cubicle shall have a separate supply and return of HVAC so that the exhausted air does not mix up with other cubicles or hospital space.

9.4.5.7 Nurse Station

Nurse station design shall be looked into so that the caregivers also maintain adequate distance. Normally, hospitals have a nurse counter, from where the patient/visitors interact with the nurse. This type of counter is more prone to spreading infection because of no barrier in between. To overcome this issue, consider going from open nurse stations to enclosing them in 'glass bubbles'. It is advised to make a proper 1829 mm high acrylic or glass partition at the top of the nurse counter so that the staffs are always on the other side of the partition while interacting with the patient/visitor. We can also use technology like Audio-Video Controlled Nurse Call System.

9.4.6 Operating Rooms

1. Often it happens that one or the other infectious patient or a patient with some kind of communicable disease has to be operated. In such cases, separate operating rooms shall be prepared for such cases.
2. Along with the infectious operating rooms, it is recommended that there shall be separate pre- and post-operative units, instruments and equipment wash areas. If possible, the entry and exit to such operating rooms shall also be separate from the non-infectious operating rooms.
3. All other services like change rooms, clean supply rooms and flash sterilization rooms can be common for infectious and non-infectious operating rooms.

9.4.7 Diagnostic Laboratories

1. It is recommended for pathological laboratories that a separate room shall be identified for the infectious patients who use a separate set of instruments and disposables.
2. While collecting blood samples of a patient, the staff has to come in close proximity with the patient; hence staff is more prone to infection. To avoid this, we can think of some type of acrylic or glass screen between the patient and staff. A barrier shall be designed in such a manner that the patient can take out only his/her arm from the window/opening in the acrylic/glass screen.

9.4.8 Radiology

1. For Radiological diagnosis, nothing much needs to be done except slight changes in the operating system.

9.4.9 Staff and Administrative Workplaces

COVID-19 or alike infectious diseases pose an occupational health risk to healthcare workers. It has been noticed that several healthcare workers in the world have already been infected by this disease. Therefore, preventing intra-hospital transmission of communicable disease shall be considered to be an important issue and shall be handled efficiently and at priority. In a hospital, the administrative staff is not directly exposed to patients; however, it is always better to take precautions to protect the staff from getting infected. Some of the measures can be:

1. **Limiting shared staff spaces**

   Designing staff spaces shall be reconsidered, including the size and separation of workstations, the number of people in an office at any moment of time and the number of people sharing each workstation. A workstation shall not be overcrowded and designed to place the seats at a suitable distance to avoid the spread of infection.
2. The staff entrance to the hospital shall be separate from the general entrance of patients.
3. The entrance shall be provided with a thermal scanning station, sanitization dispenser and mask/gloves/shoe cover dispensing stations.
4. Change rooms with lockers shall be provided to each and every staff separately so that the clothes worn in are left in the lockers to avoid the spread of infection.
5. The staff space shall be well and cross-ventilated with the induction of fresh air.
6. Large, shared lunch rooms, restrooms and locker rooms shall be changed with smaller, more discrete and private spaces.

7. Administrative departments may be moved away from the infected areas or otherwise work-from-home arrangements may be devised to reduce the staff in the hospital premises.
8. The number of students and vendors inside the hospital premises at a given point of time may be limited.
9. More storage spaces and stores shall be planned for storing additional required supplies due to increased utilization.
10. This pandemic has shown that there is a need for giving healthcare workers a place to rest in between hectic shifts, especially the staff like nurses and physicians who find it more tiring.
11. Proper handwashing facilities, sanitizer dispensers, donning and doffing rooms for PPE kits, Masks/gloves and shoe cover dispensers shall be provided at all the required stations.

9.5 Acceptance of the New and Improved Building Materials Which Seems to Be More Appropriate as Per the New Building Designs or Which Can Ease Out the Concept of the New and Better-Designed Building

Infection control is one of the most important considerations for any hospital as patients and staff both require a clean and safe working environment. A hospital space designed to support infection control makes healthcare providers' job much easier and saves more lives. Therefore, while taking the design decisions this important factor shall be addressed too. For this, the designer may have to reshuffle some of the spaces, upgrading the materials and the addition of motion sensors to doors and sinks can be implemented through renovations to existing facilities. These modifications can also be adopted in future hospital designs for better infection control.

A few of the issues that the designer can take care of while designing a hospital are:

9.5.1 Antimicrobial Finishes and Materials

The adoption of materials and finishes that are easy to sanitize or are naturally germ-resistant, make it easier to maintain a high level of cleanliness and hygiene necessary in a hospital environment. Any material or finish used in a hospital shall be nonporous and nonreactive when exposed to common disinfectants such as bleach, alcohol and ammonium compounds.

9.5.2 Use of Antibacterial Materials

Antibacterial materials like copper-based products need to be considered for elevators, handrails, doorknobs etc. as these would be frequent touchpoints. Few manufactures have already invented and introduced antimicrobial coatings on floorings, facades, paints and furniture.

9.5.3 Use of Non-porous Materials

The products that are non-porous, wipeable and cleanable are not affected by regular fumigation and spraying of disinfectants. The products that can be used are PVC, UPVC, Glass, Polycarbonate, high-pressure laminates etc.

9.5.4 For the Furniture

Use of cloth fabric for furniture upholstery and curtains shall be avoided rather, easy-to-clean and sanitize, synthetic materials can be used.

9.5.5 Touch-free Controls

Focus shall be given more to ensure minimum hand contact with either the patients, amongst the staff and various other touchpoints. Hence sensors and touch-free technology shall be preferred, like touch-free control of lights operations, thermal controlled sensors for air conditioners, detecting overcrowding, sensor-based taps in washrooms and other handwashing stations.

9.5.6 Automatic Doors and E-switchable Privacy Glass

In place of conventional doors, automatic sensor-based sliding doors or swing doors can be used in high footfall areas. Similarly, foot-operated handles, stoppers and latches can easily be used in the hospital.

9.5.7 Smart Facade Glazing

Smart facade glazing that allows occupants to electronically control the quantity and quality of daylight into the rooms can be used. Such glass technology allows avoiding fabric blinds that harbour germs and are not easy to clean and sanitize.

9.5.8 Prefabricated Materials

Products under the prefabricated item range shall be extensively used as they provide more flexibility to quickly modify spaces during epidemic outbreaks.

9.5.9 Paints

Instead of normal wall paints, antibacterial washable paints shall be preferred as there are fewer chances of bacterial and viral growth and accumulation on such surfaces. Also, it is easy to clean these surfaces.

9.5.10 Flooring

For flooring, it is recommended that instead of porous material like marble, glazed tiles shall be used, which are easier to clean and sterilize. Moreover, nowadays certain floor tiles are available which are acid, chemical and scratch resistant.

9.5.11 Clean Rooms with HEPA Filters

For the hospital spaces that are more prone to infection, the concept of a cleanroom can be adopted. Clean rooms are basically airtight rooms with smooth walls having no corners, coated with antibacterial paint and provided with a HEPA filter for air sterilization and air exchange.

9.5.12 Dehumidification

In some spaces where the humidity is more than the required levels, portable dehumidifiers can be used to control the humidity, hence safeguarding the medical equipment that works properly at a defined humidity level.

9.5.13 Contactless Office

The concept of 'contactless office' shall be adopted where employees could avoid the need to press communal buttons and rather use their smartphone to send a command to the elevator, coffee machine or any other such machine.

9.5.14 Conference Rooms

Conference rooms could be fitted with voice-activated technologies to control lighting, audio and visual equipment.

9.5.15 Automation

Passing through doors or flushing the toilet would require a simple touch to operate. Instead of self-service in office kitchens, automation or a dedicated host shall be used.

9.5.16 Automatic Body Thermal Scanner

Automatic body thermal scanners shall be installed at the entrance of crowded places, which beeps if anyone has a temperature beyond the accepted range while standing in front of it.

9.6 Temporary Conversion of Space in the Hospital into Treatment Units, Emergency Suits, ICUs and Isolation Units to Handle Surges in the Number of Patients due to Pandemics

Till today, hospitals are often designed without having any flexibility or arrangements to accommodate a sudden surge of patients. Some hospitals may have slight flexibility but are still not able to fulfil the surging demand. During the COVID-19 pandemic, it was felt by all the hospitals that they are running out of spaces and resources to treat COVID-19 patients with severe symptoms, while at the same time handling those patients having mild symptoms or are totally asymptomatic, who may infect healthcare workers and other patients.

As COVID-19 cases filled up the emergency rooms and intensive care units across the world, both in Government hospitals and in Private COVID hospitals, the management and the Government officials have been rushing to convert hotels, convention centres, stadiums and parks into new hospital spaces.

Spaces like conference halls, lecture theatres, seminar halls and library are a part of the hospital but not meant for patient use. Apart from these are spaces like parking lots (basements or multi-level car parks), cafeterias and administrative rooms. All these spaces can be temporarily converted to patient spaces in case of emergency.

However, these spaces are not designed to become hospitals; hence there is severe pressure on the medical staff to follow stringent protocols to avoid infectious spread, especially in temporarily converted places. Many of these structures may not have adequate washrooms, and if there are toilets, then bathrooms might not be there. Lifts and staircases to these spaces may not have been designed for the movement of stretchers and hospital equipment. The AC ducts and vents are not built as per hospital protocol. Other services like medical gas pipe system, kitchen, laundry, general and pharmacy stores and toilets had to be added to these facilities to make them comprehensive for accommodating the patients. If some of these services do exist, they have to be augmented to meet the demand and make the stay of patients comfortable. It is relatively easy to locate physical space, but more difficult to design the needed privacy and create a clinical environment. Parking areas could be designed in a way that they could be easily converted to a containment zone or holding areas. If there are car parking garages, they can be converted into temporary COVID treatment spaces.

Some hospitals ended up placing extra beds in Private Rooms, which is not recommended because it may pose a problem of cross-infection. Some tried to set up beds in the lobbies and conference rooms. These temporary hospital spaces are more likely to support isolation and medical care for mild COVID-19 patients than to replicate a permanent ICU fully. There are many services required for the treatment of patients in ICU like monitoring systems, the supply of medical gases, proper air conditioning systems and availability of emergency medical equipment. Hence, it is not advisable to convert any general or vacant space to an ICU.

In converted buildings, you cannot have hospital-like compliance, standards and airflows. One limitation is that the air conditioning, heating and ventilation of converted buildings cannot be provided in such hospital isolation rooms. But converted sports arenas and hotels could function as quarantine centres for mild COVID-19 cases so that hospitals can focus more and more on the seriously sick patients, who require critical care and strict isolation.

Therefore, it is insisted that future hospital designs shall have more flexibility to handle such pandemics and other such events that create temporary surges and demand.

On the other hand, it is also true that under such circumstances, the management is left with no other alternative but to compromise on the quality of services required in these spaces. The following services are generally required and can be quickly redesigned:

9.6.1 Wall Finishes

Some of the spaces like parking lots may not have the proper wall finishes, resulting in the spread or accumulation of infection. For this, we recommend affixing wallpapers or panelling of PVC material, which not only takes less time but is also easy to clean and aesthetically looks decent.

9.6.2 Flooring

If the flooring of any of these spaces is rough, Vinyl floorings can be laid down in a very short time. Such floorings are found to be hygienic and easy to clean.

9.6.3 Electrical Points

Temporary exposed electrical lines can be planned. For this, PVC conduit can be fixed on the walls (at a height, out of reach by hand) and wires and cables shall pass through such conduit. Wherever required a drop can be given and switches/sockets can be given on the exposed gang boxes. To ensure safety, proper circuits shall be prepared and safeguarded with the MCBs and circuit breakers. If medical equipment has to be operated with these temporary electrical lines, a provision for stabilizers and/or UPS shall be provided.

9.6.4 Medical Gases

It is essential to provide medical gases like Oxygen and Vacuum for the treatment of patients suffering from an illness like COVID-19. In temporarily created patient spaces, this facility can be provided from the existing central supply line of medical gases. The network of HP tubing can be created by inserting a brass Tee's in between, and the flow meter can be fixed at the patient end. To control the pressure and accidents in such temporary lines Area Line Pressure Alarms, Isolation Valves and Regulators shall be provided at the start point of such an HP Tube network.

9.6.5 Bed and Hospital Furniture

Most hospitals are equipped with regularly required hospital furniture. If extra spaces have to be converted into patient treatment or quarantine spaces bed and bedside lockers shall be provided. Firstly, it is difficult to get hospital furniture in such a short period and secondly, a huge investment has to be planned to acquire the furniture. The remedy to this is Corrugated Cardboard furniture. It can be made available and assembled quickly and is cheap compared to steel furniture.

9.6.6 Partitions

The partitions between the bed, nursing station and other services can be temporarily modular and expandable and can be created with material like ICRA Panels or by using the frame of lightweight extruded aluminium panels fitted with Vinyl laminated or PVC Panel Sections. The erection of this type of partition is cheap and time-saving (Fig. 9.2).

9.6.7 Washrooms

There are a lot of options for setting up temporary washrooms, one of them is Prefabricated toilet cabins made out of various materials like FRP, Steel, RCC and Sandwich puff panel. Other options can be Rented Toilet Trailers or Chemical Toilets.

9.6.8 Air Conditioning

In extremely hot and cold countries, air conditioning is usually required even in temporary patient spaces to comfort patients. The type of air conditioning will depend on various factors like the area to be covered, the temperature required,

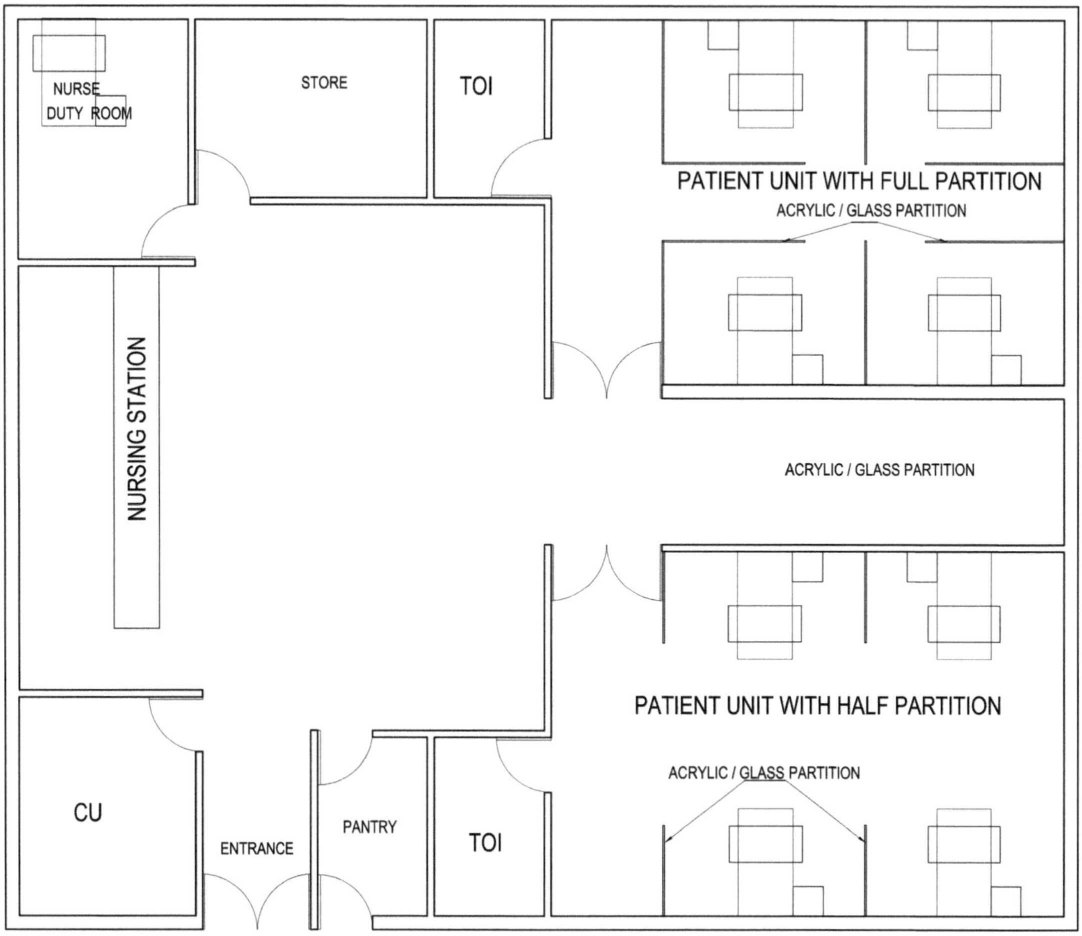

Fig. 9.2 Sample drawing of different types of bed partitions

thermal losses and humidity in the area. As designing and fixing the HVAC system is a costly affair and time consuming, we feel that by diverting some air from the pre-existing AHUs (by splitting the air ducts), the extended space can be air conditioned. Though it will not be as comfortable as a designed HVAC system but can be accepted. However, for large spaces, this method shall not work out. For small rooms, one option is portable air conditioners.

9.6.9 Nurse Call Systems

It is a difficult and costly affair to install a proper nurse call system. But wireless, infrared or Bluetooth-controlled nurse call systems can be installed. The remote with a pre-designated ID in the system can be given to the patient, and as soon as he/she activates a call, the ID number is displayed at the nurse station.

9.7 Modification and Adoption of Improved Working Systems and SOPs Which Are in Consensus with the New or Modified Design of Healthcare Facility

9.7.1 Health Worker's Safety and Support

A healthcare worker is foremost in healthcare. All other components, equipment, technologies, tools, workspaces, facilities, environment, remuneration and organizational conditions provided to the healthcare workers are secondary.

Therefore, any measures to strengthen the safety and support must be worker focused to facilitate acceptance and implementation. Some of the recommended steps that shall be adopted are:

(a) Health workers treating infected and suspected patients, and those treating non-infected patients shall be segregated altogether. This shall help in minimizing the risk of cross-infection of patients and healthcare workers.
(b) The highest risk tasks to which healthcare workers are exposed are aerosol-generating procedures like intubation, airway suctioning and bronchoscopy. Health workers treating infectious and suspected patients shall be provided with personal protective tools and gadgets. The main is donning full PPE kits, including eye protection, disposable gown, gloves and either an N95 mask or powered air purifying respirator.
(c) Daily temperature monitoring of all healthcare workers shall be made mandatory to identify those who are unwell and prevent intra-hospital propagation of infection. Healthcare workers whose temperature readings are found to be higher than 37.5°C shall be immediately be referred for further evaluation.
(d) All the healthcare workers shall be encouraged to work only for one primary institute and shall not be allowed to work in any other hospital.
(e) Mealtimes for healthcare workers shall be staggered.
(f) Training, teaching and departmental meetings shall be conducted using video conferencing. These measures are necessary as part of risk mitigation and to maintain the hospital's working continuity.
(g) Policies and infrastructure shall support clear, proper and timely communications with healthcare workers. This will facilitate effective cascading of information to frontline staff members enabling their work and facilitating their interactions with the patient and public. Daily routine instructions can be triggered through emails, Facebook, WhatsApp messages, SMS or other social media.
(h) All hospital staff should undergo the antibody test, and only those with antibodies (and hence with some immunity) should serve in ICUs and Coronavirus wards.
(i) Hand hygiene shall be performed regularly and after using the toilets, blowing nose, coughing, sneezing, before eating, before and after changing dressings or bandages and while entering or leaving rooms.
(j) You may be asked to wear a surgical mask when leaving your room.
(k) Turn away from other people in the room.
(l) The entire hospital shall be sanitized as per time to time guidelines and protocol issued by the management. If required fumigation shall also be done as per protocol.
(m) There shall be clearly defined protocols, systems, procedures and policies for entire hospital cleaning and sterilization/sanitation. All the surfaces such as working and reception counters, tables and ledges shall also be cleaned as per the written protocol.
(n) Limit the number of staff who is exposed to infectious patients by posting dedicated staff in dedicated units.
(o) Try to utilize overtime and long duty shifts for staff in the infectious units to limit the number of staff required.
(p) When possible, use staff who are already immune (recovered) from infectious diseases.
(q) Vaccinate all staff for infectious diseases to reduce the burden of that disease.
(r) Arrange for in-house childcare centres for the wellness of the children of healthcare workers if schools are closed. This can be done with the help of screened volunteers.
(s) Provide medical day care for sick family members.

9.7.2 Entrance

It is important to screen the patient just at the entry point of the hospital. The effective methods for doing this are:

(a) Wheelchairs and stretcher trolleys kept outside the entrance hall shall be sanitized and sterilized regularly.

(b) Face mask and shoe cover dispenser shall be made available at the entrance gate, and it shall be made mandatory for all visitors, patients and health workers entering the hospital.
(c) The amount of clutter that is located at the entrance, corridors and in waiting lobbies shall be minimized.
(d) Hospitals shall have a mandate to set up a facility to screen all the patients and visitors of the hospital via a window-protected interview, before allowing them into the hospital. This facility shall be set up outside the hospital entrance lobby. It is important to segregate the infectious and non-infectious patients. Those reporting any suspicious symptoms (even the mildest) should be redirected to where they can be tested for any infectious disease like COVID-19.
(e) Open walk-in access to OPDs should be banned.
(f) Visitors and outpatients may be the potential carriers of infectious pathogens in the hospital. To minimize this risk, arrangements shall be made so that all the visitors and outpatients shall undergo a questionnaire survey of travel and contact history. Along with this, they shall also undergo thermal scanning for fever before they are allowed into the hospital premises.
(g) Discourage using the services of the inquiry counter or help desk. Instead, encourage online inquiry and online help.
(h) Encourage the use of kiosk kept in the entrance hall of the hospital.
(i) Tools such as crowd detection and thermal scanning shall be used to identify critical spots and segregate potential disease carriers.
(j) Waiting in the entrance halls shall be discouraged and unnecessary waiting shall be avoided. The waiting chairs in the entrance hall shall be very limited and reserved for sick, elderly persons or pregnant women. Others shall be encouraged either to wait outside or move to the concerned sub-waiting lobbies.
(k) Each outpatient/in-patient shall be allowed only ONE accompanying person when attending the outpatient clinic or staying with the patient indoors.

9.7.3 Waiting Lobbies

As recommended to opt for sub-waiting lobbies instead of one large lobby, the waiting lobbies shall be small with limited seating capacity. Some issues which need consideration are:

(a) The patients and visitors shall be encouraged to just arrive at the time of appointment so that the time of waiting is minimized.
(b) Proper mask and shoe covers shall be worn while seated in the waiting lobby.
(c) Distance is essential and visitors or patients shall not be allowed to shift or move his/her chair close to another chair.
(d) Use the token system to help the patient or visitors know about their turn easily.
(e) Discourage wandering here and there in the waiting lobby.
(f) Limit the use of lavatory and washrooms. Use only if necessary.
(g) Discourage littering waste material and promote the use of provided dustbins. Also, keep the lobby smoke and noise free.
(h) No outside food shall be allowed in the waiting lobbies.

9.7.4 Out Patient Department

Out Patient Department (OPD) is a place where the health workers and the patient come in close proximity to each other. Further one can never know if anyone out of patients and visitors is infected or not. Therefore, care and distancing are necessary. The following steps are recommended, which may help in controlling the spread of infection:

1. To avoid the rush and gatherings at reception and waiting areas, it is recommended that Registration and Scheduling Appointment for Consultation shall be promoted. Hence, the following shall be followed:
   (a) Online registration and scheduling an appointment shall be introduced. Patients are made aware of online registration and appointment scheduling.

(b) The payment of the consultation can also be made online.
(c) If the patient still walks into the hospital without an appointment, he/she shall be discouraged from going to the reception and shall be encouraged to use the kiosk placed in the entrance lobby.
(d) On receiving the patient's online request for an appointment, the hospital shall give a particular date and time of appointment, with a request to the patient to be on time for the appointment; otherwise, the appointment might be cancelled.

2. Visitor or patient shall sanitize hands before entering the doctor's cabin.
3. OPD consultation rooms shall be sterilized and disinfected by UV-C light on a regular basis. Care should be taken that the UV light is switched off before anybody enters the OPD consultation room.
4. Only one person shall be allowed to enter the doctor's cabin with the patient.
5. Specialists (Doctors) shall use the necessary personal protective tools and gadgets like PPE kits, eye protection face shields, disposable gowns, gloves and either an N95 mask or powered air purifying respirator while providing consultation in the OPD.
6. Audio-Video consultation shall be encouraged. This can either be done by the patient right from his/her home. In case a patient has to come to the OPD, the doctor shall avoid being in close proximity to the patient. Few steps that can be taken while consulting are:
   (a) The doctor shall remain seated in the covered acrylic/glass partition and the patient should be seated on the other side of the partition.
   (b) The doctor shall use two-way audio communication kept in the OPD for conversing with the patient.
   (c) The patient shall not try to enter the doctor's cabin unless advised.
   (d) Promote the use of touch-free and wireless substitutes for gadgets like BP apparatus, Pulse Oximeter and Stethoscope.
   (e) Physical examination shall be avoided unless necessary.
   (f) Printed prescriptions and reports shall be avoided; rather, they shall be sent to the patient's registered mobile or email.
   (g) An online request shall be sent to the concerned department if an investigation is prescribed, like laboratory or radiology, and the patient should be guided to the concerned department.

9.7.5 Indoor and Isolation

In-patients who stay for a longer duration in the hospital are more prone to spread or acquire infections. Therefore, it is recommended that:

(a) The zoning concept shall be followed strictly. The patient/visitors of one zone must be restricted to enter another zone unless allowed.
(b) Separate staff shall take care of such patients in each zone. For this, separate staff will be needed for isolation cabins, intensive care units, and other indoor units. Further in each unit, separate staff shall be deputed for infective and non-infective spaces.
(c) Each in-patient shall be restricted to only ONE specified visitor to be allowed during the tenure of the hospitalization of the patient. These measures can contribute to reducing the likelihood of introducing infection from the community into the hospital environment.
(d) Equipment that is not being used should be placed in storage areas with the utmost care and precautions.
(e) One of the factors for the spread of infection in the hospital can be the face-to-face patient/visitor interaction with the nurse in indoor units. Hence, this face-to-face interaction shall be restricted and other means of interaction such as intercom, mobile or audio-visual communication must be implemented.
(f) There will be an integration of technology with digital infrastructure. Also, with the use of video calls and a virtual contact can be established between patients in quarantine, isolation or intensive care with nurses, doctors and their loved ones to minimize contact and yet create comfort.

9.7.6 Emergency Department

For the Emergency Department, the following needs to be taken care of:

(a) All patients/visitors entering the emergency shall undergo a questionnaire survey of travel and contact history, as well as thermal scanning for fever before they are allowed entry into the hospital premises.
(b) Ensure that after proper screening, suspected/infected patients must enter the emergency from a separate entry. Non-infected shall enter from a separate entry.
(c) Waiting in the emergency spaces shall be discouraged and unnecessary waiting shall be avoided. The waiting chairs in the emergency shall be very limited. Visitors shall be encouraged to wait outside.
(d) Each patient in an emergency shall be allowed only ONE accompanying attendant.
(e) The health workers in an emergency shall strictly adhere to the laid down norms of personal protection and shall always use personal protective tools and equipment.
(f) The common passage connecting any other spaces with the infective emergency shall be either closed or strictly guarded.

Further Reading

Albutt K, Luckhurst C, Alba G, Hechi M, Mokhtari A, Breen K, et al. Design and Impact of a COVID-19 Multidisciplinary Bundled Procedure Team. Ann Surg. 2020 May 1;Publish Ahead of Print:1.

Cousins S. Rethink: How will Covid-19 affect healthcare design? [Internet]. [cited 2021 Jun 14]. Available from: https://www.ribaj.com/intelligence/future-of-healthcare-design-in-post-pandemic-world

COVID-19: The Impact on Hospital Design - Architecture [Internet]. Healthcare Facilities Today. [cited 2021 Jun 14]. Available from: https://www.healthcarefacilitiestoday.com/posts/COVID-19-The-Impact-on-Hospital-Design%2D%2D25623

COVID-19's Impact on Healthcare Design and Construction - HCO News [Internet]. [cited 2021 Jun 14]. Available from: https://hconews.com/2020/09/15/covid-19s-impact-on-healthcare-design-and-construction/

Giacobbe A. How the COVID-19 Pandemic Will Change the Built Environment [Internet]. Architectural Digest. [cited 2021 Jun 14]. Available from: https://www.architecturaldigest.com/story/covid-19-design

HCD Mag [Internet]. [cited 2021 Jun 14]. Available from: https://healthcaredesignmagazine.com/trends/perspectives/implications-of-covid-19-on-healthcare-design/

Hospitals After COVID-19: How Do We Design For An Uncertain Future? | WSP [Internet]. [cited 2021 Jun 14]. Available from: https://www.wsp.com/en-GL/insights/hospitals-after-covid-19-how-do-we-design-for-an-uncertain-future

How COVID-19 is transforming hospital design [Internet]. Express Healthcare. 2020 [cited 2021 Jun 14]. Available from: https://www.expresshealthcare.in/covid19-updates/how-covid-19-is-transforming-hospital-design/422712/

How the Covid-19 Pandemic May Reshape U.S. Hospital Design [Internet]. Undark Magazine. 2020 [cited 2021 Jun 14]. Available from: https://undark.org/2020/04/16/covid-19-modified-hospital-design/

How the Pandemic is Changing Healthcare Design [Internet]. Facilitiesnet. [cited 2021 Jun 14]. Available from: https://www.facilitiesnet.com/healthcarefacilities/article/How-the-Pandemic-is-Changing-Healthcare-Design%2D%2D19098

Muller AE, Hafstad EV, Himmels JPW, Smedslund G, Flottorp S, Stensland SØ, et al. The mental health impact of the covid-19 pandemic on healthcare workers, and interventions to help them: A rapid systematic review. Psychiatry Res. 2020 Nov 1;293:113441.

What You Should Be Reading: Articles About the Impact of Covid-19 on Facility Design [Internet]. Sara Marberry. 2020 [cited 2021 Jun 14]. Available from: https://www.saramarberry.com/articles-impact-of-covid-19-on-facility-design/

10 Site Plan

A site plan is an architectural plan, a landscaped document prepared by an architect, which shows the bird's eye view of a property that is drawn to a particular scale. It shows the arrangement of buildings, roadways, landscape, garden, travel ways, utilities, parking, topography, water features, vegetation, building footprint, drainage facilities, sanitary sewer lines, water lines, trails, and lighting elements.

Once the schematic design is approved by the promoters, the next step is to prepare the site plan. Site planning begins by surveying and assessing a potential site for development through site analysis. This involves measuring the size, shape, slope of the land, and gaining information about the soil, hydrology, vegetation, orientation etc. are assessed and mapped. This analyzed information is then drawn on the architectural drawing, which marks the allowed land coverage area, where the main building will be constructed. The remaining area can be used for roadways, parking, landscape, gardening, or other hospital services that can be placed outside the building such as Transformer Room, Generator space, Bio-Medical Waste storage, STP/ETP Tanks, Liquid Oxygen Plant, Security huts, Lawns with waiting areas etc. (Figs. 10.1 and 10.2).

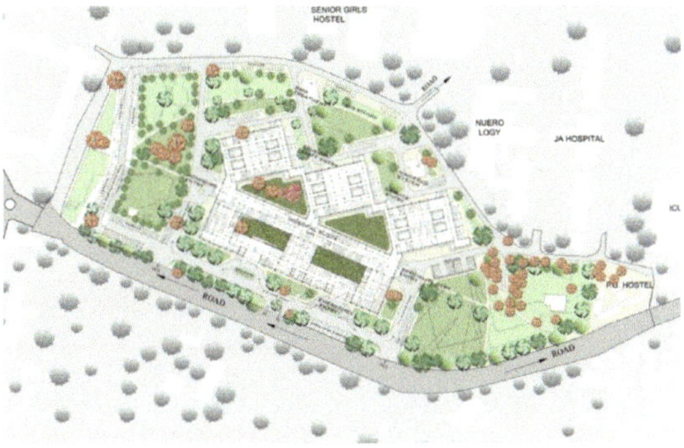

Fig. 10.1 Sample drawing of site plan

10.1 Contents of Site Plan

1. It should be an architectural drawing that is drawn to a particular scale.
2. Each and every dimension must be clearly mentioned in it.
3. It has to show property lines.
4. It must show the necessary existing structures on the land if any.
5. It must show the distance between buildings and property lines.
6. It has to show the roads, walking pathway and ramps to go to the basement.
7. It has to show the landscape and gardens.

A. Garg, A. Dewan, *Manual of Hospital Planning and Designing*,
https://doi.org/10.1007/978-981-16-8456-2_10

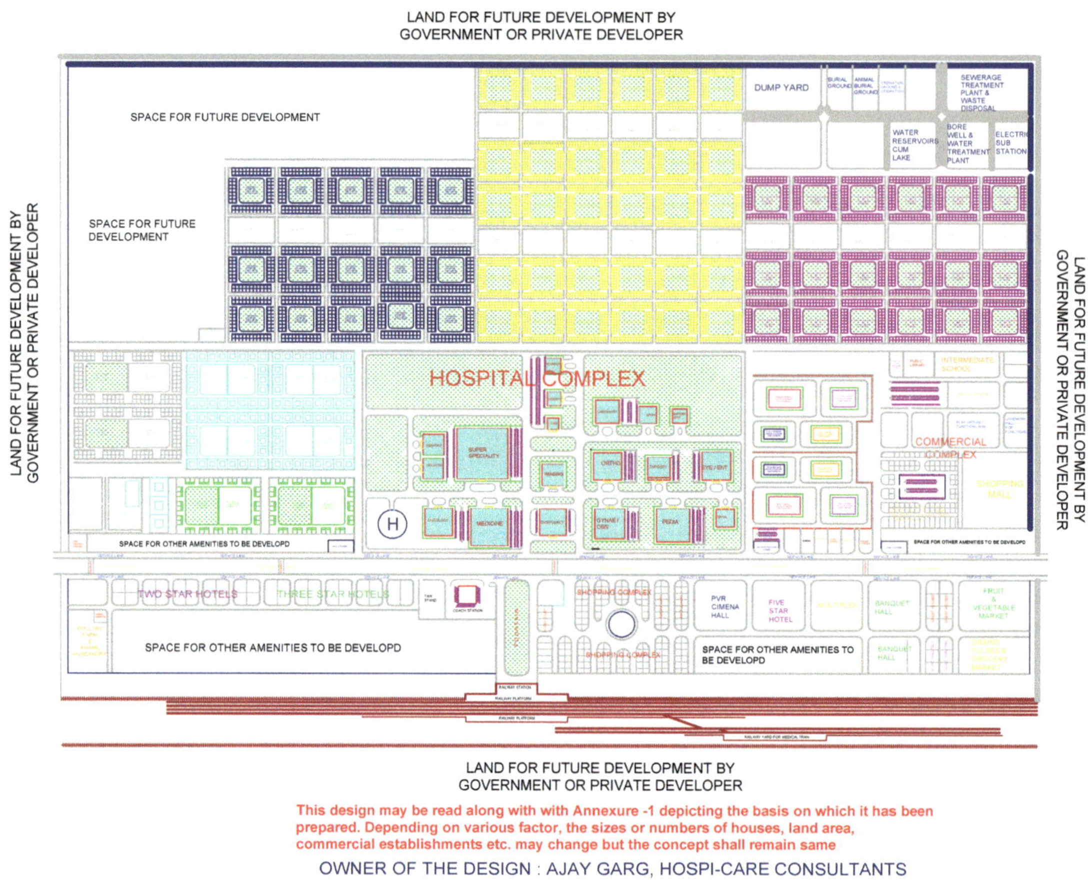

Fig. 10.2 Sample drawing of site plan

8. It must show large trees on the land if any.
9. It has to show Existing and Proposed Conditions.
10. It has to show construction limits and lay down areas.
11. It has to show parking.
12. It has to show the surrounding streets and ground sign locations.
13. It has to show fire hydrants.
14. Clearly show the location of the other services which are being planned outside the building like Transformer Room, Generator space, Bio-Medical Waste storage, STP/ETP Tanks, Liquid Oxygen Plant, Security huts and Lawns with waiting areas.

This site plan shall then be submitted to the promoters for finalization. Once the site plan is finalized, it is then submitted to the authorities for initial approval. Once it is approved, it will serve as a layout map for further designing of the floor plans.

Another factor is soil analysis. As the structure of the hospital depends a lot upon the soil condition, the soil analysis must be performed by a reputed agency to check the load-bearing capacity, type of soil etc. before designing the structure of the building.

Further Reading

Ayeni D, Olalusi C, Tukur R. Sustainable Site Planning and the Architects' Role. Acad J Sci. 2017 Jul 6;07:47–55.

Johnson BJ. Site Planning for Planners: The View from the Other Side. J Educ Built Environ. 2009 Jul 1;4(1):31–56.

Lai R. Site Planning Scheme of Hard Landscape. Kai Tak Commer [Internet]. [cited 2021 Jun 14];

Available from: https://www.academia.edu/39332540/Site_Planning_Scheme_of_Hard_Landscape

Lin JJ-C, Yang C-E, Hung W-H, Kang S-C. Accessibility evaluation system for site layout planning – a tractor trailer example. Vis Eng. 2013 Dec 9;1(1):12.

Marcus CC. Site Planning, Building Design and a Sense of Community: An Analysis of Six Cohousing Schemes in Denmark, Sweden, and the Netherlands. J Archit Plan Res. 2000;17(2):146–63.

Site planning | landscaping [Internet]. Encyclopedia Britannica. [cited 2021 Jun 14]. Available from: https://www.britannica.com/topic/site-planning

The Importance of Landscape and Site Design [Internet]. CWG Architecture. 2018 [cited 2021 Jun 14]. Available from: https://cwg-architects.com/2018/06/12/the-importance-of-landscape-and-site-design/

11 Detailed Engineering Drawings

Architectural drawings are the technical representation of a building made before the beginning actual process of construction. They are the AutoCAD drawings made with projections and are based on a defined scale. There are two fundamental architectural drawings. One is the 'Planning drawing', and the other is the 'Detailed drawing'.

Planning drawing is putting the concept, appearance and layout design in a drawing. These drawings are output from the briefing, sketching, designing and developing stages set in a shape of the drawing. They are primarily used to file the proposal to the concerned authorities to seek permission for construction.

Whereas in the Detailed Drawings, the technical side of construction information is provided. Once the designer starts preparing the detailed drawings; he/she has to consider all the minute technical details and issues that may be required for actual construction or even for estimating the cost of a building. The detailed drawings consists of different set of drawings, some of which are as follows:

11.1 Concept Drawings

They are the first draft of project drawings and do not involve many details. They act as rough sketches of the building and are mainly used to describe an overall view of the building (Fig. 11.1).

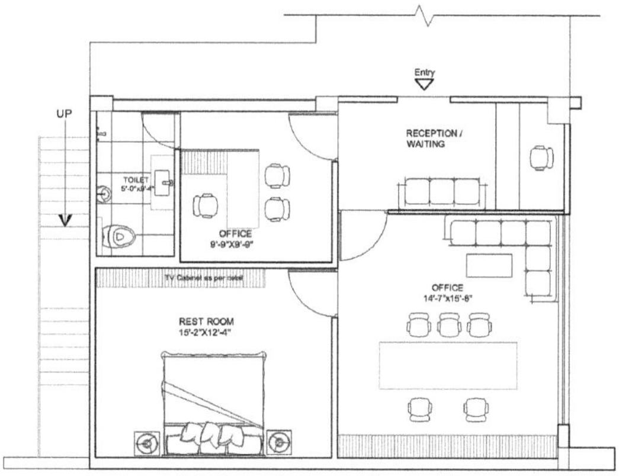

Fig. 11.1 Sample of concept drawing

11.2 Floor Plan Drawings

It depicts the layout and placement of different rooms, services and functionalities on a particular area or a floor of the building. This is an in-depth version of the room layout. It helps to analyze different issues like:

- Efficiency in the movement of men and material.
- Whether the spaces provided are sufficient for working?
- Whether the ancillary rooms have been properly placed?
- Is the infection control properly taken care of?
- Are the toilets properly placed?

A. Garg, A. Dewan, *Manual of Hospital Planning and Designing*,
https://doi.org/10.1007/978-981-16-8456-2_11

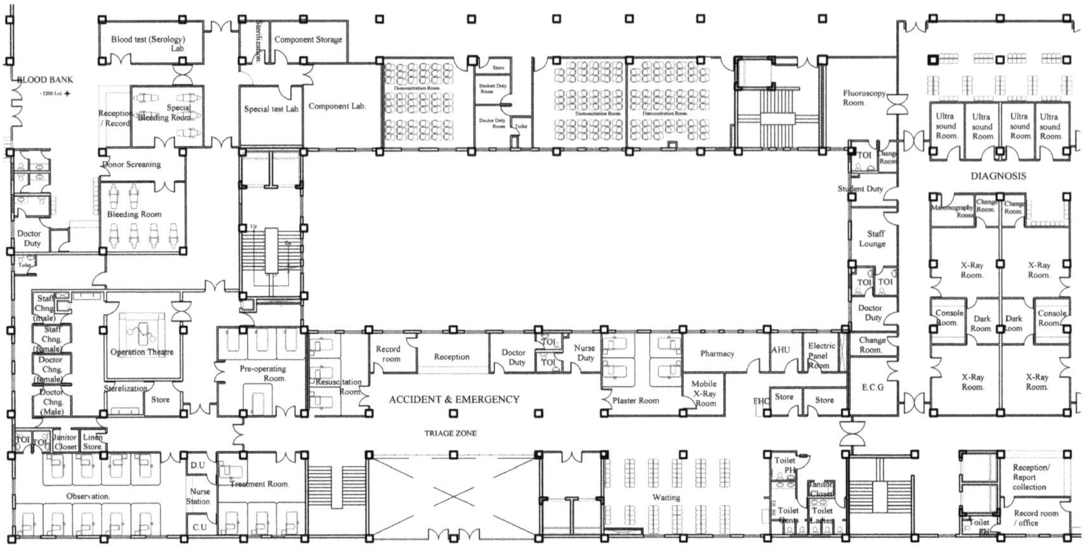

Fig. 11.2 Sample of floor plan drawing

- Are the shafts for services provided properly?
- Are the movement spaces sufficient?
- Is the fire escape root approachable?
- Is the provision of natural light and cross air ventilation properly taken care of?
- Are the doors and windows properly placed?
- Is there any possibility to reshuffle the room layouts for better design?
- (Fig. 11.2).

11.3 Cross Section Drawings

This drawing allows to look at the different components of a building vertically. In this drawing, all the floors of the building are shown vertically. These two-dimensional drawings are useful to provide an overview of both the visible and the non-visible components, fittings and structure of the building (Fig. 11.3).

11.4 Elevation Drawings

They are the drawings of the exterior of the building and the exterior surfaces of the building. This shall include the location of windows and beautification of the exterior surfaces using stones, paints, glass, grills etc. These drawings also provide information about the height of the building and the external and internal markings, such as doors and windows along with the sizes that will look from outside. It helps a designer understand which direction the building will be facing, the direction of the sun and wind corresponding to the building. Even the promoters prefer to have a 3D look on the elevation to see how the building will look from outside (Figs. 11.4 and 11.5).

11.5 Landscape Drawings

It depicts the external aesthetics of the building and the aerial view of the whole area in which the building is to be built. It shows how the open spaces of the land will be beautified. It includes spaces designated for paths, roads, pavements, parking areas, trees, street lights, parks, pools, gardens, bushes, hedges, external services and everything else (Fig. 11.6).

11.6 Finishing Drawing

It contains smaller details for finishing of the building spaces. It includes the details of types and dimension of the finishing part of the spaces like

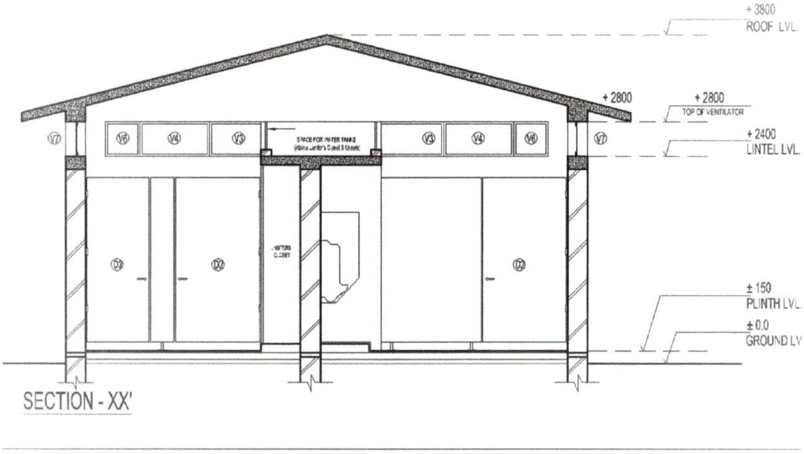

Fig. 11.3 Sample of cross section drawing

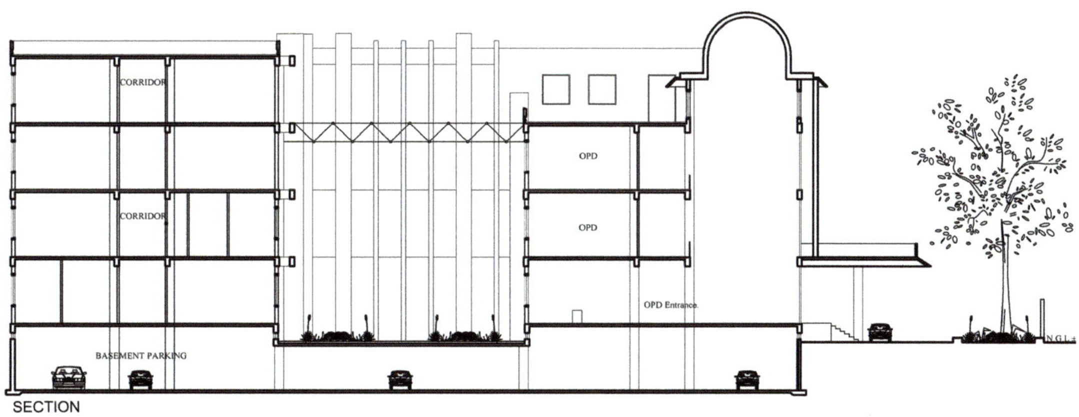

Fig. 11.4 Sample of elevation drawing

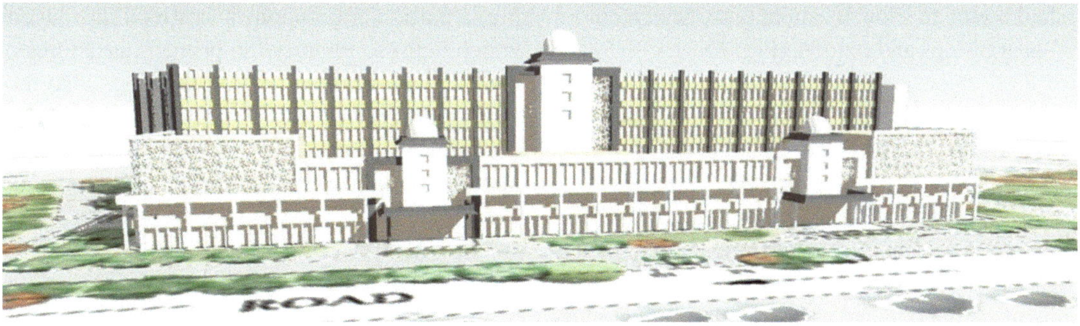

Fig. 11.5 Sample of elevation drawing

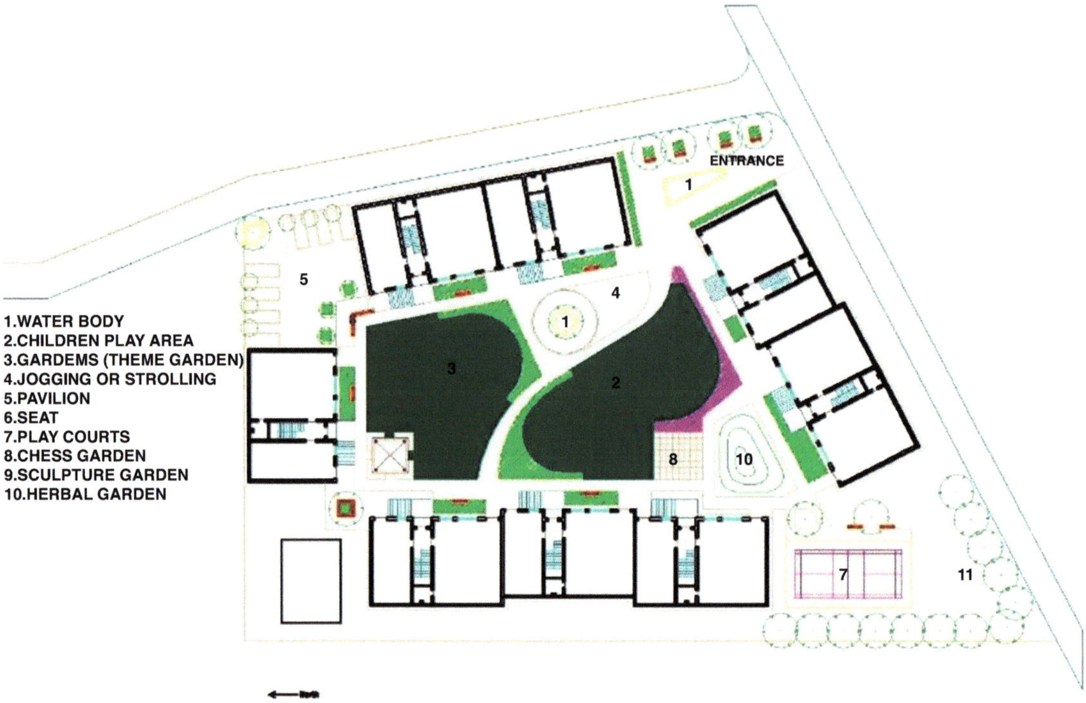

Fig. 11.6 Sample of landscape drawing

flooring, false ceiling, paints, colours, plaster, textures, doors, toilet fittings, electrical fixtures and window designs. Depending on the requirements, these drawings can be further divided into different drawings pertaining to one or more items. For example, a separate drawing can be prepared which will show the type, pattern, design, material, size etc. of doors and windows. Similarly, for electrical fittings and fixtures, there can be separate drawing to show location, type, design colour of such fittings and fixtures (Fig. 11.7).

11.7 Working Plan Drawings

The working plans or also called construction plans are for the contractors to help them in understanding the scope of work of the project. The benefits of such a plan are to facilitate the contractors to calculate and access the construction material to be used according to the overall design. The legend provided in the working drawings provides information about the different components of the drawings to the contractors. It shall incorporate the exact measurement and dimensions of each and every component. If required, the enlarged drawings of a particular component shall be depicted in the final working plan (Fig. 11.8).

11.8 Section Drawings

They show the structure in a sliced form, meaning, a particular component is sliced into layers, which helps to identify the primary structures of the building. Further, section drawings also provide information for the types of materials to be used during construction and how to erect such material during construction (Fig. 11.9).

11.9 Structural Drawings

They are the engineering drawings focused on the structural part of the building like columns, beams, foundation and slab casting. The design of the structure is a crucial part of the building design as the building's strength depends on the structure.

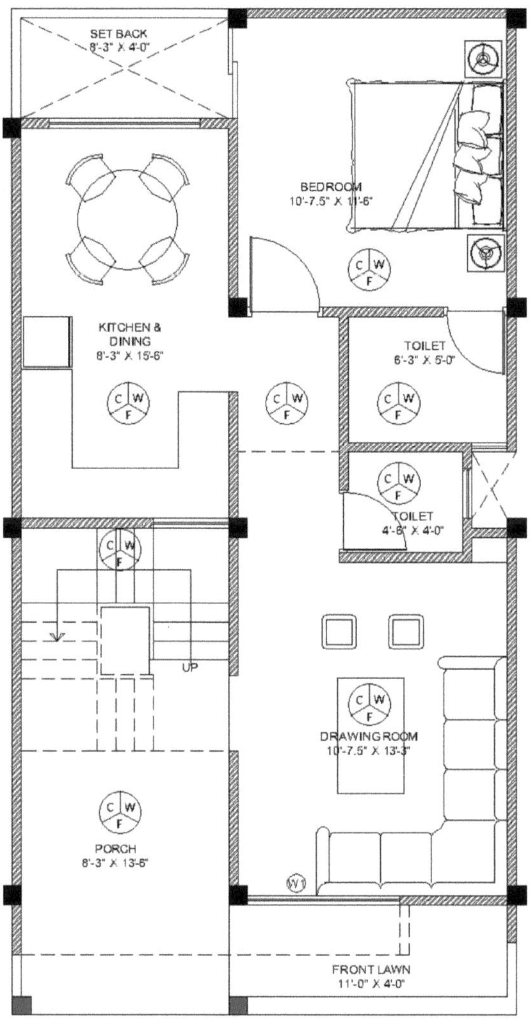

Fig. 11.7 Sample of finishing drawing

These drawings are generally prepared and certified by the Structure Engineers. Based on the floor plans, the engineer locates the position of the columns and designs the structure. While designing, the engineer has to consider the issues related to the earthquake, wind velocity, torpedo, soil analysis, flood and load in the building. They also provide details of the reinforcement and the composition of the concrete mix to be used (Fig. 11.10).

11.10 Column Layout Drawings

It depicts the design and location of the columns in the building. This drawing is a part of Structural Drawing. As the size of the column goes on reducing from floor to floor, this plan is prepared floor-wise and demarcates the exact size and distance between each and every column of the building and also marks the location of each column (Fig. 11.11).

11.11 Plinth Beam Layout Drawings

Plinth beams are the beams usually at the lower level of the structure to bind the columns in a building. The plinth beam layout drawings show the exact position, length and sectional design of the plinth beams (Fig. 11.12).

11.12 Lintel Beam Layout Drawings

Lintel beams are support structures that are made above the doors and windows to hold the construction work above the doors and windows. As the lower surfaces of door and windows are vacant and there is no brickwork, the lintel beams are used to hold the walls above the doors and windows. In these drawings, the positions, dimensions, design and number of lintel beams are shown (Fig. 11.13).

11.13 Roof Beam and Shuttering Layout Drawings

This is the drawing of the shuttering to be done for casting upper beans and the slab of the floor (Fig. 11.14).

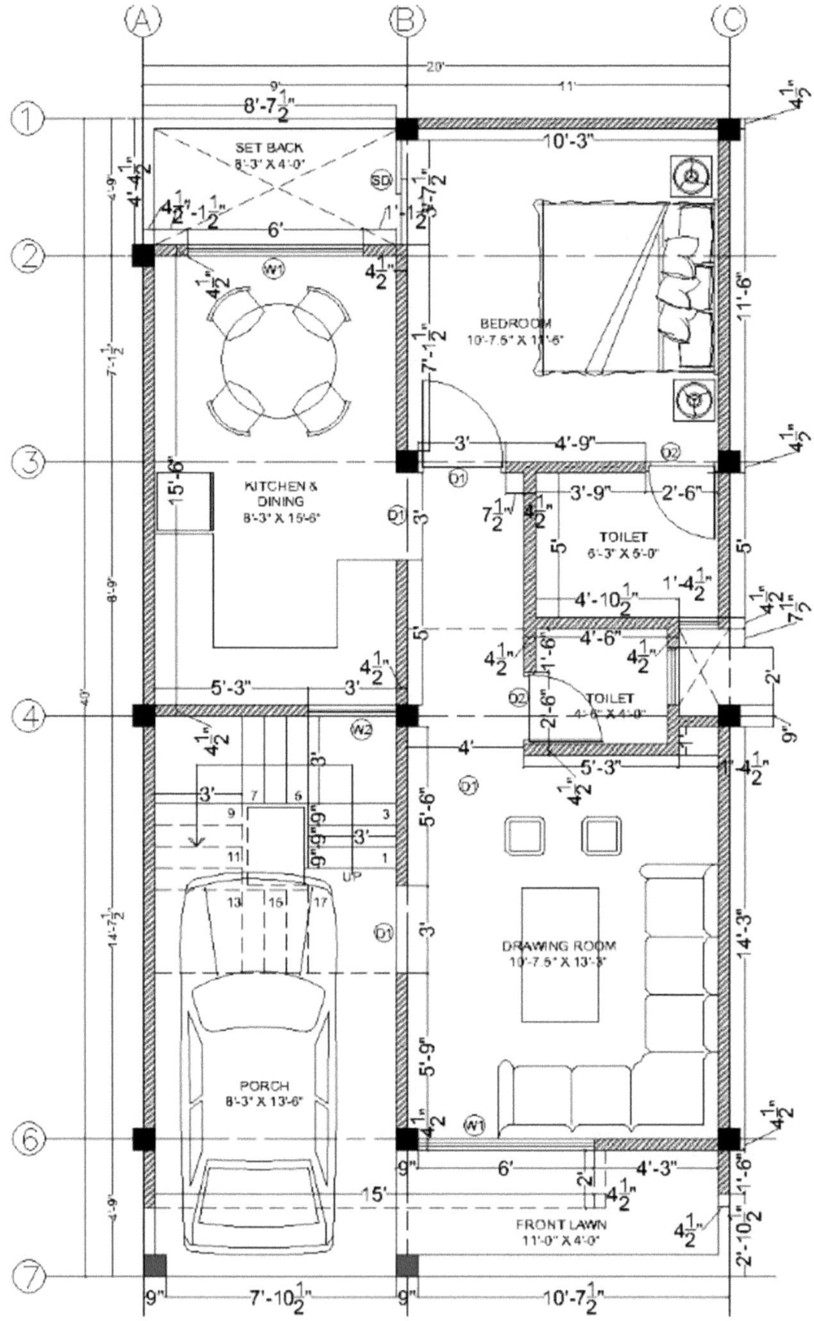

Fig. 11.8 Sample of working plan drawing

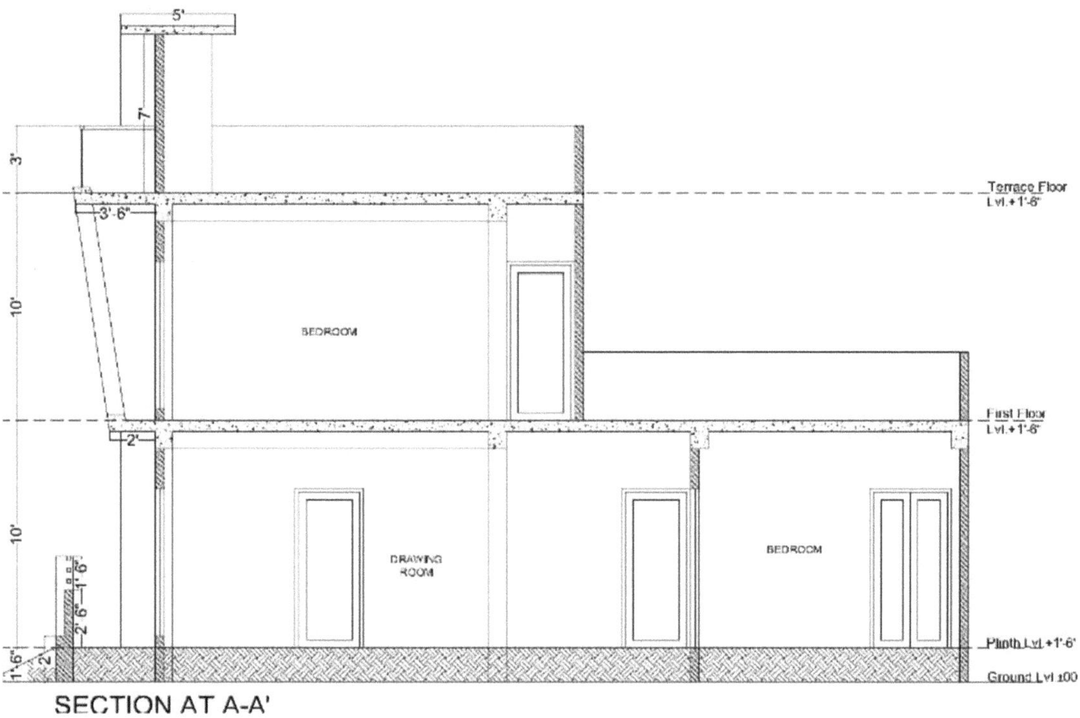

Fig. 11.9 Sample of section drawing

11.14 General Note

It is not a specific drawing in itself but contains detailed information about the by-laws, legends, mapping forms, construction type, codes, length, abbreviations and anything else that may be required for actual construction process.

11.15 Excavation Drawings

These are the details of excavation to be done for starting the construction of the building. In case there is a basement, this drawing depicts the details of basements and the excavation to be done. Also, this drawing shows the details of excavations to be done for the foundations of the building. The foundations can be individual footing columns or a generalized raft. It shows the length, depth and the width of the area to be excavated and provides information about the extent of excavation, process of excavation, removal and disposal of the soil. Different processes like trenching, wall shafts, tunnelling and complete removal are used for excavation (Fig. 11.15).

11.16 Electrical Drawings

The hospital requires a system of power and electricity to run the building. This drawing is generally prepared by the Electrical Engineer. It depicts the electrical planning for the Transformer, Energy metre, Main Panel, Floor Panel Circuit Diagrams, Line layout, Distribution Boxes, Switch Boards, Earthing etc. The drawing also

Fig. 11.10 Sample of structural drawing

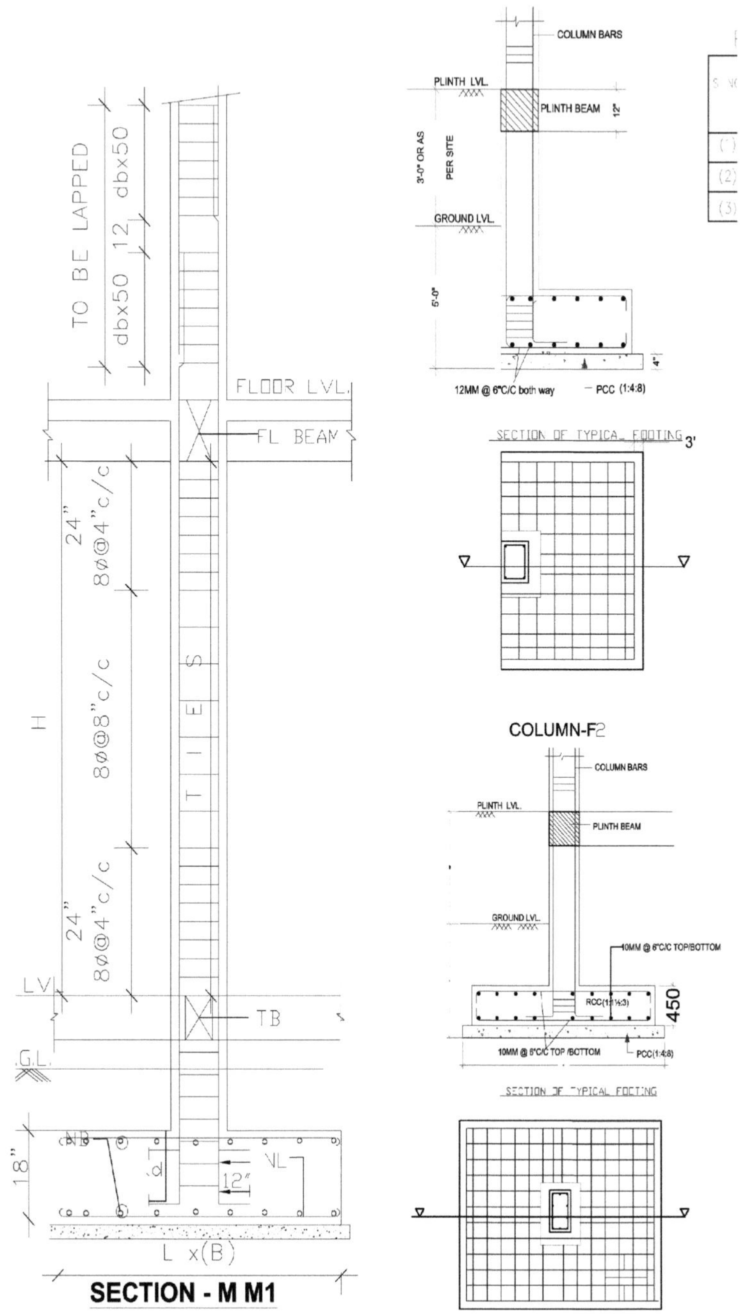

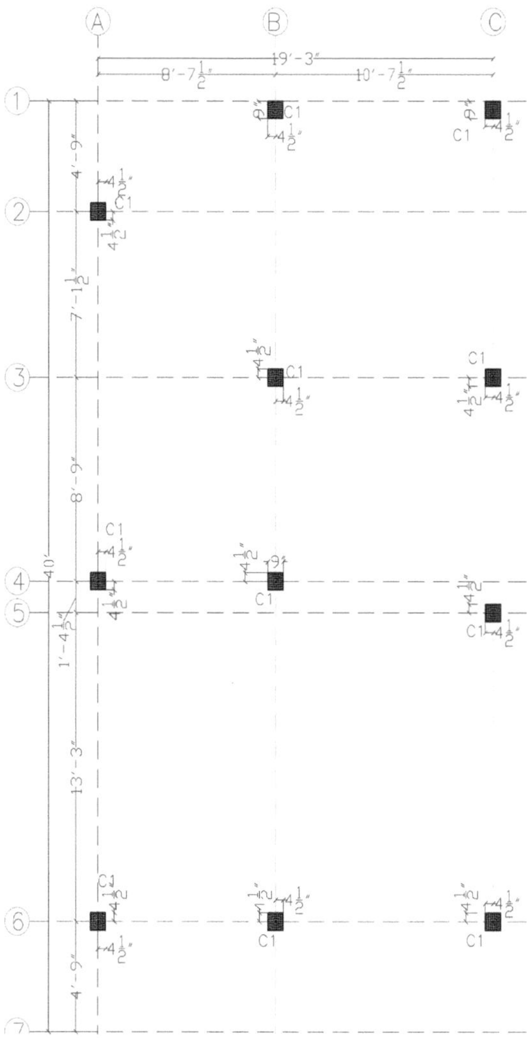

Fig. 11.11 Sample of column layout drawing

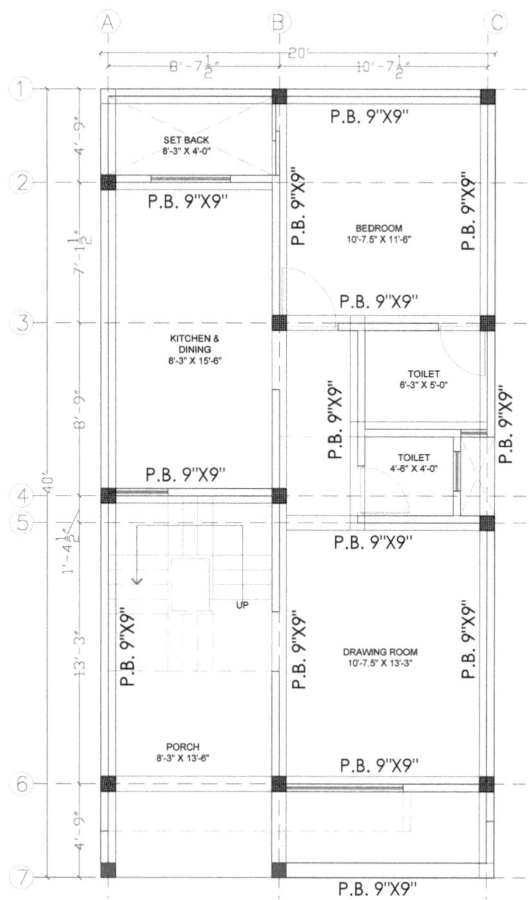

Fig. 11.12 Sample of plinth bean layout drawing

shows the location of the electrical fittings and fixtures. Along with the layout, the capacity, design and the bill of quantity is also calculated (Fig. 11.16).

11.17 Plumbing Drawings

It relates to the supply of water and drains water to and from the building. This drawing depicts the water supply layouts of bore wells, Government supply line points, overhead tanks, roof tank, the layout of the supply lines in the building and sanitary fittings. Similarly, for drainage, the drawing is prepared for the drain pipelines, main holes, STP/ETP tanks and connection to the main sewerage line. Also, the layouts for the rainwater harvesting are shown in this drawing (Fig. 11.17).

11.18 Firefighting and Detection Drawings

It relates to the setup of firefighting, fire detection and fire escape route. Firefighting drawing depicts the details and location of the fire water storage tank, pump room, water supply line, yard hydrants, sprinkler line layout, sprinkler points, rooftop tank layout for down comers, and hydrant location in the building, and upward hydrant pipeline layout. Similarly, for the fire detection system, the drawings are prepared for the control panel location, smoke detectors, hooters and

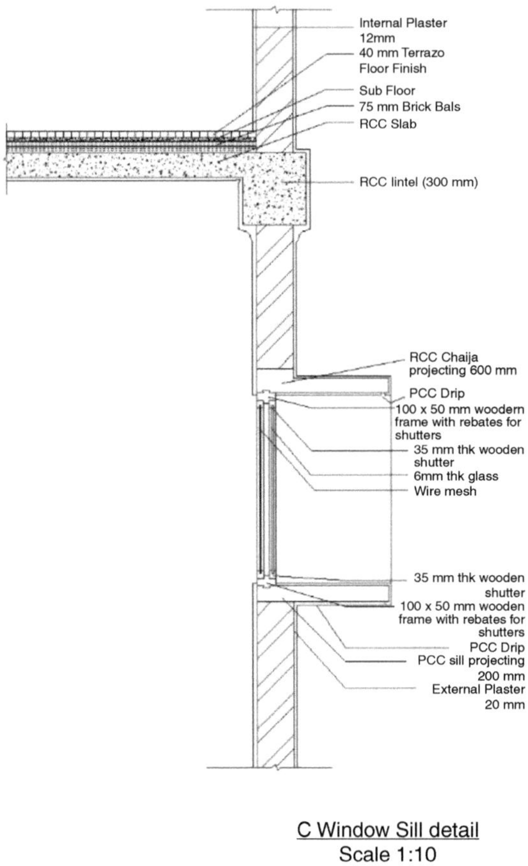

Fig. 11.13 Sample of lintel beam layout drawing

switches. Also, the escape route drawings in case of fire have to be drawn showing the routes along with the staircases, ramps, fire doors and the signage location. The drawings also show the location of the pressurizing system for lift wells, lift lobbies and staircases (Figs. 11.18 and 11.19).

11.19 Shop Drawings

These are the construction designs depicting how an object has to be installed, fitted or manufactured. These drawings are generally prepared for services like Air Conditioning, MGPS, CCTV network, EPABX network, IT network, Public Address System network and PTS (Pneumatic Tube System). They are detailed line diagrams depicting the location of the machines and the line of the system. For example, in the case of MGPS, the drawing shall show the routing of the pipelines, location of the gas points, design of the manifold room, the pump room etc. Similarly, for air conditioning, the layout plan of ducts, chilled water pipelines, AHUs, Plant room and cooling towers are set in the drawing. Mostly, the shop drawings are prepared by contractors or subcontractors to whom the work has been or would be

Fig. 11.14 Sample of roof beam and shuttering layout drawing

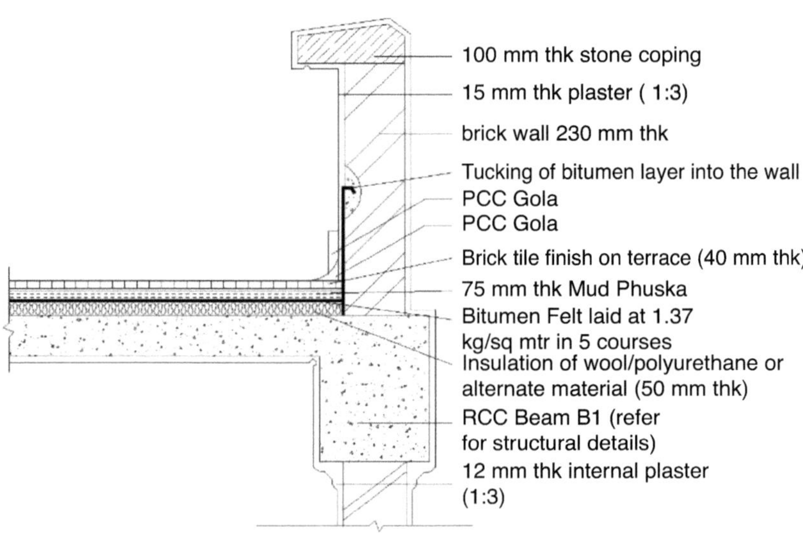

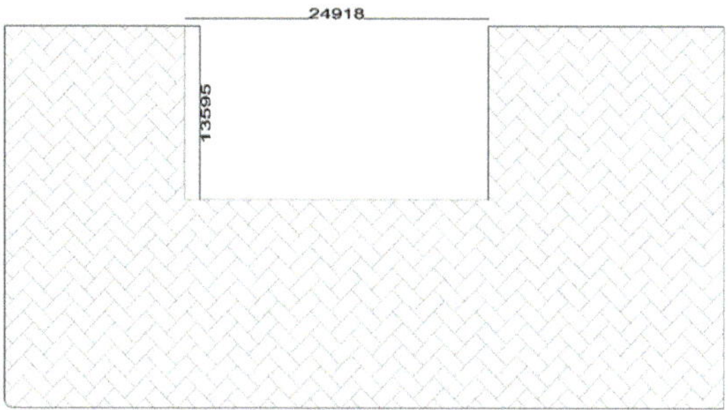

Fig. 11.15 Sample of excavation drawing

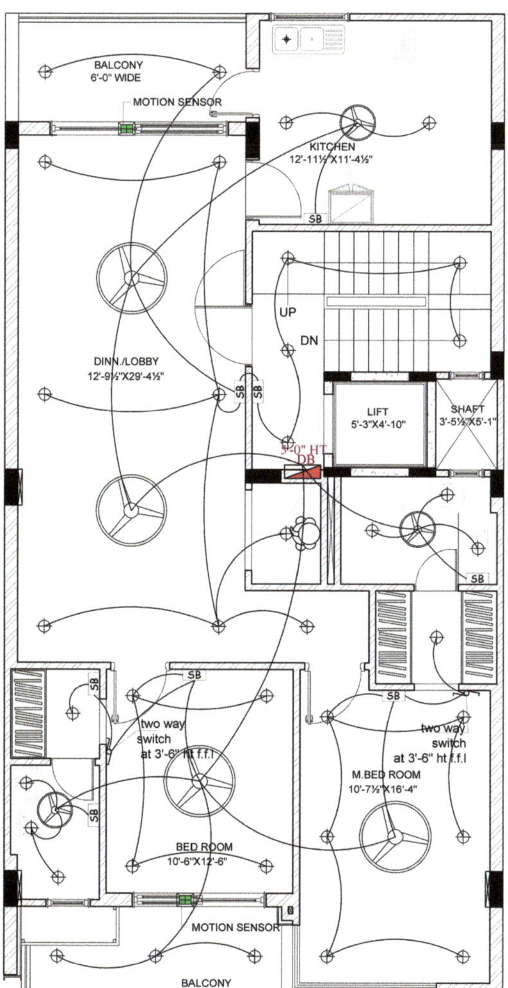

Fig. 11.16 Sample of electrical drawing

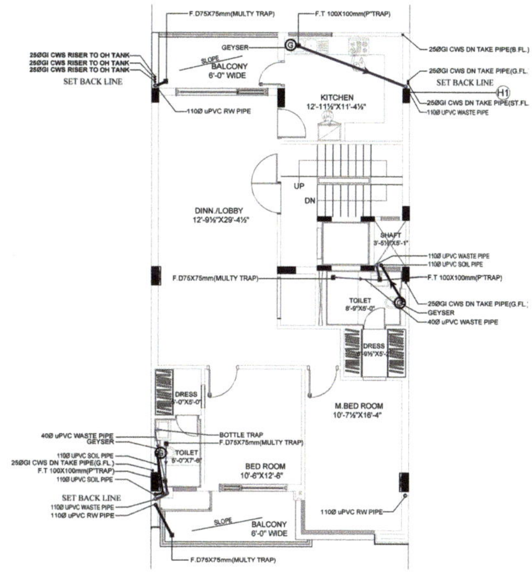

Fig. 11.17 Sample of plumbing drawing

allotted. Also, suppliers, manufacturers and fabricators can also prepare these drawings. However, these drawings shall be in compliance with the original design and specifications of the object and provided by the designer (Figs. 11.20 and 11.21).

11.20 Furniture Layout Drawings

A hospital's requirement of furniture varies from room to room including patient furniture and office furniture. The patient furniture involves patient bed, side trolley, wheelchairs, stretcher trolley, over bed table crash cart, instrument trolley, dressing trolley etc. Similarly, the office furniture involves waiting chairs, office tables, office chairs, cupboards, examination couches etc. Similarly, the size of the office furniture may vary in some rooms as compared to other rooms. This drawing depicts the layout of the furniture in each and every room and space of the hospital along with the size and dimensions of the furniture (Fig. 11.22).

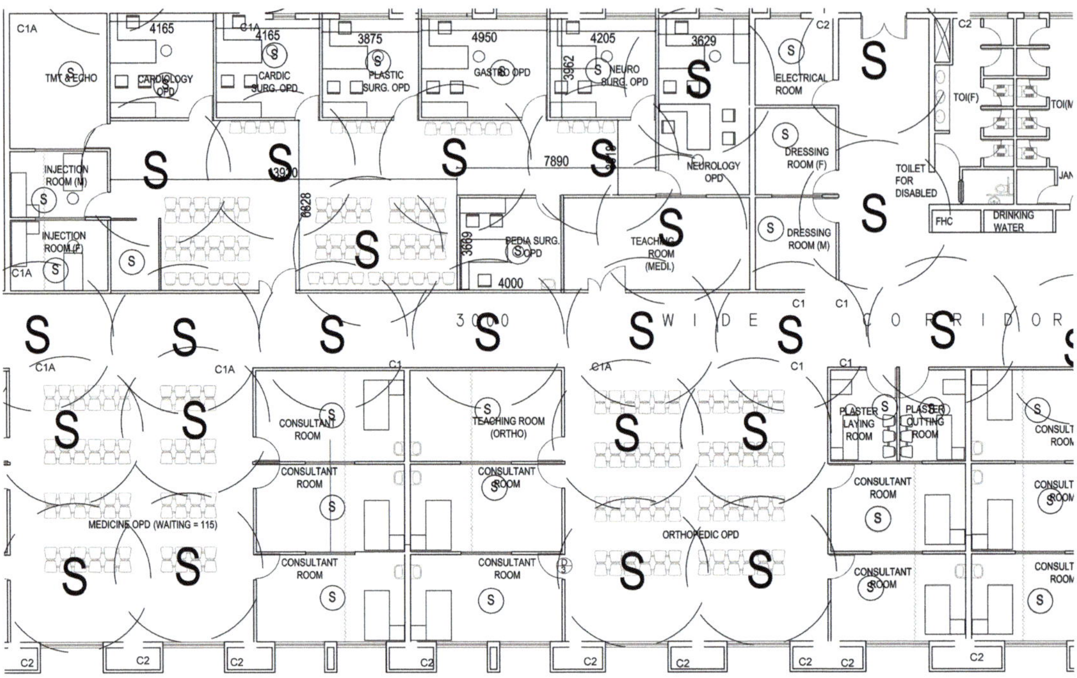

Fig. 11.18 Sample of firefighting drawing

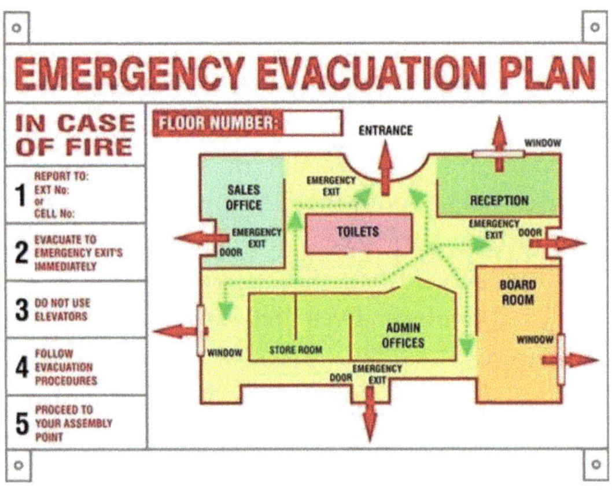

Fig. 11.19 Sample of fire escape plan drawing

11.21 Furniture Design Drawings

Most often, patient furniture has fixed size and design, whereas the office furniture is tailored according to the needs. Based on the sizes and dimensions provided by the Furniture Layout Drawing, the design of the furniture has to be worked out. The furniture design drawings describe the sizes, design, material and fittings to be used for manufacturing such furniture. This drawing is also used to work out the estimated cost of furniture.

11.22 Hospital Signage Drawings

Designing and providing signage in the hospital is a typical task, which requires careful designing. Finding signage location and design is even more important. The signage location has to be such which gives an uninterrupted view of the signage to the people. This drawing depicts the location of the signage along with its design at various locations. The design of the signage may change from one location to other. Therefore, the signage drawing is prepared separately for each floor.

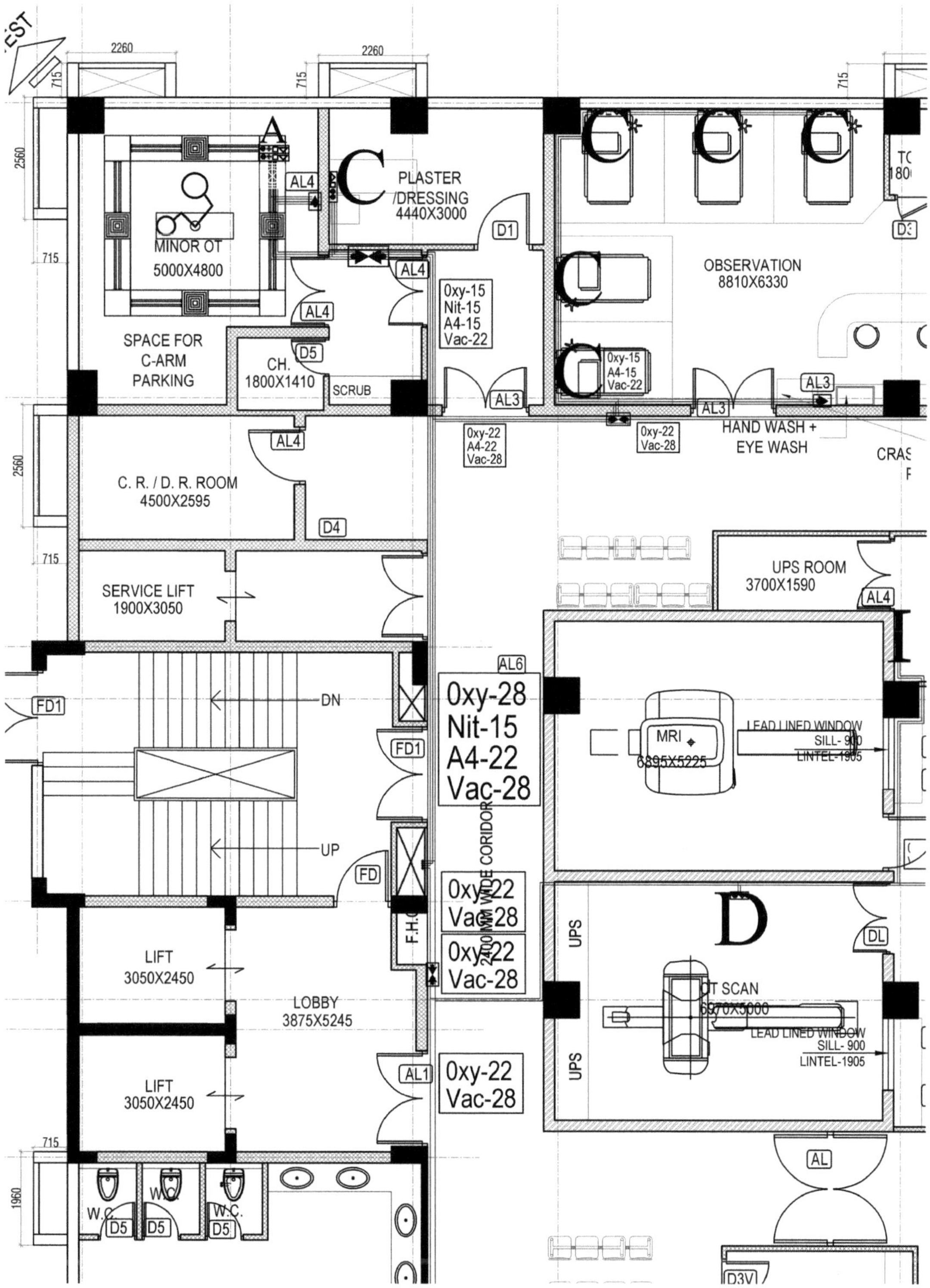

Fig. 11.20 Sample of shop drawing of MGPS

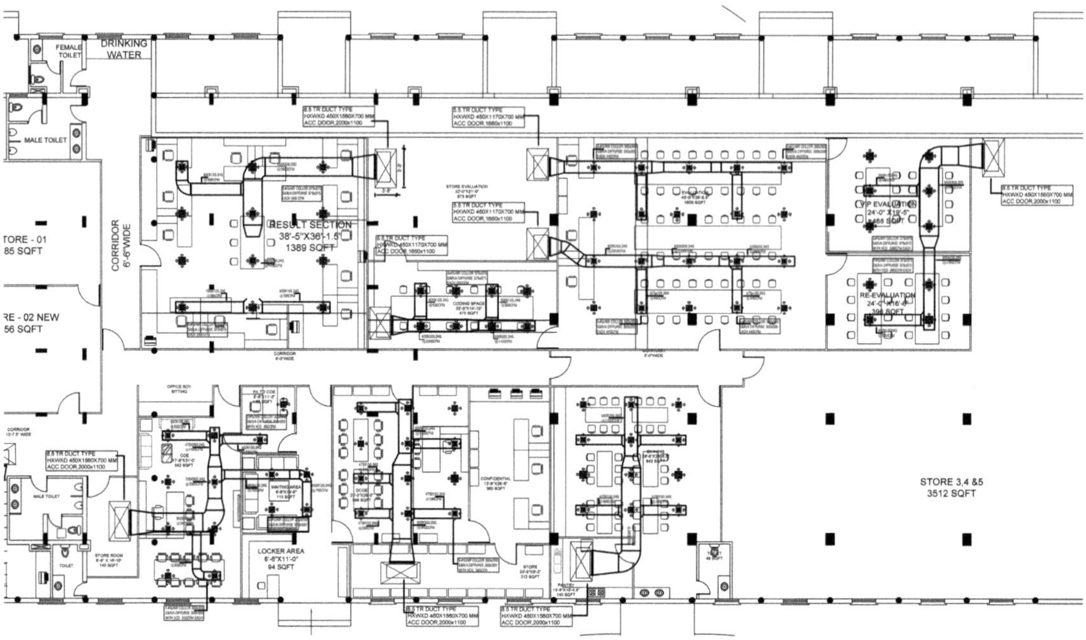

Fig. 11.21 Sample of shop drawing of HVAC

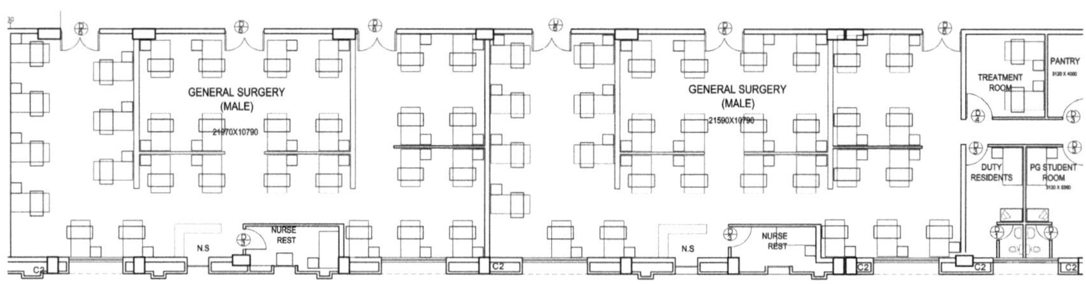

Fig. 11.22 Sample of furniture layout drawing

11.23 As-Built Drawings

At times it happens that during construction, due to some unavoidable circumstances or due to changes in the decision, the construction pattern and design may have to be changed as compared to what was planned in the working drawing or the floor plan. If it so happens, As-built drawings are prepared either during the construction process or after the construction is complete. These drawings are prepared for comparison between what has been actually been built versus the original plan to trace out the changes that have taken place during construction.

11.24 PERT Charts

It is a chart depicting the time frame for the completion of the project. It states when the activity has to be started and when to be completed. Sometimes it happens that the start of a particular activity depends on the completion of the other activity. This issue is also depicted in the PERT chart. It is an important tool for the management to know the progress of the project on regular basis.

Further Reading

Construction drawing [Internet]. https://www.designingbuildings.co.uk; [cited 2021 Jun 14]. Available from: https://www.designingbuildings.co.uk/wiki/Construction_drawing

INC U-B. 42 Types of Drawings Used in Building Design- Comprehensive Guide [Internet]. [cited 2021 Jun 14]. Available from: https://www.united-bim.com/a-comprehensive-guide-42-types-of-drawings-used-in-building-design/

Jamal H. List of Drawings Required for Building Construction | Floor Plan, Elevation, Section, Electrification, PLumbing [Internet]. [cited 2021 Jun 14]. Available from: https://www.aboutcivil.org/list-drawings-buildings.html

TreisTek. Types of Drawings Used in Building Construction [Internet]. TreisTek. 2020 [cited 2021 Jun 14]. Available from: https://www.treistek.com/post/types-of-drawings-used-in-building-construction

Types of drawings for building design [Internet]. https://www.designingbuildings.co.uk; [cited 2021 Jun 14]. Available from: https://www.designingbuildings.co.uk/wiki/Types_of_drawings_for_building_design

Types of Drawings used in Building Construction - Building Technology Guide [Internet]. The Constructor. 2018 [cited 2021 Jun 14]. Available from: https://theconstructor.org/building/drawing-types-construction/24524/

Part III

Construction Documents

Preparation of Construction Documents

12

Now, as the set of detailed drawings is ready, we move on to the next phase of construction. This phase is to engage contractors for starting the construction work; however, some documents are required for the contractor to understand before he/she gives his/her rates and quotation. It is this set of construction documents.

12.1 Definition of Construction Documents

It is a set of documents containing the general and supplementary conditions, owner's special requirements, drawings, specifications, details, change orders and other documents prepared by the designer or his/her consultants. Contraxct Documents describes the scope, type, quality of materials, supplies, equipment, systems and other elements required to construct a project and accepted by the promoter.

In any hospital, there are different contractors for different activities. For each and every activity, a separate contractor may have to be engaged. Therefore, each of these contractors may require a separate set of construction documents relating to their activity. Generally, for a hospital, construction documents are required for the following activities:

1. Soil analysis.
2. Excavation of land.
3. Civil Construction.
4. Reinforcement steel binding.
5. Electrical and Power.
6. Plumbing and Sanitary.
7. Firefighting.
8. Air Conditioning.
9. Information Technology (Computerization).
10. CCTV System.
11. Public Announcement System.
12. Door Windows.
13. Painting and Polishing.
14. False Ceiling.
15. Flooring.
16. Elevation.
17. Staircase Railing.
18. Site Development and Landscaping.
19. Elevators/Lifts.
20. MGPS.
21. Modular OT.
22. Signage.
23. Curtain track system.
24. Nurse Call System.
25. General Furniture.

A. Garg, A. Dewan, *Manual of Hospital Planning and Designing*,
https://doi.org/10.1007/978-981-16-8456-2_12

12.2 Contents of Construction Document

12.2.1 General Information About the Hospital Project

This document contains general information about the site, size of the land, project size, owners of the project, the mission of the project, services to be provided by the hospital, total covered area of the hospital etc. This document helps the contractor to understand the background of the project.

12.2.2 Construction Contract Agreement

This is the agreement that shall be entered between the construction contractor and the hospital owner when finalizing the contract. This agreement is to make the contractors aware of the terms and conditions entered in the agreement.

12.2.3 Scope of Work

This document clearly defines the scope of work (SOW) involved during the construction period and after the construction work to rectify the defect. It is prepared separately for all the activities involved during the construction and helps the contractor understand the work he/she has to perform before submitting the bid.

SOW should define and elaborate all the work to be done, the person responsible for such work, how the work has to be performed, i.e. techniques to be used, the sequence of the work and details of the materials to be used. This document should also define the terms and conditions regarding any change during the construction process.

12.2.4 Construction Schedule

The construction schedule is a document that contains the schedule of working like the expected start date of work, expected date of work completion, terms and conditions about leverage to be offered and penalties to be levied in case of delay in the project schedule.

12.2.5 General Conditions

The General Conditions such as the right, responsibilities and relationships between the owner and contractors shall be laid down. It shall offer a legal framework for the overall construction contract and includes dispute resolution clauses.

12.2.6 Special Conditions

The Special Conditions document should specify the conditions and clauses that may pertain to a specific activity or a specific portion of the job.

12.2.7 Specifications

The Specifications section of a contract document contains all the technical data, specifications and requirements of the activity to be performed. This section should contain detailed information about the materials to be used, sizes, make, model, quality, warranty terms etc. Information should also be provided regarding the techniques, equipment and tools to complete such activity. The biding contractor should be made free to seek clarification on these specifications in case of any doubt. This section also contains the terms and conditions of leverage to be offered in case of changes in the specifications during the construction process.

12.2.8 Bill of Quantities

This document contains the details of the itemized materials to be used in the contract along with the quantity of the individual item.

12.2.9 Cost Estimate

This part of the construction documents provides a breakdown of all the items to be incorporated into the construction project. It also includes an itemized list on the estimated costs of materials, parts and labour in the construction project. The total cost estimate can be worked out by multiplying the quantity (as stated in the bill of quantity (BOQ)) with the estimated costs and then adding the labour or erection charge.

12.2.10 Drawings

The Construction documents shall also include a set of simple drawings that can provide a graphic representation of the scope, extent and character of the work that will have to be performed by the contractor. This is to make the contractor understand the work in drawings.

12.2.11 Other Documents

Depending on the requirements, the construction documents may or may not include the following documents:

1. Information about liens.
2. Staff requirements.
3. Supervision requirements.
4. Safety instructions.
5. Safe work method statements.
6. Contractor Pre-qualifications terms.
7. Defect management and liability clauses.
8. Test requirement and terms.
9. Inspection and test plans.
10. Environmental monitoring system.
11. Site meetings.
12. Quality monitoring terms and conditions.
13. Terms for Extension of time.
14. Materials ordering and inspections terms.
15. Daily reporting system.
16. Disposal of wastage.

These contract documents are given to the contractors who qualify for the pre-bidding qualifications. The bidder is then allowed to visit the site and seek clarification. Generally, the last date for bidding is fixed, and the bidders are advised to bid on or before the last date. The bid has to be submitted in a sealed envelope under receiving from the owner.

On the pre-decided date, the envelopes are opened in front of the bidders. The comparative sheet is prepared to work out the lowest bidder, and rounds of discussions are carried out with the bidders. Owners shall satisfy themselves about the work experience, the capability of the bidder to perform the task, bidder's earlier experience, availability of the manpower, tools with the bidder etc.

Once the management is satisfied with all these issues, the agreement's final terms and conditions are re-discussed and finalized. Last is the negotiation on the price and costs. The terms of payment are also agreed upon and documented in the contract agreement.

Once the terms and conditions and cost are agreed upon, the contract agreement is signed off by both the parties and the work order is issued.

Further Reading

10 Documents Must Be Included on Every Construction Project [Internet]. Construction Tuts. 2016 [cited 2021 Jun 14]. Available from: https://www.constructiontuts.com/documents-for-construction-project/

10 Documents to Include in Your Construction Contracts [Internet]. The Balance Small Business. [cited 2021 Jun 14]. Available from: https://www.thebalancesmb.com/contract-documents-for-every-construction-project-844919

Construction Contract Documents | A Guide to Common Contract Parts [Internet]. Levelset. 2019 [cited 2021 Jun 14]. Available from: https://www.levelset.com/blog/construction-contract-documents-guide/

Construction Document Preparation – Architect Helper [Internet]. [cited 2021 Jun 14]. Available from: http://www.architecthelper.com/our-services/construction-document-preparation

Construction documents checklist: Ensure you have the docs you need [Internet]. Sitemate. 2019 [cited 2021 Jun 14]. Available from: https://sitemate.com/uk/resources/articles/construction/construction-documents-checklist/

Contract documents for construction [Internet]. https://www.designingbuildings.co.uk; [cited 2021 Jun 14]. Available from: https://www.designingbuildings.co.uk/wiki/Contract_documents_for_construction

Preparing Individual Construction Documents | UCOP [Internet]. [cited 2021 Jun 14]. Available from: https://www.ucop.edu/construction-services/facilities-manual/volume-4/vol-4-chapter-4.html

Searchable platform for building codes [Internet]. UpCodes. [cited 2021 Jun 14]. Available from: https://up.codes/s/preparation-of-construction-documents-and-reports

Types of Drawings used in Building Construction - Building Technology Guide [Internet]. The Constructor. 2018 [cited 2021 Jun 14]. Available from: https://theconstructor.org/building/drawing-types-construction/24524/

Part IV

Design & Development

13 Designing Details of Individual Department or Spaces of the Hospital

As the hospital is an institute providing varied types of services in varied departments through various means and equipment, each department's requirements or space shall be separate. No two requirements can be alike. For example, the ICU and patient room, both are meant to admit the patient in-house and provide treatment, but the setup requirements are totally different.

Similarly, the requirement of different OPDs may be different from each other. Hence, every department or space faces unique challenges, and there is no single design solution for any specific department or space.

The designer has to develop an understanding of a department or space key requirements to effectively plan and design an efficient and patient-friendly environment of that particular department or space.

Also, it is true that if the requirement of a particular department or space is not met or designed properly, it may not provide the services effectively, resulting in compromised quality.

In the following few chapters, we will discuss the layouts, placement of equipment, internal designing, finishing and furniture etc. of some of these departments and spaces.

A. Garg, A. Dewan, *Manual of Hospital Planning and Designing*,
https://doi.org/10.1007/978-981-16-8456-2_13

14 Design of the Main Entrance Gate to the Hospital

The hospital's main entrance is the main gate through which the patients or visitors walk into the hospital premises. This main gate is a connecting gate between the public road and the hospital road. While designing the main gate, the following issues shall be considered (Fig. 14.1):

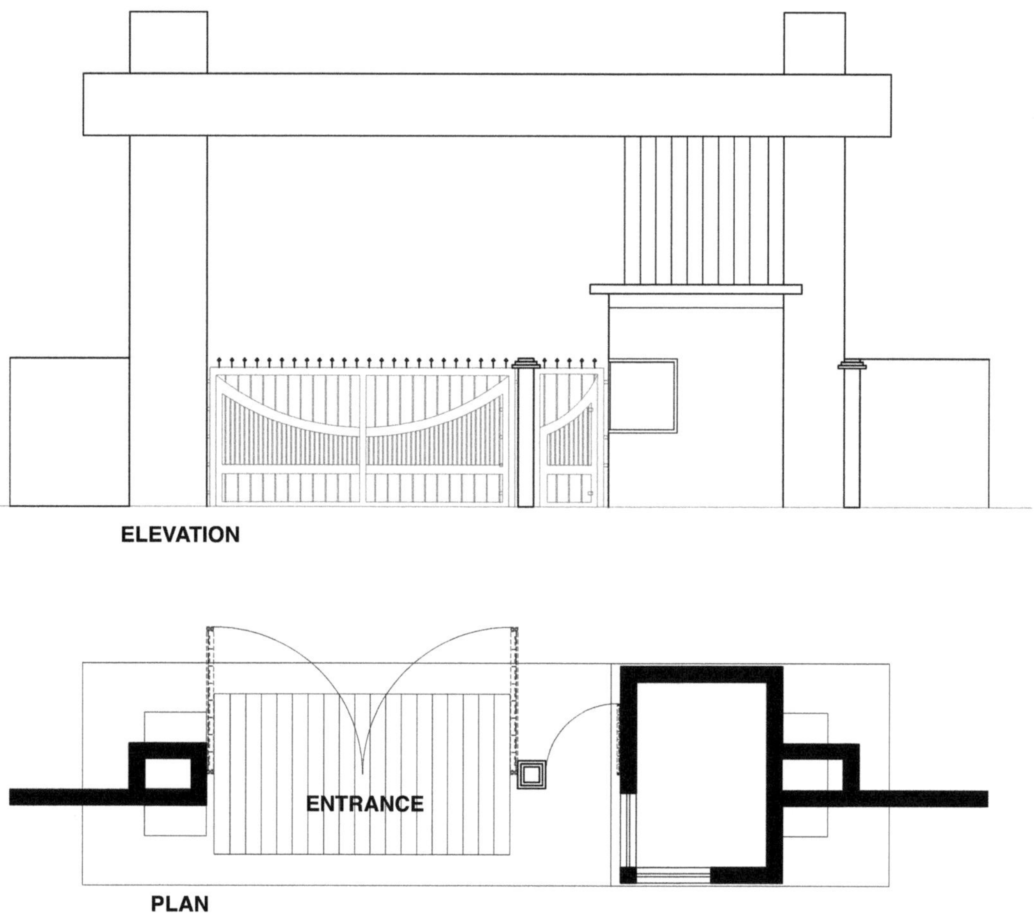

Fig. 14.1 Sample of main entrance gate drawing

A. Garg, A. Dewan, *Manual of Hospital Planning and Designing*,
https://doi.org/10.1007/978-981-16-8456-2_14

1. Usually, the main gate is fixed in the boundary wall of the hospital.
2. Normally, the hospital shall have at least two or more such main gates. One for entrance and the other is for exit.
3. The width of the gate shall be at least 20 ft. connected to the internal road of 20 ft.
4. Be careful that there shall be no hump or speed breaker at the main gate.
5. On one side of the gate, a small additional gate shall be provided for the pedestrians.
6. Inside the hospital premises, a security post shall be provided to guard the gate for 24 h.
7. Preferably the gate shall be fabricated from such material which is rustproof. Use of Stainless Steel is recommended for the fabrication of the gate.
8. To involve technology, automated gates or automated barriers are also used these days.
9. The provision for checking the vehicles shall also be provided at the main gate.
10. The guard shall be trained to guide the driver of the vehicle about the landing bay and parking.
11. The guard at the gate shall also be trained about the Gate Pass system.

Further Reading

Before You Walk through the Door: Site Design for Healthcare|HDR [Internet]. [cited 2021 Jun 18]. Available from: https://www.hdrinc.com/insights/you-walk-through-door-site-design-healthcare

NHS Estates. The design of hospital main entrances. London: H.M.S.O.; 1993.

Designing of the Entrance Lobby of the Hospital

15

The entrance lobbies are the first place where the patients, workers and visitors land into. Entrance lobbies in hospitals are more than a transitional space between the outside and the inside of the building. This is the starting point in a hospital to provide quality healthcare services. As it is said, 'the first impression is the last impression', and it is this lobby that reflects the first impression of the hospital.

This is the place from where onwards the segregation, distancing and infection control begin. Normally, services like Reception, Inquiry desk, Help desk, Registration, Admission and Discharge desk and Cash Counter are provided in the entrance lobby.

15.1 Location of the Entrance Lobby

The Entrance lobby shall be located on the ground floor of the building and shall be placed just near the main hospital building entrance. It must be placed at a prominently visible location from outside as soon as the patient/visitor approaches the main hospital building. The approach way to the lobby shall be marked with the signage's so that the visitor/patient can easily reach the entrance lobby.

15.1.1 The Infrastructure of the Entrance Lobby (Fig. 15.1)

Entrance Lobby	Trolley Park
	General Waiting
	Public Utilities
Reception	Enquiry Counter
	Registration Counter
	Queuing Tracks
	Records
	Admission Counter
	Discharge Counter
	Cash Counter
	Health Insurance Counter
	Empanelled Patients counter
Pharmacy	Storage and Disbursing Hall
	Bulk Storage
	Cold Room
	Expiry Medicine Room
	Costly Medicine Room
	Cut Strip Sorting Room
	Pharmacist Office
	Public Utility for Staff
Arcade	Temple
	Snack Counter
	Book Shop
	Gift Shop
	Other Shop—1
	Other Shop—2
	ATM

A. Garg, A. Dewan, *Manual of Hospital Planning and Designing*,
https://doi.org/10.1007/978-981-16-8456-2_15

Control Rooms for	Security
	Housekeeping
	Fire Safety
	Water Supply
	Electrical Safety
	Ambulance
Service/Staff Entrance	**Staff Utilities**
	Lockers
	Change Rooms
	Time Keeping

15.2 Services in the Lobby

Lobbies must include a range of activities apart from their integral functions to act as a first point of contact. It shall have:

- Information centre and a small waiting area
- Reception
- Inquiry desk
- Help desk
- Registration
- Admission and Discharge desk
- Cash Counter
- Cafeteria
- Pharmacy
- Banking facilities
- Shops
- Public and Accessible Toilets separate for males and females
- Parenting/Baby Change facilities
- Prayer Rooms
- Back office for administrative support
- Store for the use of the reception and registration
- Strong room for cashier
- Florist
- Gift Shop
- Book Shop
- Newspaper reading deck
- ATM of bank

15.3 Reception and Enquiry Counter

As soon as the patient/visitor enters the entrance lobby, he/she has the first view of the reception and enquiry counter. So, these counters shall be just opposite to the main entrance gate of the lobby. Further, the Reception counter should have a direct view of the Main Entry and the Waiting Areas. The reception counter's size shall depend on the expected number of patients/visitors likely to use the services of reception. It is recommended that space shall accommodate two receptionists to be seated. Hence, the ideal size of the reception shall be about 3048 mm–4572 mm long. The counter can be made out of civil work with an aesthetic look, and granite of other material can make it more

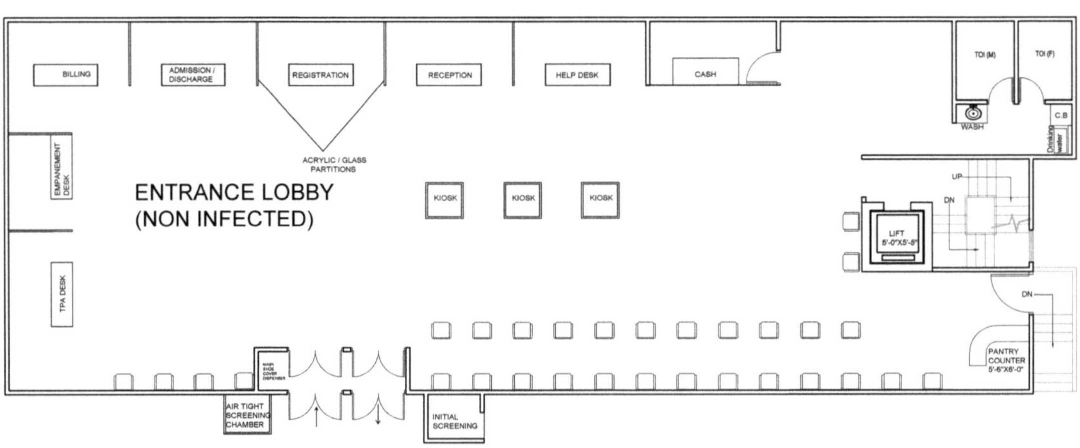

Fig. 15.1 Sample layout drawing of the entrance lobby

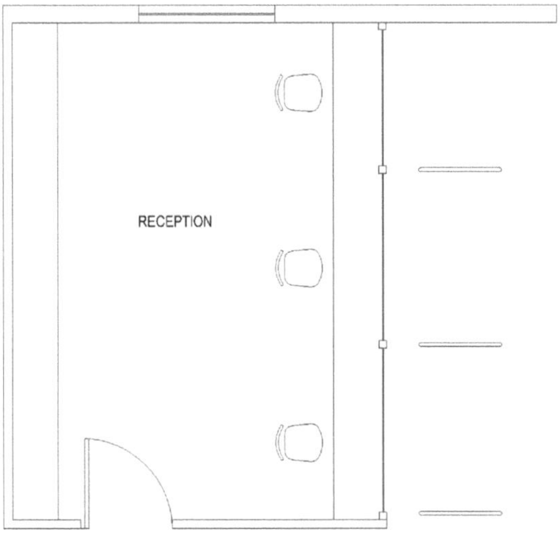

Fig. 15.2 Sample of reception drawing

appealing. Alternatively, a counter made out of wood can also be provided.

A storeroom shall be provided behind the reception, where the receptionist can keep general items like stationery, forms, documents and discharged files. This room shall have only one door that shall open in the reception. The size of this room can be about 3657 mm × 3048 mm. The required racks and cupboards shall be provided in the storeroom (Fig. 15.2).

15.3.1 Furniture at the Reception

1. The counter's front side shall be about 1524 mm in height to let a person stand comfortably while talking to the receptionist. On the other side of the counter, a 610-mm broad and 762 mm high working top shall be provided for the receptionists.
2. Two chairs for the receptionists.

15.3.2 Electrical and Other Points at the Reception

1. At least six 6 Amp Switches/Sockets on the counter wall at the height of about 152 mm from the working top. These points shall be used for connecting the computers and the printers.
2. Two 15 Amp Switch/Socket shall be provided on the wall behind the reception counter for other appliances.
3. Two RJ 45 points for Computer networking.
4. Two RJ 11 for Intercom and extension line.
5. Two USB points for charging mobiles or for other uses.

15.4 Help Desk, Registration and Admission and Discharge Counters

Along with the Reception and enquiry counters, on either side of the Reception, or other convenient places in the lobby, the Help Desk, Patient Registration and Admission Discharge counters shall be placed. But these counters shall be separate and at some distance so that these services' users shall not intermingle with each other. These counters' size shall again depend on the expected number of patients/visitors likely to use the services. Still, space shall be provided for two staff members to be seated on each counter. Hence, the ideal size can be about 2438 mm–3657 mm long. The counters can either be made out of civil work with an aesthetic look, and the granite of other material can be used to make it more appealing. Alternatively, the counters made out of wood can also be provided.

15.4.1 Furniture at Help Desk, Registration, Admission and Discharge Counters

1. The counter's front side shall be about 1524 mm in height to let a person stand comfortably while talking to the staff. On the other side of the counter, a 610-mm broad and 762 mm high working top shall be provided for the staff.
2. Two chairs for the staff on each counter.

15.4.2 Electrical and Other Points at Help Desk, Registration and Admission and Discharge Counters

1. Each counter shall have at least six 6 Amp Switches/Sockets on the counter wall at the height of about 152 mm from the working top. These points shall be used for connecting the computers and the printers.
2. Each counter shall have two 15 Amp Switches/Sockets shall be provided on the wall behind each counter for other appliances.
3. Each counter shall have two RJ 45 points for Computer networking.
4. Each counter shall have two RJ 11 for Intercom and extension lines.
5. Each counter shall have two USB points for charging mobiles or for other uses.

15.5 Cash Counter

If the registration and admission/discharge counter is provided in the lobby, the cash counter shall also be provided in the lobby because these two counters work simultaneously to provide services related to financial transactions. Hence, providing a cash counter nearby shall make it easy for the patient/visitors to deposit cash. The cash counter shall be located separately from other counters and need not be near the other service counters. The cash counter's size shall depend on the expected number of patients/visitors likely to use cash deposit services. Still, space shall be provided for two cashiers to be seated. Hence, the ideal size can be about 2438 mm–3657 mm long. The counter can either be made out of civil work with an aesthetic look, and the granite of other materials can be used to make it more appealing. Alternatively, a counter made out of wood can also be provided.

Attached to the Cash Counter, a small substantial room shall also be provided, where the cashier can keep safe, and as and when required, the cash can be kept in the safe. This room shall have only one door which shall open in the cash counter. However, if the hospital has a system of collecting the cash timely (say at least twice a day), this room may not be required (Fig. 15.3).

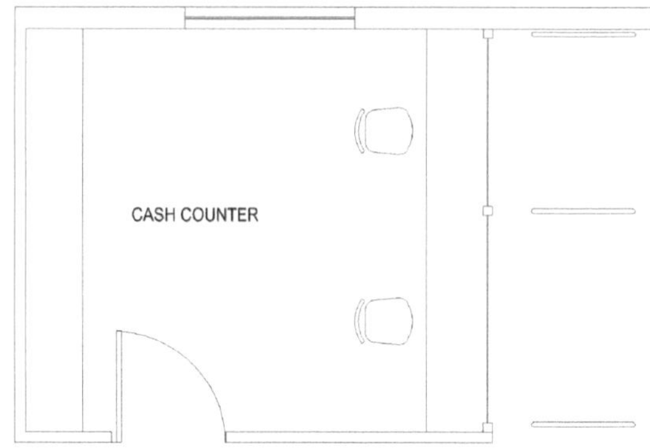

Fig. 15.3 Sample of cash counter drawing

15.5.1 Furniture at Cash Counter

1. The counter's front side shall be about 1524 mm in height to let a person stand comfortably while talking to the cashier. Above the counter, there shall be a glass partition up to the height of about 1219 mm from the top of the counter with a cut window on the lower side of the glass. On the other side of the counter, a working top shall be provided, which shall be about 610 mm in width and 762 mm in height.
2. Two chairs for the cashiers.

15.5.2 Electrical and Other Points at Cash Counter

1. At least six 6 Amp Switches/Sockets on the counter wall at the height of about 152 mm from the working top. These points shall be used for connecting the computers and the printers.
2. Two 15 Amp Switches/Sockets shall be provided on the wall behind the cash counter for other appliances.
3. Two RJ 45 points for Computer networking.

4. Two RJ 11 for Intercom and extension lines.
5. Two USB points for charging mobiles or for other uses.

15.6 Cafeteria

Due to a large number of visitors landing in the hospital, the facility of cafeteria shall be provided at the corner of the lobby, where visitors can have refreshment. It shall be at a visible location inside the lobby and have a separate entrance door. The size of the cafeteria shall be sufficient to accommodate at least 30 people. Hence, the size of the cafeteria shall not be less than 9144 mm × 6096 mm.

The cafeteria shall have a proper service counter which shall be located on one side. The counter shall be made out of the civil work with the granite tops. On the wall behind the counter, the working top shall be provided to keep the appliance like Microwave Oven, Induction Plate and Tea/Coffee machine.

It shall have a proper seating arrangement with tables and chairs. Along with the seating, some standing tables can also be provided.

There shall be a proper provision of handwash in the cafeteria with the necessary water supply and drain lines.

The cafeteria shall also have one back door, to bring in the eatables without entering into the main lobby.

Proper ventilation shall be provided to remove the smell of the eatables so that it does not enter the lobby.

Cafeteria must have waste bins in all corners and other required places to facilitate adequate food and other waste disposals (Fig. 15.4).

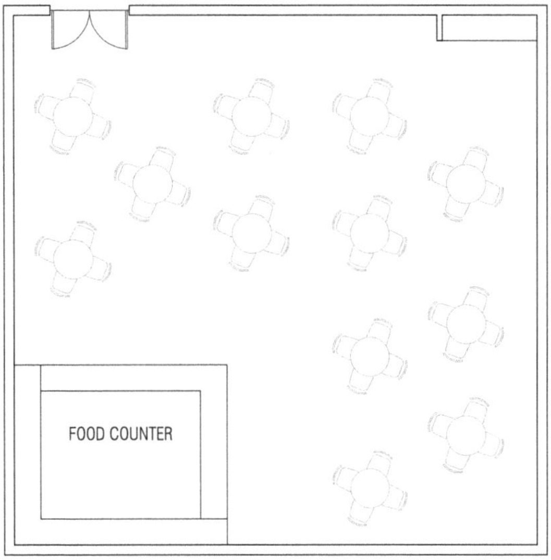

Fig. 15.4 Sample layout drawing of the cafeteria in entrance lobby

15.6.1 Furniture in the Cafeteria

1. The service counter's front side shall be about 1524 mm in height to easily stand and place an order and take delivery of the eatables. On the other side of the counter, a working top shall be provided with about 610 mm width and 762 mm height.
2. Two chairs for the cafeteria staff.
3. Dining tables with chairs.
4. Standing dining tables.

15.6.2 Electrical and Other Points in the Cafeteria

1. Main Switchboard at the entrance wall of the cafeteria (other than the wall on which door will open) for controlling the fan and lights of the room along with one 6 Amp Switch/Socket.
2. Air Conditioning Control button with temperature adjustment.
3. At least six 15 Amp Switches/Sockets on the back wall at the height of about 305 mm from the working top. These points shall be used for connecting the cooking appliances.
4. At least six 6 Amp Switches/Sockets on the counter wall at the height of about 152 mm from the working top. These points shall be used for connecting the computers and the printers.
5. Two 15 Amp Switches/Sockets shall be provided on the wall behind the cash counter for other appliances.
6. Two RJ 45 points for Computer networking.

7. Two RJ 11 for Intercom and extension lines.
8. Sufficient Power/USB points for charging mobiles in the dining area.

15.7 Pharmacy

As the outpatient generally prefers to purchase medicines from the in-house pharmacy counter, the pharmacy shall be preferably located in the lobby only. Some important points to be considered are:

- Pharmacy needs to be at a visible location from the exit point of the out-patient department.
- Proper showcases and signage's shall be provided in the pharmacy.
- A prescription explanation desk shall be provided to make the customer understand the prescribed medication dosage and side effects.

For more details on Pharmacy, please refer to the chapter of 'Pharmacy' (Chap. 28) of this book (Fig. 15.5).

15.8 Other Service Counters in the Entrance Lobby

Depending on the space, need of the patient/visitors, space may also be allocated for the services like Banking facilities, General shops, Florist, Gift Shop, Book Shop, ATM and Newspaper reading deck. The size of these spaces shall be decided depending on the requirement and space availability. As far as the electrical points and other connectivity points are concerned, it shall be as per the concerned shop's demand.

15.9 Public Utility for Patient/ Visitors

Along with the entrance lobby, the toilet facility shall be provided. The toilets shall be separate for males and females. They shall have the provision for handwash, and proper sanitary fittings shall be provided. The size of the toilet shall be about 6096 mm × 4572 mm.

Proper ventilation must be ensured to facilitate exhaust of the toilet air in order to keep the lobby odour free.

Further, at least one Accessible toilet shall be provided with the main toilet block to be used by the physically disabled or elderly patient/visitors. This toilet shall have a proper provision of handrails and grab bars.

Along with the toilet, on one corner, a parenting/baby change facility shall be provided with a space for disposal of the baby's soiled diapers. The provision shall be made for the foldable baby change counter either made out of wood or stainless steel.

Also, at some distance from the toilets, the facility of drinking water shall be provided. It

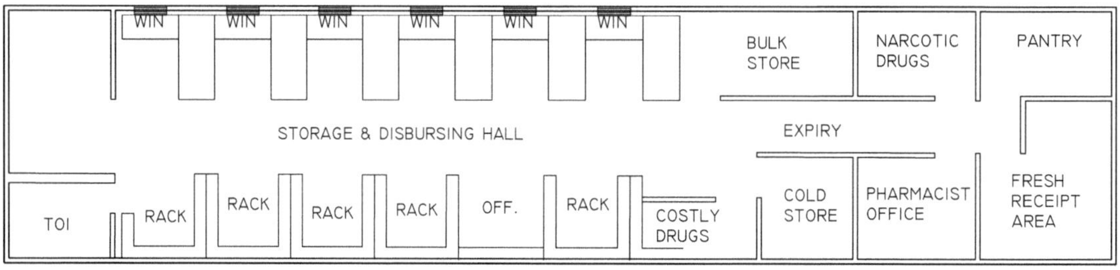

Fig. 15.5 Sample layout of the pharmacy in entrance lobby

will still be better if the tea/coffee vending machine is also placed in this area.

15.10 Prayer Room/Meditation Spaces

Disturbed family members of the patient usually are under fear and often seek blessings from the Almighty. Therefore, it is advised to provide Prayer Rooms on one side of the entrance lobby for prayer, meditation, reflection and spiritual contemplation. Particular attention should be paid while designing the space, especially considering that adequate space is available for all/different religions.

15.11 Self-Service Kiosks

Self-service kiosks can help expedite processes like hospital registration, Enquiry and Healthcare Information. Patients can increasingly do the work that could have been done at counters without having to come in contact with anyone. This can help with staff savings while increasing patient comfort. Automated kiosks can assist patients with paying co-pays, checking identification, signing paperwork and other registration requirements.

15.12 Interiors of the Entrance Lobby

1. Enlivened by the creation of art galleries or exhibition spaces.
2. Wide range of materials, colours and textures shall be used to make it attractive.
3. Adequate windows provision to bring in natural light and offer views of nature.
4. Spaces for indoor plants.
5. Private space for visitors to discuss their health and payment issues with receptionists and other personnel at the counters.
6. Play areas for children, if possible.
7. Interactive displays.
8. Designated area for working on laptops with the provision of charging points.
9. Mobile charging points in the lobby.
10. Free Internet or Wi-Fi.
11. Sound-absorbing materials shall be used on the walls, floors and ceilings.
12. Selected floor finish shall be able to reduce the risk of slips and falls of visitors, patients and staff.
13. Proper handrails at the staircase and other areas.
14. Good internal lighting.
15. The lobby shall be provided with television, fish tanks, magazines, movies/DVDs etc.
16. Food and Drinks vending machines.

15.13 Entrance Gates to the Lobby

1. The lobby shall have two sets of doors, one for entrance and the other for exit.
2. Single door set shall be at least 2438 mm wide with two doors open on both sides.
3. For automation, the sensor-operated glass doors can also be opted for.
4. An Airlock space connecting the external areas with internal areas shall be provided. This can be done by providing two doors at a distance of say 1829 mm from each other. The purpose is to decrease the infection rate and to maintain air conditioning, temperature and air pressurization from internal to external areas.
5. Measure shall be provided to prevent outside air contaminants, such as dust entering the building and therefore the air curtain can be provided.

15.14 Signage and Wayfinding in the Lobby

Proper Signage shall be provided, which will allow visitors to understand the layout of the lobby.

Provide simple and clear wayfinding solutions. This can be done either with proper signage or design and material solutions, such as colour-coordinating paths or accent lighting.

15.15 Acrylic or Glass Partitions

It is believed that despite automation, some patients/visitors will be using the counters and service desks. Under such circumstances, there are chances of the staff getting infected. To overcome this issue, it is advised to make a good 1219 mm high acrylic or glass partition at the top of the counter or desk so that the staff is always on the other side of the partition.

15.16 General Issues Related to Entrance Lobby

1. Inside the lobby, the spaces shall be clearly demarcated into visual zones and visual pathways.
2. A security checkpoint shall be located in close proximity to the entrance of the lobby.
3. Security barriers that can be locked in case of emergencies shall be provided.
4. Size of the lobby shall be decided based on the number of service counters to be provided, the size of the counters, waiting spaces to be provided, the number of visitors expected in the lobby etc.
5. Security features like CCTV shall be provided in this area and shall not be visible and noticeable to the visitors.
6. Security features such as hooters and alarms shall be provided.
7. Security to the Reception Desk shall be provided to prevent unauthorized access behind counter areas.
8. The cashier shall also be provided with appropriate barrier for safety.
9. Provision for proper heating and air conditioning shall be provided.
10. A wheelchair-accessible reception booth should be provided for disabled patients.

15.17 Outside Entrance Lobby

Outside of the lobby, there shall be a Landing bay for dropping and picking up the visitors. This landing bay shall preferably be provided with a Porch at the entrance gate as a shelter from inclement weather. The porch shall be wide enough to allow two vehicles to pass easily at a time. The height of the porch shall be at least 4572 mm from the road level.

There shall be a clear traffic pattern outside the lobby.

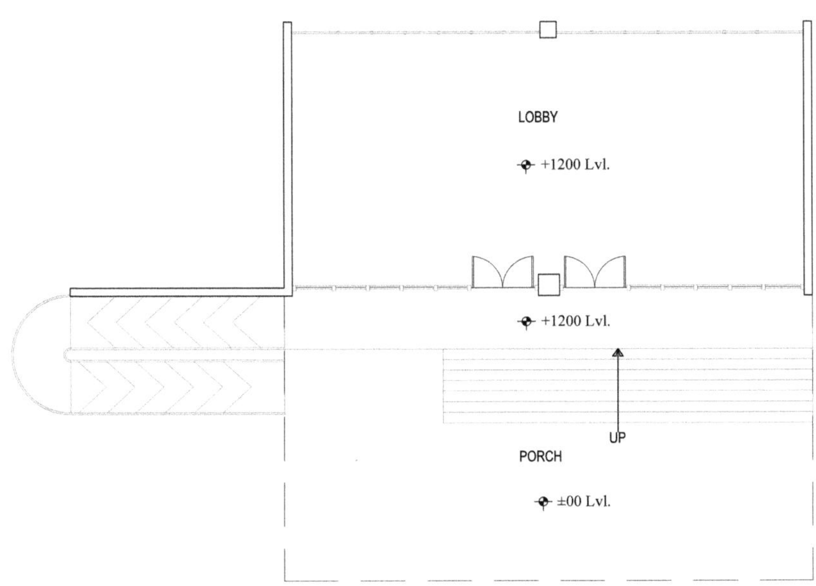

Fig. 15.6 Sample of porch drawing

The emergency department's entrance lobby has to be separate and shall not conflict with the main entrance lobby (Fig. 15.6).

The trolley bay shall be provided outside the lobby for parking of wheelchairs and stretcher trollies so that the patients dropping in the porch can use them.

15.17.1 Screening Areas

It is recommended to provide a screening area at the Hospital entrance and any other main public entry to perform screening through questionnaires and measurement of body temperature and other basic vitals. For this, isolated screening cabins can be used. It is a closed chamber with a provision of negative pressure and UV sterilization with a glass partition on the front side. There are two holes in the glass to fix the long elbow gloves. A healthcare worker sitting in the cabin can examine the patient standing on the other side of the glass through the gloves. This can help to sort out infectious patients at the entry point. This allows hospital workers to easily trace out the infectious and contagious patients and isolate them or restrict their access to the Hospital.

15.17.2 Hand Wash/Sanitizer Stations

Hospitals should place handwash stations or hand sanitizer dispensers at doors and entrances and encourage staff, patients and visitors to use them more frequently. Before placing the handwash stations or sanitizer stations, analysis of the building's layout for other accessible locations should be done.

15.17.3 Face Masks /Shoe Covers Dispensers

Hospitals should also make arrangements for placing the Face Mask/Shoe Cover dispensers at the hospital's doors and entrances. Any staff, patients and visitors entering the Hospital shall be encouraged to use them regularly. As in the case of Hand Wash and Sanitizer stations, before placing the dispensers, an analysis of the building's layout for other accessible locations should be done.

15.18 Reduction of People Landing in the Entrance Lobby

It is recommended that the entrance, waiting, gathering and sitting areas in the entrance lobby should be reduced to a possible extent.

1. The arrangement should be made to provide such services through technology like online registrations, admissions and discharges over the phone etc.
2. There shall be no sitting provision in the lobby (if essential few people can be allowed with proper distancing, used majorly for disabled, pregnant ladies or sick patients).
3. As the patients are increasingly becoming more and more technology savvy, the portal helps them do most of the hospital-related bits of help and tasks. Portals can ease the registration, collection of reports, inquiry, bookings etc. easily without visiting the Hospital.

Further Reading

Adams A, Theodore D, Goldenberg E, McLaren C, McKeever P. Kids in the atrium: Comparing architectural intentions and children's experiences in a pediatric hospital lobby. Soc Sci Med. 2010 Mar;70(5):658–67.

Building for Everyone: A Universal Design Approach.:88.

Cho Y. Wellness Design Evaluation Criteria for the Main Entry Lobby in a Healthcare Facility. 2017 Nov 30

Healthcare Waiting Room Designs & Patient Research [Internet]. Steelcase. [cited 2021 Jun 18]. Available from: https://www.steelcase.com/spaces-inspiration/health-spaces-transition-waiting/

Hospital Lobby Design Trends and Their Place in Design | Thought Leadership [Internet]. HMC Architects. 2020 [cited 2021 Jun 18]. Available from: https://hmcarchitects.com/news/hospital-lobby-design-trends-and-their-place-in-design-2020-05-06/

Emergency Services 16

The Emergency Department provides urgent diagnostic and therapeutic care to patients with:

1. Injuries by accidents.
2. Sudden attacks of illness or exacerbation of the disease.
3. Illness during non-OPD hours or holidays.

As this department is the window or can say door of the hospital from where the patients enter the hospital, the emergency department should provide the first impression on the patients, relatives and friends who come along with the patient. With the quick response in handling the emergency's patient and friendliness environment, the patients or their relatives and friends can form their opinion about the care they will receive. Quick and efficient care can save lives and also reduce the severity and duration of illness. This department should have adequate accommodation, and care should be taken to avoid cross infection.

The patients landing in the emergency department are usually major trauma patients, patients with physical and mental disabilities, patients with mental health issues, elderly patients, children and adolescents, domestic violence, custodial patients, sexual assault patients, victims of child abuse, patients with infectious diseases or who are immunocompromised and patients affected by chemical, biological or radiological contaminants etc.

The staff in the emergency department should be professionally expert in performing their jobs. Also, the supporting departments should be adequate with good communication facilities. The emergency department should have a close relationship with all other departments and units of the hospital.

16.1 Objectives of the Emergency Department

The treatment in the emergency department should be immediate and competent. The word 'EMERGENCY' is derived from the Latin word 'URGENS', which means 'pinches', i.e. what is urgent must be done without delay. If the condition of the patient is serious, it can make a difference between life and death. Hence, the motive of the emergency department should be 'effective and immediate treatment to the patients'. The other objectives of the emergency department are as below:

1. Provision of immediate relief and management of patients arriving in the department with acute medical and surgical emergencies. Examples include injury, poisoning, shock, myocardial infarction, gunshot and roadside accidents.
2. Attending to the medico-legal cases and coordinating with the local police for the same.

A. Garg, A. Dewan, *Manual of Hospital Planning and Designing*,
https://doi.org/10.1007/978-981-16-8456-2_16

3. Providing first-aid and/or providing the required treatment to the patients.
4. Screening patients for admission and providing OPD care during the non-OPD hours or on the holidays.

16.2 Location of Emergency Department

The hospital's emergency department should be located on the ground floor, in front of the hospital with a separate entry. The emergency shall be easily identifiable using signboards by the patients and the vehicles coming into the hospital. The department should be near to other investigative departments like laboratory and radiology.

16.3 Signage of the Emergency Department

An emergency is an important department and patients or visitors landing in this department are usually disturbed and in a hurry. Thus, an effective signage system allows them to easily identify their way for treatment. The following idea must be considered while designing signages for the emergency department:

1. The hospital entrance must be well sign-posted with illuminated signboards.
2. Signboards with proper directions should be displayed at the entrance gate of the hospital compound and emergency department.
3. Signboards with proper direction for all the rooms in the Emergency department should be displayed at the reception and waiting lobby.
4. Clear way-finding paths for movement in an Emergency Department shall be provided for easy movement of the staff, patients and visitors in the department. This can be done with the colour-coded strips on the floor or the walls of the department.
5. Clear signage for facilities toilets, drinking water and refreshments areas shall be provided.
6. Signage for visually impaired patients and visitors shall also be planned.
7. All the signage shall be Multilingual, and one language shall be the local language of the area.
8. Signage of the fire exit shall be prominent at the places.
9. Fire escape route maps shall be provided at the prominent places.
10. Staircases and ramp shall have luminated signboards.
11. Lifts shall have proper signboards.
12. Room numbers shall be allotted for each room and also the signage of room number/name shall be displayed on the door.
13. Signboard of all the room details with room numbers shall be displayed at the reception.
14. Signboard of precautions to be taken in the department shall be provided.
15. List of do's and don'ts shall also be provided in the department.

16.4 Size of the Emergency Department

The overall size of the Emergency depends on the volume and scope of services provided in the department. It is not the overall department floor space that is important, but the space critical to the services' efficient functioning. To decide the size of the emergency department and about services to be provided in the department, various factors influence the decision, few of them are:

1. The area in which the hospital is located and the type of patients received in the emergency department. For example, suppose the hospital is situated on a roadside or in an industrial area, accidents cases are always expected to be more, but if the hospital is in a residential area, more patients with cardiac, gastrointestinal or pulmonary diseases will be seen.

2. Academic activities being undertaken in the department.
3. Analysis of the data pertaining to:
   (a) Number of patients attended in the emergency and pattern of diseases.
   (b) The overall length of patient's stay.
   (c) Indoor admission rates of the hospital.
   (d) Number of accident patients attended in the emergency.
   (e) Number of head injury patients.
   (f) Number of patients with an acute emergency like cardiac and gastroenterology patients.
   (g) Number of fracture cases.
   (h) Number of medicine cases.
   (i) Medico-Legal cases attended.
   (j) Turnaround time for radiological, pathological and other investigations.
4. Space required for the stretchers, stretcher trolleys and wheelchairs for wheeling the patient to and from the emergency department.
5. Space for proper reception and waiting areas.
6. Open spaces around the building to make the department airy, well lightened and ventilated.
7. Space required for toilets for the use of patients and attendants.
8. Space for a minor and major operation theatre complex.
9. Space for Triage and Observation ward.
10. Space required for handling disasters such as mass casualties, train/bus accident and fire.
11. Therefore, the emergency department's total spaces shall be calculated after summing up the individual room requirement.

16.5 Areas Required for Emergency Department (Fig. 16.1)

Entrance Lobby	Trolley Park
	General Waiting
	Public Utilities
Reception	Enquiry Counter
	Registration Counter
	Queuing Tracks
	Records
	Admission Counter
	Cash Counter
Attached Rooms	Procedure Rooms
	Plaster Room
	Clean Utility
	ECG Room
	Medico-Legal specimen and record
	Dirty Linen
	Store
	Portable X-ray Room
	Disaster Storage Room
Triage	Examination resuscitation
	Waiting
	Examination Cubicles
	EMO Duty Room
	Public Utility for Faculty
	Public Utility for Patients and Attendants
Minor Operating Suite	Minor OT
	Scrub/Gowning
	Dirty Utility
Staff Accommodation	Nurse Duty
	Doctors Duty
	Ambulance Driver/ Nursing assistant
Emergency Operation Theatre Complex	Operation Theatre
	Pre-operative Room
	Post-operative Recovery
	Sterilization
	Clean Storage
	Toilet
	Sluice Room
	Instrument/Linen Wash
	Store
	Change Room Doctors—Male
	Change Room Doctors—Female
	Change Room Staff – Male
	Change Room Staff—Female

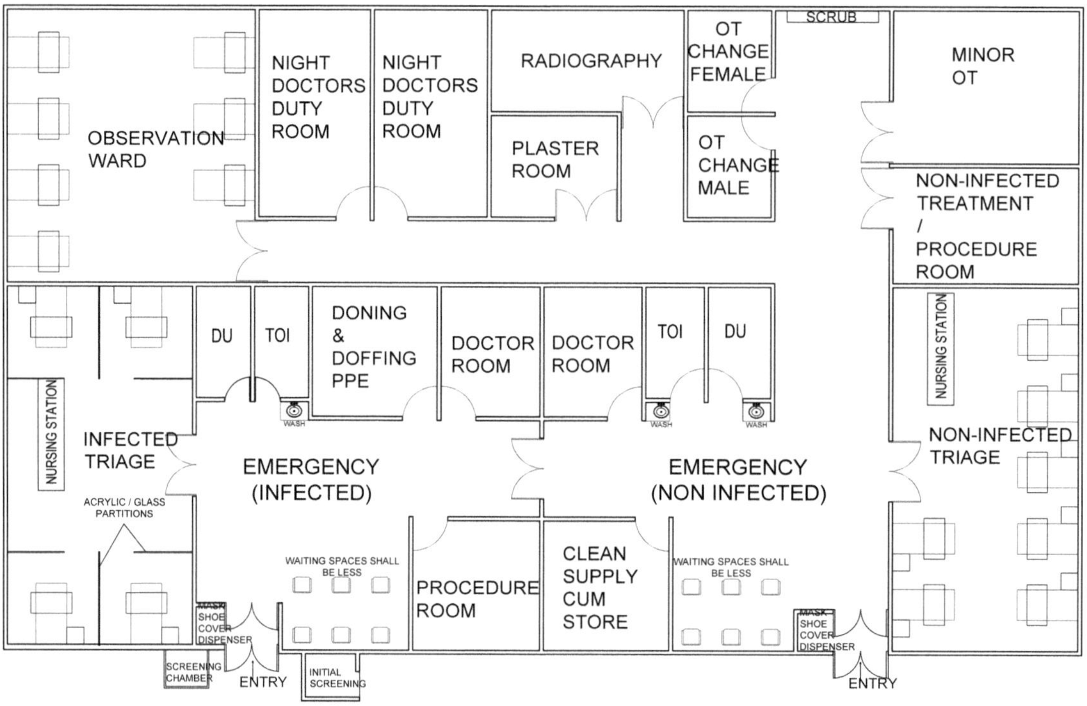

Fig. 16.1 Sample layout drawing of emergency

16.6 The Entrance of the Emergency Department

16.6.1 Main Gate

The emergency department's main entrance gate shall preferably be separate and shall not be combined with the gate provided general use. While designing the main gate, the following issues shall be kept in mind:

1. Usually, the main gate is fixed in the boundary wall of the hospital.
2. The width of the gate shall be at least 6096 mm unobstructed and connected to the internal road of 6096 mm.
3. Be careful that there shall be no hump or speed breaker at the main gate.
4. On one side of the gate, a small additional gate shall be provided for pedestrians.
5. This gate shall be guarded round the clock.
6. The gate shall be fabricated with rustproof material such as stainless steel.
7. To involve technology, automated gates or automated barriers can be used.
8. Free car parking spaces shall be allocated beside the Emergency Department. Apart from this, some parking spaces shall be reserved for disabled people and people carrying babies and young children.
9. Appropriate provision for ambulances to park close to the emergency entrance and allow for safe patient disembarkation.
10. Proper turning spaces shall be provided for the ambulance.
11. The guard shall be trained to guide the vehicle's driver about the landing bay and parking of emergency.

16.6.2 Entrance Door to the Emergency Department

1. The emergency shall have two sets of doors, one for entrance and the other for exit.
2. Single door set shall be at least 2438 mm wide with two doors open on both sides.
3. For automation, sensor-operated glass doors can also be opted for.
4. An Airlock space connecting external areas with internal areas shall be provided. This can be done by providing two doors at a distance of say 1829 mm from each other. The purpose is to decrease the infection rate and maintain air conditioning, temperature and air pressurization from internal to external areas.
5. Measures shall be taken to prevent outside air contaminants such as dust entering the department by providing the air curtain.

16.6.3 Outside Entrance Lobby

Entrance lobby for the emergency department has to be separate and shall not conflict with the main entrance lobby.

1. Outside of the lobby, there shall be a landing bay for ambulances to drop off patients.
2. This landing bay shall preferably be provided with a porch at the entrance gate as a shelter from inclement weather.
3. The porch shall be wide enough to ease the pass of two vehicles at a time.
4. The height of the porch shall be at least 4572 mm from the road level.
5. The ambulance disembarkation area shall be near the triage or resuscitation room.
6. The walk-in entrance should be separate from the ambulance entrance.
7. There shall be a clear traffic pattern outside the emergency entrance.
8. The trolley bay shall be provided outside the lobby for parking of wheelchairs and stretcher trollies to be used for the patients dropping in the porch.

16.6.4 Screening Areas

It is recommended to provide a screening area at the Emergency entrance to perform screening through questionnaires and measurement of body temperature and other basic vitals. For this, isolated screening cabins can be used. The screening chamber is a closed chamber with negative pressure and UV sterilization with a glass partition on the front side. There are two holes in the glass to fix the long elbow gloves. A healthcare worker sitting in the cabin can examine the patient standing on the other side of the glass through the gloves. This can help to sort out infectious patients at the entry point. This allows hospital workers to easily identify infected and contagious patients and isolate them or restrict their entry to the hospital.

Ensure that after proper screening, suspected/infected patients must enter the hospital from a separate entry than non-infected patients.

16.6.5 Handwash/Sanitizer Stations

Outside the Emergency Entrance, space shall be provided for handwash stations or hand sanitizer dispensers.

16.6.6 Face Masks/Shoe Covers Dispensers

Entrance gate shall also have provision for Face Mask/Shoe Cover dispensers.

16.6.7 Decontamination Area

1. Emergency department shall be free from any type of contaminations like chemical, biological or radiation hazards.
2. The decontamination area shall be located near the entrance.
3. If possible, a tiled shower area may be provided to decontaminate patients exposed to chemicals, pesticides or radiation.

16.6.8 General Waiting

During an emergency, patients are usually accompanied by their attendants. As the attendants are in a disturbed state of mind and fear, they need to be handled tactfully. The following issues relating to the waiting area in the emergency department shall be considered:

1. Each patient in an emergency shall be allowed only ONE accompanying attendant.
2. For the attendants, waiting area shall be provided at the entrance of the emergency. They shall not be allowed inside the triage. This is because, firstly, the emergency department can be infectious. Secondly, the patient can be in pain, or some painful procedure is needed to be performed, seeing which the attendants may get disturbed.
3. The waiting area shall not be huge, and social distancing must be followed.
4. There must be basic facilities available such as telephones and public address system to call attendants of patients to provide information about patients' conditions.
5. Near the waiting area, separate toilets shall be provided for males and females. Drinking water dispense machine shall be provided.
6. Mobile charging points shall also be provided in the waiting area.

16.6.9 Ambulance Control

Usually, hospitals have one or more ambulances. Hence, the Ambulance Control, parking and washing have to be done regularly. Therefore, the transport office is needed. Some hospitals may plan a separate transport department in the administrative area; others may plan in/or near the emergency department. As the ambulance service may be required at any time after office hours, it is better if the transport department is placed near or in the emergency department. Following points shall be considered for ambulance services:

1. As discussed earlier, a landing bay must be provided outside the emergency's main gate under the porch.
2. A separate area shall be provided for parking of ambulances when not in use. It will be better if this parking area is covered or a shed is provided.
3. The facility of cleaning and washing ambulances shall be provided near the parking area.
4. Usually, the ambulances are fully equipped. But, this equipment may not be required at all times or the hospital may provide some extra equipment for backup. Under these cases, the equipment has to be stored safely at some place. Hence, it is better to provide an ambulance equipment store, which shall be under the control of a Transport Officer.
5. Ambulance drivers are on duty round the clock, but their services may not be required all the time. Thus, the driver restroom with a toilet shall be provided where they can relax.
6. If the ambulance control is planned in or near the emergency, a transport office with a toilet and store needs to be provided.
7. If there is a demand and it is feasible, the hospital shall plan for the Air Ambulance facility. For this, the hospital needs to provide the Helipad that can either be a rooftop helipad or otherwise on the ground, if the open spaces permit and fulfils the by-laws of the Aviation Regulatory Authorities of the country.

16.7 Reception

Just at the entrance of the emergency department, a dedicated reception shall be provided. It shall take care of the patient or the attendant/visitors entering the department. The reception shall act as both Enquiry and Registration Counter. While designing a reception, the following issues shall be kept in mind:

16.7.1 The Infrastructure of Reception

1. The reception counter shall be just near the entrance of the emergency department.
2. The waiting area shall be in front of the reception, providing adequate space for social distancing.
3. Reception should be clearly visible and reachable without blocking human or trolley traffic.
4. Depending on the size and volume of the patients availing the services of the department, the size of the reception must be decided.
5. Reception can be split into two or three parts: enquiry counter, registration counter and cash counter.
6. If the emergency admission rate is high, the designer can introduce a fourth counter known as 'Admission Counter', or otherwise the registration counter can act as the admission counter.
7. A wheelchair-accessible reception booth should be provided for the disabled patients.
8. Along with the reception, a record room shall be provided to keep the reception's records and files.
9. Similarly, for securing the cash, a small strong room shall also be provided.
10. There shall be adequate space to allow queuing of the people desirous to avail the services of the reception.

16.7.2 Furniture

The following furniture shall be placed in the reception:

1. Reception Counter.
2. Reception Chairs.

16.7.3 Tools and Instruments

Reception shall include a provision to place:
1. Computer with Printer and UPS.
2. Scanner.
3. Public Announcement system.
4. Cash Collection Box screwed to the counter.
5. Intercom and Telephone Line.

16.7.4 Electrical Points at Reception

The following electrical points shall be provided at the reception:

1. At least six 6 Amp Switches/Sockets on the counter's wall at the height of about 152 mm from the working top. These points shall be used for connecting the computers and the printers.
2. Two 6/16 Amp Switches/Sockets on the wall near to the reception counter at the height of 18″ above the floor level. One pair shall be connected to UPS supply.
3. Two 6 Amp Switches/Sockets on the wall at a counter height near the counter.

16.7.5 Other Communication Points at Reception

The following communication points shall be provided at the reception:

1. RJ 45 point for Computer networking.
2. RJ 11 for Intercom and extension line.
3. HDMI point for computer display at other locations.

16.8 Triage and Resuscitation

This is the most important area and the heart of the emergency department. A triage acts as the first evaluation area, where a patient's condition and degree of urgency to provide treatment is assessed. Depending on the patient assessment outcome, if immediate care is required, the patient will be resuscitated. If required, the patient will be shifted to the Intensive Care Unit after resuscitation, or if there is a separate treatment cum resuscitation room attached to the emergency, the patient is shifted there. If the condition of the patient is not critical but requires indoor admission, he/she shall be sent to the ward. Otherwise, the patient shall be given first-aid and discharged.

16.8.1 Location of Triage

The following shall be considered while deciding the location of a Triage:

1. It shall be immediately near to the entrance and reception.
2. It should not be far off from the other support services like Radiology.
3. It shall have an uninterrupted entry and follow a single corridor from the entrance to triage.

16.8.2 Size of Triage

The size of Triage depends on a lot of factors which are given below:

1. How many patients are expected in Triage per Day?
2. How many of them may require immediate attention?
3. Is the hospital located near the main road or industrial area, because if it is so, the number of accidental cases can be more?
4. Whether separate resuscitation/treatment area has been provided?
5. What shall be the average length of patient stay in triage?
6. Time taken for investigations.
7. The admission rate of the patients.
8. Number of patients of accidents or head injury.
9. Number of patients of acute emergency like cardiac and gastroenterology.
10. Medico-Legal cases attended per day.
11. Turnaround time for radiological, pathological and other investigations.

Apart from this, the triage size also depends on the number of beds to be placed in triage and the numbers of partitions that have to be done in the triage to break it into areas like Isolation rooms. Once the number of beds to be placed has been decided, the area required by triage is calculated considering the standard layout plan of beds and services. However, per bed area in the triage shall not be less than 120 sq. feet.

However, depending on the load factors of the Emergency department more than one triage area can be considered. If more than one triage is planned, each triages can also be designated for different departments. Like one for Medicine, one for Gynae and Obs, one for Orthopaedic, one for Surgery etc.

16.8.3 Issues Related to Infrastructure of Triage

The following issues shall be kept in mind while deciding the infrastructure of Triage:

1. The Triage shall be in a single hall. However, separate triage can be planned for infectious patients.
2. In a single Triage hall, not more than 10 beds shall be placed. If more patients are landing or expected, the second hall of triage shall be planned.
3. The Triage shall have a single entry door.
4. The Room of the Emergency Doctor shall be attached to Triage, and a door connecting both shall be provided.
5. The Support Services like X-Ray, Ultrasound, Minor OT shall be attached to Triage as far as possible.
6. Twenty-five percent of the total bed in Triage shall be Isolation beds for infected patients.
7. Toilet shall be attached to Triage.
8. Plaster Room shall be attached to Triage.
9. Treatment Room shall be attached to Triage.

10. Nursing Station of the Triage shall be located in the centre of the hall.
11. Attached to Triage shall be the Clean Utility, Dirty Utility, Equipment Store, Medicine Store, General Store and Nurse duty room.

16.8.4 Bed Layout in Triage

The bed in the triage shall be laid out in such a fashion, that it allows easy and smooth working all around the bed, also the inter-bed spaces shall be appropriate for easy working and reduce cross-infection rate. The following issues shall be kept in mind while laying down a bed in Triage:

1. The head end of the Bed shall be at least 610 mm away from the wall.
2. The Head support panel of the bed shall be removable.
3. A clear space shall be about 1524 mm on the foot end so that the stretcher trolley can be easily turned around, and the patient can be transferred from/to bed.
4. Most important, distance from bed to bed shall not be less than 1829 mm.

16.8.5 Isolation Room/Units/Area in Triage

Triage is the area where all the patients land. Triage shall have the provision for normal beds and a few beds for infected patients called Isolation cabin. Infected patients arriving in the Triage shall be placed separately from the non-infected patients.

Therefore, it is recommended that air-tightened and negative pressure isolation rooms shall be created in the Triage. The isolation room/units shall have a separate entry than the normal entry of the triage. It is recommended that about 25% of the triage bed be fixed for isolation bed/room/unit. Isolation rooms should have attached toilet. Separate staff shall take care of the patients in isolation cabins. In case of shortage of space, a few normal beds can be converted to isolation beds in the triage using collapsible shutters around the bed or fixing temporary acrylic partitions.

For Negatively pressurizing the isolation room/unit/bed please refer to the chapter of 'HVAC' (Chap. 38) of this book.

16.8.6 Resuscitation Rooms in Triage

As mentioned earlier in this chapter, depending on the patient load and management policies, the Resuscitation Room may or may not be created. If the Resuscitation area is created, the setup will be more or less the same except for the following differences:

1. Normally, the resuscitation room has a single bed. If it has more than one bed, it will act as a triage.
2. The resuscitation room aims to provide extensive care and treatment to the patient at a place away from the other patients.
3. The individual room shall be equipped with gadgets for extensive monitoring like ECG, NIBP, Oxygen saturation, core temperature, invasive monitoring, CO2 monitoring and defibrillator.
4. Each room shall have a facility for invasive and non-invasive ventilation.
5. Each room shall have an emergency crash cart equipped with medicines, material for intubation, catheters, cannulization and external pacing facilities.
6. Each room shall have a separate washbasin for hand wash.
7. Good quality portable OT light shall also be provided in the room.
8. Two portable ventilators shall be provided for all the rooms put together for patient transfer to imaging and other clinical facilities or other indoor units like ICU.
9. If needed, the patient warming system shall be provided.

16.8.7 Furniture in Triage

16.8.7.1 Patient Furniture

Patient Bed (Multi-positional ICU Bed on lockable wheels with bedside safety rails)	Step Stool
Bed Side Locker	Scrub Station
Over Bed Table	IV Stand
Examination Table	IV Rod
Wheel Chair	Crash Cart
Stretcher Trolley	Oxygen Cylinder Trolley
Dressing Trollies	Back Rest
Instrument Trollies	Patient Transfer System

16.8.7.2 Office Furniture

Nursing Counter	Filing Cabinet
Office chairs	Visitor Chairs etc.
Almirah/Cupboard	Stools

16.8.8 Equipment in Triage

Multi-para Vital Sign Monitor	Suction Machine
Invasive Mechanical Ventilator	Portable X-Ray Machine
Non Invasive Ventilator	Blood Gas Analyzer
High Flow Nasal Canula	Cardiac Marker Analyser
Infusion Pump	B.P. Apparatus
Nebuliser	Glucometer
Defibrillator	Laryngoscope
ECG Machine	Oxygen Cylinders with Masks
View Boxes	Ambu bag

16.8.9 Tools and Instruments

Sterilizing Drums	Torches
Walkers/Crutches	Examination Light
Splints	Chetal Forceps
Extension Cord and Boxes	Forceps of all styles and sizes
Operating Light	Needle Holders
Refrigerator	Tray of all styles and sizes
Instrument Boxes	Scissors of all styles and sizes
Proctoscope	Suture Sets
Weighing Machine	All other required instruments

16.8.10 Doors

The Door of the Triage shall not be less than 1829 mm wide, unobstructed. The door shall be openable on both sides in and out.

16.8.11 Windows

The windows shall be preferred in the room, but direct sunlight shall be avoided. As the bed head panels have to fix on the wall above the patients, the window's bottom shall not be less than 1829 mm from floor level. The window glass can be tinted, or the curtains/blinds shall be provided.

16.8.12 Hand Washing

For handwash, a single bay scrub shall be provided, which shall be operational with sensors and foot.

16.8.13 Central Piped Medical Gas Supply

As critical patients arrive in the Triage, they usually need oxygen. For some patients, invasive or non-invasive ventilation may be required. Hence, the supply of Piped Centralized Medical Supply is a must. The gases supplied shall be:

- Oxygen.
- Compressed Air.
- Wall-mounted Suction.
- Nitrous Oxide.

In Triage, the supply (except Nitrous Oxide, which is used in OTs) lines shall be provided on each bed. In some hospitals, the outlets of these gases are fixed on the wall itself.

Nowadays, the bed head panel is used for this. Bed Head panel is a 1524-mm panel made of extruded sections of aluminium. This panel has a provision of fixing the gas outlets and electrical points. This panel also has a service railing on which the IV rod, tray, and utility basket can be fixed. This panel is fixed at a height of 1524 mm above the floor level and goes up to 1829 mm.

Other options can be the ceiling suspended pendant. This has the same facilities as a Bed Head Panel but is fixed on the ceiling and is suspended below so that the bottom of the pendant shall be 1524 mm above the floor level.

In Triage each bed shall have the following outlets:

1. 2 outlets for Oxygen
2. 1 outlet for Compressed Air
3. 2 outlets for Suction.

Suitable electrical and communication points and ports shall be provided on the bed head panel or the pendant as the case may be.

16.8.14 Electrical Points in Triage

1. The main switchboard shall be at the entrance wall for controlling fan and lights of the hall along with one 6 Amp Switch/Socket.
2. Air conditioning control button with temperature adjustment.
3. At least 3 pairs of 6/16 Amp switches/sockets on each bed and these shall be on UPS supply.
4. In the centre of two beds, a pair of two 6/16 Amp switches/sockets shall be provided at the height of 457 mm from the floor level. Out of these two, one pair shall be on UPS.
5. Two 6/16 Amp switches/sockets at the height of 1219 mm shall be provided on the wall near or behind the nursing counter for View Box or charging the medical equipment.
6. Two 6 Amp Switches/Sockets shall be given on the Nursing Counter.

16.8.15 Other Communication Points in Triage

The following communication points shall be provided at each Bed of Triage:

1. Point for Nurse Call device.
2. RJ 45 point for Computer networking.
3. RJ 11 for Intercom and extension line.
4. HDMI point for monitor display at other locations.

Similarly, at the Nursing Station, the following points shall be provided:

1. Point for Nurse Call Control Console.
2. RJ 45 point for Computer networking.
3. RJ 11 for Intercom and extension line.
4. HDMI point for monitor display at other locations.

16.8.16 Curtain Partitions

All the bed in the Triage shall be provided with hanging curtain partitions. However, the following issues relating to curtain partitions must be taken care of:

1. The Bed shall be placed in front of one wall of the Triage.
2. The Bed shall have a curtain on all other three sides of the patient bed.
3. The ceiling suspended curtain track is fixed at 2134 mm above the floor level.
4. Curtains shall be hanged on these tracks and shall be moveable and collapsible.
5. The bottom of the curtain shall be about 457 mm above the floor to allow easy cleaning.

16.8.17 Doctors Duty Rooms in Triage

Generally, depending on the size of triage, level of the emergency department and the volume of patients, there may be a need to place physicians from different disciplines in the emergency department to provide immediate care to the patients landing the emergency. In that case, a few extra doctors' duty rooms have to be provided in the emergency department. The following issues shall be considered while providing duty rooms in the triage:

1. The physicians to be placed are usually from the department of:
   (a) Medicine.
   (b) General Surgery.
   (c) Orthopaedics.
   (d) Paediatric.
   (e) Gynaecology and Obstetrics.
   (f) Neuro Surgery.
   (g) Cardiology.
2. Physicians of other departments like Eye, ENT and Pulmonology can be on call.
3. One room for the physicians of each department has to be allotted.
4. The room shall be of the size 4572 mm × 4267 mm.
5. Rooms shall have a provision of an attached toilet.
6. Furniture wise, the room shall have one office table, chair, bed and cupboard.
7. The room shall have points for a computer with an Internet connection and intercom point apart from the light and fan.
8. The room shall be air-conditioned and the control button with temperature adjustment shall be provided in the room.

16.9 Treatment/Procedure Room/ Minor Operation Theatre

Out of the patients landing in Triage, some may require minor procedures like catheterization, suturing of small wounds, dressing and bandaging. At times it becomes difficult to do these procedures in the triage due to chances of getting infected, the privacy of the patient or the procedure requires anaesthesia. Therefore, a separate room must be dedicated for this purpose. One can call such room as 'treatment room', 'procedure room' or 'Minor OT'. The only difference between the three is, that administration of anaesthesia is easier in a Minor OT, and thus it is recommended to have one in a triage.

Here, we shall discuss some important features of a Minor OT as the other two (treatment rooms and procedure rooms) are similar.

16.9.1 Location of Minor OT

It shall be either attached or near to a triage. Also, it should not be far off from the other support services like Radiology etc.

16.9.2 Size of Minor OT

It shall not be less than 4572 mm × 4572 mm. All other ancillary areas to Minor OT shall be over and above this size.

16.9.3 The Infrastructure of Minor OT

Attached to Minor OT shall be:

1. Separate changing room for males and females.
2. Scrub Room.
3. Store Room.
4. Clean Supply Room.
5. Dirty Utility.
6. Equipment Store.

16.9.4 Issues Related to Infrastructure of Minor OT

1. It shall be in a single complex and shall be a sterilized area.
2. It shall have a single OT table.
3. It shall have a single entry door.

16.9.5 Furniture in Minor OT

16.9.5.1 Patient Furniture

OT Table	Step Stool
Stretcher Trolley	Scrub Station
Dressing Trollies	IV Stand
Instrument Trollies	IV Rod
Wheel Chair	Crash Cart
Patient Transfer System	Oxygen Cylinder Trolley

16.9.6 Equipment

Basic Boyle's Machine with a vaporizer	Alternately if required, Anaesthesia Work Station can be provided
Multi Para Vital Sign Monitor	Suction Machine
Operating Light Single or Double Dome	Operating Loupe
Surgical Cautery	Laryngoscope
Infusion Pump	Oxygen Cylinders with Masks
Defibrillator	Ambu bag
ECG Machine	View Boxes

16.9.7 Tools and Instruments

Sterilizing Drums	Torches
Extension Cord and Boxes	Examination Light
Instrument Boxes	Chetal Forceps
Forceps of all styles and sizes	Scissors of all styles and sizes
Needle Holders	Suture Sets
Tray of all styles and sizes	All other required instruments

16.9.8 Doors

The Door of the Minor OT shall not be less than 1829 mm wide, unobstructed. The door shall be openable on both the sides in and out.

16.9.9 Windows

A window need not be provided in the Minor OT.

16.9.10 Handwashing

For handwash, a double bay scrub shall be provided, which shall be operational with sensors and foot.

16.9.11 Central Piped Medical Gas Supply

As surgical interventions have to be done in the Minor OT, the following gases shall be supplied:
Oxygen.
Compressed Air.
Suction.
Nitrous Oxide.

The Minor OT shall also have the following outlets:

1. 2 outlets for Oxygen
2. 2 outlets for Compressed Air
3. 2 outlets for Suction
4. 2 outlets for Nitrous Oxide.

A ceiling suspended pendant should be fixed and suspended so that the height of the pendant is 1524 mm above the floor. On this pendant, both electrical and communication points and ports shall be provided.

16.9.12 Electrical Points in Minor OT

The following electrical points shall be provided in the Triage:

1. The main switchboard at the entrance wall for controlling fan and lights of the hall along with one 6 Amp switch/socket.
2. Air-conditioning control button with temperature adjustment.
3. On the surface of the hanging pendant, at least 3 pairs of 6/16 Amp switch/socket shall be provided. These points shall be on UPS supply.
4. In the centre of each of the three walls of the Minor OT (leaving the wall on which a door is provided), a pair of two 6/16 Amp switches/sockets is to be provided at the height of 457 mm from the floor level. Out of these two, one pair shall be on UPS.

16.9.13 Other Communication Points in Minor OT

The following communication points shall be provided in the Minor OT at any convenient place/wall:

1. RJ 45 point for Computer networking.
2. RJ 11 for Intercom and extension line.
3. HDMI point for computer display at other locations.

For other details of Operating Room, please refer to the chapter of 'Operation Theatre Suite' (Chap. 19) of this book.

16.10 Procedure and Diagnostic Setup

For effective care, resuscitation and treatment of the patients landing in the emergency, the investigations like Radiology, Pathology and few others are crucial. Without the support of these investigations, diagnosis and treatment are not possible.

Depending on the size of the emergency, the following departments may/may not be provided in the emergency department:

1. ECG Room.
2. Sample Collection Room.
3. X-Ray Room.
4. Ultrasound Room.
5. CT Scan.
6. MRI Room.
7. Portable X-ray Room.

Out of the above-listed diagnostic investigation, the following are necessary to be placed in the emergency department:

1. ECG Room.
2. Sample Collection Room.
3. Ultrasound Room.
4. Portable X-ray Room.

If the size of the emergency department is not big, or the patient load or investigation load is less, the other investigation rooms can be located in the department of Radiology.

16.10.1 Location of Investigation Rooms

The following shall be considered while deciding the location of the investigation rooms:

1. These rooms shall be located in the Emergency Department, but need not be located in the front.

2. These can be located in the backside of the department but connected through a proper corridor.
3. Corridor shall be wide enough to easily move the stretcher or the patient bed without any interruption.

For other details of the Radiology Department and Pathology Department, please refer to the chapters of 'Radiology' (Chap. 22) and 'Clinical Pathology' (Chap. 23) of this book.

16.11 Emergency Operation Theatre Complex

At times, some patients arriving in the emergency department may require major surgery and have to be operated immediately.

Depending on the emergency department's size, the volume of patients and the number of patients requiring major surgeries, the management can plan to locate the Major OT complex in the emergency department.

Secondly, the Major OT complex must be established as per the norms of different countries or regulating bodies/authorities. For example, in India, the Medical Council of India regulates the medical college and has established the norms to establish a major OT complex in the Emergency Department. Hence, establishing OT complex in the Emergency Department or not shall be the hospital's management's decision.

If the Major OT complex has to be established in the Emergency Department, the set up of the OT complex shall be the same as any major OT.

For other details of Major Operation Theatre Complex, like Size of Rooms, Infrastructure of OT Complex, Furniture, Equipment, Instruments and Tools, Doors, Windows, Central Medical Gas Supply, Electrical Points and Other Communication Points, please refer to the chapter of 'Operation Theatre Suite' (Chap. 19) of this book.

16.12 Day-Care Observation Ward

A day-care ward shall be provided in the Emergency Department to admit a patient who needs to be kept under observation for a small period. For example, after giving necessary treatment to an asthmatic patient in the emergency department, he/she will need to be kept under observation for a few hours in a day-care ward. During follow-up, if the patient is stable, he/she will be discharged from this ward.

16.12.1 Location of Observation Ward

Observation Ward shall be near the emergency department but connected through a corridor. The following shall be considered while deciding the location of the Observation Ward:

1. It shall have an uninterrupted entry and a single corridor from Triage to Observation Ward.
2. Corridor shall be wide enough to move the stretcher or the patient bed.

16.12.2 Size of Observation Ward

It depends on the number of patients that are expected to be shifted to the ward per day. It is recommended that the ward shall have not less than 10 and not more than 30 beds. Also, the per bed area in the ward shall not be less than 8.36 sq. mtr.

16.12.3 The Infrastructure of Observation Ward

Observation Ward	Ward
	Store
	Examination and Treatment room
	Nurses Duty Room
	Ward Pantry
	Resident Doctors and Student Duty Room
	Night Duty Room for Junior Residents
	Public Utility for Faculty
	Public Utility for Patients and Attendants

16.12.4 Issues Related to Infrastructure of Observation Ward

1. It shall preferably be in a single hall.
2. It shall have a single entry door.
3. Support services like X-Ray, Ultrasound and Minor OT shall not be far from the Observation Ward.
4. Twenty-five percent of the total beds in the Observation Ward shall be treated as Isolation beds for the infected patients.
5. Separate male and female toilets shall be attached to Observation Ward.
6. Nursing Station of the Observation Ward shall preferably be located in the centre of the hall.
7. Attached to Observation Ward shall be the Clean Utility, Dirty Utility, Equipment Store, Medicine Store, General Store and Nurse duty room.
8. Resident doctors' duty room shall also be provided near the Observation Ward.

16.12.5 Bed Layout in Observation Ward

The bed layout should allow easy and smooth working, along with enough inter-bed space to reduce cross-infection rate. Some of the following issues shall be considered while laying down beds in an Observation Ward:

1. The head end of the bed shall be at least 305 mm away from the wall.
2. The head support panel of the bed shall be removable.
3. A clear space of about 1524 mm shall be kept near the foot end to allow easy stretcher trolley movement for patient transfer.
4. Inter-bed space shall not be less than 914 mm.

16.12.6 Isolation Room in the Observation Ward

Out of all normal beds, the ward shall have about 25% beds for infected patients called Isolation cabin. For this, negatively pressurized and air-tightened isolation rooms shall be created with an attached toilet in the Observation Ward. These isolation rooms shall not be mixed with other beds in the same hall, but shall be a separate zone with a barrier in between. Separate staff shall take care of the patients in isolation cabins.

In case of a shortage of space for separate rooms, few beds in the observational ward can be converted to isolation cabins. This can be done using collapsible shutters around the bed or by fixing temporary acrylic partitions.

For negatively pressurizing the isolation room/bed, please refer to the chapter 'HVAC' (Chap. 38) of this book.

16.12.7 Furniture in Observation Ward

16.12.7.1 Patient Furniture

Patient Bed (Multi-positional ICU Bed on lockable wheels and bedside safety rails)	Step Stool
Bed Side Locker	Oxygen Cylinder Trolley
Over Bed Table	IV Stand
Wheel Chair	IV Rod
Instrument Trollies	Crash Cart
Stretcher Trolley	Back Rest
Dressing Trollies	Patient Transfer System

16.12.7.2 Office Furniture

Nursing Counter	Filing Cabinet
Office chairs	Visitor Chairs etc.
Almirah/Cupboard	Stools

16.12.8 Equipment

Multi-Para Vital Sign Monitor	Suction Machine
Non -invasive Ventilator	ECG Machine
High-flow Nasal Canula	Oxygen Cylinders with Masks
Infusion Pump	B.P. Apparatus
Nebuliser	Glucometer
Defibrillator	View Boxes

16.12.9 Tools and Instruments

Sterilizing Drums	Torches
Extension Cord and Boxes	Chetal Forceps
Refrigerator	Forceps of all styles and sizes
Instrument Boxes	Needle Holders
Weighing Machine	Tray of all styles and sizes
All other required instruments	Scissors of all styles and sizes

16.12.10 Doors

The door of the Observation Ward shall not be less than 1829 mm wide, unobstructed. The door shall be openable on both sides.

16.12.11 Windows

They shall be preferred in the room, but direct sunlight shall be avoided. As the bed head panels have to be fixed on the wall above the patient, the bottom of the window shall not be less than 1829 mm above the floor level. The window glass can be tinted, or the curtains/blinds shall be provided.

16.12.12 Handwashing

Washbasin shall be provided near the nurse station.

16.12.13 Central Piped Medical Gas Supply

Patients in the Observation Ward may require oxygen. Hence, Piped Centralized Medical Supply is a must on each bed. The gases supplied are:

- Oxygen.
- Wall-mounted Suction.

In some hospitals, the outlets of these gases are fixed on the wall itself. Normally, the Bedhead panel is used for this. It is a 914-mm panel made out of extruded sections of aluminium. This panel has a provision for fixing the gas outlets and the electrical points. The bedhead panel also has a service railing on which the IV rod, tray, and utility basket can be fixed. It is fixed at a height of 152 mm above the floor level and goes up to1829 mm. Alternatively, a hanging pendant can also be provided.

16.12.14 Electrical Points in Observation Ward

1. The main switchboard shall be at the entrance wall for controlling fan and lights of the hall along with one 6 Amp switch/socket.
2. Air-conditioning control button with temperature adjustment.
3. At least 2 pairs of 6/16 Amp switches/sockets on each bed. These points shall be on UPS supply.
4. In the centre between two beds, a pair of two 6/16 Amp switches/sockets shall be provided at the height of 457 mm from the floor level. Out of these two, one pair shall be on UPS.
5. Two 6/16 Amp switches/sockets at the height of 1372 mm shall be provided on the wall near or behind the nursing counter for View Box or charging the medical equipment.

6. Two 6 Amp switches/sockets shall be given on the nursing counter.

16.12.15 Other Communication Points in Observation Ward

1. Point for nurse call device.
2. RJ 45 point for computer networking.

Also, the following points shall be provided at the nursing station:

1. Point for Nurse Call Control Console.
2. RJ 45 point for Computer networking.
3. RJ 11 for Intercom and extension line.
4. HDMI point for computer display at other locations.

16.12.16 Curtain Partitions

All beds in the Observation Ward shall be provided with hanging curtain partitions. Some issues related to curtain partitions are as follows:

1. The bed shall be placed in front of one wall of the observation ward.
2. The bed shall have a curtain on all other three sides.
3. The ceiling suspended curtain track is fixed at 2134 mm above the floor level.
4. Curtains shall be hung on these tracks and shall be moveable and collapsible.
5. The bottom of the curtain shall be about 457 mm above the floor to allow easy cleaning.

16.13 Other Issues Relating to Emergency Department

1. Emergency Ward shall always have a backup of power supply preferably with the help of auto-start generators.
2. All the rooms and corridors shall have the provision of battery-operated emergency lights.
3. **Lighting**
   Use of natural light is recommended as much as possible. All the rooms and the corridors shall be well lit with proper overlapping of the lights. No fancy lights are recommended.
4. **Temperature**
   Emergency Department shall preferably be centrally air-conditioned and maintained at a comfortable temperature. Particular attention shall be paid towards the proper return of the air, with no mixing allowed. Air-conditioning temperature control shall be provided in all rooms.
5. **Cross Ventilation**
   Cross ventilation must be encouraged without mixing return air.
6. **Space for a patient brought dead**
   When a patient is declared dead on arrival, no treatment is carried out and the body needs to be handed over either to the police or to the relatives for further disposal. The procedural formalities involved in such cases are likely to take some time till the body is disposed of. However, in the meantime, it is unreasonable to send the body to the mortuary and it is kept at a place that is not otherwise visible to other incoming patients/visitors.
7. **Calming colours**
   Bright colours shall be avoided in the emergency department. It is advisable to use pastel or other soothing colours.
8. Artwork, pictures, posters murals and images shall be provided wherever possible in the department, as it can help to reduce stress and anxiety in patients.
9. The flooring of the department shall be non-slippery. The level of the floors shall be at Zero for all the rooms and corridors. If tiles are fixed on the floor, they should be jointless and no spacers shall be used for fixing the tiles.

16.14 Disaster Plan

Major accidents and the furies of nature can impose a sudden and unexpectedly heavy load of casualties on a hospital. The hospital, therefore, has to be prepared to meet such contingencies. At the same time, it is not practically possible for a hospital to keep a huge amount of equipment, staff and supplies at all times to deal with such mass casualties as such incidents may occur rarely. However, with a prepared plan to deal with such a situation, it should be possible for the existing staff to accept the challenge and provide quality patient care effectively, without confusion.

This plan aims to enable the hospital to arrange for collection and treatment of casualties arising from major accidents and disasters like air/train crash, major industrial or traffic accidents, fire, hurricane, earthquake and flood.

16.14.1 Factors for Disaster Plan

1. A warning rarely precedes disasters of the type envisaged above. Such accidents can occur anywhere at any time of the day or night.
2. The number of casualties is unpredictable. For this plan, we assume that there will be about 50 casualties, mainly surgical (including burns).
3. Under such circumstances, Observation Ward shall be originally designed in a manner so that it can be converted into a Triage when needed.
4. A separate room shall be located in the Emergency Department, which shall store the material, consumables, instrument and tools for any such disaster.
5. Many casualties are likely to succumb to serious haemorrhage at the accident scene if prompt first-aid is not provided. Hence, there shall be a provision of providing first-aid immediately on arrival of the patient.
6. The sudden arrival of a large number of casualties could throw a heavy strain on the hospital's resources. For example, there may not be an adequate number of vacant beds to receive the casualties and the available staff might need to work overtime. Also, there may be a sudden demand for large quantities of sterile dressings, syringes, splints or drugs like morphine, pethidine, anti-tetanus serum, anti-gas gangrene serum and antibiotics, or fresh blood and plasma expanders. General supplies like beds, mattresses, blankets, linen, stretchers and refreshments may fall short. Inter-department communication may become difficult due to overload on available telephones. Available transport may not be enough for speedy evacuation. Hence, while designing an emergency department all these issues shall be addressed, and facilities provided beforehand.
7. Besides the above problems, the arrival of mass casualties along with anxious relatives and curious spectators may create security issues related to cash and valuables belonging to disabled patients.

Further Reading

Abdelsamad Y, Rushdi M, Tawfik B. Functional and Spatial Design of Emergency Departments Using Quality Function Deployment. J Healthc Eng. 2018 Nov 14;2018:e9281396.

Designing the Future, Engineering Reality: Prototyping in the Emergency Department [Internet]. [cited 2021 Jun 18]. Available from: https://iris.unimore.it/handle/11380/1169020#.YMxhe2hKg2x

Door Gasketing for Hospitals-Challenges Expectations and Innovations.:5.

Emergency Department Design for a More Efficient and Safe ER | Thought Leadership [Internet]. HMC Architects. 2019 [cited 2021 Jun 18]. Available from: https://hmcarchitects.com/news/emergency-department-design-for-a-more-efficient-and-safe-er-2019-02-27/

Emergency Department Design [Internet]. Huddy HealthCare Solutions. [cited 2021 Jun 18]. Available from: https://huddyhealthcare.com/service/emergency-department-design/

Emergency Department Infrastructure and Design [Internet]. [cited 2021 Jun 18]. Available from: https://dialremedy.com/blog/emergency-department- infrastructure-and-design

Finefrock SC. Designing and Building a New Emergency Department: The Experience of One Chest Pain, Stroke, and Trauma Center in Columbus, Ohio. J Emerg Nurs. 2006 Apr 1;32(2):144–8.

Hospital Planning: Emergency Departments - Design Collaborative [Internet]. [cited 2021 Jun 18]. Available from: http://www.designcollaborative.com/design-blog/hospital-planning-emergency-departments/

Hospital swinging-door requirements [Internet]. [cited 2021 Jun 18]. Available from: https://www.hfmmagazine.com/articles/3401-hospital-swinging-door-policy
In and Out of the Emergency Room | Streamlined design of patient flow [Internet]. [cited 2021 Jun 18]. Available from: https://www.asianhhm.com/facilities-operations/emergency-department-streamlining
Marsh RH, Chalmers KD, Checkett KA, Ansara J, Rimpel L, Edmond MC, et al. Emergency Department Design in Low- and Middle-Income Settings: Lessons from a University Hospital in Haiti. Ann Glob Health. 2020 Jan 20;86(1):6.
New strategies in ED design [Internet]. [cited 2021 Jun 18]. Available from: https://www.hfmmagazine.com/articles/1451-new-strategies-in-ed-design
Wang T, Zhang S, Bai X. Study on the Design of Emergency Entrances for Hospitals Evidence from extremely cold regions -- Urban healing transition space. 2017;6.
What's The Future Of Emergency Department Design? [Internet]. DuvaSawko. 2018 [cited 2021 Jun 18]. Available from: https://www.duvasawko.com/emergency-department-design/

17 Outpatient Department

The Outpatient Department (OPD) Unit, also known as Ambulatory Care Unit, is the department in a hospital where consultation is given to the ambulatory patients by specialists or super-specialists. Patients who do not have to remain in the hospital overnight are attended to in OPD.

The main purpose of OPD is to avoid the rush in the indoor department and to provide follow up management of the indoor patient after discharge. This is an arrangement of mutual advantage to all concerned, i.e. the doctor, the patient, the society and the hospital.

The OPD provides the following functions:

1. Consultation with medical specialists and super specialists.
2. Physical examination and investigations.
3. Providing treatment on a day-care basis.
4. Performing Minor procedures.
5. Follow up consultation and ongoing case management.
6. Pre-operative screening of the patient.
7. Providing health education and counselling of the patients and families.
8. Referring the patients to other specialities or super-specialities for second opinion or ongoing care and treatment.
9. Refer the patient for admission to a hospital for inpatient services.
10. Good centre for providing the training and education to the students.
11. A connecting chain between the community and the hospital and helps in providing the knowledge and education to the community at large regarding health awareness and prevention of the diseases and promotion of public health.

17.1 Location of the OPD

Location wise, the OPD should be located on the ground floor, easily approachable and preferably should have a separate entry. In some cases, because of the shortage of space, it becomes evident that the upper floors are also used for OPD. In such cases the upper floors should be reserved for the examination rooms and the ground floor should be preferred for the Reception, Registration and Waiting etc.

Further, all the OPDs should be located near to each other, so that the patients can easily be referred to other doctors for cross-reference. Ideally, if possible a separate OPD block should be provided.

A good arrangement of the OPD is that a main waiting hall should be made in the centre and the OPDs should be made around that hall, otherwise, there should be the main corridor running through the centre of the clinical section, side corridors giving access to and separating the different units. Wherever required the OPD rooms should be provided with an examination room, and if the space permits, a dressing room.

A. Garg, A. Dewan, *Manual of Hospital Planning and Designing*,
https://doi.org/10.1007/978-981-16-8456-2_17

All facilities for investigation and supply of medicine should be provided in the outpatient's departments. Further, the outpatient's department of the hospital should be planned in such a way that all the specialists and facilities to the outpatients can be carried out here only.

The Diagnostic services and the commercial section should be approachable from the OPD. The most common diagnostic and commercial services are Radiology, Pathology, Minor Operation Theatre, Injection/Dressing room, the Medical Record section etc.

If the resources allow, the way to the OPD should be marked with signs so that an illiterate patient can also reach the respective OPD easily. Normally, the best signage for the hospital is by putting coloured stripes on the walls and providing signs in the local language at various places.

Outpatients should, as far as possible, be discouraged from moving into the in-patients area to avoid disturbance to the Inpatients who are more seriously ill. Uncontrolled traffic of outpatients in wards and departments of the inpatients' block is undesirable from all points of view. Even if it has to be done the common gate between the OPD and the Inpatients Department should be guarded in such a way that the movement of the OPD patients to the area of the Inpatients is as minimum as possible.

Further, some of the other hospital facilities and the backup services like accounting, housekeeping and maintenance services should not be duplicated and the same facilities serving in the indoor can take care of the work in the OPD.

In the OPD, the main attention should be paid to the reception, the doctor's chamber and the examination room.

Generally, there are two designs based on which the OPD can be located:

1. **Centralized Outpatient Services**
   In this design, all services are provided in a single compact area which along with the consultation chambers, also includes diagnostic and therapeutic facilities to be provided at the same place.
2. **Decentralized Outpatient Services**
   Where the services are provided in the respective departments.
3. **Separate Block**
   Under this type of layout, the OPD block is located separately in the annexure building/block or wing.

17.2 Schemes of the Layout of the OPD

Generally, there are two designs based on which the OPD can be located:

17.2.1 Single Corridor OPD

In this design, the OPDs are located on both sides of a single corridor with the waiting and reception common for all. The waiting can be in between the OPDs or it can be common for all the services. The disadvantage is the rush of visitors and patients in a single corridor. The same corridor shall be used for in and out.

17.2.2 Double Corridor OPD

In this design, the OPDs are located on both the sides of double corridor side by side. The waiting and reception are common for all. The waiting can be in between the OPDs or it can be common for all the services. The advantage is that one corridor can be used for IN and the second can be used for OUT.

17.2.3 Clustered OPD Block

In this scheme, the OPD are located side by side around the hall and the waiting and reception are in the centre of the hall. The only issue in this type of scheme is the privacy of the patient.

17.3 Infrastructure Requirements in the OPD

The following are the infrastructures in the OPD department (Fig. 17.1):

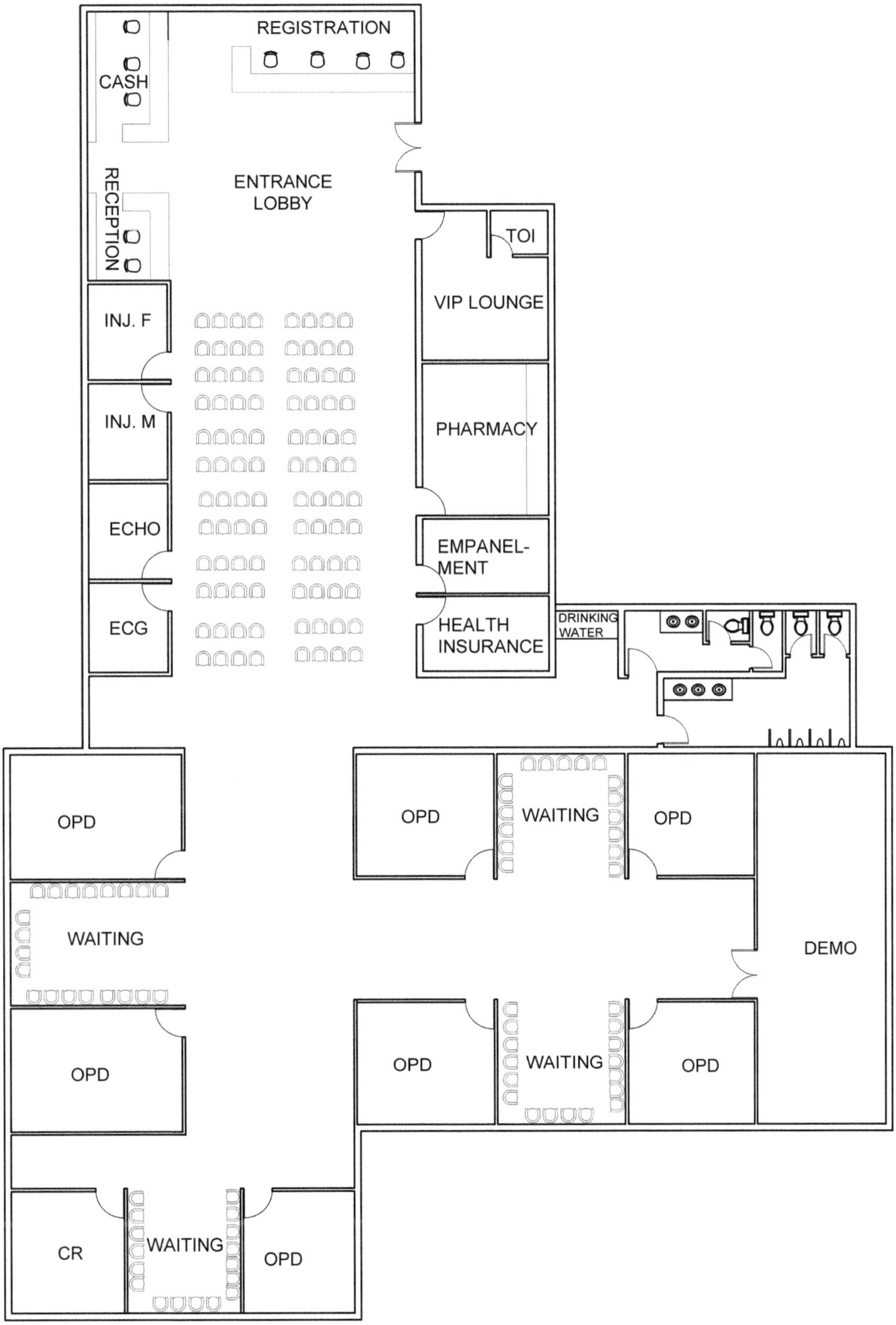

Fig. 17.1 Sample layout drawing of the OPD infrastructure

17.4 Reception and Enquiry Counter

Immediately after the arrival of the patient in the OPD department, this is the first area of contact. The reception provides the required information to the visitors, guides the visitors to the required place, books an appointment etc. Hence, the reception counter has to be placed just at the entry of the OPD Block. The reception of the OPD should be at such a place that is easily approachable.

The size of the reception counter shall depend on the expected number of patients/visitors likely to use the services of reception. It is recommended that space shall be provided for two receptionists to be seated. Hence, the ideal size of the reception shall be about 3048 mm–4572 mm long. The reception and enquiry counters can be either made out of civil work with an aesthetic look or granite of other material can be used to make it more appealing. Alternately, a counter made out of wood can also be provided.

17.4.1 Furniture at the Reception

1. The Front side of the counter shall be about 5 ft. in height so that the person can easily stand and talk to the receptionist. On the other side of the counter, the working top shall be provided which shall be about 610 mm in width and 762 mm in height.
2. Two chairs for the receptionists.

17.4.2 Electrical and Other Points at the Reception

The reception counter shall have:

1. At least six 5 Amp Switches/Sockets on the wall of the counter at a height of about 152 mm from the working top. These points shall be used for connecting computers, printers and other similar devices.
2. Also, two 15 Amp Switches/Sockets shall be provided on the wall behind the reception counter for other appliances.
3. Two RJ 45 point for Computer networking.
4. Two RJ 11 for Intercom and extension line.
5. Two USB points for charging mobiles or for other use.

17.5 Registration Counter

Next to the reception counter, the registration counter has to be located. The Registration counter registers the patient for OPD, prepares OPD consultation form, receives payment for OPD Consultation, issues Token number etc. In some hospitals, the case records are retained and stored with the registration department and patients are given a small card containing his/her registration number. Every time the patient visits the hospital, the case record has to be taken out and sent to the physician for consultation. This job has to be done by the registration counter.

The size of this counter shall again depend on the expected number of patients/visitors likely to use the services of this counter. Still, space shall be provided for two staff members to be seated on each counter. Hence, the ideal size can be about 2438 mm–3658 mm long. The registration counters can be either made out of civil work with an aesthetic look or granite or other material can be used to make it more appealing. Alternately, counters made out of wood can also be provided.

17.5.1 Furniture at Registration Counter

1. The Front side of each counter shall be about 1524 mm in height so that the person can easily stand and talk to the staff. On the other side of the counter, the working top shall be provided which shall be about 610 mm in width and 762 mm in height. If the Registration counter deals with the cash also, then above the counter there shall be a glass partition up to

the height of about 1219 mm from the top of the counter with a cut window on the lower side of the glass.

2. Two chairs for the staff on each counter.

17.5.2 Electrical and Other Points at Registration Counters

Each of these counters shall have:

1. At least six 6 Amp Switches/Sockets on the wall of the counter at a height of about 152 mm from the working top. These points shall be used for connecting computers, printers and other similar devices.
2. Also, two 15 Amp Switches/Sockets shall be provided on the wall behind each counter for other appliances.
3. Two RJ 45 point for Computer networking.
4. Two RJ 11 for Intercom and extension line.
5. Two USB points for charging mobiles or for other use.

17.6 Waiting Lobby/Hall

After getting registered for OPD consultation, patients need to wait for their turn for consultation. Waiting area shall have drinking water and toilet facilities. Hospitals may have a temple or meditation room in the waiting hall. Pre-COVID era, there was a concept to create more and more spaces for waiting lobbies to make it comfortable for patients and attendants to wait. The design was such to accommodate more and more chairs for seating. Now post COVID-19, all public spaces including waiting areas, lobbies and dining hall shall be carefully planned and designed to create a better physical separation between people and the system of appropriate queuing shall be introduced. Few of the concerned issues are:

1. The foremost principle to be followed is that individual seats shall be provided in a fashion to maintain appropriate social distancing.
2. **Sub-waiting lobbies**

   It is recommended that instead of large waiting lobbies, hospitals shall be designed for small and sub-waiting lobbies, e.g. instead of providing a large lobby with a seating capacity of 200 in the OPD block, a separate sub-waiting lobby of around 30 seats serving one or two OPD rooms shall be created. However, such measures may not be practical in all situations, especially for small hospitals, nursing homes, clinics etc. The number of people who shall be allowed to wait in hospital lobbies shall be limited to a defined number of persons that shall be maximum allowed with a specified minimum spacing between their seats. So, future waiting lobbies could be smaller and in scattered clusters (Fig. 17.2).
3. **Minimize Interaction with others**

   The concept of a smaller enclave waiting space that separates the sick from other patients or the visitors shall be preferred. The seating also has to be in the clusters of small numbers of chairs, say 2–3 chairs per cluster. Further, each cluster shall be portioned from the other with at least 1524 mm acrylic or glass partition to reduce exposure with other patients/visitors.
4. **Outside waiting**

   Patients and families shall be advised to wait outside or in their car instead of waiting in the lobby.
5. **Adopting a Token system**

   To reduce the crowd in waiting lobbies, a token system shall be introduced. With this system, the patient or visitor is issued a token at the time of registration so that he/she is well aware of his/her turn. He/she need not be in the waiting lobby near the service room but can be waiting somewhere else. For information about the status of the token, LCDs can be provided at various places of the hospital wherein a token holder can see the status of his/her token number. We can further use SMS services where a notification will be sent to the registered mobile number of the token holder as and when his/her turn arrives.

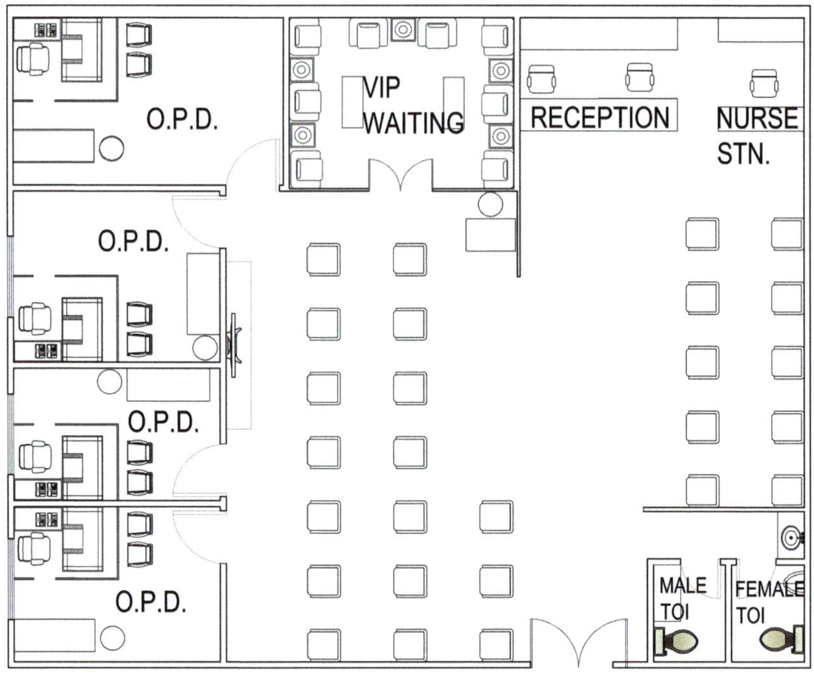

Fig. 17.2 Sample layout of waiting areas

17.7 Examination Rooms

The examination/consultation rooms can be of two types. First is the Combined Multi-Disciplinary Consultation room and the second is the Separate Consultation Room.

17.7.1 Combined Multi-Disciplinary Consultation Room

Under this design, several physicians of different disciplines share the same room at different points of days or time. In this type of scheme, the equipment required for that particular speciality is brought into the room when needed and stored again when not in use. The benefits of this type of scheme are that it can be used for consultation of different specialities and saves floor spaces.

17.7.2 Separate Consultation Room

Under this type of design, an individual room is allotted to a single speciality and no other speciality can use this room. The benefit of this type of arrangement is that every time the equipment need not be removed from the room, resulting in low wear and tear.

17.8 Procedure/Treatment Rooms

There are some OPDs that require procedure/treatment rooms, e.g. Surgery OPD requires Dressing Room, Minor OT; Ophthalmology requires, Refraction, Orthopty, Dark Room, Dressing Room rooms; ENT requires Audiometry, ENG Lab Speech Therapy Rooms; Gynae Obs. require D&C Room, Antenatal Clinic, Family Welfare Clinic, Cancer Detection Clinic and Colposcopy Room etc.

Preferably, this procedures/treatment shall be placed near their respective OPD. Locating them in a cluster at a particular location is not recommended, as it results in the wastage of physicians' time and unnecessary movement of the patients.

The total list of such rooms is provided in this book in the chapter of 'Area Requirement and Planning' (Chap. 7).

17.9 Support Rooms

These rooms though do not directly provide consultation but give backup and support the consultants conducting the OPD. Some of these rooms are like:

1. It is a practice to take the vitals of the patients like Blood Pressure, SPO2, Pulse, Weight and Height, before the patient moves to the consultation chamber of the physician. Hence, the Vital signs examination room shall be given near to the registration counter.
2. Also, the Sample collection room shall be provided to take the blood and other specimens of the patient for clinical laboratory investigation.
3. Provision shall be made for Interview/meeting/counselling rooms in the OPD.
4. Clean Store Room.
5. Dirty Utility Room.
6. General Store.
7. Record room.
8. Equipment storage room.
9. Medicine and Drug Store room.
10. Staff room with beverage and food storage facilities.
11. Pharmacy for patient medications.
12. Rehabilitation Unit for patient.
13. Toilets for Patients and Visitors.
14. Drinking Water facility.
15. Storage facilities for patient belongings.

17.10 General Issue While Designing the OPD

1. Transfer of noise and sound between the consultation rooms should be minimised to improve the concentration of the physician and to reduce miscommunication, disruptions and staff errors.
2. Waiting rooms and play areas should be located away from consultation and treatment rooms as these areas are generally more noisy.
3. Natural Light/Lighting shall be maximized.
4. Windows are desirable in waiting areas and consultation rooms.
5. Careful consideration shall be paid for privacy and comfort of the patient to reduce discomfort and stress of patients.
6. For interior decor colour, textures, surface finishes, fixtures, fittings, furnishings and artworks shall be used.
7. Colours should be used in combination with lighting to ensure that they do not mask skin colours as this can create a problem to the physician to examine the patient.
8. The Unit shall have suitable seating and provisions for bariatric patients.
9. Entire OPD block shall be lockable when not in use.
10. All the individual rooms in the OPD shall be lockable.
11. Medical gases may be provided within Consultation/Procedure/Treatment rooms where ever required.
12. Bio-Medical Waste Management shall be introduced in all Consultation, Procedure and Treatment rooms.
13. Support services like laboratory, radiology, billing, registration, enquiry, medical record department and pharmacy shall be situated near OPD.
14. The design must consider that the patients coming from different areas and the direction shall ordinarily move only in one direction.

17.11 Number of OPDs Required

The number of OPDs required depends on many factors such as:

1. Number of physicians who will be conducting OPD at a particular moment of time.
2. Type of OPD-like system of whether Combined Consultation room or Separate Consultation Room. Naturally, if the management opts for Single Consultation room concept, the requirement of OPD consultation rooms will be more.
3. The size of the population served by the unit and demographic trends.

4. Expected number of patients to attend OPD.
5. The average duration of the consultation.
6. Timing of the OPD. If the OPDs are being conducted throughout the day, the chamber sharing system can be adopted, hence less number of OPDs will be required.
7. The number of referrals and transfers from other regions or hospitals.

17.12 Consultation Room

17.12.1 Size of the OPD Room

The exact size of the consultation room depends on factors like expected visitors, the policy of the hospital and Furniture to be placed in the consultation room. But the ideal size shall not be less than 4267 mm × 3658 mm with arrangements of the running water.

17.12.2 Doors

The Door of the OPD Room shall not be less than 1219 mm wide, unobstructed. The door shall be on the other side of the examination couch to avoid patient exposure in Consultation and Treatment rooms.

17.12.3 Windows

The windows shall be preferred in the room, but direct sunlight shall be avoided. The window glass can be tinted or curtains/blinds shall be provided.

17.12.4 Hand Washing

A Hand Basin shall be provided in the room.

17.12.5 Furniture

The following furniture shall be placed in the consultation room:

Doctors table with Side Rack	Two Attendants Chairs
Doctors Chair	Examination Couch
Height adjustment revolving stool for patient	Step Stool

17.12.6 Instruments and Equipment

All the necessary equipment and gadgets shall be provided like.

B.P. Apparatus	Tongue depressor
Stethoscope	Weighing machine
Torch	Finger Pulse Oximeter
Knee hammer	Intercom
View Box	Computer with a Printer and UPS
Special equipment required for different types of OPDs should also be provided.	

17.12.7 Electrical Points in Consultation Room

The following electrical points shall be provided in the consultation chamber:

1. Main Switchboard at the entrance wall (other than the wall on which door will open) for control of fan and lights of the room along with one 6 Amp Switch/Socket.
2. Air Conditioning Control button with temperature adjustment.
3. One point on the wall 610 mm above the examination table for examination light along with the switch.
4. Two 6 Amp Switches/Sockets above on the wall 1 ft. above the doctor's table shall be provided. Also, one 15 Amp Switch/Socket shall be provided adjoining this.
5. Three 6 Amp Switches/Sockets above on the wall 1 ft. above the doctor's side rack for the computer and printer. Also, one 15 Amp Switch/Socket shall be provided adjoining to this for other equipment or heater.

17.12.8 Other Communication Points in OPD

The following communication points shall be provided in the consultation chamber:

1. RJ 45 point for Computer networking.
2. RJ 11 for Intercom and extension line.
3. HDMI point for computer display at other locations.

17.12.9 Curtain Partitions

The examination table in the OPD shall be provided with hanging curtain partitions. Following should be kept in mind when using curtain partitions:

1. The couch shall be placed in front of one wall of the OPD.
2. The couch shall have a curtain on all the other three sides.
3. The ceiling suspended curtain track is fixed at 2133 mm above the floor level.
4. Curtains shall be hung on these tracks and shall be moveable and collapsible.
5. At the bottom of the curtain, there shall be a clear area of about 457 mm from the floor for cleaning of the floor.

17.13 Design of OPD

The design of an OPD shall have the provision to maintain distancing and avoid direct contact with patients. For this, some type of acrylic or glass partitions can be used, wherein on one side the staff will be seated and on the other side of the partition the patient. For communication between the two, a two-way audio-visual system shall be preferred for easy interaction. Doctors can see the patient remotely on video, conduct examinations remotely using IoT-enabled devices (Fig. 17.3).

17.13.1 Use of Touch-free Medical Devices

To avoid direct and close contact with the patient, it is advised to use wireless and touch-free medical devices to replace the current BP apparatus, Stethoscope, Pulse Oximeter, Thermometer etc.

17.13.2 OPD Consultation Rooms with Videoconferencing Solutions

It is evident that in the near future, patients would avoid going to hospitals until and unless it is really necessary. This would result in patients adopting more and more video consultations rather than OPD visits, thereby allowing OPDs to be less crowded. This would completely change the layout and design of the OPD consultation rooms, which would now need to incorporate more elements for videoconferencing solutions.

17.13.3 Creating Virtual OPD

We recommend adopting and introducing the concept of Virtual OPD, wherein IT infrastructure shall play a major role in designing. The patient to doctor communication interface and doctor-to-staff communication will be carried out through AV controls. In today's world, the widely available technologies such as video chat and virtual reality headsets will have to be incorporated to help patients stay connected to friends and family.

17.13.4 Sterilization and Pressure

A provision shall be made to protect the OPD by UV-C light disinfection and sanitization from time to time. Also, the OPD should be positively pressurized.

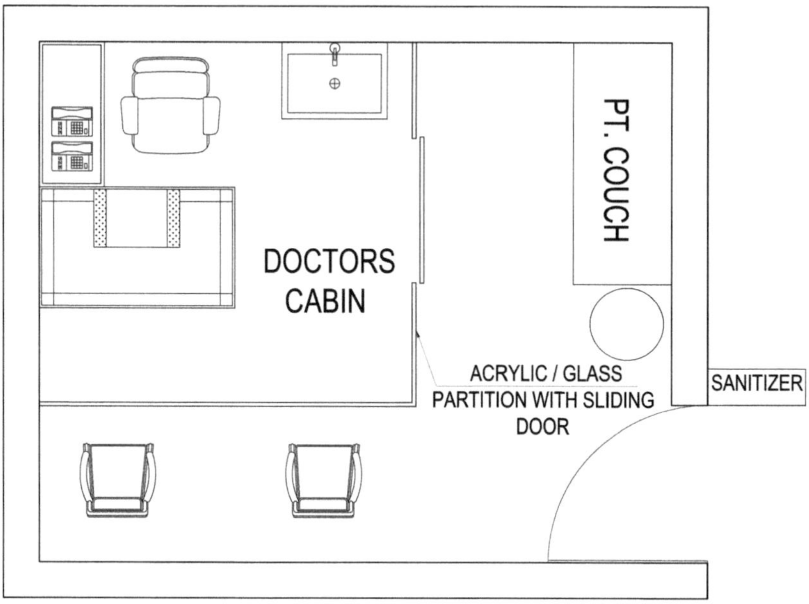

Fig. 17.3 Sample layout of consultation chamber in OPD

17.13.5 Telemedicine Impact on the Facility

Telemedicine has boomed during this crisis of COVID-19 era, thus forcing healthcare workers to perform routine check-ups and treat patients without putting either doctor, staff or patient at risk. The technology of telemedicine is relatively cheap and enables physicians to see more patients in less time, and virtually requires no space. Increased use of telemedicine could possibly increase number of patients. Also, it may give chances to increase the medical tourism for international patients because it will be easy for the patients sitting at far off places to connect to the doctors. Initial consultations can be done over videoconferences and test reports can be shared likewise. Only the patients requiring procedural intervention could come down to the hospital. All tests are done in the hospital within 15 minutes using Point of Care diagnostics and medicines are dispensed automatically using a combination of machines.

17.13.6 Mobile Health

Mobile health is becoming more and more popular these days as the elimination of wires and cords and enabling physicians and patients to check healthcare processes online. Smartphones and tablets allow healthcare providers to freely access and send information to the desired. Physicians and service providers can use Mobile Health tools for orders, documentation or to simply search for more patient information.

17.14 Procedure /Treatment Room

17.14.1 Size of the Procedure/ Treatment Room

The exact size of the procedure/treatment room shall depend on factors like equipment to be placed in the room, numbers of persons required in the room, movement spaces required to perform the procedure etc. But the ideal size shall not be less than 4267 mm × 3658 mm. However, the size may be increased as per requirement.

17.14.2 Doors

The Door of the procedure/treatment room shall not be less than 1524 mm wide, unobstructed for easy movement of the wheelchair/stretcher trolley. The door shall be on the other side of the procedure table to avoid patient exposure in procedure and treatment rooms.

17.14.3 Windows

The windows can be avoided to maintain the privacy of the patients until and unless essentially required. If provided, direct sunlight shall be avoided. The window glass can be tinted or the curtains/blinds shall be provided.

17.14.4 Handwashing

A Hand Basin shall be provided in the room and arrangements of the running water shall be made. Similarly, proper drainage of water shall be provided.

17.14.5 Furniture

The following furniture shall be placed in the procedure/treatment room:

Procedure table	Step Stool
Small Writing Table	Scrub Station
Doctors Chair	IV Stand
Height adjustment revolving stool	IV Rod
Instrument Trollies	Crash Cart
Stretcher Trolley	Oxygen Cylinder Trolley
Dressing Trollies	

17.14.6 Instruments and Equipment

All the necessary equipment and gadgets as required by the respective departments or respective procedures shall be provided.

17.14.7 Electrical Points in Procedure/Treatment Room

The following electrical points shall be provided in the procedure/treatment room:

1. The main switchboard at the entrance wall (other than the wall on which door will open) for control of the fan and lights of the room along with one 6 Amp Switch/Socket.
2. Air Conditioning Control button with temperature adjustment.
3. One point on the wall 610 mm. above the procedure couch for examination light along with the switch.
4. Three 6/16 Amp Switches/Sockets on the wall where the procedure couch is located, 457 mm above the floor level for equipment. One pair shall be connected to the UPS supply.
5. Three 6/16 Amp Switches/Sockets on the sidewall of procedure couch, 1457 mm above the floor level for equipment. One pair shall be connected to the UPS supply.
6. Two 6 Amp Switch/Socket above on the wall 305 mm above the writing table shall be provided. Also, one 15 Amp Switch/Socket shall be provided adjoining to this.

17.14.8 Other Communication Points in Procedure/ Treatment Room

The following communication points shall be provided at the reception:

1. RJ 45 point for Computer networking.

2. RJ 11 for Intercom and extension line.
3. HDMI point for computer display at other locations.

Further Reading

10 hospital design changes, post COVID [Internet]. Health Care Radius. [cited 2021 Jun 18]. Available from: https://www.healthcareradius.in/projects/26279-10-hospital-design-changes-post-covid

Athula Wijewickrama A K., Soemon Takakuwa. Designing outpatient appointment systems with patient characteristics: a case study. Int J Healthc Technol Manag. 2012 Jan 1;13(1–3):157–69.

Broberg O, Edwards K. User-driven innovation of an outpatient department. Work. 2012 Jan 1;41(Supplement 1):101–6.

Contributor G. Healthcare Facilities Design After COVID-19 [Internet]. Facility Executive - Creating Intelligent Buildings. 2020 [cited 2021 Jun 18]. Available from: https://facilityexecutive.com/2020/06/healthcare-facilities-design-after-covid-19/

COVID-19: Smart OPDs To Help Keep Our Doctors Safe [Internet]. Moneylife NEWS & VIEWS. [cited 2021 Jun 18]. Available from: https://www.moneylife.in/article/covid-19-smart-opds-to-help-keep-our-doctors-safe/60092.html

Design and application of a new doctor workstation system in outpatient department-- 《Information of Medical Equipment》 2006年09期 [Internet]. [cited 2021 Jun 18]. Available from: https://en.cnki.com.cn/Article_en/CJFDTotal-YLSX200609011.htm

Donnellan F, Hussain T, Aftab AR, McGurk C. Reducing unnecessary outpatient attendances. Int J Health Care Qual Assur. 2010 Jan 1;23(5):527–31.

Fleming RW. outpatient care: Design of outpatient areas. Hosp Top. 1973 Oct 1;51(10):45–9.

Madsen NB. Framework for Layout Design Supporting Patient Flow in Outpatient Departments.:144.

Tabish SA. outpatient services in a hospital. In 2011.

The patient-centered new outpatient building process design-- 《Journal of Medical Postgraduates》 2009年04期 [Internet]. [cited 2021 Jun 18]. Available from: https://en.cnki.com.cn/Article_en/CJFDTotal-JLYB200904022.htm

Vahdatzad V, Griffin J. Outpatient clinic layout design accounting for flexible policies. In 2016. p. 3668–9.

Zhao Y, Mourshed M. Patients' Perspectives on the Design of Hospital Outpatient Areas. Buildings. 2017 Dec;7(4):117.

18 Intensive Care Units

An Intensive Care Unit (ICU) is a specially designed, equipped, staffed, furnished separate and self-contained area of a hospital dedicated to the management of patients with critical and life-threatening illnesses. With close monitoring and observation, this unit provides specialized expert care and facilities for the support of vital functions and uses the skills of medical, nursing and other personnel experienced in the management of such problems.

Designing an intensive care unit (ICU) to handle the needs of critically ill patients is really a difficult job. Before going for planning and designing of ICU, the designers first of all need to understand how many ICUs including advanced like ICU, PICU, Neuro-intensive care, Cardiac Intensive Care and Trauma units are required and with how many beds in each unit.

18.1 Types of ICUs

There can be different types of ICU depending on the severity of the illness to be treated or otherwise, the ICUs can be designed department wise. The following ICUs can be planned:

1. Medical ICU
2. Surgical ICU
3. Interventional Cardiac ICU
4. Intensive Coronary Care Unit (ICCU)
5. CTVS ICU
6. Pulmonology ICU
7. Respiratory ICU
8. Neuro ICU
9. Neurosurgery ICU
10. Psychiatry ICU
11. Transplant ICU
12. Nephrology ICU
13. Urology ICU
14. Robotic Surg. ICU
15. Endocrinology ICU
16. Endocrine Surgery ICU
17. Gastro ICU
18. Gastro Surgery ICU
19. Bariatric Surgery ICU
20. Burn ICU
21. Vascular Surgery ICU
22. Gynae ICU
23. Ortho ICU
24. Pedia ICU
25. Pedia Surg. ICU
26. Neonatal ICU
27. Ophthalmology ICU
28. ENT ICU
29. Derma ICU
30. Geriatrics ICU
31. Oncology ICU etc.

However, all the hospitals do not need to have all these ICUs. Before planning the type, the number of ICUs or the number of beds in each ICU, three questions have to be answered, What, Why and How Many. The answers to these have

A. Garg, A. Dewan, *Manual of Hospital Planning and Designing*,
https://doi.org/10.1007/978-981-16-8456-2_18

to be collected by the management before planning the ICUs. The answers will come from the data about the number of patients expected; with which disease and how many such patients; the physicians, nurses and paramedical staff required to treat them etc.

Based on the answers, it has to be decided which all ICUs have to be planned, how many beds in each ICU are to be planned and what facilities and equipment are to be provided in each ICU.

At times, the designers also design the ICU of different levels like Level-1, Level-2 and Level-3. These levels are based on the number of beds in ICU, Equipment facility and the staffing pattern of ICU.

18.2 Number of Beds in a Single Unit of ICU

Once the number of ICUs and types of ICUs to be established has been decided, the next question that arises is 'How many beds in each unit of ICU?'. As stated earlier, the management has to assess the number of patients expected to arrive in each ICU. While assessing the number of patients the management shall also assess the expected increase in the number of patients in future. Also, the assessment has to be done regarding the average duration of a patient's stay in ICU. Accordingly, a final decision has to be made about the number of beds to be placed in ICU.

Another important factor to be considered is that there are few departments in which the patient turnover ratio is very high as compared to others, e.g. the patient's turnover in Medical ICU, Surgical ICU shall be very high as compared to others. For these types of ICUs, the bed strength can be somewhere between 10 and 15 in each ICU unit of Medicine and Surgery.

Then there are departments that may have a moderate turnover of patients like Cardiology, Neurology, Neuro Surgery, Paediatric and Respiratory. The ICUs of these departments can be planned with a bed strength of about 6 to 10 each.

Last are the departments which rarely use the ICU. Hence the ICUs for these departments shall be planned if unavoidable. The patients of these departments shall be adjusted with other ICUs. But still, if ICUs for these departments have to be provided, the bed strength shall not be more than 5.

Also, it shall be noted that more than 20 beds in each ICU are not recommended in any case, otherwise, the required care cannot be provided and justified.

18.3 Location of Intensive Care Units

There are two schools of thought relating to the location of ICUs. First recommends that all the ICUs should be at a centralized place so that they are readily accessible to one another. The reason is that hygiene can be maintained much more effectively, control of visitors shall be more effective and if the patient develops any complications suddenly, the specially trained professionals and equipment are immediately available to patients from other ICUs.

The second school of thought favours that the location of such intensive units shall be dependent on the type of disease or patient. For example, the surgical ICU should be close to the operating theatre while the medical ICU should be in close proximity to the medical ward to facilitate easy follow up for progressive care.

We can agree with both the thoughts as there are pros and cons for each thought. However, we suggest that if one to five sets of ICUs are required and the hospital is in a single block of the building, it is better if the ICUs are located at a centralized place and on one floor, referred to as the 'Intensive Care Floor'.

If the design of the hospital is spread in multiple buildings and different departments are placed in different buildings, then it is better to build the ICU of that particular department in the building or the floor where the parent department is located.

But one thing for sure is that, whatever be the location of ICUs, it has to exclude through-traffic and strong provision of infection control shall be provided. Particular care has to be taken about the movement and access of ICUs to the public and visitors. ICUs being restricted areas, the access and movement of visitors and the public should be very restricted.

Regarding the floor at which the ICU shall be located, again there are different opinions. Some people prefer to have ICUs on the top floor of the building. The reason stated behind this thought is that the traffic can be controlled effectively and the chances of infections are reduced. The other thought is that the ICUs shall be sandwiched between two floors somewhere between the buildings. The reason is that due to heavy thermal losses on the top floor, the air conditioning has to be more effective resulting in higher operational costs.

Another factor to be considered while deciding the location of the ICUs is that it should be adjacent to and not far off from Emergency, Operating Room, Radiology etc.

As the diagnostic department and Emergency are mostly on the ground floor, hence this can be one justification to locate ICU somewhere on the second or third floor of the building.

18.4 Infrastructure of ICU

ICU mainly consists of four major zones, each zone housing a particular function or set of interrelated functions. The Zones are (Fig. 18.1):

1. Patient Care Zone
   This zone consists of Patient Rooms, Isolation Rooms and adjacent areas and its main function is direct patient care only.
2. Clinical Support Zone
   This Zone consists of functions closely related to direct patient care.
3. Unit Support Zone
   This is a Zone from where the administrative, materials management and staff support functions shall be provided.
4. Family Support Zone
   This is the zone designed to support families and visitors.

The following are the room/areas required for an ideal setup of ICU:

Patient Care Zone	Intensive Care Beds
	Isolation Rooms
	Examination and Treatment room
	Nursing Station
	Public Utility for Patients
Clinical Support Zone	Clean Utility
	Dirty Utility / Sluice Room
	Medication Rooms
	Equipment Park / Store
	Radiology
	Sample Collection Room
Unit Support Zone	Change Room—Male
	Change Room—Female
	Resident Doctors and Student Duty Room
	Nurses Night Duty Room
	Night Duty Room for On-Call Junior Residents
	Staff Lounge
	Staff Restrooms
	Ward Pantry
	Lockers
Family Support Zone	Family Lounge
	Consultation Rooms
	Meditation Spaces
	Family Nourishment
	Public Utility for Attendants
	Family Laundry
	Family Sleep Rooms

18.5 Size of the ICU

Before deciding and designing the ICU, the designer has to understand in depth the equipment to be placed in ICU; support functions to be provided; the movement of men and material; inventory of tools, instruments, consumables and supplies; staff ratio and distances from support rooms etc. This designer shall also keep in mind the current and future requirements. Ample spaces shall be planned to adjust future expansions without any major alterations.

The design shall be such that can reduce the travel distances of staff by placing mostly needed spaces and equipment as close as possible to the site of use.

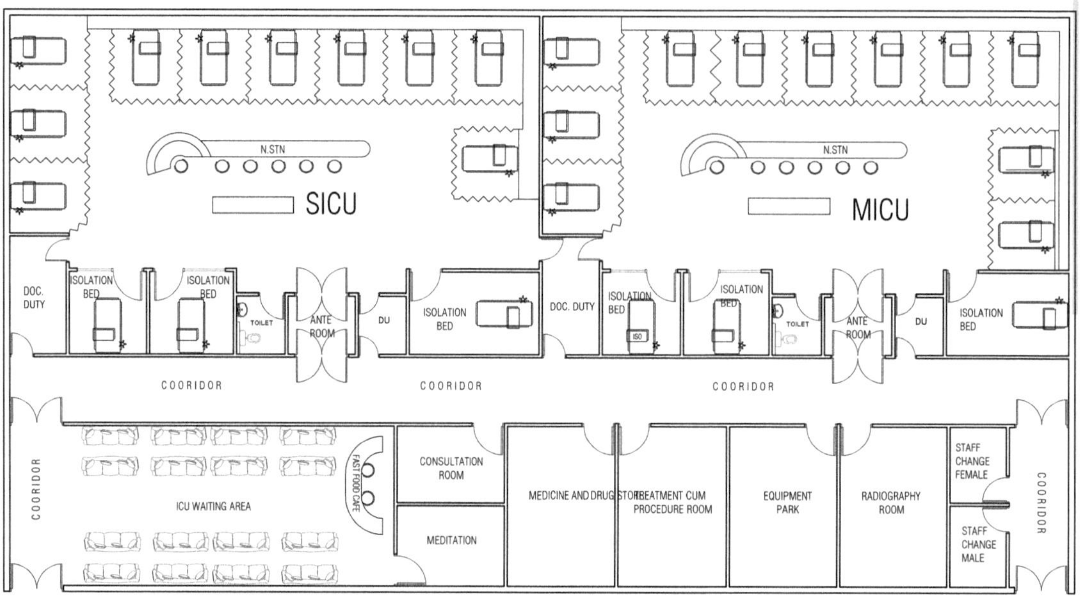

Fig. 18.1 Sample layout of ICU complex

18.6 Sizing Considerations

How much area per bed is needed in ICU along with movement spaces? How to answer this question? There are different thoughts on this issue. Even some countries or the governing bodies and regulating authorities have specified different norms for such areas.

Let us calculate the area scientifically:

- Dimensions of Bed (H × W): 1829 mm ×914 mm = 1.672 Sq. Mtr.
- The distance of the head end of the bed from wall: 610 mm.
- Free space for bed at foot end: 1524 mm.
- Left and right bed to bed distance 914 mm on each side.
- Now the total width space required: 914 + 914 + 914 = 2742 mm.
- Total Length space required: 1829 + 610 + 1524 = 3963 mm.
- Total area per bed: 3963 ×2743 mm = 10.87 Sq. Mtr.

Add at least 45% for other movement spaces including Nursing Station that has to be in the patient unit. Hence, the total area per bed in ICU shall be 10.87 Sq. Mtr. + 40% of 10.87 Sq. Mtr. = 15.24 Sq. Mtr.

Therefore, the per bed area of any ICU shall be somewhere between 13.94 and 16.26 Sq. Mtr.

This figure is always subjected to variation depending on the criticality of the patient. If very sick patients are to be treated, where more equipment, material and manpower will be required, the area can go up to 18.58 Sq. Mtr. If it is felt that the patients in any ICU will not be very sick and the requirement of equipment will be less, the area can be reduced to 13.0–13.94 Sq. Mtr.

If instead of Open ICU, a closed cubical with a single bed is planned, the area shall not be less than 23.23 Sq. Mtr. per bed. Same is the case with the isolation chamber/room.

Now about the issues of all four zones one by one.

18.7 Patient Care Zone

The Patient Care Zone is the area where direct patient care is provided and includes Patient Units/Rooms/Cubicles. It also includes immediately adjacent areas like Treatment/Procedure Room and the Nursing Counter.

18.7.1 Patient Unit

18.7.1.1 Bed Layout in ICU Hall

The bed in the ICU shall be laid out in such a fashion, that it allows easy and smooth working all around the bed, also the inter-bed spaces shall be appropriate for easy working and reduce cross-infection rate. Some issues that shall be kept in mind while laying down the beds in ICU:

1. The head end of the Bed shall be at least 610 mm away from the wall.
2. The Head support panel of the bed shall be removable.
3. On the foot end, a clear space shall be about 1524 mm so that the stretcher trolley can easily be turned around and the patient can be transferred from/to bed.
4. Most important, distance from the bed to bed shall not be less than 1829 mm, i.e. 914 mm on either side of each bed.

In case the cubicles or rooms are provided with fixed walls or partitions, please remember that the upper portion (above 914 mm from the floor) shall be made of clear glass so that the Nursing staff can have a clear view of the patient all the time. For the privacy of the patient, during a procedure, curtains can be slid which have been prefixed to cover the glass.

18.7.2 Isolation Room/Units/Area in ICU

ICU is the area where the patients are kept under intensive monitoring and patients with life-threatening diseases are provided treatment and care. Out of all the patients, there may be some patients who might be suffering from some contagious disease like Tuberculosis and COVID-19. These patients shall be placed separately from other non-infected patients to avoid the spread of the disease. Therefore, ICUs shall have the provision for normal beds and few beds for infected patients called Isolation cabin/unit/cubical.

Therefore, it is recommended that Negative pressure isolation rooms/units/cubicles shall be created in the ICU. The Isolation room/units shall have a separate entry other than the normal entry of the ICU. It is recommended that about 25% of the beds in ICU can be reserved for isolation beds/rooms/units. Isolation rooms should have separate attached toilets.

The isolation shall be properly air-tightened and negatively pressurized. These isolation cabins/rooms/units shall not be mixed up with other beds in the same hall, but shall be a separate zone with a barrier in between. Separate staff shall take care of the patients in isolation cabins. Or otherwise, if there is a shortage of space for separate rooms/units, few particular beds in the ICU can be converted to an isolation unit. For this, at some particular bed, with the help of collapsible shutters around the bed or fixing temporary acrylic partitions, an isolation bed can be created.

For negatively, pressurizing the isolation room/unit/bed please refer to the chapter of 'HVAC' (Chap. 38) of this book.

18.7.3 Furniture in ICU

The following furniture shall be placed in the ICU:

Patient Furniture

Patient Bed (Multi-positional ICU Bed on lockable wheels with bedside safety rails)	Step Stool
Bed Side Locker	Scrub Station
Over Bed Table	IV Stand
Examination Table	IV Rod
Wheel Chair	Crash Cart
Stretcher Trolley	Oxygen Cylinder Trolley
Dressing Trollies	Back Rest
Instrument Trollies	Patient Transfer System

Office Furniture

Nursing Counter	Filing Cabinet
Office chairs	Visitor Chairs etc.
Almirah/Cupboard	Stools

18.7.4 Equipment

Multi-para Vital Sign Monitor	Suction Machine
Invasive Mechanical Ventilator	Portable X-Ray Machine
Non-invasive Ventilator	Blood Gas Analyzer
High Flow Nasal Canula	Cardiac Marker Analyser
Infusion Pump	B.P. Apparatus
DVT Pumps	Pulse Oximeter
Nebuliser	Glucometer
Defibrillator	Laryngoscope
ECG Machine	Oxygen Cylinders with Masks
View Boxes	Ambu bag
Blood Gas Analyzer with Electrolytes	Cardiac Marker Analyzers
Air Mattress	Ambu Mask different sizes
Chest drainage equipment	ETO sterilization
CRRT	Fibreoptic Bronchoscope
Dialysis Machines	IABP, Intra-Aortic Balloon Pulsation
End-tidal CO_2 monitor—Capnography	Intubating Video scope
Invasive BP, SPO_2, NIBP, ECG, RR, Temp Probes with trays	Pacemaker
Spinal Board	Transport Ventilator
Computers	Ultrasound and Echo machine

18.7.5 Tools and Instruments

Sterilizing Drums	Torches
Walkers/Crutches	Examination Light
Splints	Chetal Forceps
Extension Cord and Boxes	Forceps of all styles and sizes
Operating Light	Needle Holders
Refrigerator	Tray of all styles and sizes
Instrument Boxes	Scissors of all styles and sizes
Proctoscope	Suture Sets
Weighing Machine	All other required instruments

18.7.6 Doors

The Door of the ICU shall not be less than 1829 mm wide, unobstructed. The door shall be openable on both the sides in and out.

18.7.7 Windows

As natural light helps in early recovery and avoid disorientation and sense of claustrophobia of patients, windows shall be preferred in the room but direct sunlight shall be avoided. Further, if the patient is provided with a window to have an outside view, like looking at a garden, trees, courtyard or another natural setting, may help to relieve anxiety and stress, improve care, enhance patients' comfort and improve patient orientation. As the bed head panels have to be fixed on the wall above the patients, the bottom of the window shall not be less than 1829 mm from floor level. The window glass can be tinted or curtains/blinds shall be provided.

If cost is not a criterion, even **electronic windows** that are opaque when the switch is on and transparent when switched off, can be thought of.

18.7.8 Nursing Station

Nursing is a crucial factor for the treatment of the patient in an ICU. It is the Nurse who is available to the patients most of the time. The nurse has to keep a rigorous watch on the patient and skilfully notice the vitals of the patient. Nurse, therefore, shall have a continuous watch on the patient in the unit/room.

Therefore, the proper location of the nursing station is very crucial. The location shall be such so that the nursing staff can have a continuous look at the patients in the entire unit. If we place a nursing station on one side or corner of the unit, he/she may not be able to see the patients on the other end of the unit or rooms.

Therefore, the centre of the unit is the best location for the nursing station. The nursing station shall be of the same shape as the ICU hall. If the hall is rectangular the nursing station can also be rectangular.

The design of the nursing station can be a 'U' shape counter so that the nurses can be seated on all three sides of the station and can see the patients. One of the open sides of the U shape station shall be used for movement of the nurses to/from the station.

Nursing station shall be at some height so that the nurse can easily see the patient, because if the counter is at normal floor height, sometimes it becomes difficult to see the patient while the nurse is in the sitting position. For this, a platform of about 305 mm height can be provided on which the nursing counter can be placed.

Nursing stations shall have sufficient storage facilities for instruments, tools, patient files and stationery. Sufficient electrical and communications points shall be provided. Such details are given below under the heading of electrical points and communication points. A view box shall also be fixed on a wall near the nursing station.

18.7.9 Hand Hygiene

For Hand Hygiene, in ICUs, two-way Scrub Stations shall be used and placed near the entrance. Dispensers for soap should be located near the scrub station. A paper towel dispenser and trash receptacle should be next to the scrub station. Scrub Station should enable hands-free operation. Sensor-controlled and/or foot-operated scrub stations shall be used. The Scrub station shall have the provision of both hot and cold water.

Alcohol gel/sanitizer dispensers: Alcohol gel/ sanitizer dispensers shall be located in the patient room as well as at other staff locations around the unit. In the patient room, this can be located at the foot end of the bed in a holder which can be hung from the bed.

18.7.10 Toilets

As the patients in ICU are critically sick and immobile, the relative use of conventional toilets is very less.

Generally, combined toilets are provided in the ICU unit. This toilet is also useful for cleaning bedpans and bed pots.

However, for patients with limited mobility, the use of a mobile commode chair is preferred. But the room design shall permit the space for such chairs and shall have total privacy of the patient.

For Isolation rooms, separate attached toilets shall be provided.

For bariatric and handicapped patients the handicapped toilets shall be provided with proper supports and handrails.

The toilets shall have an exhaust of appropriate size.

18.7.11 Air Conditioning System of ICUs

ICUs should be fully air-conditioned which shall allow for control of temperature, humidity and air exchanges. Suitable and safe air quality must be maintained at all times. Following issues are important while designing the Air Conditioning System:

1. For Air Conditioning of ICU, either the Chilled Water Pipe Line with AHUs can be opted, or otherwise, the Duct able Split or VRV system can be opted. All the systems have their own advantages and disadvantages.
2. Air Flow, direction and air exchanges have to be as per the norms of the industry.
3. Heating shall be done with a Water pipeline and AHUs having a hot water Generator instead of Water Chillers. Otherwise, the use of room heaters can be opted, but room heaters are not generally recommended.

4. Temperature shall be between 18 and 24 degree Celsius.
5. Depending on the type of room/unit the choice of positive or negative operating pressures has to be adopted. For the Isolation room, the concept of Negative pressure shall be adopted.

For full details on Air-conditioning, heating and air exchanges, please refer to the chapter of 'HVAC' (Chap. 38) in this book.

18.7.12 Central Piped Medical Gas Supply

As the critical patients arrive in the ICU, usually they are in need of oxygen. Also for some patients invasive or non-invasive ventilation may be required. Hence, the supply of Piped Centralized Medical Supply is a must. The gases supplied are:

- Oxygen
- Compressed Air
- Wall-mounted Suction

In ICU, the facility of supply of these lines shall be on every bed. In some hospitals, the outlets of these gases are fixed on the wall itself.

Nowadays, the Bedhead panel is used for this. Bedhead panel is 5 ft. panel made of extruded sections of aluminium. This panel has a provision for fixing the gas outlets and the electrical points. Also, this panel has a service railing on which the IV rod, tray and utility basket can be fixed. This panel is fixed at a height of 1524 mm above the floor level and goes up to 1829 mm.

Another option can be the Ceiling suspended pendant. This also has the same facilities as the Bedhead Panel. This panel is fixed on the ceiling and is suspended below so that the bottom of the pendant shall be 1524 mm from the floor. The Gas outlet points are fixed on the back wall of the pendant. On both, the side walls are the electrical points and on the front wall shall be the utility tray for bedside multi-parameter vital sign monitor and also the utility basket can be fixed on the front wall. The pendant can revolve at 270 degrees. Further, the pendant can be a single arm or dual-arm. The single-arm revolves at its own axis only, whereas the dual-arm pendant can revolve on both arms hence covering more area around the bed.

In ICU, each bed shall have the following outlets:

1. 2 outlets for Oxygen
2. 1 outlet for Compressed Air
3. 2 outlets for Suction

On the bed head panel or the pendent both, the electrical and communication points and ports shall be provided. Details are given in the electrical point and Communication point below.

18.7.13 Electrical Points in ICU

The following electrical points shall be provided in the ICU:

1. Main Switchboard shall be at the entrance wall for controlling fan and lights of the hall along with one 6 Amp Switch/Socket
2. Air Conditioning Control button with temperature adjustment
3. On each of the Bedhead Panel or Hanging Pendent, electrical points are provided. There shall be at least 4 pairs of 6/16 Amp switches/sockets on each bed, i.e. 8 points. These points shall be on UPS supply.
4. In the centre between two beds, three pairs of 6/16 Amp. Switches/sockets shall be provided on the back wall at the height of 457 mm from the floor level, i.e. 6 points. Out of these two pairs shall be on UPS supply.
5. Five 6/16 Amp Switches/Sockets at the height of 1372 mm shall be provided on the wall near or behind the nursing counter for View Box or charging of the medical equipment etc.
6. Two 6 Amp Switches/Sockets shall be given on the Nursing Counter.

18.7.14 Other Communication Points in ICU

The following communication points shall be provided at each Bed of ICU:

1. Point for Nurse Call device
2. RJ 45 point for Computer networking
3. RJ 11 for Intercom and extension line
4. Point for reading light for patient

Similarly, at the Nursing Station, the following points shall be provided:

1. Point for Nurse Call Control Console
2. RJ 45 point for Computer networking
3. RJ 11 for Intercom and extension line
4. HDMI point for computer display at other locations

18.7.15 Curtain Partitions

If not cubicles, all the beds in the ICU shall be provided with the hanging curtain partitions. Following are some issues relating to curtain partitions:

1. The Bed shall be placed in front of one wall of the ICU
2. The Bed shall have a curtain on all other three sides
3. The ceiling suspended curtain track is fixed at 2134 mm above the floor level
4. Curtains shall be hung on these tracks and shall be moveable and collapsible
5. At the bottom of the curtains, there shall be a clear area of about 457 mm from the floor for cleaning purposes

18.8 Procedure and Treatment Room

At times, some of the patients in ICU may require minor procedures like catheterization, suturing of small wounds, dressing, bandaging and bronchoscopy. At times it becomes difficult to do these procedures in the ICU due to chances of getting infected, the privacy of the patient or procedure requiring anaesthesia.

Therefore, a treatment room or procedure room is attached to the ICU.

18.8.1 Location of Treatment/Procedure Room

The following shall be the considerations for deciding the location of the Treatment/Procedure Room:

1. Treatment/Procedure Room shall be either attached to ICU or otherwise very near to ICU.
2. Treatment/Procedure Room should not be far off from the other support services like Radiology and other necessary support services.

18.8.2 Size of Treatment/Procedure Room

The size of Treatment/Procedure Room shall not be less than 4572 mm × 4572 mm.

18.8.3 Issues Related to Infrastructure of Treatment/Procedure Room

The following issues shall be kept in mind while designing the infrastructure of Treatment/Procedure Room:

1. The Treatment/Procedure Room shall be sterilized.
2. In a Treatment/Procedure Room single OT table shall be placed.
3. The Treatment/Procedure Room shall have a single entry door.
4. Attached to the Treatment/Procedure Room shall be a Gowning and Scrub Station.

18.8.4 Furniture in Treatment/Procedure Room

The following furniture shall be placed in the ICU:

Patient Furniture

OT Table	Step Stool
Instrument Trolley	Scrub Station
Stretcher Trolley	IV Stand
Dressing Trollies	IV Rod
Oxygen Cylinder Trolley	Crash Cart
Instrument Trollies	Patient Transfer System

18.8.5 Equipment

Multi Para Vital Sign Monitor	Portable Operating Light Single Dome
Infusion Pump	Laryngoscope
Suction Machine	Oxygen Cylinders with Masks
Defibrillator	B.P. Apparatus
View Boxes	Ambu bag with Mask of different sizes

18.8.6 Tools and Instruments

Sterilizing Drums	Torches
Examination Light	Needle Holders
Instrument Boxes	Chetal Forceps
Extension Cord and Boxes	Forceps of all styles and sizes
All other required instruments	Suture Sets
Scissors of all styles and sizes	Tray of all styles and sizes

18.8.7 Doors

The Door of the Treatment/Procedure Room shall not be less than 1524 mm wide, unobstructed. The door shall be openable on both the sides in and out.

18.8.8 Windows

Windows need not be provided in the Treatment/Procedure Room.

18.8.9 Handwashing

For handwash, a single bay scrub shall be provided, which shall be operational with sensors and/or foot.

18.8.10 Central Piped Medical Gas Supply

As the surgical interventions have to be done in Treatment/Procedure Room, the gases to be supplied are:

- Oxygen
- Compressed Air
- Suction

The Ceiling suspended pendant should be provided. This panel is to be fixed on the ceiling and is suspended below such that the bottom of the pendant shall be 1524 mm from the floor.

In Treatment/Procedure Room shall have the following gas outlets:

1. 2 outlets for Oxygen
2. 2 outlet for Compressed Air
3. 2 outlets for Suction

On the Pendent both the electrical and the communication points and ports shall be provided. Details are given in the electrical point and Communication point below.

18.8.11 Electrical Points in Treatment/Procedure Room

The following electrical points shall be provided in the treatment/procedure room:

1. Main Switchboard shall be at the entrance wall for controlling fans and lights of the hall along with one 6 Amp Switch/Socket.
2. Air Conditioning Control button with temperature adjustment.
3. On Hanging Pendent, electrical points are to be provided. There shall be at least 3 pairs of 6/16 Amp switches/sockets on the back wall

of the pendant. These points shall be on UPS supply.
4. On three walls of the Treatment/Procedure Room (leaving the wall on which door is provided) in the centre of each wall, a pair of two 6/16 Amp. switches/sockets is to be provided at the height of 457 mm from the floor level. Out of these two, one pair shall be on UPS.

18.8.12 Other Communication Points in Treatment/ Procedure Room

The following communication points shall be provided in the Treatment/Procedure Room at any convenient place/wall:

1. RJ 45 point for Computer networking
2. RJ 11 for Intercom and extension line
3. HDMI point for computer display at other locations

18.8.13 Other Issues on Patient Care Zone and Procedure/ Treatment Room

1. **Clear Floor Space**

   Clear floor space is a space not utilized by the patient, equipment and fixed room furnishings. As sometimes a lot of medical equipment may be required for treatment of patients, it is advisable to keep the maximum floor clear around the bed to be used for equipment like portable X-ray, echocardiography and dialysis machines. That is the reason why it is recommended to keep 1828 mm the distance between two beds.
2. **Patient Room Furnishings**

   ICU rooms or units shall have a decent and aesthetic finish and look. It helps a lot for the early recovery of the patient and leaves a long-term effect on the patient about the quality of service. Hence, the furnishing of the patient room/unit shall be designed carefully. In the room/unit, apart from the furniture as mentioned above, the room shall also be furnished with:
   (a) Soiled linen collection hamper.
   (b) The waste collection as per the norms of Biomedical Waste Management.
   (c) A Wall Clock on the foot end of the patient.
   (d) Calendar.
   (e) Tack Boards.
   (f) Whiteboards.
   (g) Horizontal surfaces to keep greeting cards and photos.
   (h) Mobile/ Laptop charging points.
   (i) Internet Connection / Wi-Fi.
   (j) Intercom with facility for an outside call.
   (k) Cabinet for storage of personal belongings.
   (l) A television, if it is a room but not in an ICU hall.
   (m) Secure storage space for patients' and family clothing and limited personal effects.
3. **Room Decor**

   Pleasant aesthetic surroundings for patients and increased comfort results in improved outcomes. The care to be taken shall be:
   (a) Good Colour schemes affect mood and stress levels. Particularly light green and blue colours decrease the stress levels of patients.
   (b) Wall furnishings shall be excellent with waterproof washable paints.
   (c) Pictures, paintings, murals and artwork shall be placed appropriately for patients, families and caregivers.
   (d) For bed-ridden patients, the ceiling is most often what is seen. The ceiling can be painted with pictures and sceneries. Even 3D laminated ceilings can be opted.

18.8.14 Lighting in the ICU

Lighting for general illumination and specific tasks has to be carefully planned. Few issues related to lighting, to be considered are:

1. The Lights shall not be too bright or too dull. Proper lumens have to be planned as per the standards.

2. Use of LED lights is always recommended because of the long life of the LEDs and lower energy consumption.
3. The lights shall be equally distributed in the unit/room.
4. Surface exposed lights shall not be used. Ceiling flush-mounted lights shall be used.
5. Wall lights are not effective, hence avoid those.
6. Fancy lights shall not be used.
7. To prevent burns, incandescent and halogen light sources should be avoided.
8. Flexible arms, if used with the light source, must be mechanically controlled to prevent the lamp from contacting linen.
9. The patient bed should be provided with an adjustable reading light that can be easily controlled by the patient.
10. Separate lighting for emergencies and procedures should be located in the ceiling directly above the patient on each bed. The LED light, of 610 mm ×610 mm ceiling flush-mounted should be fixed at a 1219-mm distance from the wall. This light shall be switched on only during any procedure.
11. Night low-level illumination shall be provided at the height of 457 mm from the floor near the bed of the patient.
12. Emergency battery operated light shall be provided in the corridors and patient unit.
13. It will be better if the light controls are done through variable-control dimmers at the user end.

18.8.15 Dialysis Equipment

1. Usually, some of the patients in ICU require Haemodialysis, for bedside renal dialysis or continuous renal replacement therapy. For this, the appropriate conditions of RO/de-iodinated water supply and drain facilities shall be provided. Water and drain connections should be separate from being used for scrub stations and toilets.
2. Provision for RRT shall be made on at least two beds of ICU.

18.8.16 Power Backup

Please take the Power backup in ICU as a serious concern. The ICU should have its own power backup, which should start automatically in the event of a power failure. First of all, it shall be ensured that the essential and lifesaving equipment has its own power backup with the internal batteries of the equipment which shall be in the standard configuration of the equipment.

Secondly, the important electrical points on all the beds shall be connected to UPS. Each ICU shall have its own UPS and a common UPS for all the ICUs is not recommended. If all the ICUs are connected to common UPS, in case of breakdown of UPS, all the ICUs will have to suffer.

Thirdly, the Intensive Care Floor shall have its own backup of Auto Start Diesel Generator. Also, provide necessary provision for the regulation of the voltage or power supplied to ICUs.

18.9 Clinical Support Zone

Clinical Support Zone relates to all the functions related to the diagnosis and treatment of patients. Some of these functions may take place within the ICU Complex, adjacent areas or elsewhere in the hospital or sometimes even outside the hospital premises.

Very careful designing of this zone has to be done by the designer. He/She has to ensure that different clinical support services/rooms are available to the patient in the least possible time. Delay may cause severe irreversible damages even to the extent of risk of the patient's life.

The main diagnostic and treatment support services in the Clinical Support zone are:

18.9.1 Rigorous Monitoring

It is correctly said that all five senses have to be applied for efficient monitoring of the patient. Every sense has its own important role. Through Sight, the patient is visualized for the position or face expressions and also to visualize the multi-parameter bedside monitor located near the patient.

Secondly, the hearing of sound, the patient can be monitored through the conversation with the patient or screams of the patient. Through touch, the temperature of skin abnormality can be monitored. Through Smell the patient can be monitored for the hygienic condition. Similarly, through taste, the food being served to the patient can be monitored. Therefore, it becomes imperative for the nurse to continuously monitor the patient.

As far as arrangements are concerned, a place and means shall be provided to fix the monitor at the bedside of the patient. This can be done by providing a monitor tray on the bed head panel or on the hanging pendant. If it is not possible, the monitor tray can be fixed on the wall by fasteners, where a monitor can be installed.

At times some physicians opt for centralized monitoring through CNS (Central Nursing Station). For this, the cabling (Cat 6) has to be laid down from all the beds individually and all the cables to end at the nursing station, where the CNS is installed.

Ever-changing technology has introduced **Remote Monitoring**. In this technology, the live data parameters are sent to the physicians online for continuous monitoring and giving necessary instructions. To facilitate this, cabling has to be done from each bed to the computer placed at the nursing station, from where the data will be transmitted to the physician.

18.9.2 Radiology

The service of the radiology department is an important service that helps to diagnose and access progress during treatment. The services of Radiology can be X-Ray, CT Scan, MRI, Ultrasound Mammography, PET CT, PET MRI etc. Similarly, the DSA has an important role in the peripheral intervention of ICU patients.

Services of Radiology therefore should be readily accessible to the ICU. As far as X-ray is concerned, a portable X-ray machine shall be placed in the ICU. Similarly, the Ultrasound cum Echocardiography machine shall also be placed in the ICU. These machines shall be for the exclusive use of ICUs only and shall be parked in the equipment room of ICU.

For all other services of imaging, the radiology department shall be located at such a place that has easy and quick access to the patients of ICU. Another issue is the report of the imaging procedures. As it takes time to print the film and send it to the ICU, the system of online transmission of images is the answer. By using PACS (software), the images from the radiology department can be easily transmitted at the computer screen placed in ICU.

18.9.3 Laboratory

ICUs must have access to clinical laboratory services round the clock. As the equipment of Central Clinical Laboratory is installed in the department at a place other than ICU and the patient need not be moved to the laboratory, it hardly matters if the laboratory is not placed in the ICU Complex.

However, a full-fledged **Sample Collection Room shall** be located near the ICU, with a facility of specimen collection, short-time storage and pre-processing of the specimen can be done here.

Apart from the routine specimens that need to be sent to the laboratory, a few lab investigations have to be done in the ICU itself, such as arterial blood gas analysis and mixed venous blood gas analysis. Hence, a convenient space shall be allotted in the ICU itself for placing such machines. This space shall fulfil all the requirements for installation like the electrical point, water supply/drain and temperature required to run the machine.

Pneumatic tube systems may be used for rapid transport of specimens to and from the laboratory.

18.9.4 Medication Rooms

While designing the ICU setup, the designer shall consider the location of the Medication Room just near the ICU. The medication room serves the purpose of storage of medicines and distribution to the patient. Considering the fact that, as most of the patients are sick in ICUs, the pharmacy services should be readily accessible and operative round the clock. The room with the approx. Size of 3658 mm × 3658 mm shall be placed near the ICU. However, the size of the room can be increased depending on the requirement. The room shall have the facility for cabinets, drawers and racks for storage of medicines. The room shall be provided with an ample countertop for disbursing medicines. If the medication room is attached to the ICU, a window can be given which shall open in the ICU, from where quick communication can be done. Also, the provision of a refrigerator shall be made in the room. Similarly, the provision of the Telephone line and intercom shall also be done. Nowadays, the automated dispensing machines are also used for dispensing medicines.

The medication room should be large enough to accommodate at least a staff of two, a nurse and a pharmacist who shall double-check the accuracy of medicines being supplied.

The medicines and drugs can be transferred from the main pharmacy store by a messenger which takes a long time. An alternative to this is Pneumatic Tube Systems (PTS). What is PTS and how it works is explained below?

18.9.5 Pneumatic Tube Systems

The PTS is an air pressure operated system having the air pump installed in the control station. This system is used as a transport system of documents, material and medicines. This is the best, accurate and quickest mode of transport of small documents, specimens, material and medicines.

In this system, at all the important points of the hospital (called stations) where the documents and specimens have to be sent or from where the material and medicines have to be transported, an outlet is installed along with a control unit. These areas can be ICUs, laboratories, sample collection rooms, pharmacy, billing and radiology. The networking of the plastic pipe is installed in the hospital which opens at the desired stations. Then there are boxes in the shape of a capsule, which carries the material and documents. These boxes run in the pipeline and carry the desired material to a specific location.

It is very easy to operate. The user has to just put the desired material to be transported in these capsules and give the command to the system and feed the station ID where the material has to be sent. In seconds, the material or document is transported to the desired location.

18.9.6 Clean Utility

The clean utility is a room attached to ICUs or any other service unit, which is used for storage of the clean linen. The sterilized material like drums and drapes is also stored in this room.

Normally, the room shall not be less than 3658 mm × 3658 mm. But depending on the requirements, the size of the room can be changed. The room is provided with closed cabinets, drawers and racks. This room shall have only one door of about 914 mm.

18.9.7 Dirty Utility/Sluice Room

The dirty utility is a room attached to ICUs or any other service units, which is used for storage of soiled linen. From here the linen is moved for pre-wash before sending it to the laundry.

Normally, the room shall not be less than 3658 mm × 3658 mm but depending on the requirements, the size of the room can be changed. The room is provided with covered linen collection hampers or containers to collect the dirty linen. This room shall have two doors of about 914 mm. One door shall open in the ICU and the other in the corridor from where the laundry staff can collect the linen and he/she need not come to the ICU for collection of linen. Instead of a door on the ICU side, an openable window can be provided. Air from this room has to be exhausted, hence exhaust fans are a must and shall be provided.

18.9.8 Equipment Park/Store

Generally, in ICU there are few medical equipment which is not always in use, but have to be kept ready all times to be used whenever required. Hence, this equipment has to be stored at a separate place in the ICU so that the floor space of the ICU is not unnecessarily occupied with this equipment. Therefore, the equipment storage room/area is provided in the ICU.

Normally, the room of size not less than 4267 mm × 4267 mm is provided attached to ICU. This area can be a closed room with a door or otherwise open area attached to ICU. The room shall have the provision of grounded electrical charging points for charging the unused medical equipment.

18.9.9 Emergency Eyewash Station

Staff working in ICUs are exposed to many hazardous fluids. Despite universal precautions, splashes of chemicals/bodily fluids can occur. Therefore, an eyewash station shall be provided near the scrub station of ICU.

18.10 Unit Support Zone

The unit support zone consists of areas where administrative, logistic and staff support functions are performed.

18.10.1 Change Room: Male/Female in ICU

ICU being a most hygienic and clean area, no outside clothes shall be allowed in the ICU. Therefore, the staff must change into sterilized clothes by changing the outside dress. The following issues shall be considered regarding Change room (Fig. 18.2):

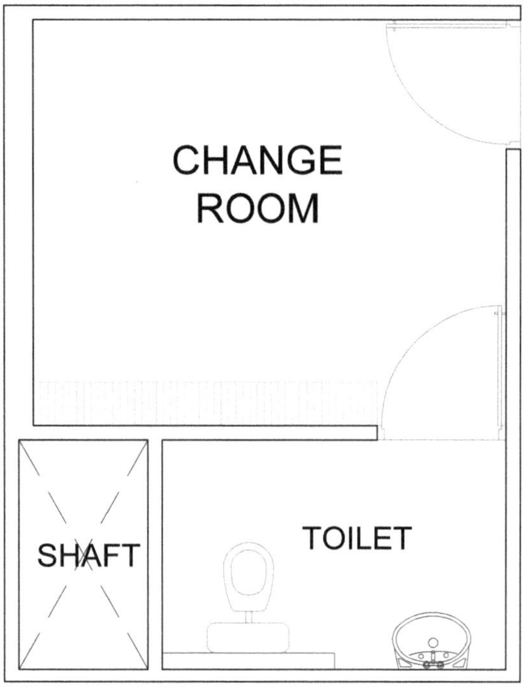

Fig. 18.2 Sample of change room drawing

1. Separate change rooms shall be provided, one for males and the second for females.
2. The room shall be of the size 4572 mm × 4267 mm.
3. The room shall have a provision of an attached toilet.
4. Furniture wise, the room shall have one chair and cupboards.
5. Almirah shall be provided with the provision for hanging clothes.
6. Apart from the light and fan, the room shall have points for Intercom.
7. Also, the room shall be Air Conditioned and the Control button with temperature adjustment shall be provided in the room.
8. In the change room, staff lockers shall also be provided where the staff can keep their personal belongings. Individual lockers shall be about 610 mm × 305 mm. These individual lockers are combined and the locker almirah can be fabricated. Each locker shall be secured separately. One such locker shall be allotted to each staff on duty.

18.10.2 Doctors Duty Rooms in ICU

Generally, depending on the size of ICU, and the number of beds in each ICU, the physicians from different disciplines shall be placed in the ICU to provide immediate care to the patients. In that case, one or more than one Doctors duty room shall have to be provided in the ICU complex. The following issues shall be considered regarding provided duty rooms in ICU:

1. One or more rooms for the physicians of each department shall be allotted.
2. The room shall be of the size 4267 mm × 3658 mm.
3. Rooms shall have a provision of an attached toilet.
4. Furniture wise, the room shall have one office table, chair, bed and cupboard.
5. Apart from the light and fan, the room shall have points for a computer with Internet connection and Intercom point etc.
6. Also, the room shall be Air Conditioned and the Control button with temperature adjustment shall be provided in the room.

18.10.3 Nurses Night Duty Rooms in ICU

At times, due to the heavy load of work in the ICU, or due to overwork, the Nurses feel tired. Otherwise, it also happens due to the shortage of nursing staff they may have to perform double duties. Under both circumstances, the nurses need to take rest. Generally, depending on the size of ICU and the number of beds in each ICU, the nurse's night duty room shall be planned. At least one such room shall be provided with each ICU. The following issues shall be considered regarding provided nurses with duty rooms in ICU:

1. The room shall be of the size 3658 mm × 3658 mm.
2. Rooms shall have a provision of an attached toilet.
3. Furniture wise, the room shall have a bed and cupboard.
4. Apart from the light and fan, the room shall have a point for Intercom.
5. Also, the room shall be Air Conditioned and the Control button with temperature adjustment shall be provided in the room.

18.10.4 Night Duty Room for On-Call Junior Doctors

During the daytime, all the physicians are in the hospital to take care of the patient in ICU, but this is not true for the night. Hence for the night, junior doctors are posted and they are supposed to be on duty in the ICU or near ICU. Hence a room has to be allotted to them for taking rest. The following issues shall be considered regarding provided duty rooms in ICU:

1. One or more rooms for the junior doctors shall be provided.
2. The room shall be of the size 4267 mm × 3658 mm.
3. Rooms shall have a provision of an attached toilet.
4. Furniture wise, the room shall have one office table, chair, bed and cupboard.
5. Apart from the light and fan, the room shall have points for a computer with internet connection and Intercom point etc.
6. Also, the room shall be Air Conditioned and the Control button with temperature adjustment shall be provided in the room.

18.10.5 Ward Pantry

As the patients admitted in ICU have to be served a full day diet, there shall be a space for storage of diet and further distribution. This space is called the Ward Pantry. It is not necessary that the diet has to be cooked in the ICU premises; the diet is prepared in the kitchen and then sent to the ward pantry for further distribution. The diet is sent in bulk from the kitchen either packed for direct distribution or otherwise in an unpacked position.

The size of the ward pantry shall be about 3658 mm × 3658 mm, with a single door opening outside in the corridor. The ward pantry shall have a countertop for packing the food. Along with the countertop, a sink with hot and cold water shall be available. The waste bin/s has to be kept in the ward pantry and a trolley for collecting soiled utensils. A microwave oven may be useful.

18.10.6 Staff Lounge

After long hours of tiring working, the staff definitely needs some rest and refreshment. Therefore, a staff lounge shall be provided near the ICU Complex. The capacity shall depend on the number of ICUs and staff. An ideal lounge shall be having a seating of about 25–30 persons. The lounge should be well ventilated to remove food smells from the ICU complex. Preferably an attached toilet shall be provided with the lounge.

Lounge shall provide a private, comfortable, spacious and relaxing environment. The lounge should have a comfortable seating arrangement, a table with chairs for dining and food storage facilities, including a refrigerator, microwave oven and coffee dispenser or maker. Additionally, a television and a computer with internet access can also be provided. In the lounge, a notice board shall be provided, as it is the best place to display any information relevant to the staff.

The staff lounge should be connected to ICU by telephone or intercom so that in case of emergency they can be contacted immediately.

18.11 Family Support Zone

Along with the patients, anxious family members or friends also usually visit the hospital. While the patient is in ICU, it is not advisable to allow these family members or friends to visit patients. But family support has been recognized as an important factor in a patient's recovery and reduced morbidity.

For this, a Family Support Zone is placed at a distance from the main ICU Complex, consisting of those spaces and functions outside of the patient room to serve family and visitors.

The Family Support Zone should have the following:

18.11.1 Family Lounge

A family and visitor's lounge should be provided adjacent to or near ICU Complex. If the ICUs are scattered at different places, a lounge shall be provided for each ICU. Lounges shall be placed at such places which do not disrupt the patient, staff and supply circulation system of the hospital.

A lounge must have a comfortable space to wait, reclining chairs to relax, the privacy of conversations, telephone and intercom facility. The Lounge shall also have basic amenities like a small snacks bar, television, newspaper and magazine stand and a small play area for children. Coffee and tea vending machines shall also be provided. Visitor access should be controlled from a separate reception area provided in the lounge itself.

Shelves, closets and secured lockers shall also be provided in the lounge to avoid scattering the personal belongings here and there around the lounge. Accessible toilets for males and females shall be close to or part of the lounge (Fig. 18.3).

18.11.2 Consultation Rooms

Family members and friends being anxious to know the position and development in the condition of the patient need to meet the treating physician and have an interaction with him. Therefore, the Consultation Rooms are provided for this purpose. This room shall be about 4572 mm × 4267 mm with a provision of a doctor's table, chairs and a sofa set. The physician goes to that room, calls for the family members of the patient and has an interaction with them.

At times there can be hot discussions between the physicians and the visitors of the patient. Therefore, some security personnel shall be

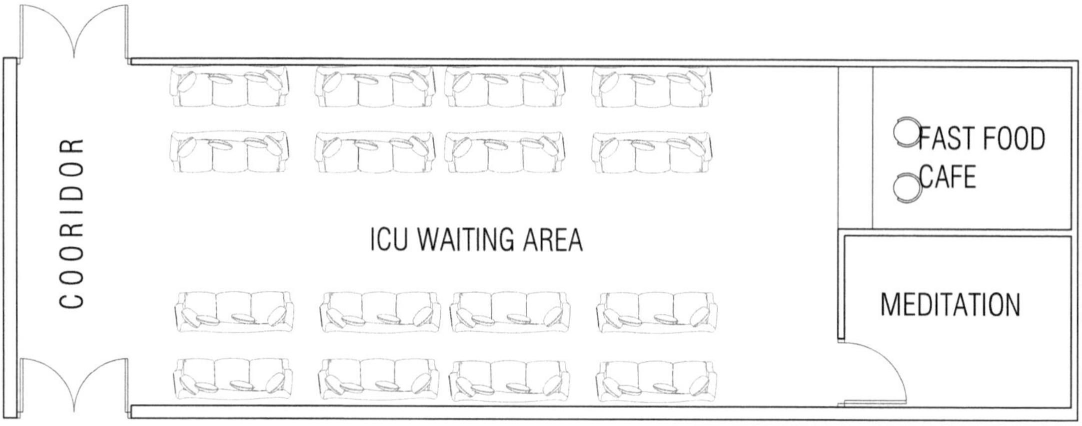

Fig. 18.3 Sample layout drawing of ICU waiting lounge

placed outside the room. Furthermore, this room shall be under CCTV surveillance from inside with audio-video recording.

18.11.3 Meditation Spaces

Disturbed family members of the patient are normally under fear and often seek blessings from the Almighty. Therefore, it is advised that near the ICU space shall be provided for a Medic Room for meditation, reflection and spiritual contemplation. Particular attention should be paid while designing the space that there shall be space for all religions and not particularly for any one religion.

18.11.4 Family Cafeteria

For the convenience of the family members, adequate provision of cafeteria shall be made in the hospital. Usually, a cafeteria is provided on the ground floor of the hospital where they can get the refreshment. Drinking fountains or another fresh water supply should be conveniently located within or near the cafeteria and lounge.

Some hospitals provide food trays to families at mealtimes. In that case, a separate space or dining hall shall be provided where the family members can be served the meals. Vending machines can also be helpful, particularly at late hours when hospital coffee shops or food services may not be available.

In both cases, care shall be taken to provide arrangements for disposal of utensils and maintain hygiene. The arrangement shall be made in such a fashion that the smell of the food does not spread in the hospital complex.

18.11.5 Family Sleep Rooms

It has been seen that some patients need to stay in ICU or other units of the hospital for a long time, maybe weeks or months. Even for some diseases, the patient may have to visit the hospital for a few hours for treatment like chemotherapy or radiotherapy. Under such circumstances, the patient and or the family members are really in a confused state of mind about where to stay. Particularly for the long-distance patients, it is not always possible to return home to rest.

It is recommended that on the availability of land, a separate guest house shall be provided, which can be allotted to family members on a paid basis. These guest houses may have all the amenities like mess, toilet, bed, TV, fridge and bedding.

If the space for a guest house is not available, the hospital can enter into an agreement with a nearby hotel to accommodate visitors and families coming from out of town, the rent of which shall be paid by the family member.

18.11.6 Family Laundry

This can be an extra facility provided to the family members of the patient, particularly the patients who have to stay long in the hospital. For such a facility, a separate counter can be dedicated where the clothes can be given to and collected from. The unwashed clothes can be sent to the central laundry of the hospital for a wash and returned to the same counter from where they were collected. This service shall be payable to the visitors.

18.12 Specialized Intensive Care Units

Apart from the generalized ICUs like Medical and Surgical ICUs, there are some specialized ICUs that are designed to provide treatment for a particular disease or discipline like Cardiology, Respiratory, Neuro Surgery, CTVS, Neonatal and Burn A few of them are as mentioned below:

18.12.1 Intensive Coronary Care Unit

Intensive Coronary Care Unit (ICCU) is designed and used mainly for cardiac patients like mayo cardiac infarction etc. This ICU is also called ICCU. While designing the ICCU care shall be taken to handle any emergency and tools like Pacemaker and Echocardiography machines are readily available. In the case of an ICCU, excessive noise and visual clutter shall be ruled out, otherwise, it can have an adverse effect on heart rates, arrhythmias and blood pressure.

18.12.2 Respiratory Care ICU

This ICU is designed to treat patients suffering from respiratory diseases like COPD and respiratory distress. Most of the sick patients of this ICU may require ventilated support. Hence the design shall give sufficient backup for the supply of medical gases. These patients may also require Arterial Blood Gas tests done occasionally. Hence, the provision for ABG machines shall be done in the ICU itself.

18.12.3 Neurosurgical Intensive Care Unit

Most of the patients in this ICU are suffering from Head Injuries which can be either conservative or post-operative. Being head injury, the chances of immediate deterioration of the patient's condition cannot be ruled out. Hence, the extensive monitoring of the vitals of patients has to be done continually.

18.12.4 Burn Unit

Burn Unit is another specialized intensive care facility for treating patients of burn. This ICU has to be very sophisticated and shall be carefully planned because this is one of the highly infected ICU. All beds in this ICU shall be the isolation beds and shall be under negative pressure. Apart from this, a shower room and sterile dressing room have to be provided along with this ICU. Even if needed, Hyperbaric Chambers are also provided in the burn ICUs.

18.12.5 Geriatric ICU

This ICU is for the treatment of elderly patients. In addition to the normal medical ICU or surgical ICU, certain features need to be added to make a geriatric ICU. Because the elderly people are short of hearing and vision, the design shall avoid unnecessary noise in the ICU and provide a system with which the patient can understand the command easily. Because of diminished vision, lighting should be such that can avoid glare. This also means reducing highly reflective surfaces to a minimum.

Another risk with the elderly is to fall down because of low muscle power or weak nerves. Hence, the bed shall be adjustable to floor level. Also, proper handrails have to be provided in the walking area. Toilets shall be handicapped toilets with proper supports and railings.

18.12.6 Neonatal Intensive Care Unit

As compared to any other ICUs, the Neonatal Intensive Care Unit (NICU) has a different setup altogether. As this ICU is to be exclusively used for newborns, there are no beds in this ICU. Instead of the bed's bassinets are provided. Nowadays, bassinets have been replaced by the Servo Controlled Radiant Heat Warmers.

The main considerations while designing the NICU are:

18.12.6.1 Location of NICU

Preferably NICU shall be located near to the department where births occur like the department of Obs. & Gynae., so that after the delivery, the baby can be shifted to NICU without much exposure to the infected atmosphere.

18.12.6.2 The Infrastructure of NICU

NICU shall have the following rooms/areas (Fig. 18.4):

1. Inside baby clean ICU

    The babies delivered in the same hospital and/or who are considered to be free from any type of infection.
2. Outside or infected baby ICU

    Babies who come from outside and the state of affairs about infection is unknown.
3. Ventilation room

    Room used for taking the baby on mechanical Ventilation and who have to be rigorously monitored.
4. Step down ICU

    For the babies who are stable or who recover from ICUs but still need to be kept under monitoring.
5. Mothers' Feeding Room

    Separate room for breastfeeding the baby by mother. Please ensure the privacy of this room and no outsider shall be allowed to visit this room when in use.
6. Nappy Wash area

    Used to wash the soiled napkins of the babies. Nowadays, this is not being used much because these days the disposable absorbent baby napkins are used.
7. Formula Room

    Used to prepare the milk and diet of the babies.
8. Store
9. Clean Supply Room
10. Dirty Linen / Sluice Room
11. Nurse Station
12. Change Room
13. Scrub Station
14. Medication Room
15. Doctors Duty Room
16. Nurses Duty Room
17. Staff Toilet

18.12.6.3 Placement of Warmers

1. Area per patient space shall be about 11.15 Sq. Mtr. per bassinet.
2. The radiant warmers are placed on the wall at a distance of about 610 mm from the wall.
3. Inter-distance between two warmers shall be about 1219 mm for easy working of the staff.
4. Each warmer shall be supplied with Medical gas points as has been described above in case of ICU.

18.12.6.4 Equipment of NICU

Following are the main equipment used in NICU:

Multi-para Vital Sign Monitor	Slow Suction Machine
Neonatal Mechanical Ventilator with a low Tidal Volume starting from 5 to 10 onwards	Servo Controlled Radiant Heat Warmer mounted with the baby trolley
Non-invasive Ventilator	Paediatric B.P. Apparatus
High-flow Nasal Canula	Defibrillator
Infusion Syringe Pump	Skin Sensor Thermometer
Electronic Weighing Machine Basket type	Oxygen Cylinders with Masks
Phototherapy unit on the stand—Upper Surface	Ambu bag with Pediatric Masks
Phototherapy unit on the stand—Under Surface	Laryngoscope
Humidifiers	Transport Incubator
View Boxes	Bilirubin meter
Oxygen Hoods of various sizes	Vein Finder
Other small tools and instruments required	Resuscitation Units for Delivery Suites

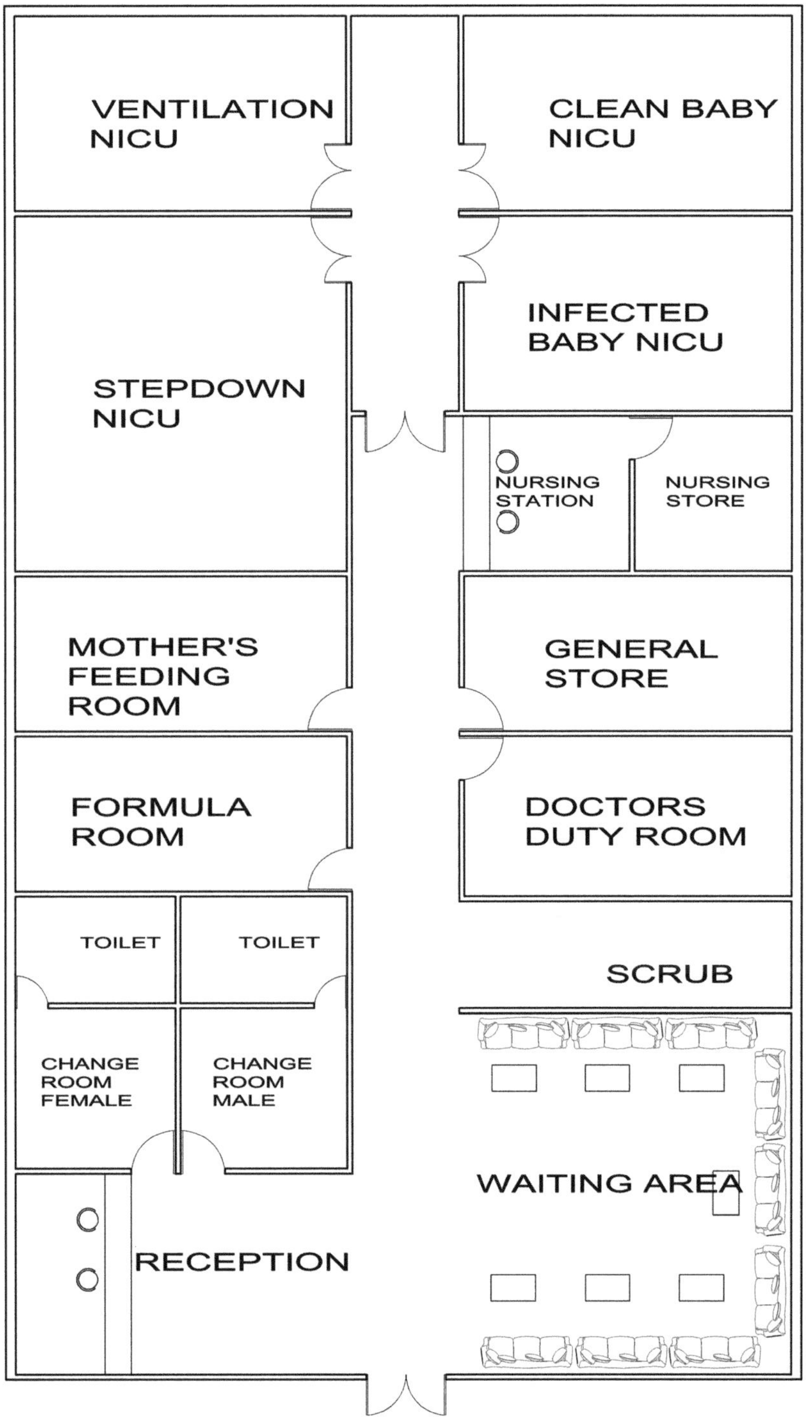

Fig. 18.4 Sample layout drawing of neonatal ICU

18.13 Common Design Considerations

18.13.1 Signage and Way Finding

Signage in the ICU Complex shall be clearly visible to the visitors. The multilingual signboard with arrow markers shall be used. For the ICU floor, a different colour coding can be used. Other techniques like landmarks, art and floor patterns may be considered. Public notices, rules and regulations for public and facilities available to the visitors etc. shall be affixed in the Visitors Lounge. Patient room number or Bed number shall be clearly marked. Directional signage should be easy to read, understand and follow.

18.13.2 Security and Access Control

ICU Complex shall have a limited and dedicated entrance which shall be guarded properly with the provision of surveillance with CCTV. Only authorized visitors with official passes shall be allowed to enter the ICU complex. The entrance shall be provided with the proper communication systems like Intercom or Mobile to allow communication between the ICU staff. Even the entrance from visitors lounge to the ICUs shall be guarded so that unrequired movement of visitors to and from ICUs shall be controlled. If due to financial restraints, it becomes difficult to place guards round the clock, an option is to provide the visitors with a Card-key to open the door.

18.13.3 Patient Safety Technology

This technology is basically used to identify the actual and right patient for medications, blood transfusion, investigations, procedures etc. Therefore, technologies such as barcoding or radio frequency identification shall be used. The designers have to just ensure to make provision of such technologies to be adopted.

18.13.4 Communications

For efficient treatment and patient safety, the communication system has to be very effective. The communication with other ICUs, patient rooms or modules, physician on-call rooms, conference rooms, supply room, diagnostic departments, administration, security, blood bank, pharmacy, the staff lounge etc. has to be quick and perfect. Communication systems like Intercom, telephones and technologies such as pneumatic tube stations and dumbwaiters shall be used.

18.13.5 Storage

The ICU design should provide adequate storage for all equipment, supplies, consumable materials, medical disposables and other items currently being used. The designer shall also consider future requirements while designing the storage space. Storage is needed for personal items belonging to staff, patients and visitors. Equipment and supplies storage shall be designed to be stored as close as possible to point of use. The storage shall be lockable as far as possible and shall be free from humidity, termite proof and fire safe. Particular care shall be taken for storage of medicines and injectable etc. and shall be properly marked and under the strict control of an authorized person.

18.13.6 Relationships with Other Departments

Intensive care units should be as close as possible to the areas like emergency, Operation Theatre Suite, Pathology and Radiology. It is evident that most of the admissions in ICUs are either through the emergency department or from the operating rooms following major surgery. These departments shall not be too far from the ICU complex as patients may have to be transferred to any of these departments as and when required. Close/easy proximity is also desirable to diagnostic facilities, blood bank, pharmacy etc.

18.13.7 Central Nursing Station

- This is the nerve centre of ICU, hence with the changing technologies, the design of nursing stations also changes from time to time.
- Most important is the location of the nursing station in the ICUs. Preferably the nursing station shall be located such that all or nearly all monitors and patients must be observable from there, either directly or through the central monitoring system.
- Ensure that there is enough space and chairs to meet the requirement of the staff. The space shall also be available to accommodate computer terminals and printers.
- In case of space constraint, collapsible desktops or shelves that can flip up on the wall can be planned.
- Sufficient cupboards shall be provided to keep the necessary items that may be required for nursing care. All these cupboards should be labelled and lockable.
- By the bedside of the patient, over-bed tables shall be able to accommodate vital charts and cupboards shall be sufficient to store medicines, disposables investigations and records of the patient.
- If the concept of the sub-nursing station is followed, provisions shall be made that each nursing substation should be capable of providing most, if not, all functions of a central station.
- There must be adequate overhead and task lighting, and a wall-mounted clock should be present.

18.13.8 Patient Records

Adequate space and seating shall be provided for the physicians and nurses to sit and complete medical record charting Shelving, file cabinets and other storage for medical record forms must be located nearby so that they are readily accessible by all personnel requiring their use.

18.13.9 X-ray Viewing Area

Some physicians or the management prefer a separate room or distinct area near ICUs for viewing and storage of patient radiological films. An illuminated viewing box of appropriate size shall be provided in this room for viewing X-ray films.

18.13.10 Reception Area

The ICUs should have a reception area to control visitor access. Ideally, the reception shall be located at such a place that visitors must pass by this area before entering the ICU complex. The receptionist should be connected with the ICUs by telephone and/or other intercommunication systems.

18.13.11 Corridors in ICU Complex

An ICU complex shall have:

1. A separate corridor for entrance and movement of the visitors and shall be separate from that being used by healthcare professionals.

2. Healthcare workers and the patients may have the same corridor for entrance and movement.
3. A separate perimeter corridor with easy entrance and exit can be provided for supplying and servicing each ICU. Removal of soiled items and waste should also be accomplished through this corridor. But generally, this concept is now not adopted anywhere.
4. The corridor should be at least 2438 mm in width. Doorways, openings and passages into each ICU must be a minimum of 1829 mm in width to allow easy and unobstructed movement of equipment and supplies.

18.13.12 Administrative Offices

It is desirable to have a space for administrative offices adjacent to the ICU(s) for medical and nursing management and administrative personnel. This can also be the requirement of an interdisciplinary team like office for management, education and clinical speciality purposes. Office spaces should be large enough to accommodate necessary equipment and shall have comfortable furnishings and to permit meetings and consultations with ICU team members and/or patients' families. Also providing a Multipurpose Conference Room can be thought of which shall be capable of accommodating educational/training conferences, multidisciplinary staff meetings. This conference room shall have a provision of audio-visual equipment and high-speed Internet connections. It should have provision to access hospital/health information system, picture archiving, communication system monitors, emergency cardiac arrest alarms and a telephone or other intercommunication systems linking to the ICU.

Further Reading

Bartley J, Streifel AJ. Design of the environment of care for safety of patients and personnel: Does form follow function or vice versa in the intensive care unit? Crit Care Med. 2010 Aug;38:S388.

Bazuin D, Cardon K. Creating Healing Intensive Care Unit Environments: Physical and Psychological Considerations in Designing Critical Care Areas. Crit Care Nurs Q. 2011 Oct 1;34:259–67.

Chen H-L, Chen C-H, Wu C-C, Huang H-J, Wang T-M, Hsu C-C. The Influence of Neonatal Intensive Care Unit Design on Sound Level. Pediatr Neonatol. 2009 Dec 1;50(6):270–4.

Ferri M, Zygun DA, Harrison A, Stelfox HT. Evidence-based design in an intensive care unit: End-user perceptions. BMC Anesthesiol. 2015 Apr 25;15(1):57.

HealthManagement.org. Radiology Management, ICU Management, Healthcare IT, Cardiology Management, Executive Management [Internet]. HealthManagement. [cited 2021 Jun 18]. Available from: https://healthmanagement.org/c/icu/issuearticle/future-icu-design-return-to-high-visibility

Journal of Marine Medical Society - Planning a modular intensive care unit for patients of the COVID-19 pandemic: Download PDF [Internet]. [cited 2021 Jun 18]. Available from: https://www.marinemedicalsociety.in/downloadpdf.asp?issn=0975-3605;year=2020;volume=22;issue=3;spage=51;epage=56;aulast=Narayan;type=2

Katirci Y, Şafak T, Aydemir S. A Review of Design Features of Intensive Care Unit in General Terms.:8.

Kesecioglu J. Improving the patient's environment: the ideal intensive care unit. Réanimation. 2015 Jan 1;24(2):341–3.

Rashid M. A decade of adult intensive care unit design: a study of the physical design features of the best-practice examples. Crit Care Nurs Q. 2006 Dec;29(4):282–311.

Rashid M. Environmental Design for Patient Families in Intensive Care Units. J Healthc Eng. 2010;1(3):367–98.

Robinson J. The design and function of an intensive care unit. Br J Anaesth. 1966;

Rungta DN, Govil DD, Nainan DS, Munjal DM. ICU Planning and Designing in India – Guidelines 2010. :26.

Rungta N, Zirpe KG, Dixit SB, Mehta Y, Chaudhry D, Govil D, et al. Indian Society of Critical Care Medicine Experts Committee Consensus Statement on ICU Planning and Designing, 2020. Indian J Crit Care

Med Peer-Rev Off Publ Indian Soc Crit Care Med. 2020 Jan;24(Suppl 1):S43–60.

SALUS - Article - Critical care design of tomorrow: how technology fits in [Internet]. [cited 2021 Jun 18]. Available from: https://www.salus.global/journal/view/article/critical-care-design-of-tomorrow-how-technology-fits-in-1

Sessler CN. Evolution of ICU Design: Smarter Is Better. CHEST. 2014 Feb 1;145(2):205–6.

Technology and the Future of Intensive Care Unit Design [Internet]. [cited 2021 Jun 18]. Available from: //www.nursingcenter.com/journalarticle?Article_ID=1236265&Journal_ID=54003&Issue_ID=1236032

Thompson DR, Hamilton DK, Cadenhead CD, Swoboda SM, Schwindel SM, Anderson DC, et al. Guidelines for intensive care unit design*. Crit Care Med. 2012 May;40(5):1586–600.

Tripathy S, Acharya SP, Sahoo AK, Mitra JK, Goel K, Ahmad SR, et al. Intensive care unit (ICU) diaries and the experiences of patients' families: a grounded theory approach in a lower middle-income country (LMIC). J Patient-Rep Outcomes. 2020 Jul 23;4(1):63.

Valentin A, Ferdinande P, ESICM Working Group on Quality Improvement. Recommendations on basic requirements for intensive care units: structural and organizational aspects. Intensive Care Med. 2011 Sep 15;37(10):1575.

White RD, Smith JA, Shepley MM. Recommended standards for newborn ICU design, eighth edition. J Perinatol. 2013 Apr;33(1):S2–16.

19 Operation Theatre Suite

Operating Theatre (O.T.) is a place where the operations, surgical procedures and other invasive interventions are carried out. It offers a sterile environment, with all personnel wearing protective clothing including shoe covers, masks, caps, eye shields and other coverings to prevent the spread of germs and microorganisms. The environment is brightly lit, and the temperature and humidity are maintained as per requirements.

However, only the Operating Theatre does not complete the definition of the 'Operating Theatre Suite/Complex'. It is more like a set of different rooms located in different zones of the whole complex.

19.1 Location of Operating Theatre (O.T.) Complex

While finalizing the location of the O.T. complex, the following points shall be considered:

1. It shall be in a restricted area, where the general movement is not allowed.
2. Complete O.T. complex shall be located at the same place as a cluster, ideally on the same floor. Avoid scattering it into different areas.
3. This complex shall be somewhere in the middle of the building and shall be sandwiched between two floors. There is often an argument that O.T. complex should be on the top floor of the hospital. But considering the thermal losses because of the high temperature in summers, the Air Conditioning has to be much more powerful, resulting in more operational costs. Another drawback by O.T. complex being on the top floor is that this complex will be away from other support services like pathology, radiology and Blood Bank.
4. Two connected corridors opposite to each other shall be available—one which can be used as an entry to O.T. complex and the other to be used as an exit from the O.T. complex.
5. Elevators and lifts shall be available near the O.T. complex.
6. Lesser the outer wall in the O.T. complex, better it will be.
7. Intensive Care Units (ICU) shall be in close proximity to the O.T. complex.

19.2 Zones in O.T. Complex

Normally, the O.T. complex is divided into four zones:

19.2.1 Unsterile Zone

This is a zone that is normally unsterile and the movement is allowed without any change.

A. Garg, A. Dewan, *Manual of Hospital Planning and Designing*,
https://doi.org/10.1007/978-981-16-8456-2_19

19.2.2 Protective Zone

This zone is comparatively more sterile and the movement is restricted, but not always. The area can be assessed only by changing the shoes.

19.2.3 Clean Zone

This area is more sterile and mainly for the exit of the change room, the supply of materials and services, and the spaces forwards like pre- and post-operative wards.

19.2.4 Sterile Zone

This area is extremely sterile and aseptic, is and reserved for the actual surgeries and interventions. None other than people actually involved in performing the surgery or assisting in surgery should be allowed to enter.

One significant issue is that the **O.T. complex shall have separate entry and exit doors connected to corridors. The O.T. complex movement has to be one way, i.e. backward movement is not allowed under any circumstances.** The movement can be clockwise or anticlockwise as per design.

19.3 Infrastructure of O.T. Complex

Following is the zone-wise list of different rooms in the complex (Fig. 19.1):

Unsterile Zone	Administrative area
	Operation theatre in-charge or manager
	Head of the anaesthesia department
	Surgeons room for office work
	Frozen section biopsy laboratory
	Entry door for changing room
	Trolley bay
	Shoe changing area
	Linen pre-wash room
	Instrument washroom
	Waiting area for attendants
	Public utility for attendants
Protective Zone	Staff changing technicians with toilet—males
	Staff changing technicians with toilet—females
	Staff changing class IV with toilet—males
	Staff changing class IV with toilet—females
	Students changing with toilet—males
	Students changing with toilet—females
	Doctors change room with toilet—males
	Doctors change room with toilet—females
	Lockers
	Entry gate of the pre-operative ward
	Unsterile store for equipment storage
	Store for medicines, consumables and disposables
	Pantry
Clean Zone	Pre-operative room
	Exit gate of the pre-operative ward
	Surgeons restroom
	Restroom for staff—males
	Restroom for staff—females
	Exit doors of all change rooms
	Dirty utility
	Pre-anaesthetic check-up room (PAC)
	Preparation room
	Post-operative recovery ward
	Public utility for patients
Sterile Zone	Main operating theatres
	Septic operation theatre
	Endoscopy room
	Scrub station
	Instrument trolley lay-up
	Clean supply room
	Sterilization room

19.4 Unsterile Zone

This area of the O.T. complex is unsterile, and the movement is allowed to all those who need to provide services or material, or require any communication with the O.T. staff. This area is located at the entry gate of the O.T. complex and is connected through the entry corridor. Details of rooms located in this zone are:

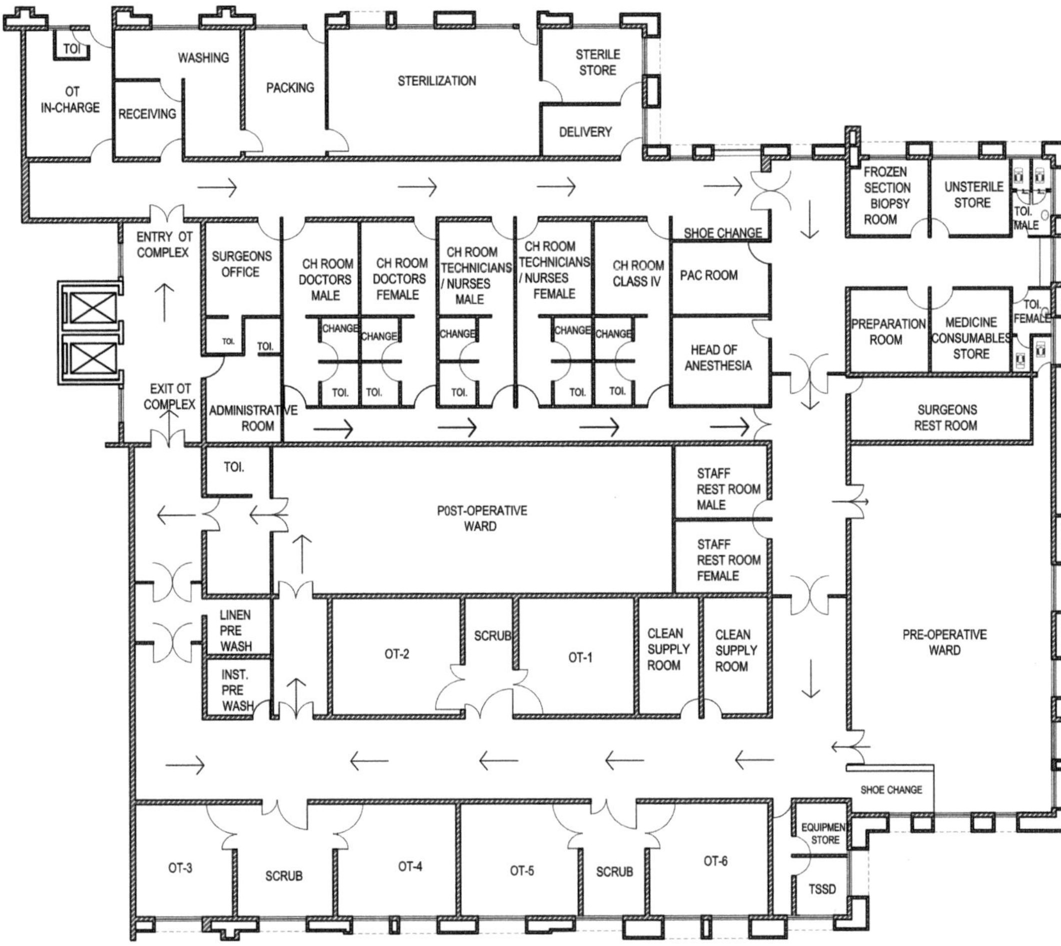

Fig. 19.1 Sample layout drawing of a standard operating theatre complex

19.4.1 Administrative Area

This is for the general administrators and clerical staff managing the O.T. complex. The staff can be from the H.R., Purchase, Stores, Sterilization, Housekeeping and Nursing department. The size of this room shall be about 4572 mm × 6096 mm, but depending on the requirement and number of persons likely to sit, the size can be increased or decreased. The room shall have an adequate arrangement of cabinets, drawers and racks for smooth working. Office tables and chairs shall also be provided. Preferably, the room shall have an attached toilet. If required, a separate store shall be attached to this room. The room shall also have proper arrangements for electrical points, intercom connection, I.T. network, CCTV surveillance and air conditioning.

19.4.2 Operation Theatre In-charge or Manager

This room is for the In-charge of O.T. complex and shall again be located at the entry of the O.T. complex. As he/she is the person who manages the entire non-medical operations of the complex, naturally he/she will have a lot of visitors and staff. The size of this room shall be about 4572 mm × 4267 mm. The room shall include an arrangement of office tables, executive chair, visitor chairs and side rack. The room shall have an attached toilet. The room shall also have an attached P.A. room for a clerk to be seated. If required and long working hours are expected, a small restroom/lounge can also be provided with this room. The room shall have proper arrangements for electrical points, intercom connection, I.T. network and air conditioning.

19.4.3 Room for Head of Anaesthesia

Officially, the anaesthetist being the medico person is also treated as the in-charge of the O.T. complex. However, his/her scope of work is limited to the medical administration. The non-medical administration is left to the manager. This room shall be located adjacent to the manager's room. The size of this room shall be about 4572 mm × 4267 mm. The room shall contain an arrangement of office tables, executive chair, visitor chairs, side rack etc. The room shall have an attached toilet. The room shall also have an attached P.A. room for a clerk to be seated. If required and long working hours are expected, a small restroom/ lounge can also be provided with this room. The room shall have proper arrangements for electrical points, intercom connection, I.T. network and air conditioning.

19.4.4 Surgeons Room for Office Work

This room is for the surgeons and their assistants to carry out the official work of the surgeries performed, to prepare notes of surgery etc. An O.T. register is usually kept here for daily entry. This room shall be located adjacent to the anaesthetist room. The size of this room shall be about 4572 mm × 4267 mm. The room shall contain an arrangement of office tables, executive chair, visitor chairs, side rack etc. The room shall have an attached toilet. The room shall also have an attached P.A. room for a clerk to be seated. The room shall have proper arrangements for electrical points, intercom connection, I.T. network and air conditioning.

19.4.5 Trolley Bay

An area shall be provided in this zone, which shall be reserved for the stretcher trollies and wheelchairs allotted to the O.T. complex. Normally these stretcher trollies are used to move out the patient from O.T. complex after surgery. As far as bringing the patient to the O.T. complex is concerned, usually, the patient is brought by the staff of the concerned ward or ICU. He/She uses the stretcher trollies allotted to his/her own ward. After dropping the patient in the Pre-operative ward, he/she takes the stretcher trollies or wheelchairs back to his/her own ward. Hence, the stretcher trollies and wheelchairs are generally not required at the entry point of O.T. complex. Therefore, this trolley bay is located in the unsterile zone at the exit point of the O.T. complex.

19.4.6 Frozen Section Biopsy Laboratory

It is the lab where the biopsy sample is quickly frozen and the histopathological findings can be reported. Usually, it takes only half an hour for the total process. At times it happens that while performing the surgery, the surgeon is not sure about the disease and desires re-confirmation of the diagnosis. For example, in the case of Mastectomy, the surgeon wants to be sure that the patient is a confirmed cancer case before completely removing the breast. Therefore, while performing the surgery, he/she takes a small specimen of the part as a biopsy and sends it to the frozen section lab for a confirmed diagnosis. While the investigation is in process, the patient is kept anaesthetized. Once the confirmed report is received, the surgeon can take the final decision. As an immediate report is required under such circumstances, the sample is not sent to the central lab to avoid wastage of time.

The Laboratory shall be provided with a countertop for working and placing the equipment and shall have an arrangement of lab sink and sufficient electric points.

19.4.7 Shoe Change Area

Space shall be provided in this zone for changing shoes. The staff desirous of entering the complex has to remove the outside shoes and change with the sleepers/shoes kept for use in the O.T. complex. This area shall be provided with a sufficient number of shoe racks and a chair for sitting while removing or wearing shoes.

19.4.8 Entry Door for Changing Room

In the O.T. complex, different types of change rooms are provided for Doctors, Technicians, Nurses and class four workers required to work in the sterile zone of the complex. The change rooms have to be separate for males and females. The number of the change room to be provided depends on the size of the O.T. complex and the number of staff required in the complex. It is recommended that the change room should have dual doors—one for entry and the other for exit. The philosophy behind this is, that after the change, the staff shall not come to the unsterile zone. Hence, the entry door of a change room is provided in this zone.

19.4.9 Waiting Area for Attendants

This area is for the attendants and family members of the patient undergoing surgery/intervention in the O.T. The family members being very curious, do not prefer to be seated at a faraway place and always want to sit near the O.T. complex. Therefore, the waiting area shall be provided outside the main entry door of the O.T. complex. The waiting area shall be provided with chairs for a comfortable sitting of the family members. This area shall have a speaker connected to the mike system placed in the O.T. complex for listening to the announcements made from the O.T. This area shall also have an Intercom facility so that the O.T. staff can contact the family members in case of requirement. This area shall be guarded by the security to control the unnecessary movement of family members in the O.T. complex and shall be under CCTV surveillance.

19.4.10 Public Utility for Attendants

Along with the waiting area for the family members, the facility of toilets shall be provided. If possible, separate toilets shall be provided for males and females. The facility of drinking water shall also be provided. It will still be better if the tea/coffee vending machine is placed in this area.

19.4.11 Linen Pre-wash Room

This room is used to give a pre-wash to the soiled linen used in the O.T. before sending them to the laundry. As said earlier, no back movement is allowed in the O.T. complex, the used linen has to move out from the exit gate or the corridor behind the O.T. complex. Therefore, this room has to be provided near the exit gate of the O.T. complex or the exit of the corridor behind the O.T. A room shall be provided with the sink, drainboard and a low-height water tap to wash the clothes. Special care shall be taken about the slope in this room so that the water does not spill outside the room.

19.4.12 Instrument Wash Room

This room is used to give a pre-wash to the soiled surgical instruments used in the O.T. before sending them to the CSSD for sterilization. As no back movement is allowed in the O.T. complex, the used instruments have to move out from the exit gate. Therefore, this room has to be provided near the exit gate of the O.T. complex. The room shall be provided with a large size sink, drainboard and a countertop for drying up the instruments.

19.5 Protective Zone

This zone is a bit more sterile as compared unsterile zone and the movement is restricted, but not always. The area can be assessed only by changing the shoes or wearing the shoe covers. The clothes need not be changed for going to this area. This area is located just after the unsterile zone and shall be separated from the unsterile zone with the help of a door which shall be guarded. Details of rooms located in this zone have been provided below:

19.5.1 Changing Rooms

The changing rooms are provided in the O.T. complex to enable the doctors and staff to remove the outside clothes and change them to the O.T. clothes. It is a set of the pre-sterilized dress (normally full-length bottom pants and half-sleeved long top) kept in the change rooms. The dresses of different sizes are stitched for different staff members. Some hospitals also prepare the dress for individual staff members and it is tagged with the name of the staff member. Different change rooms are provided for different categories of staff members. Also, the change rooms for males are separate from females. Following change rooms are generally provided in the O.T. complex (Fig. 19.2):

1. Doctors Change Room—Males.
2. Doctors Change Room—Females.
3. Technicians Change Room—Males.
4. Technicians Change Room—Females.
5. Nurses Change Room—Males.
6. Nurses Change Room—Females.
7. Class IV Staff Change Room—Males.
8. Class IV Staff Change Room—Females.
9. Students Change Room—Males.
10. Students Change Room—Females.

Infrastructure wise:

1. Each change room shall be of the size of approximately 4572 mm × 4267 mm.

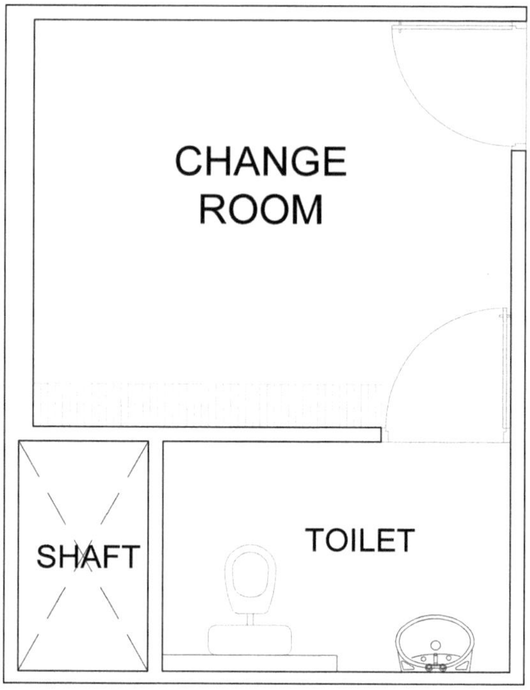

Fig. 19.2 Sample of change room drawing

2. Along with the change room, an attached toilet with bath facility shall also be provided.
3. The room shall have adequate provision of the personal lockers to keep the personal belongings.
4. There shall be adequate hooks on the wall to hang clothes.
5. A hanger rod shall be provided with hangers to hang clothes.
6. There shall be a cabinet to keep the sterilized O.T. dresses.
7. A large bin for dirty linen shall also be provided in the change room.

19.5.2 Entry Gate of Pre-operative Ward

To maintain the sterility of the O.T. complex, it is advised that the Pre-operative ward shall have dual gates. One for the entry and other for the exit of the patient. The entry gate shall be in this Protective Zone. The patient is wheeled from the main entry door of the O.T. complex and then through the entry gate of Pre-operative Ward. The width of the door of the pre-operative ward shall be 1829 mm.

19.5.3 Unsterile Store for Equipment Storage

O.T. is a highly sensitive place and requires extra equipment and instruments to be stored. These are not generally used but are kept in stock for providing a backup of the main equipment and instruments. The store shall be at least 4572 mm × 6096 mm in size. Adequate lockable cupboards, racks and drawers shall be provided in the store. The store shall also have multiple electric points to charge the equipment when not in use. This store shall be in charge of the store-keeper of O.T. complex.

19.5.4 Store for Medicines, Consumables and Disposables

During surgery, a surgeon can raise demand for medicines, consumables and disposables depending on the patient's condition. As the surgeon will not be in a waiting position, his/her requirement has to be fulfilled immediately. To avoid any untoward incident, generally, all the required medicines, consumables and disposables are stocked in the O.T. complex. A separate store shall be provided to keep such items in the protective zone of the O.T. complex. The room shall be at least 4572 mm × 6096 mm in size. Adequate lockable cupboards, racks and drawers shall be provided in the store. The store shall also have a countertop to prepare the drugs if required. This store shall be in charge of the storekeeper of O.T. complex.

19.5.5 Pantry

Pantry is provided in the O.T. complex to facilitate the staff to have tea/coffee whenever there is a break from surgeries. This pantry can also serve the requirements of the doctor's lounge or the staff lounge. Apart from tea/coffee, it can have the provision of pre-cooked light snacks and biscuits. Infrastructure wise, the pantry shall be about 3658 mm × 3658 mm in size. It shall be provided with the countertop slab for cooking and to place gas burners or inductions. The provision of a sink with a drainboard shall be made for washing utensils. A microwave and refrigerator shall also be provided in the pantry. A sufficient number of electric points shall be provided to operate these machines.

19.6 Clean Zone

This area is cleaner than the protective zone and the entry to this zone shall be more restricted. Entry into this zone shall be allowed after the change of outside clothes. This area is located just after the protective zone and shall be separated from the protective zone with the help of the door which shall be guarded. Details of the rooms located in this zone are:

19.6.1 Pre-operative Room

The pre-operative ward is the area where the patient is kept for examination before taking him to the operation theatre. Depending on the requirement, a few beds can be placed in this ward. As the stay of the patient is very less in this ward, a large number of beds are not required. Normally, one to two beds per O.T. room shall be placed.

The size will depend on the number of beds to be placed. Generally, 7.43–9.29 Sq Mtr. space per bed is sufficient. Not all but a few beds shall have the provision for the supply of Medical Gas Pipeline mounted on the bed head panel. Each bed shall be provided with at least two electrical points to connect the medical devices. Along with the Pre-operative ward, an adjoining toilet shall be provided. The ward shall also have a cloth changing room, where the patient can change to the O.T. dress. This ward shall have two doors, entry and exit. As mentioned earlier, the entry door shall be in the protective zone and the exit gate in this clean zone.

19.6.2 Preparation Room

Though instructions are given to the wards to prepare a patient before sending him/her to the O.T., sometimes it is found that the patient has not been properly prepared, for example the patient has not been shaved, the dress has not been changed etc. Therefore, a preparation room is provided in this zone to complete the formalities of preparation before sending the patient to the O.T. This room shall be about 3658 mm × 3658 mm in size, with an examination couch. The room shall have a cabinet to keep the necessary items, a sink and a portable O.T. light.

19.6.3 Surgeons Rest Room

This area is also called the ‘Surgeons Lounge’. Usually, in a running hospital, the surgeries are planned in a series which can range between 2 and 5 in a single O.T., by the same or different surgeons. Once the surgery is performed in an O.T., the patient has to be transferred from the O.T., it has to be cleaned and disinfected, a fresh set of sterilized instruments and linen has to be kept, and the new patient has to be shifted in the O.T. All these activities take about 30 min to an hour. Till that time, the surgeon can relax in the lounge and complete the patient file, prepare operative notes and post-operative prescriptions. The lounge shall be provided with an attached toilet and a provision of tea/coffee, which can be served from the pantry.

Size-wise the lounge shall be about 6096 mm × 4572 mm, with a sofa set and a centre table. On the request, a single bed can also be placed in the lounge for surgeons to lay down for some time (Fig. 19.3).

19.6.4 Restroom for Staff: Males and Females

As in the case of surgeons, a lounge shall also be provided for the staff. But the lounge for males and females shall be separate. The size of the room shall depend on the requirement and number of staff members to be accommodated at any particular moment of time. All other facilities as provided in the surgeon’s lounge shall also be provided here.

19.6.5 Exit Doors of all Change Rooms

The exit of all change rooms shall be in the clean zone. The logic is that, after a change, the staff is

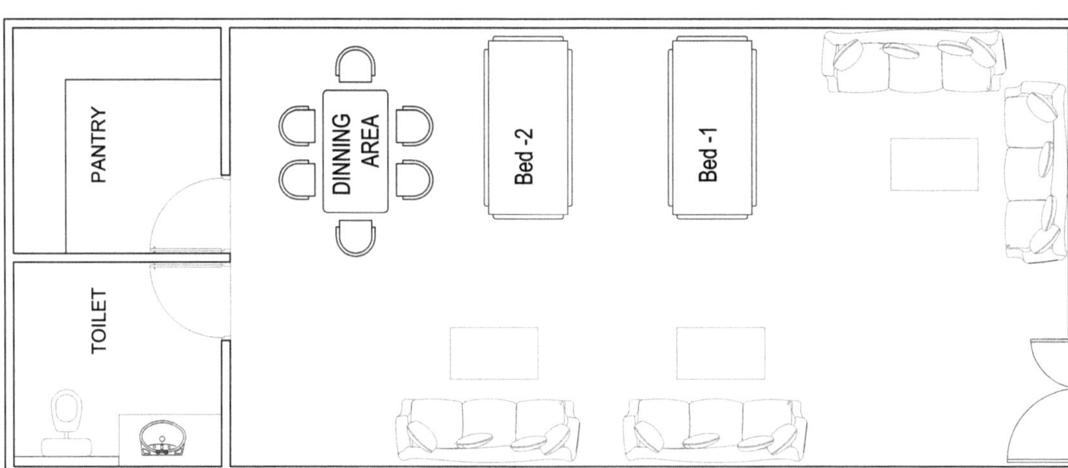

Fig. 19.3 Sample layout surgeons rest room

in sterilized dress and shall not be allowed to go back to the unsterile areas. From here, the staff and surgeon either move forward to the sterile zone or remain in this zone. The exit doors shall be 914 mm wide and swing type so that it closes automatically.

19.6.6 Pre-anaesthetic Check-up Room (PAC)

PAC is a check-up performed on a patient by the anaesthetist to ensure that the patient is fit to administer anaesthesia. He/She performs different investigations like blood tests, X-rays or sometimes echocardiography. Usually, it is performed in the ward, a day before the surgery, but at times, re-examination is required before administering the anaesthesia. This is the place where it shall be done. This room shall be about 3658 mm × 3658 mm in size, with an examination couch. The room shall have a cabinet to keep the necessary tools and instruments, a sink and a portable O.T. light.

19.6.7 Dirty Utility

After completion of the surgery, a lot of used items like linen, instruments, covers of disposables, soiled drapes, cotton and gauze have to be removed. Out of this, the linen is sent to linen pre-wash area and instruments to the instrument washroom. Therefore, this dirty utility room is provided at the exit end of the O.T. complex. The room shall be about 3048 mm × 3048 mm and provided with bins as per the biomedical waste management rules for other waste products.

19.6.8 Post-operative Recovery Ward

Once the surgery is complete, the patient is moved to the Post-operative Recovery Ward. This ward is used to provide specialized care to the patient until he/she is out of anaesthesia. The location of the Post-operative Recovery Ward shall be at the exit end of the O.T. complex. After the recovery of the patient, he/she is transferred to the respective ward or ICU as the case may be.

The number of beds in the Post-operative Recovery Ward shall be in proportion to the operating room. For each O.T., there shall be two recovery beds. The Post-operative Recovery Ward shall have a setup exactly as per the ICU, i.e. the beds shall be placed at an appropriate distance, all beds shall have the provision of Central Medical Gas Pipeline, and there shall be electric points similar to ICU. The ward shall have a nursing station in the centre, attached general store, medicine store, clean utility room, dirty utility room and a toilet. The size of the Post Operative Recovery ward shall depend on the number of beds to be placed in the ward.

19.7 Sterile Zone

This is the most sensitive zone in the whole O.T. complex. This area has to be totally sterile and aseptic. It is separated from the Clean Zone by providing a swing-type door that shall not be less than 1829 mm wide. These doors shall be sealed so that any unwanted organisms cannot enter the sterile zone. On the exit side of this zone, similar doors shall be provided. The movement in this zone shall be strictly restricted and only authorized persons shall be allowed in this zone that too after a proper change and with caps and masks. Just at the entry of this zone, a shoe rack is placed which contains sterilized shoes or slippers to be worn before entering this zone. At the exit end of this zone, a double door with air lock shall be provided to transfer the patient out of the recovery room. If possible, one exit shall be given in the corridor which connects to the ICU complex so that the patient can be moved to the ICU directly with any outside atmosphere exposure. The details of rooms located in this zone are as follows:

19.7.1 Clean Supply Room

This room is also termed as Clean Store. This room is mainly used to store the instruments and linen received from CSSD after proper sterilization. It is also used for storing sterile consumables and disposables that are normally used in the Operating Rooms (OR). This room shall be located near the OR so that it can serve the needs effectively. Better if it is placed somewhere in the centre of all the OR. The access to this room shall be strictly restricted.

This room shall be about 4572 mm × 3658 mm in size with a single entry and the door shall be swing type openable on both sides. It is still better if the door is hermetically sealed door operational with sensors. The room shall not have any window; however, if the window is not avoidable, it shall be a sealed with double glazing glass. There should be no water supply or drain in this room.

The room shall have stainless steel racks divided into bins, to store the sterilized material stacked set wise of surgery wise or OR wise. The sterilized material is brought into this room through sterilized covered carts and the material is unloaded in the racks. From here, the stored material shall either move directly to OR or otherwise to the Instrument Trolley Lay-up room.

19.7.2 Instrument Trolley Lay Up

This room is for preparing the trolley for a particular type of surgery or a particular OR. As the requirement of the linen and instruments is different for different surgeries, this room eases out the preparation of the trolley. The material is brought in this room from the Clean Supply Room and laid on the trolley which in turn shall move to the concerned OR. The trollies for layout are also wheeled from the same OR where it has to go back after lay-up.

This room shall be about 3658 mm × 3658 mm in size with a single entry and the door shall be swinging type openable on both sides. The door shall be a sealed door. The room shall not have any window; however, if the window is not avoidable, it shall be sealed with double glazing glass. There should be no water supply or drain in this room.

19.7.3 Scrub Station

The scrub station is used for washing up before entering the OR to perform a surgery or intervention. Every person involved in the surgery shall be scrubbed in this area. This area should be adjoining to the OR. The scrub station can be either in an open area or in a closed room. If it is in a closed room, the doors of this room shall be able to easily swing in either direction just by the tap of the foot and should have a see-through glass in the middle.

The scrub area shall be provided with a stainless steel scrub station which could be operated by foot and/or sensors. Hand-operated taps are not allowed in the scrub station. It shall have a minimum of two bays, with the provision of both hot and cold water to wash hands. The number of scrub stations depends on the number of OR in the complex. It is better if each OR has its own scrub station. No more than two OR can share one scrub station.

The water outlet of the scrub station shall be designed to allow the water to fall in the centre of the scrub and not spill around. There shall be a provision for dispensing the soap using a wall hanging soap dispenser, which shall be elbow operated. Similarly, an elbow-operated wall-hung antiseptic solution dispenser shall be provided with the scrub station. A nail brush should be provided, along with a nail cutter and a nail file.

19.7.4 Sterilization Room

Proper sterilization is the backbone of any O.T. complex, thus special care needs to be given to the sterilization department. The main sterilization jobs are carried out in the Central Sterile Supply Department (CSSD) located somewhere in the vicinity of the O.T. complex, or at any other convenient place with a proper transport facility, like goods lift, to transport the sterilized material to O.T. complex. In CSSD, bulk sterilization is carried out to cater to the needs of the O.T. complex and other departments of the hospital.

At times during surgery, the surgeon may require some instrument or if accidentally some instrument drops down and gets contaminated, it has to be quickly sterilized to send it back to the surgeon. Therefore, a small sterilization room is provided in the Sterile Zone of the O.T. complex which is usually called **Theatre Sterile Supply Unit (TSSU)**. This room is located near the OR clean supply room. The size of the room shall be about 3658 mm × 3658 mm. It shall have a quick steam sterilizer, a hot air oven, and a formalin chamber. The room shall have a proper supply of soft water to be used in the sterilizer and the required drain. The room shall have adequate arrangements for exhaust and air exchanges. It shall also be provided with the required electrical point to connect the machines. A compressed air point shall also be provided to remove the debris from the instruments if required.

19.7.5 Operating Theatres/Rooms

It is this room where the actual surgeries/interventions are carried out. This room has to be the most sterile and aseptic area in the whole of the hospital. No person is allowed in the Operating Theatres/Rooms (OR) without wearing protective clothing, including shoe covers, masks, caps, eye shields and other coverings to prevent the spread of germs.

19.7.6 Number of OR

How many OR are to be made? This is the question normally faced by the owners. There is no thumb rule to decide the number of OR to be made. It will entirely depend on factors like:

1. How many surgical departments does the hospital plan to have? Like General Surgery, ENT, EYE, Gynae & Obs, Orthopaedic, Urology, Neurosurgery, CTVS, Pedia Surgery, G.I. Surgery, Onco Surgery etc.
2. How many surgeons will be operating simultaneously?
3. What will be the timings of O.T.?
4. Will the OR be common to all or will it be dedicated to a OR, i.e. will a particular OR be reserved for a specific department?
5. How many surgeries are expected per day? (Both Major and Minor).
6. How many patients are generally referred to this hospital for surgeries/interventions per day?
7. What is the load of trauma patients per day?
8. Does the hospital plan for specialized surgeries like robotic surgeries or organ transplants?

Ideally, a hospital of 500 beds shall have a set of 10 OR, i.e. one OR for every 50 bed. This is not a standard, but the practical experience recommends the same. Out of these, one O.T. can be reserved for advanced surgeries, one for Robotic Surgery, one for Organ Transplant, one for CTVS, one for Obs and one for Eye Surgery. The balance OR shall be common for other departments.

But if the departments performing surgeries/interventions are more, the number of OR shall be increased, which can even go up to 20 or more.

19.7.7 Location and Layout of the ORs

The location of the OR shall be in the most sterile and restricted zone. This is the last zone of the O.T. complex.

The layout of the OR can be in different designs. The first can be that in the centre of this zone there shall be a corridor and OR can be provided on both ends of the corridor. The second design is that all the OR can be on one side of the corridor and the services on the other side. The third design can be the cluster of OR in a specific area connected through small corridors. Despite all three designs being acceptable, the first act is the best. In this case, the corridor shall be at least 3048 mm wide.

The doors can open either directly in the corridors or side opening can also be considered. The disadvantage of opening the doors directly in the corridor is that there will be no barrier in between and any person moving in the corridor shall have direct access inside the OR. Therefore, the designer shall design the OR in such a way that there shall be a gallery between two OR, and doors of both these OR shall open in that gallery. Another advantage is that at the end of such a gallery, a common scrub station for both these OR can be fixed.

19.7.8 Types of Operating Rooms

Based on the requirements and technological development, the construction of OR has undergone a tremendous improvement over the years. The modern OR are supposed to be sterile and have proper environmental conditions inside the OR. There are different types of OR as follows:

1. Simple room OR.
2. Pre-fabricated Modular OR.
3. Semi-Modular OR.
4. Modular OR.
5. Hybrid OR.

Now little more detail on all these types of ORs.

19.8 Simple Room OR

In earlier days, these types of OR were commonly constructed. Even today, some small hospital setups opt for this type of OR. These are the simplest type of OR with no specific provision of sterility, no environmental consideration, and no air exchanges. In these OR:

1. The walls are all just simply plastered.
2. On the walls, either washable paint or glazed tiles are affixed.
3. The ceiling is normally plastered or at the most POP false ceiling is used.
4. Flooring can be of normal marble stone or glazed tiles.
5. The doors can be of normal wood door or aluminium.
6. For Air Conditioning, Split Air-conditioners are used.
7. In the centre of the room, an O.T. light is fixed at the ceiling.
8. The O.T. table is just placed in the centre of the room.
9. Proper pipeline for medical gases is not laid down.
10. There is no specific size of such OR.

19.9 Pre-fabricated Modular OR

These are the most commonly used OR types. They are developed inside a room having walls and a concrete ceiling. These OR fulfil most needs of an ideal OR like Sterility, Environment, Temperature, Humidity, Air Exchanges, Cleanliness, Air Flow and Internal Pressure. The details of these OR are as follows:

19.9.1 Size of the OR

The standard size of these OR shall be 6096 mm × 6096 mm, i.e. 37.16 Sq Mtr. However, for specialized surgeries such as Cardiac, Neuro and Robotic Surgery, the size shall be about 46.45 Sq Mtr. For transplant surgeries, the area shall be about 74.32 Sq Mtr.

19.9.2 Walls of the OR

These walls are artificially created in front of the pre-constructed brick walls. First of all, the prefabricated panels are prepared at the site or in the workshop. For preparing the panels, the structure is fabricated using a welded frame made of Mild Steel or Stainless Steel. This frame is about 25–50 mm in width. On both sides of the frame, a sheet is fixed to create the panel. This height and width of the panel depend on the design. On the side facing the wall, normally a G.I. sheet is used. On the other side which will be exposed in the room, a G.I. or S.S. sheet is used as per the choice of the owners.

In an empty area between both the sheets, a puffing of polyurethane is filled up to make it a puff panel. This makes the panel tough to protect itself from any dents and reduces thermal loss. Due to financial restraints if any, the asbestos sheet can also be filled in between two sheets of the panel.

These panels are then arranged on the walls and fixed with rod fasteners about 152 mm to 254 mm away from the wall, creating a vacuum between the wall and the panel to further reduce the thermal losses. Please note that the corners are kept empty for fixing the return air duct. Space shall be about 305 mm on both sides of the corner.

Now all the panels are welded to each other so that no space is left in between the panels. The extra welding spots are ground to smoothen the panel surface.

In this panel, no corners are allowed, so at the bends, the panels are welded at an angle of 45 degrees instead of 90 degrees.

19.9.3 Ceiling of the OR

The ceiling of these OR is also fabricated from the puff panel as discussed earlier. First of all, the centre of the OR is marked on the ceiling. Then a Plenum is hung from the ceiling with the help of screw rod fasteners. The Plenum is a box-like structure measuring 2400 mm × 2400 mm × 305 mm, open from the bottom, and is made out of a G.I. sheet. It is used to provide HEPA (High-Efficiency Particulate Air) filters for air conditioning and also the centre lights. Just at the centre of the Plenum, a round cut-out is given to hang the O.T. light from the ceiling. On the outer sides of the Plenum, cut-outs are provided to fix the air-conditioning supply ducts.

As no sharp corners are allowed in the ceiling, slanted panels are provided on the vertical panels to join the same with the ceiling panels. The slanted panels which are about 630 mm wide, are fixed at the angle of 45 degrees on the top of wall panels fixed earlier to avoid corners. Then all these slanted panels are welded to each other and also welded to the wall panel. The required grinding is done.

The space left in between the slanting panel and the plenum is filled up with the straight puff panel by hanging these panels from the ceiling using screw rods. These panels are welded to each other. Also, the welding of these straight panels is done with the slanting panel and the plenum.

19.9.4 Corners of OR

All four corners of the OR shall be covered. First of all, the return air duct, which is a vertical duct made of Aluminium sheet, is fixed with clamps screwed to the wall on all the four corners. The leftover corners, where the wall panels were not fixed earlier, are covered with the same type of puff panel as was fixed to the wall, and all panels are welded to each other. These corner panels shall also be installed at a 45-degree angle to avoid corners.

19.9.5 Door of the OR

Normal doors made of wood or aluminium are not recommended in the pre-fabricated modular OR. Instead of that, a pre-fabricated puff door shall be installed. The width of the door shall be at least 1524 mm. This door is a hermetically sealed door, which seals all the surfaces of the door and wall, and does not allow any leakage of air in or out of OR. These doors are either manually operated with a handle or are motor driven. Motor-driven doors are called automatic door and are operated and controlled with sensors. The sensors are either foot sensor, infrared hand sensor or both. This door slides on the railing fixed on top of the door opening. It has a computerized control fixed in the hood above the door opening near the sliding rail. In the door at eye level, a sealed glass is also provided to peep in the OR.

19.9.6 Window in OR

There are various arguments regarding providing a window in the OR. One thought says not to provide windows as it distracts the surgeon and can also be a source of infection in the OR. The second thought is to provide windows as it relieves the surgeon from stress due to long hours of surgery. But nowadays, the designers prefer to provide windows in OR.

The window in the OR is fixed in the outer wall of the OR. The size of the window can be 610 to 1000 mm in width and about 610 mm in height. The windows shall be a fixed type and not openable. The glass of the windows shall be double-glazed glass with a vacuum in between. In the vacuum space, between two layers of glass, vanishing blinds can be fixed, which shall be motorized and controlled by a switch button or remote. The glass can also be tinted and coated so that no direct sunlight or ultraviolet rays can enter the OR.

19.9.7 Control Panel

The control panel is recessed in the panelled wall next to the entrance of the OR. This panel is used to control the functioning of the entire OR. It can have 6 or 9 tiles. The tiles here mean the module which performs a particular function that can be controlled through that tile. Normally, the control panel can control functions like:

1. O.T. Light.
2. Peripheral Lights.
3. Plenum Lights.
4. Time Elapsed.
5. Clock.
6. Hand-free Intercom.
7. Medical Gases Pressure.
8. Music System.
9. Temperature Meter.
10. Humidity Meter.

19.9.8 View Box

The LED view box is recessed in the panelled wall, which will be in front of the surgeon while operating. Usually, the surgeons operate from the right-hand side of the patient, so this view box shall be fixed on the wall which is on the left hand side of the patient. The bottom height of the view box shall be about 4 ft. so that it reaches the surgeon's eye level. Both single film and double film view boxes are available, but it is recommended to use a double film view box as it has a dimmable LED white light. The control of the view box is given on the view box itself.

19.9.9 Writing Board

A Magnetic White Writing Board is also recessed in the panelled wall adjoining the view box. The bottom height of the board shall be about 4 ft. so that it reaches the surgeon's eye level.

19.9.10 Pressure Relief Damper (PRD)

In this type of OR, a particular pressure is to be maintained (further details related to this shall be discussed later in this chapter). At times it happens, that the pressures in the OR increases beyond the defined pressure. Under such circumstances, the excess pressure has to be reduced by pushing the air out of the OR. This function is performed by PRD. It is a set of Stainless Steel Fins connected together at a particular distance and a Stainless Steel weight is welded on one of the fins. This system is enclosed in a box-type structure. This box is fitted at the bottom in the cut-out of a wall of the OR. The cut-out on the wall has to be throughout the brick wall. The bottom height of the PRD shall be about 305 mm from the floor level.

19.9.11 Peripheral Lights

In the straight panel of the ceiling of the OR, peripheral lights are recessed. These are the 610 mm LED lights packed in a unit and have the facility of a dimmer. Normally, 8 such lights are fixed, two on each side of the OR. Their purpose is to provide light in the OR generally when surgery is not in progress. While surgery, as per the choice of the surgeon, these lights can be dimmed or switched off. These lights are controlled by the control panel provided in the OR.

19.9.12 Plenum

As stated earlier, the plenum is a box-type structure hung from the ceiling. Its main purpose is to fix HEPA Filters for air filtration and form a unidirectional flow of air. The plenum is closed from the bottom either by fixing a framed silken fabric or by a Stainless Steel sheet which has multiple holes for passage of the air. In both the cases, it has to be ensured that the air coming from the HEPA filter passes through without any hindrance.

19.9.13 Plenum Lights

These are 1219 mm LED tube lights fixed in the plenum. At the bottom of the plenum, an aluminium frame is fixed, and about 32 such tube lights are fixed in the frame. These lights give an excellent look and the OR brighten up when these lights are switched on. During the surgery, as per the surgeon's choice, these lights can be dimmed or switched off. These lights are controlled from the control panel provided in the OR. In some OR, as per the design, if the plenum is covered with a Stainless Steel sheet, these lights are not fixed.

19.9.14 Pass-through Windows/ Hatch Boxes

These are provided in the OR to pass clean supplies and material without opening the doors. It can also be used for passing soiled linen and instruments during or after the surgery. Design-wise, this window has two doors opening on both the sides and the doors shall be at a distance of 305 mm from each other, hence creating a space in-between. Special consideration shall be taken about the fact that only one door can be opened at a time. If somebody wants to pass the material, he/she will open the door and keep the material in the window. Once he/she closes the door, only then the door on the opposite side can be opened.

19.9.15 Electrical Points

Sufficient number of electrical outlets shall be provided in the OR for connecting the medical appliances. It is, therefore, recommended that at least two dual sets of 6/16 amp (it means 4 outlets) switches/sockets are provided on each wall of the OR. Power in most of these outlets shall be supplied through UPS. These points shall be fixed at a height of 305 mm from the floor level.

19.9.16 Anaesthetist Pendant

On the left-hand side of the patient, an anaesthetist pendant is hung from the ceiling. This pendent shall be hung at a distance of 610 mm from both sides of the corner so that the pendant can easily revolve up to 270 degrees. Please ensure that the pendent shall not touch the wall of OR, else the walls will be damaged.

These are available as single arm and double arm pendants. Single-arm pendants cover less area as compared to the double-arm pendants. At the lower end of the pendant, a box-type structure called the body of the pendant is fixed. The size of this body is about 610 mm × 305 mm × 305 mm.

On the back wall of the pendant body, the outlets of medical gases are fixed. Two outlets of each supply, i.e. Oxygen, Nitrous Oxide, Compressed air and Vacuum are provided. On both, the sidewalls of the body of pendant, electric and communication ports are provided. On the front wall of the pendant body, a service tray and drawers are provided. Also, a railing is provided for fixing the utility basket. The pendants also have a provision for fixing the IV rod.

19.9.17 Surgeon Pendant

On the right-hand side of the patient, a surgeon pendant can be given, if required. This is generally a fixed arm pendant that can only revolve on its own axis. This pendant is mainly used by the surgeon and has electrical outlets on the side-walls and 2–3 trays.

19.9.18 Flooring

These OR have an anti-static flooring, i.e. they have adequate earthing properties. It is a PVC flooring with a layer of carbon coating at the bottom. It is available in form of tiles (610 mm × 610 mm) and rolls. While fixing the flooring, a copper strip is pasted on the corners, which is ultimately connected to the earthing wire. After that, the PVC tile or roll is glued to the flooring of the OR. A skirting of about 3 inches is also made from the same tile or roll. To ensure that there are no 90-degree corners, plastic corners are fixed and the tile or roll is pasted above that. Once the tile or roll is glued, the joints are thermo welded with a PVC cord to fill any gaps in the flooring.

19.9.19 Painting

All surfaces (walls and ceiling) of the OR are painted. First of all, a coat of primer is applied. Then the metal putty is applied to fill any gaps. Once the putty dries up, the surfaces are scrubbed with sandpaper. If needed, a second coat of putty can be applied. This is followed up with at least two coats of washable antibacterial and antifungal paint. Please make sure that the colour of the OR is light and attractive. Dark colours shall be avoided.

19.9.20 Air Conditioning and Environment of ORs

The OR should be fully air-conditioned, allowing control of temperature, humidity and air exchanges. Suitable and safe air quality must always be maintained in the OR. Following issues are important while designing the Air Conditioning System in the OR:

1. Either opt for Chilled Water Pipe Line with AHUs (Air Handling Units), or if the number of OR is less than opt for Ductable Split system.
2. Air Flow, direction and air exchanges have to be as per the industry norms.
3. Heating shall be done using water pipeline and AHUs having hot water generator instead of water chillers. Also, room heaters can be opted; however, they are generally not recommended to be used in the OR (Fig. 19.4).

19.9.21 Supply Air Ducts

The AHU shall push out clean, sterilized and cool air at a particular velocity and quantity. This air has to be carried to the HEPA Filters and ultimately in the OR. This job is done with the help of air ducts which are insulated aluminium ducts fabricated as per the design. This duct on one end is connected to the AHU and on the other end to the HEPA filters. The main duct is split into a number of ducts equal to the number of HEPA Filters. The air then passes through the HEPA Filters in the plenum. As an equal number of HEPA Filters are placed opposite to each other, the airwaves coming from both directions hit each other and the final stream bends down and is released from the plenum. Thus, forming a unidirectional flow of air in the shape of an umbrella, which then rushes towards the return air duct fitted in the corners of the OR.

19.9.22 Return Air

In all four corners of the OR, vertical return air ducts are provided with a vent on the lower end of the duct. The air thrown in the OR from plenum is forcefully rushed towards the return air duct. This happens because the air is continuously being induced in the OR which increases the air

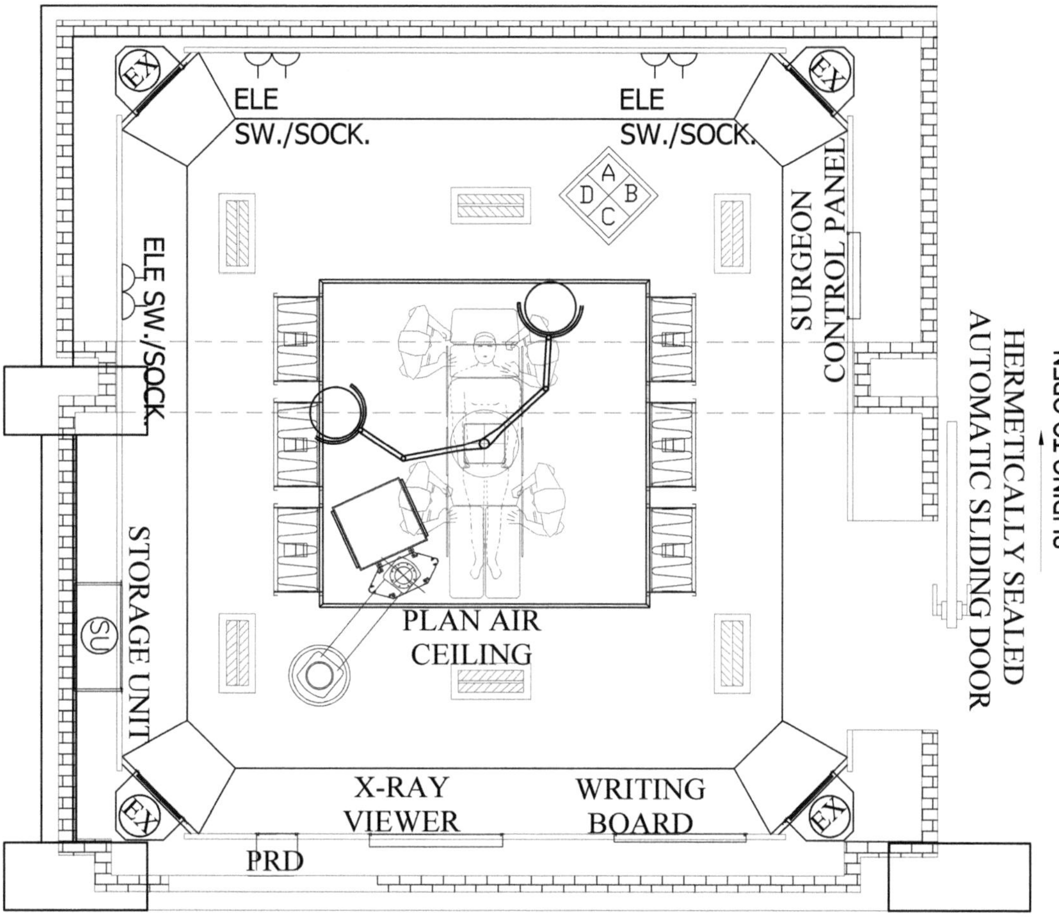

Fig. 19.4 Sample layout drawing of modular OR

pressure inside the OR, and ultimately the excess air has to exhaust to maintain a particular pressure. The air which moves to the return air duct is sent to the AHU, filtered, mixed with fresh air, cooled and again released from the AHU into the OR, and the same process continues.

19.9.23 Special Air Requirements for OR

19.9.23.1 Air Changes Per Hour

Minimum total air changes should be 20 based on biological load and the location.

The minimum fresh air component of the air change shall be a minimum of 4 out of 20 air changes.

If the designer chooses to have a 100% fresh air system, then appropriate energy saving devices like heat recovery wheel and run-around pipes should be installed.

19.9.23.2 Air Velocity

The airflow needs to be unidirectional and downwards on the OR table. The air face velocity of 25–35 FPM (feet per minute) from non-aspirating unidirectional laminar flow diffuser/ceiling array is recommended.

19.9.23.3 Positive Pressure

The minimum positive pressure recommended is 2.5 Pascal (0.01 inches of water). It has to be ensured that positive pressure differential between the OR and the adjoining areas shall be maintained to prevent outside air entry into the OR. Positive pressure shall always be maintained in OR (operational and non-operational hours).

19.9.23.4 Air Handling in the OR Including Air Quality

Air shall be supplied through Terminal HEPA filters in the ceiling. The HEPA filters can be at AHU level or at the terminal level inside the OR. The minimum size of the filtration area should be extended to one foot on all sides of the OR table.

19.9.23.5 Air Filtration

AHU is the air purification and filtration unit. There must be two sets of washable flange-type filters of efficiency 90% down to 10 microns and 99% down to 5 microns with aluminium/stainless steel 304 frames within the AHU.

The AHU of each OR should be a dedicated one and should not be linked to the air conditioning of any other area in the OR and surroundings. One AHU for multiple OR is permitted, provided there is a contingency plan to accommodate surgeries in another OR in case of failure of infection control in one of the OR.

The AHUs can either be a floor model or ceiling suspended. The designer has to decide the place for AHUs depending on the size of the AHU or the ceiling height of the building.

AHU blower shall be operational round the clock (maybe without temperature control). Variable frequency devices (VFD) may be used to conserve energy. Air changes can be reduced to 25% during non-operating hours through VFD, provided a positive pressure relationship is not disturbed during such period.

The location of outdoor air intake for an AHU must not be located near potentially contaminated sources like D.G. exhaust hoods, lab exhaust vents and vehicle parking areas.

19.9.23.6 Service Panels to Be Provided for Servicing the Filters, Motors and Blowers

HEPA filters of efficiency 99.97% down to 0.3 microns or higher efficiency are to be provided. Air quality at the supply end, i.e. at the grill level should be Class 100 at rest condition, which means a cubic foot of air should not have more than 0.5 microns or larger.

19.9.23.7 Temperature and Relative Humidity

Temperature should be maintained at 21 degree Celsius ±3 degree Celsius (except for joints replacement where it should be 18 degree Celsius ±2 degree Celsius) with corresponding relative humidity between 20 and 60%, though the ideal relative humidity is considered to be 55%. Appropriate devices to monitor and display these conditions inside the OR may be installed.

19.9.23.8 Window and Split AC

These should not be used in any type of OR because they are pure re-circulating units and have pockets for microbial growth which cannot be sealed.

19.9.24 Other Communication Points in OR

The following communication points shall be provided in each OR, either at the walls, control panel or the pendant:

1. R.J. 45 points for Computer networking.
2. R.J. 11 for Intercom and extension line.
3. Point for reading light for patient.

19.9.25 Equipment in OR

The list of Equipment to be placed in the OR is exhaustive and the need varies from one discipline to other. However, generally, the following equipment shall be placed in the OR:

Anaesthesia ventilator	Mobile Ultrasound
Anaesthesia work stations/ Boyle's machine	Morcellator
Blood pressure Apparatus	Multi Para Monitor with ET Co_2
Cryogun	Navigators for Hip / Knee
Cryophthalmic Unit	Nephroscopes
CUSA	Nerve Stimulator
Defibrillator	Operating Instruments
ECT Machine	Operating light
Electro Surgical Cautery	Operating Microscope
Emergency light	Operating table attachments
Femto Lasix	Ophthalmic Laser
Fetal Doppler	Phaco- fragmentation Unit
Head Light	Pneumatic Tourniquet Electrical
Heart-Lung Machine	Portable O.T. Light
Heating Block	Sternum Saw Operation table
Holmium Laser	Saw, Drill and Remer Sets
Hysteroscopy Pump	Suction machine electrical
Hysteroscope	Telescopes
Image Intensifier (C-Arm)	UPS 10 Kva
Intra-Aortic Balloon Pump	Uretero-Renoscope
Laparoscope set	Vaporizer
Lithotripter	Vitreous Aspiration

19.9.26 Furniture OR

The following furniture shall be placed in the OR:

1. Instrument Trolleys.
2. Mayo stand.
3. Swab rack.
4. Steel bucket with lid Footstool.
5. Doctor stool.
6. I.V. stand.
7. Sterilization drums.

19.10 Septic Operation Theatre

It is the OR where infected cases are operated. The construction, specifications and design of this OR are the same as any other. However, the equipment and furniture of this OR are separate, and shall not be used in the normal OR.

19.11 Endoscopy Suite

It is used for the Upper G.I. endoscopy, colonoscopy and other related procedures like ERCP. Some hospitals keep the endoscopic suites in the O.T. complex, whereas others keep it outside the O.T. complex. Irrespective of the place, the design and requirements of the suite remain the same. A complete endoscopy suite shall have the following:

19.11.1 Endoscopy Room

It is an OR like structure where the endoscopy procedure is actually performed. This room has an operating table placed in the centre. On the right-hand side of the patient is a monitor and the processing unit of the endoscope. The doctor/ technicians perform the procedure from the left hand of the patient and the images captured by the camera (in the scope), and processed by the processor, are displayed on the monitor. All the design, parameters and specifications of a prefabricated modular OR shall be followed for this room. Apart from this, an endoscope storage cabinet shall be provided in the room, which is specially designed to hang the endoscopes saving them from being damaged.

19.11.2 Endoscope Washroom

After every procedure, the endoscope needs to be washed and disinfected. Therefore, an endoscope washroom shall be provided with the endoscopy room. This room has a long and deep sink with a drainboard. The size of the sink shall be about 914 mm in length, 610 mm in width and 305 mm deep.

19.11.3 Store

It is given along with the endoscopy room to store consumables and other items which may not be frequently used.

19.11.4 Change Room

This room is provided to allow physicians and technicians to change their clothes before entering the endoscopy suite. This room is provided only if the endoscopy room is out of the O.T. complex.

19.11.5 Recovery Room

This room is used by post endoscopy patients till they are stabilized. This room is provided only if the endoscopy room is out of the O.T. complex.

19.11.6 Consultation Room

This room is used for consultation and interaction with the family members of the patient. This room is provided only if the endoscopy room is out of the O.T. complex.

19.12 Semi-modular OR

At times due to some financial constraints, it is not possible to provide a full-fledged pre-fabricated OR. In such cases, a semi-modular OR can be designed. In these OR, the modular wall structure is avoided. Also, all other fittings like control panel, reassessed view box, whiteboard, PRD, window and hermitical door are avoided. Only the ceiling structure with the proper plenum and HEPA filters with proper AHU are provided so that the unidirectional flow of the air can be achieved.

19.13 Modular OR

For this type of OR, a vacant hall is provided which has no walls except the outer walls. For these OR, a complete structure is fabricated with channels, angles and other specialized sections made of either Mild Steel or Stainless Steel. These fabricated structures then are assembled to give the shape of a room-like structure. Thereafter, the wall panels and ceiling panels are fixed in these fabricated structures to make it a room.

All other design parameters and specifications of a pre-fabricated modular OR shall be followed for this OR. It shall have the control panel, view box, whiteboard, PRD, window, hermitical door, pendants, plenum, HEPA Filters etc. and shall comply with environment control norms.

19.14 Hybrid OR

It is an OR where multi-disciplinary integration is done by combining advanced imaging diagnostics and surgery, which allows the surgeons, radiologists and other healthcare providers to use real-time images for guidance and assessment during complex surgeries. Before Hybrid OR, mobile imaging equipment was used, but it does not produce high-quality images that are required for delicate procedures. This allows conducting more accurate, safe and less invasive surgical procedures, leading to quicker patient recovery. If an emergency arises during an interventional procedure, it can quickly be revised to an open procedure since the room is set up as a fully functional OR. No critical time is lost in changing equipment or transporting the patient to a different operating room.

As different types of procedures such as cardiac, vascular and neurosurgery are performed in a hybrid OR, it requires a variety of imaging equipment to be used. Some examples of commonly installed imaging equipment in a hybrid OR are Angiography Equipment (Cathlab), Computed Tomography (CT) Scanners, Magnetic

Resonance Imaging (MRI) Scanners, C-arm, X-ray and Digital Subtraction Angiography System (DSA).

When designing these types of facilities, it is critical to determine the primary use of the hybrid OR. It shall be at least 1.5 times larger than a normal OR, i.e. about 55.74 Sq Mtr. However, if a CT scan or MRI has to be integrated into the Hybrid OR, the space requirement can go up to 74.32 Sq Mtr. An ancillary room for these modalities shall also be provided, which may require additional space. Some examples of the ancillary room are control room, UPS room and machine panel room.

As far as the shape of the hybrid OR is concerned, it is more of a rectangular shape as compared to the regular OR, which is almost square in shape. Even the length may vary from 7620 mm to 9144 mm. The reason is that both the imaging equipment and the actual operating table are in length to each other. Considering the movement area of staff, such length is required in the hybrid OR.

Construction-wise, the hybrid OR shall follow similar norms to a pre-fabricated modular OR, i.e. walls, ceiling, doors, windows, air-conditioning and control panel.

Acknowledgement I am grateful to Dr. Rohit Varshney for his great support in compiling this chapter. I wish to convey my thanks and gratitude to him for the time and efforts he has put in.

Further Reading

Agnew GH. Designing the Operative Suite. Can Med Assoc J. 1965 Nov 13;93(20):1071–9.

Blowers R, Crew B. Ventilation of operating-theatres.*. Epidemiol Infect. 1960 Dec;58(4):427–48.

Chow TT, Kwan A, Lin Z, Bai W. Conversion of operating theatre from positive to negative pressure environment. J Hosp Infect. 2006 Dec 1;64(4):371–8.

Different Types of Operating Rooms: Hybrid, Integrated, Digital O.R. [Internet]. Brainlab. [cited 2021 Jun 21]. Available from: https://www.brainlab.com/journal/hybrid-integrated-digital-o-r-differences-similarities/

Essex-Lopresti M. Operating theatre design. The Lancet. 1999 Mar 20;353(9157):1007–10.

Gupta S, Bharti AA. Interior designing for general operation theater (An architectural approach). 2018;05(11):6.

Harry. General Operating Theatre Design [Internet]. Hospital Design Tips. [cited 2021 Jun 21]. Available from: https://hospitaldesigntips.com/2017/12/07/general-operating-theatre-design/

Harsoor SS, Bhaskar SB. Designing an ideal operating room complex. Indian J Anaesth. 2007 May 1;51(3):193.

HCD Mag [Internet]. [cited 2021 Jun 21]. Available from: https://healthcaredesignmagazine.com/architecture/integrated-operating-room/

Humphreys H. Infection control and the design of a new operating theatre suite. J Hosp Infect. 1993 Jan 1;23(1):61–70.

Indmedica - Journal of the Academy of Hospital Administration [Internet]. [cited 2021 Jun 21]. Available from: https://www.indmedica.com/journals.php?journalid=6&issueid=72&articleid=907&action=article

Kameel R, Khalil E. Energy Efficient and Hygienic Operating Theatres' Hvac Airside Design: Architectural and Engineering Consideration. In: first International Energy Conversion Engineering Conference (IECEC) [Internet]. American Institute of Aeronautics and Astronautics; [cited 2021 Jun 21]. Available from: https://arc.aiaa.org/doi/abs/10.2514/6.2003-5997

Kavic MS. Operating Room Design: "The Devil is in the Details". JSLS. 2001;5(4):297–8.

Krupka D, Sandberg W. Operating room design and its impact on operating room economics. Curr Opin Anaesthesiol. 2006 May 1;19:185–91.

Kumar S. Designing an ideal operating room complex. [cited 2021 Jun 21]; Available from: https://www.academia.edu/29223685/DESIGNING_AN_IDEAL_OPERATING_ROOM_COMPLEX

B. T. Mayes M.V.O. Frcog MB,BS,FRCSE,FRACS. Inst allations in Operating Theatres. Archit Sci Rev. 1961 Mar 1;4(1):2–5.

Ng I. Integrated Intra-operative Room Design. In: Pamir MN, Seifert V, Kiris T, editors. Intraoperative Imaging [Internet]. Vienna: Springer; 2011 [cited 2021 Jun 21]. p. 199–205. (Acta Neurochirurgica Supplementum). Available from: https://doi.org/10.1007/978-3-211-99651-5_31

Planning and constructing a hybrid operating room: Lessons learned [Internet]. Building Design + Construction. [cited 2021 Jun 21]. Available from: https://www.bdcnetwork.com/blog/planning-and-constructing-hybrid-operating-room-lessons-learned

Sánchez-Barroso G, García Sanz-Calcedo J. Evaluation of HVAC Design Parameters in High-Performance Hospital Operating Theatres. Sustainability. 2019 Jan;11(5):1493.

Smylie HG, Dudley HAF. Some Principles in Operating Theatre Design. Scott Med J. 1961 Dec 1;6(12):588–96.

Weldon S-M, Korkiakangas T, Bezemer J, Kneebone R. Music and communication in the operating theatre. J Adv Nurs. 2015;71(12):2763–74.

20 Delivery Room/Labour Room

The Delivery Suite or the Labour Room is a place where childbirth takes place. It is also termed as 'Birthing Unit'. This unit provides facilities for safe prenatal care, delivery and immediate post-natal care of mothers and infants. For a better understanding of this chapter, we will refer to this as '*LDR*' (Labour, Delivery and Resuscitation).

20.1 Location of LDR Complex

While finalizing the location of the LDR, the following points shall be considered:

1. It shall be in a restricted area, where the general movement is not allowed.
2. Complete LDR complex shall be located at the same place as a cluster, ideally on the same floor. Avoid scattering it into different areas.
3. As LDR is a part of the Maternity Unit or Obstetric Unit, it shall be located near to the Obstetric department.
4. It shall be near the NICU (Neo-Natal Intensive Care Unit).

20.2 Zones in LDR Complex

The LDR complex is divided into the following three zones:

20.2.1 Unsterile Zone

This is a zone that is normally unsterile and the movement is allowed without any change.

20.2.2 Protective Zone

This zone is comparatively more sterile and the movement is restricted, but not always. The area can be assessed only by changing the shoes. This area is mainly for change rooms, the supply of materials and services and the spaces for pre-labour room/ward and post-labour room/ward.

20.2.3 Delivery Zone

This area is extremely sterile and aseptic, and is reserved for the actual birth and resuscitation of the babies.

20.3 Infrastructure of LDR Complex

Following is the zone-wise list of different rooms in the complex (Fig. 20.1):

A. Garg, A. Dewan, *Manual of Hospital Planning and Designing*,
https://doi.org/10.1007/978-981-16-8456-2_20

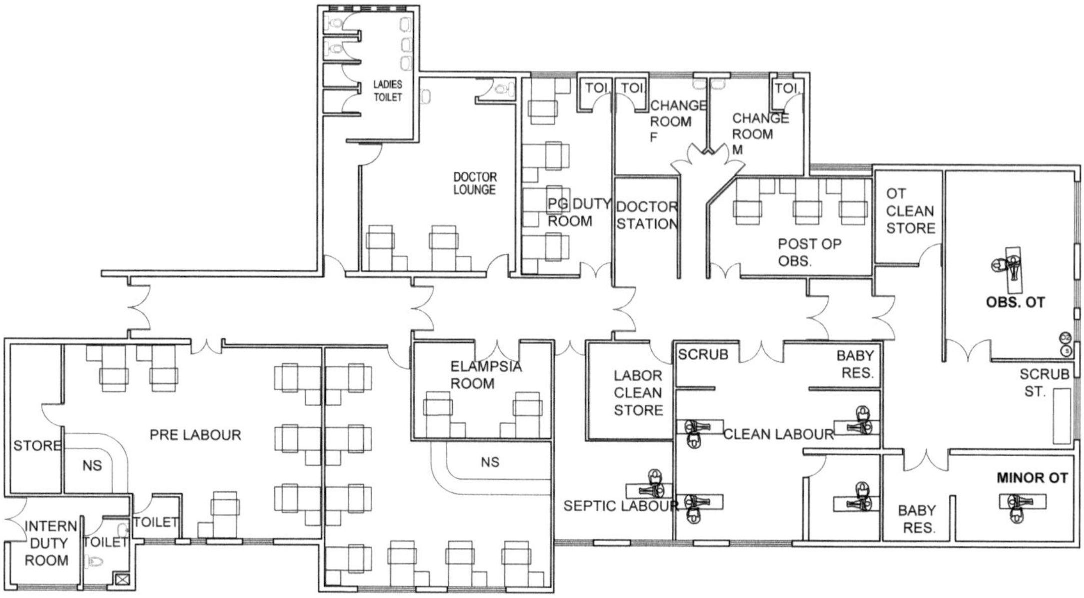

Fig. 20.1 Sample layout drawing of delivery suite with Obs. OR

Unsterile Zone	Administrative area
	Labour room in-charge
	Gynaecologist room for office work
	Entry door for changing room
	Trolley bay
	Shoe changing area
	Linen pre-wash room
	Instrument washroom
	Waiting area for attendants
	Public utility for attendants
Protective Zone	Nursing station
	Pre-labour patient beds
	Eclampsia beds
	Exam/prep
	Postnatal recovery
	Public utilities for patient
	Nurses change room with toilet—males
	Nurses change room with toilet—females
	Class IV change room with toilet—males
	Class IV change room with toilet—females
	Doctors change room with toilet—males
	Doctors change room with toilet—females
	Lockers
	Unsterile store
	Doctors duty room—males
	Doctors duty room—females
	Surgeons restroom

Delivery Area	Delivery room
	Scrub/gowning
	Clean utility
	Baby bath and resuscitation area
	Dirty utility
	Store

20.4 Unsterile Zone

This area of the LDR Complex is an unsterile area, and the movement is allowed to all those who need to provide services or material, or require any communication with the LDR staff. This area is located at the entry gate of the LDR complex and is connected through the entry corridor. Details of rooms located in this zone are:

20.4.1 Administrative Area

This room is for the general administrators and clerical staff managing the LDR Complex. The staff can be from Stores, Sterilization, Housekeeping and Nursing department. The size of this room shall be about 3658 mm × 4572 mm, but depending on the requirement and number of persons likely to sit, the size can be increased or decreased. The room shall have an adequate arrangement of cabinets, drawers, and racks for smooth working. Office tables and chairs shall also be provided. Preferably the room shall have an attached toilet. If required, a separate store shall be attached to this room. The room shall also have proper arrangements for electrical points, intercom connection, I.T. network, CCTV surveillance and air conditioning.

20.4.2 Labour Room In-Charge

This room is for the In-charge of LDR Complex and shall again be located at the entry of the LDR Complex. The size of this room shall be about 4572 mm × 4267 mm. The room shall include an arrangement of office tables, executive chair, visitor chairs and side rack. The room shall have an attached toilet. The room shall also have an attached P.A. room for a clerk to be seated. The room shall have proper arrangements for electrical points, intercom connection, I.T. network and air conditioning.

20.4.3 Gynaecologist Room for Office Work

This room is for the Gynaecologists and their assistants to carry out the official work of the deliveries performed, to prepare notes of delivery etc. The LDR register and the birth register are usually kept here for daily entry. The size of this room shall be about 3658 mm × 4267 mm. The room shall have an arrangement of office tables, executive chair, visitor chairs, side rack etc. The room shall have an attached toilet. The room shall have proper arrangements for electrical points, intercom connection, I.T. network and air conditioning.

20.4.4 Trolley Bay

The is the area reserved for the stretcher trollies and wheelchairs allotted to the LDR Complex. Normally these stretcher trollies are used to move out the patient from LDR Complex after delivery.

20.4.5 Shoe Change Area

Space shall be provided in this zone for changing shoes. The staff desirous of entering the complex has to remove the outside shoes and change with the sleepers/shoes kept for this purpose. This area shall be provided with a sufficient number of shoe racks and a chair for sitting while removing or wearing shoes.

20.4.6 Entry Door for Changing Room

In the LDR Complex, different types of change rooms are provided for Doctors, Technicians, Nurses and class four workers who are required to work in the delivery zone of the complex. The change rooms have to be separate for males and females. The number of the change room to be provided depends on the size of the LDR complex and the number of staff required in the complex. It is recommended that the change room should have dual doors—one for entry and the other for exit.

20.4.7 Waiting Area for Attendants

This area is for the attendants and family members of the patient undergoing the delivery in LDR. The family members being very curious, do not prefer to be seated at a faraway place and always want to sit near the LDR Complex. Therefore, the waiting area shall be provided outside the main entry door of the LDR complex. The waiting area shall be provided with chairs for a comfortable sitting of the family members. This area shall have a speaker connected to the mike system placed in the LDR complex for listening to the announcements made from the LDR. This area shall also have an Intercom facility so that the LDR staff can contact the family members in case of requirement. This area shall be guarded by the security to control the unnecessary movement of family members in the LDR complex and shall be under CCTV surveillance.

20.4.8 Public Utility for Attendants

Along with the waiting area for the family members, the facility of toilets shall be provided. If possible, separate toilets shall be provided for males and females. The facility of drinking water shall also be provided. It will still be better if the tea/coffee vending machine is placed in this area.

20.4.9 Linen Pre-wash Room

This room is used to give a pre-wash to the soiled linen used in the LDR before sending them to the laundry. The room shall be provided with a sink, drainboard and a low height water tap to wash the clothes. Special care shall be taken about the slope in this room so that the water does not spill outside the room.

20.4.10 Instrument Wash Room

This room is used to give a pre-wash to the soiled surgical instruments used in the LDR before sending them to the CSSD. The room shall be provided with a large size sink, drainboard and a countertop for drying up the instruments.

20.5 Protective Zone

This zone is a bit more sterile as compared unsterile zone and the movement is restricted, but not always. The area can be assessed only by changing the shoes or wearing the shoe covers. The clothes need not be changed for going to this area. This area is located just after the unsterile zone and shall be separated from the unsterile zone with the help of a door that shall be guarded. Details of rooms located in this zone have been provided below:

20.5.1 Changing Rooms

The changing rooms are provided in the LDR Complex to enable the doctors and staff to remove the outside clothes and change them to the LDR clothes. It is a set of the pre-sterilized dress (normally a full-length bottom pants and half-sleeved long top) kept in the change rooms. The dresses of different sizes are stitched for different staff members. Different Change rooms are provided for different categories of staff members. Also, the change rooms for males shall be separate from females. Following change rooms are generally provided in the LDR Complex.

1. Doctors Change Room—Males
2. Doctors Change Room—Females
3. Nurses Change Room—Males
4. Nurses Change Room—Females
5. Class IV Staff Change Room—Males
6. Class IV Staff Change Room—Females

Infrastructure wise:

1. Each change room shall be of the size of approximately 4267 mm × 4572 mm.
2. Along with the change room, an attached toilet with a bath facility shall also be provided.
3. The room shall have adequate provision of personal lockers to keep the personal belongings.
4. There shall be adequate hooks on the wall to hang clothes.
5. A hanger rod shall be provided with hangers to hang clothes.
6. There shall be a cabinet to keep the LDR dresses.
7. A large bin for dirty linen shall also be provided in the change room.

20.5.2 Store for Equipment, Medicines, Consumables and Disposables

To avoid any unwanted incident, generally, all the required extra equipment, instruments, medicines, consumables and disposables are stocked in LDR Complex. To store these items, a separate store shall be provided in the protective zone of LDR Complex. The room shall be at least 4572 mm × 6096 mm in size. Adequate lockable cupboards, racks and drawers shall be provided in the store. The store shall also have multiple electric points to charge the equipment when not in use. The store shall also have a countertop to prepare the drugs if required. This store shall be in charge of the storekeeper of LDR Complex.

20.5.3 Pre-labour Room/Ward

The pre-labour room/ward is the area where pregnant women are kept during the labour pain until the cervix is dilated, and the patient is ready for delivery. The definite time of stay in this room is very difficult to access, therefore, there shall be a sufficient number of beds in the ward/room. Based on experience, it is recommended to have four beds per labour table. However, it is advised not to keep more than four beds in one ward, and if more beds are required, an additional ward/room shall be provided.

At times the patient may not like to stay in the ward along with other labour patients and may demand a single room. Also, if the patient is in unrest and disturbing other patients, she should be shifted to a single room. Therefore, a better combination will be to provide a ward of three beds and a single room for each labour table.

If we consider three beds in one ward, size-wise, generally, 7.43–9.29 sq.m space per bed is sufficient, i.e. the room size can be 4572 mm × 6096 mm. For a single bedroom, the size shall be about 4267 mm × 3658 mm.

The room/wards shall also have the following provisions:

1. Supply of Medical Gas Pipeline mounted on the bed head panel on a few beds.
2. Each bed shall be provided with at least two electrical points to connect the medical devices.
3. An adjoining toilet and bathroom with bath and shower facility shall be provided.
4. Individual nurse call button shall be provided on all beds.
5. The facility of foetal monitoring such as cardiotocograph (CTG) monitors should be located to provide ready access to the patient and the monitor.
6. Provisions within the room to support a variety of pain relief methods such as bean bags, alternative seating areas and shelves for patients to lean on at standing and sitting heights.
7. Space for patients to walk around the room with sufficient support.
8. Designated areas for the mother's belongings, gifts and flowers.
9. Provision of soothing music or aromas.
10. Provision of grab rails for patients.
11. Temperature control within the room.

20.5.4 Eclampsia Room

The pre-labour eclampsia room shall be provided in the LRD. Some designer believes in having a single ward with 2–3 eclampsia bed. As the eclampsia patient is very disturbed, it is recommended to have a single bed eclampsia room instead of a single ward with multiple beds. Number wise, one eclampsia room shall be provided with each labour table. Size-wise the room size shall be about 4267 mm × 3658 mm. The facilities in the room shall be similar to the pre-labour room.

20.5.5 Examination/ Preparation Room

This room is used to examine the patient during labour pain for cervix dilation and bleeding. This room shall also work as a Preparation Room to complete the formalities of preparation before sending her to the labour room. This room shall be about 3658 mm × 3658 mm in size, with an examination couch. The room shall have a cabinet to keep the necessary items, a sink and a portable light.

20.5.6 Surgeons Rest Room

This area is also called as the 'Surgeons Lounge'. This room is used by the gynaecologists to relax, complete the patient file, prepare labour notes and post-labour prescriptions. The lounge shall be provided with an attached toilet and a provision of tea/coffee, which can be served from the pantry.

Size-wise the lounge shall be about 3658 mm × 4572 mm, with a sofa set and a centre table. On the request, a single bed can also be placed in the lounge for gynaecologists to lay down for some time.

20.5.7 Dirty Utility

After the delivery, a lot of used items like linen, instruments, covers of disposables, soiled drapes, cotton and gauze have to be removed. Out of this, the linen is sent to linen pre-wash area and instruments to the instrument washroom. Therefore, this dirty utility room is provided at the exit end of the LDR complex. The room shall be about 3048 mm × 3048 mm and provided with bins as per the biomedical waste management rules for other waste products.

20.5.8 Post-labour Recovery Ward

Once the delivery is complete, the mother and the baby have to be sent out of the labour room, and usually the mother is shifted to the post-labour ward/room. This ward is used to provide specialized care to the mother until she is stable. Generally, two beds per labour table are sufficient. However, at times the patient may not like to stay in the ward along with other patients and may demand a single room. Therefore, the provision shall be provided for a single bed post-labour room.

Size-wise, if we consider three beds in one ward, generally, 7.43–9.29 sq.m space per bed is sufficient, i.e. the room size can be 4572 mm × 6096 mm. For a single bedroom, the size shall be about 4267 mm × 3658 mm.

If the baby is normal and stable, he/she may be shifted to the mother's side, or if sick he/she shall be transferred to NICU. Thus, a provision for keeping the baby shall also be provided in the post-labour recovery ward. Bassinets can be used along each bed for this purpose.

The Nursing station shall be provided in the centre of post-labour recovery ward or outside the rooms in case of the single bedroom.

The post-operative recovery ward shall have an attached general store, medicine store, clean utility room, dirty utility room and a toilet. Also, it shall have all other facilities as is provided in the pre-labour room.

After the recovery of the patient, she is transferred to the respective ward or ICU as the case may be. Thus, the location of the post-operative recovery ward shall be at the exit end of the LDR complex.

20.5.9 Doctors Night Duty Rooms

As LDR has to be operative round the clock, there is a need to post a doctor on duty day and night. Hence, a doctor duty room is required in the LDR complex. Separate rooms shall be provided for the males and females. The room shall be of the size 3658 mm × 4267 mm, with an attached toilet. Furniture-wise, the room shall have one office table, chair, bed and cupboard. Apart from the light and fan, the room shall have points for computer with Internet connection and intercom. Also, the room shall be air-conditioned and the control button with temperature adjustment shall be provided in the room.

20.6 Delivery Zone

This is the zone where the actual vaginal birth takes place. This is the most sensitive zone in the LDR Complex. This area has to be totally sterile and aseptic. Delivery zone is separated from the protective zone by providing the swing-type doors, which shall not be less than 6 ft wide. These doors shall be sealed so that any unwanted organism cannot enter this sterile zone. On the exit side of this zone, similar doors are provided. The movement in this zone shall be strictly restricted and only authorized persons shall be allowed, that too after the proper change, with cap and masks. Just at the entry of this zone, a shoe rack is placed which contains sterilized shoes or slippers to be worn before entering this zone. At the exit end of this zone, a double door with air lock shall be provided to transfer the patient out of the post labour recovery room. Details of the rooms located in this zone are as follows:

20.6.1 Clean Supply Room

This room is also termed as Clean Store. This room is mainly used to store the instruments and linen received from CSSD after proper sterilization. It is also used for storing sterile consumables and disposables that are normally used in the labour room. This room shall be located near the labour room so that it can serve the needs effectively.

This room shall be about 4572 mm × 3658 mm in size with a single entry and the door shall be swing type openable on both sides. It is still better if the door is hermetically sealed door operational with sensors. The room shall not have any window; however, if the window is not avoidable, it shall be sealed with double glazing glass. There should be no water supply or drain in this room.

The room shall have stainless steel racks divided into bins, to store the sterilized material. The sterilized material is brought into this room through sterilized covered carts and the material is unloaded in the racks. From here the stored material shall either move directly to LDR or otherwise to the Instrument Trolley Lay-up room.

20.6.2 Instrument Trolley Layup

This room is for preparing the trolley for delivery. The material is brought in this room from the Clean Supply Room and laid on the trolley which in turn shall move to the concerned Labour Room. The trollies for layout are also wheeled from the same Labour Room where it has to go back after lay-up.

This room shall be about 3658 mm × 3658 mm in size with a single entry and the door shall be swing type openable on both sides. The door shall be a sealed door. The room shall not have any window; however, if the window is not avoidable, it shall be sealed with double glazing glass. There should be no water supply or drain in this room.

20.6.3 Scrub Station

The scrub station is used for washing up before entering the labour room for delivery. Every person involved in the delivery process shall be scrubbed in this area. This area should be adjoining the Labour Room. The scrub station can be placed either in an open area or in a closed room. If it is in a closed room, the doors of this room shall be able to easily swing in either direction just by the tap of the foot and should have a see-through glass in the middle.

The scrub area shall be provided with a stainless steel scrub station, which could be operated by foot and/or sensors. Hand-operated taps are not allowed in the scrub station. It shall have a minimum of two bays, with the provision of both hot and cold water to wash hands. The number of scrub stations depends on the number of labour rooms in the complex. It is better if each labour room has its own scrub station. No more than two labour rooms can share one scrub station.

The water outlet of the scrub station shall be designed to allow the water to fall in the centre of the scrub and not spill around. There shall be a provision for dispensing the soap using a wall hanging soap dispenser, which shall be elbow operated. Similarly, an elbow-operated wall hung antiseptic solution dispenser shall be provided with the scrub station. A nail brush should be provided, along with a nail cutter and a nail file.

20.6.4 Sterilization Room

At times during delivery, the surgeon may require some instrument or if accidentally some instrument falls down and gets contaminated, it has to be quickly sterilized to send it back to the surgeon. Therefore, a small sterilization room is provided in the Sterile Zone of the LDR complex which is usually called the Theatre Sterile Supply Unit. This room is located near the LDR clean supply room. The size of the room shall be about

3658 mm × 3658 mm. It shall have a quick steam sterilizer, a hot air oven and a formalin chamber. The room shall have a proper supply of soft water to be used in the sterilizer and the required drain. The room shall have adequate arrangements for exhaust and air exchanges. It shall also be provided with the required electrical point to connect the machines. A compressed air point shall also be provided to remove the debris from the instruments if required.

20.6.5 Delivery Rooms

This room is where the actual vaginal deliveries are carried out. This room has to be the most sterile and aseptic area in the whole of the LDR complex. No person is allowed in the LDR without wearing protective clothing, including shoe covers, masks, caps, eye shields and other coverings to prevent the spread of germs.

20.6.5.1 Number of Delivery Rooms

How many Delivery Rooms shall be required? This is the question normally faced by the designers. There is no thumb rule to decide the number of Delivery Rooms to be made. It will entirely depend on factors like:

1. How many patients of delivery are expected per month? (This figure can be judged from the OPD of the Gynae. and Obs.).
2. How many obstetric patients are generally referred to this hospital per day?

Based on the expected deliveries per month, the number of Delivery Rooms can be planned as follows:

- <20 Deliveries/ month—one Labour Room
- 20–99 Deliveries/ month—two Labour Rooms
- 100–199 Deliveries/ month—four Labour Rooms
- 200–499 Deliveries/ month—six Labour Rooms

If more than 500 deliveries per month are expected, there can be an increase of two labour rooms per 100 deliveries.

20.6.6 Location and Layout of the Delivery Rooms

The location of the delivery rooms shall be in the most sterile and restricted zone. This is the last zone of the LDR Complex.

Design-wise, in the centre of this zone there shall be a corridor and delivery rooms can be provided on both ends of the corridor. In this case, the corridor shall be 3048 mm–3658 mm wide. The delivery room must ensure privacy, and thus the doors shall open on the sidewall of the delivery room. Therefore, there shall be a gallery between two delivery rooms, and doors of both these delivery rooms shall open in that gallery. Another advantage is that at the end of such a gallery, a common scrub station for both these delivery rooms can be fixed.

20.6.7 Types of Delivery Rooms

Based on the requirements and technological development, the construction of delivery rooms has undergone a tremendous improvement over the years. The modern delivery rooms are supposed to be totally sterile and have proper environmental conditions inside the delivery rooms. There are different types of delivery rooms as follows:

1. Simple Room Delivery Rooms
2. Pre-fabricated Modular Delivery Rooms
3. Semi-modular Delivery Rooms
4. Modular Delivery Rooms

The construction and designing of all types of delivery rooms are exactly as per OR. Thus, for further detail on this topic, please refer to the chapter 'Operation Theatre Suite'.

20.6.8 Equipment in Delivery Rooms

Suction machine electrical	Multi-para Monitor with ET CO_2
Defibrillator	Blood pressure apparatus
Electrosurgical cautery	Surgical instruments
Tools for assisted deliveries	UPS 10 KVA

Foetal doppler	Portable O.T. Light
Labour table	Portable Ultrasound
Operating light	A clock with seconds hand on the wall
Emergency light	Baby Resuscitation Unit

20.6.9 Furniture Delivery Rooms

Instrument Trolleys	Doctor stool
Mayo stand	I.V. stand
Swab rack	Sterilization drums
Steel bucket with lid Footstool	

20.6.10 Other Issues Relating to the Delivery Room

1. Lighting in birthing rooms should be dimmable for patient comfort.
2. Privacy is essential for both the assessment and the birthing rooms. Avoid direct views into the room from the outside, through the windows and doors, i.e. do not provide door viewing panels and a privacy curtain should be allowed.
3. The foot end of the labour table should be facing away from the door or the access point.
4. Walls should include a sound-deadening material to prevent noise transfer between rooms.

20.6.11 Septic Delivery Room

It is the room where infected cases are delivered. The construction, specifications and design of this delivery room are the same as any other. However, the equipment and furniture of this delivery room are separate, and shall not be used in the normal delivery room.

20.7 Baby Resuscitation Area

Space for infant resuscitation/stabilization shall be provided within delivery rooms. At times, the baby resuscitation area is separated within the delivery room with a partition in between. In such cases, windows and doors shall be designed for visual and acoustical privacy and shall allow easy exchange of an infant between personnel. When an delivery room is equipped with a pass-through window or door, it shall have a positive pressure so that air flows out to the infant room when the window or door is opened. The ventilation system for each delivery and resuscitation room shall be designed to control the ambient temperature between 72 and 78 °F (22–26 °C) during the delivery, resuscitation and stabilization of the newborn.

Following equipment are normally placed in the baby resuscitation area:

1. Radiant warmer
2. Resuscitation kit with functional bag and mask
3. Mucus extractor
4. Pre-warmed baby receiving towels
5. Shoulder roll
6. Paediatric stethoscope
7. An oxygen cylinder

A minimum clear floor area of 7.43 sq.m shall be provided for infant space. This space may be used for multiple purposes including resuscitation, stabilization, observation, examination, sleep or other infant needs.

A total of 2 oxygen, 2 air, 2 vacuum and 12 simultaneously accessible electrical outlets shall be provided for the infant in addition to the facilities required for the mother.

The infant space may not be omitted from the delivery room even if a separate infant resuscitation/stabilization room is provided.

20.8 Other Important Issues to be Considered While Designing LDR

20.8.1 Labour Table Specifications

1. Adjustable side rails.
2. Facilities for Trendelenburg/reverse positions.
3. Facilities for height adjustment (hydraulic pump or Electric).

4. Stainless steel IV rod.
5. Mobility: swivelling castor wheels and brakes.
6. The mattress should be washable, waterproof, seamless, divided into three parts, have thin cushioning at the joints, detachable at the perineal end and a spare set shall be kept.
7. Disposable draw sheet.
8. Steel basins attachments.
9. Calf support, handgrip and leg support.

20.8.2 Shifting Baby to NICU

Preterm infants are at greater risk and often require additional personnel, equipment and time to optimize resuscitation and stabilization, thus requiring care as per the NICU standards. Such babies shall be immediately shifted to NICU just after the resuscitation. For shifting a 'Transport Incubator' shall be kept near the delivery room.

20.8.3 Access to the Operating Room

At times it may happen that during the vaginal delivery, the patient suddenly gets serious and immediately requires a Caesarean Section. Therefore, the approach and access to the Obstetrics operating room shall be quick. Hence, it is advised that the Obstetrics Operating Room shall be in the LDR Complex.

To increase the safety of newborns, the use of electronic tagging may be implemented immediately after birth. This involves a combination of the infant wearing a tag around the ankle and sensor panels located at every access and exit point to the unit and possibly the entire hospital.

Acknowledgement I am grateful to Dr. Rohit Varshney for his great support in compiling this chapter. I wish to convey my thanks and gratitude to him for the time and efforts he has put in.

Further Reading

12VAC5-410-442. Obstetric service design and equipment criteria. [Internet]. [cited 2021 Jun 22]. Available from: https://law.lis.virginia.gov/admincode/title12/agency5/chapter410/section442/

Atmaca H. Patient Centered Approaches in Labor and Delivery Room Design in Hospitals: Case Study in Dokuz Eylül University Hospital. 2013;130.

Austin N, Kristensen-Cabrera A, Sherman J, Schwandt D, McDonald A, Hedli L, et al. Analyzing the heterogeneity of labor and delivery units: A quantitative analysis of space and design. PLOS ONE. 2018 Dec 26;13(12):e0209339.

ECG | Obstetrics Unit Labor and Delivery Design: LDR Vs. LDRP [Internet]. [cited 2021 Jun 22]. Available from: https://www.ecgmc.com/thought-leadership/articles/obstetrics-unit-labor-and-delivery-design-ldr-vs-ldrp

Esfeh B, Kazemi A, Shamsaie A. Designing architecture of soothing labor–delivery–recovery–postpartum unit: a study protocol. Reprod Health. 2020 Dec 10;17.

Jullien JM. Planning the Labor-delivery Unit in the General Hospital. U.S. Department of Health, Education, and Welfare, Public Health Service, Division of Hospital and Medical Facilities, Architectural and Engineering Branch; 1964. 28 p.

Wrønding T, Argyraki A, Petersen JF, Topsøe MF, Petersen PM, Løkkegaard ECL. The aesthetic nature of the birthing room environment may alter the need for obstetrical interventions – an observational retrospective cohort study. Sci Rep. 2019 Jan 22;9(1):303.

21 Intermediate Care Area (Patient Rooms)

In any hospital setup, the importance and utility of the Patient Rooms cannot be ignored. It is a zone where a patient is admitted for the required treatment and recovery. This is also one of the places where the patient or family members get to know about the quality of care and services provided by the hospital.

Patients rely on staff to respond quickly to an emergency situation, check them frequently and ensure a full recovery. However, the staff can treat patients effectively only when they perform their tasks efficiently and have adequate equipment and supplies that are easily accessible. Thus, the design, interiors, comfort, cleanliness and safety of the room, and alertness and care provided by the nursing staff are the main factors contributing towards patient satisfaction.

One of the greatest challenges faced by the designers while designing a hospital room is the need to accommodate the following three important functions. First, the room shall be comfortable and calming for the patient. Second, health workers must be able to navigate the space, quickly and efficiently. And finally, family members and other visitors must have an area where they can comfortably sit or sleep without disrupting the staff workflow or the patient's recovery. This may not always be possible for small hospitals; however, the designer shall always try to accommodate such spaces.

Such designs not only streamline the staff workflow but also help to improve patient recovery rate, leading to higher patient satisfaction. This, in turn, results in the increased business of the hospital.

General issues to be considered while designing the Patient room/ward in the hospital

21.1 Improve Patient and Staff Safety

While designing the patient room spaces, the safety of the staff and patients shall be the priority. The staff shall be able to protect themselves and the patient in case of any adverse condition. The following measures shall be taken while designing or constructing such spaces:

1. If a patient is deemed to be at a higher risk for self-harm, self-injury or suicide, the room shall be designed in such a way that each corner of the room is visible from the outside corridor. This allows nurses and other hospital staff to continuously watch the patient.
2. One-on-one observation by the staff or the patient's attendants shall be arranged.
3. CCTV can be used for surveillance of the patient inside the room.
4. There shall be no hiding places, sharp-edged furniture or tools for patient to use any equipment or furnishings in the room, as a weapon against staff or self.

A. Garg, A. Dewan, *Manual of Hospital Planning and Designing*,
https://doi.org/10.1007/978-981-16-8456-2_21

5. Curved angles, hidden and pull-out equipment and furniture in the room can greatly reduce the risk of using them as weapons to harm staff or self.
6. Glass shall be avoided in the room; however, if it cannot be avoided, tempered glass shall be used instead of normal glass.
7. Plastic silver-coated mirrors shall be used rather than glass mirrors.
8. Bottom height of the windows shall be more so that the patient cannot jump out of the windows.
9. Double glazing or grills shall be fit on all windows.
10. Ceiling fans shall be avoided.
11. Curtain rod or cloth hanging rods shall be avoided.
12. Shower rod and showerheads shall be short with no weight-bearing capacity.
13. The flooring of the room and the bathroom shall be non-slippery and at zero levels.
14. Bathroom shall be provided with the proper grab bars.
15. Since most of the falls occur between the bed and the toilet, designers shall try to reduce this distance. Grab bars shall be added in this distance.

21.2 Increase Patient and Staff Satisfaction

One of the most important factors in a hospital setup is the satisfaction level of the patients, which helps to increase the business. Above this, is the staff satisfaction level. If they are satisfied, they will give more input, and efficiency, resulting in good patient care and treatment. This care will again increase patient satisfaction, and this vicious cycle will continue. The following factors in a patient room contribute to increased patient and staff satisfaction:

1. The room shall have excellent facilities and shall be pleasant looking.
2. Environmental conditions such as the temperature of the room shall not be too high or too low.
3. Similarly, humidity shall be kept at average as higher humidity levels will cause suffocation to the patient.
4. The room shall be silent and free from unwanted sounds and noise.
5. The room shall be designed to allow cross ventilation and be odourless.
6. The room shall have sufficient natural lighting. However, glaze shall be minimized in the room. As natural light shifts throughout the day (and throughout the year), proper sun shades shall be provided to the building.
7. The room shall be provided with windows through which natural landscapes like trees, gardens etc. are visible.
8. Single-patient rooms with private toilets shall be preferred.
9. The room shall have a provision for the patient's family and friends to be seated comfortably.
10. The room shall be designed to allow easy cleaning. For example, provide wipeable surfaces, washable paints, easy-clean flooring and a proper garbage disposable system in the rooms.
11. The room shall provide entertainment facilities like television or small indoor/board games like Ludo, Playing Cards and Chess.
12. The room shall have attractive wall paintings, wall arts and sceneries.
13. The hospital can also think of providing free Internet facility to patients with a smartphone or laptop.
14. The hospital can also think of providing portable electronic media to allow patients to make an audio-video call to his/her family members.

21.3 Provide Amenities and Comfort for the Family

Often anxious family members/friends visit a hospital with the patient. Moreover, the family's support plays a significant role in the patient's recovery and reduces morbidity. For this reason, a Family Support Zone shall be placed near the patient rooms. This zone shall have the following facilities:

21.3.1 Family Lounge

A family and visitor's lounge should be provided adjacent to the patient room. For a few rooms put together, a single-family lounge can be created. It must have a comfortable waiting area with reclining chairs, privacy during conversations and a telephone/intercom facility. It shall also have basic amenities like a television, newspaper and magazine stand and a small play area for children. Snack, tea and coffee vending machines shall also be provided. Visitor access should be controlled from the receptionist area. Shelves, closets and secure lockers shall also be provided to avoid scattering personal belongings around the lounge. Accessible toilets for males and females should be reasonably close to, or a part of, the lounge.

21.3.2 Consultation Rooms

Anxious family members often need to see the treating physician to obtain an update on patient condition/recovery. Therefore, consultation rooms shall be provided in the patient rooms area. One such room for 20–30 beds is sufficient. This room shall be about 4572 mm × 4267 mm with the provision of a table, chairs and a sofa set. At times there can be hot discussions, thus, a security personnel shall be placed outside the room. Further, this room shall be under CCTV surveillance.

21.3.3 Meditation Spaces

Disturbed family members of the patient are often under fear and seek blessings from the Almighty. Therefore, it is advised to provide a room near the patient rooms for meditation, reflection and spiritual contemplation. It should be noted that while designing this space, there shall be an area dedicated to all religions and not particularly any one religion.

21.3.4 Family Cafeteria

Usually, a cafeteria is provided on the ground floor of the hospital, from where the family members can obtain refreshments. Drinking water fountains or other freshwater supply facilities should be located within or near the cafeteria and lounge. Some hospitals provide food trays to the family members at different meal times. In such cases, a separate space or dining hall shall be provided, where the family members can be served their meals. Vending machines can also be helpful, particularly at late hours when the hospital coffee shops or food services may not be available. However, in both the cases, care shall be taken to provide arrangements for adequate disposal of used utensils and maintain hygiene standards.

21.3.5 Family Sleep Rooms

At times, a family member needs to stay with the patient for providing special care. Therefore, it is recommended that an individual patient's room shall have a provision for a family member to stay. If that cannot be provided, then a separate guest house shall be arranged, which can be allotted to the family members on payment. These guest houses may have the amenities like bed, bedding, toilet, TV, fridge and mess. The hospital can also enter into an agreement with a nearby hotel to accommodate visitors and families, the rent of which shall be paid by the family member.

21.3.6 Family Laundry

This can be an extra facility provided to the family members of the patient, particularly the patients who have to stay longer in the hospital. For this, a separate counter shall be dedicated where clothes can be given. The unwashed clothes can be sent for washing to the central laundry of the hospital and returned to the same counter from where they can be collected. This service shall be payable by the family member.

21.4 Increase Staff Efficiency

The hospital staff is under a great deal of tiredness and pressure as they have to run throughout the day to provide care and treatment to patients. The following factors can help reduce staff run-around and increase their efficiency:

1. Decentralizing the supply of consumables, instruments, medicines and equipment by making it available within or near the patient rooms.
2. Nursing counter shall be placed near the patient rooms.
3. Nurse Call System shall be provided between the patient room and the nurse station. An audio-visual system can also be provided near the patient for easy communication. This can be done with the help of a call activation button hanging near the patient bed, which shall be in reach of the patient. As soon as the patient presses the button, the audio and video system shall get activated. The video camera can be fixed on the ceiling, at the patient head side. Once the call is activated, the nurse can see the patient's video on the screen fitted in the nurse control unit. He/she can then have a conversation with the patient and can also see the patient's condition. If needed, the patient can be given proper instructions via the call, else the nurse can visit the patient's room for assistance.
4. Providing proper support room for the staff near the nursing stations allows for more efficient working. These rooms shall be like nurses duty room, staff change rooms, medication store for patient medicines, clean store, dirty utility, pantry, separate toilet for the staff, janitor etc.
5. Charting can be choreographed through a touch screen monitor placed beside the patient's bed. This will save physicians and nurses from writing notes in the charts, bringing the chart to the patient room and turning the pages to see the chart. It is even better if the physicians' instructions are immediately recorded in the system through the same monitor. Another advantage is that the access to lab reports, vital signs and medications throughout the course of the patient's treatment and other details of the patient shall be immediately available to the physicians on the monitor next to the patient's bed.

21.5 Patient Room Furnishings

Patient rooms or units shall have a decent and aesthetic finish. It helps in early recovery of the patient and leaves a long-term effect on the patient about the quality of service. Hence, the furnishing of the patient room/unit shall be designed carefully. Apart from the furniture, the room shall also have the following:

1. Soiled linen collection hamper.
2. The waste collection as per the norms of Biomedical Waste Management.
3. A Wall Clock on the foot end of the patient.
4. Calendar.
5. Tack Board.
6. White Board.
7. Horizontal surfaces to keep greeting cards/photos.
8. Mobile/Laptop charging points.
9. Internet Connection/Wi-Fi.
10. Intercom with facility for outside calls.
11. Cabinet for storage of personal belongings.
12. Television (not applicable for ICU).

21.5.1 Room Decor

Pleasant and aesthetic patient surroundings, along with increased comfort, results in improved outcomes. For this, the following can be done:

1. Good colour schemes, particularly, light green and blue colours shall be chosen as they decrease stress levels in patients.

2. Wall furnishings shall be excellent with waterproof and washable paints.
3. Pictures, paintings, murals and artwork shall be placed appropriately for patients, families and caregivers.
4. The ceiling is the most often observed space by a bed-ridden patient. Thus, it can be painted with pictures and sceneries. Even 3D laminated ceilings can be opted for.

21.5.2 Lighting in the Patient Room

Lighting for general illumination and specific tasks has to be carefully planned. Following issues related to the lighting shall be considered:

1. The lights shall not be too bright or too dull. Proper lumens have to be planned as per the standards.
2. Use of LED lights is always recommended because they offer a longer usage life and lower energy consumption.
3. The lights shall be equally distributed in the unit/room.
4. Surface exposed lights shall not be used. Instead, ceiling flush-mounted lights shall be used.
5. Avoid wall lights as they are not effective.
6. Avoid fancy lights.
7. Avoid incandescent and halogen light sources to prevent burns.
8. Flexible arms, if used with this light source, must be mechanically controlled to prevent the lamp from contacting linen.
9. The patient bed should be provided with an adjustable reading light that can be easily controlled by the patient.
10. Separate lighting for emergencies and procedures should be located in the ceiling directly above the patient on each bed. An LED light of 610 mm × 610 mm ceiling flush-mounted should be fixed at a 1219-mm distance from the wall. This light shall be switched on only during any procedure.
11. Night low-level illumination shall be provided at the height of 18 in. from the floor, near the patient's bed.
12. Emergency battery operated light shall be provided in the corridors and patient unit.
13. It will be better if the light controls are done through variable-control dimmers at the user end.

21.5.3 Ceiling Finishes

The ceilings in patient rooms/units/wards shall be smooth, able to be scrubbed with chemicals, non-absorptive and without crevices. If the false ceiling is provided, it shall have securely tightened service windows. The paint of the ceiling shall be elegant and pleasing.

21.6 Types of Patient Rooms in the Hospital

There are different types of wards in a hospital such as Family Suites, Deluxe Rooms, Single bed (Private) Rooms, Sharing beds (Semi-private) Rooms, General Ward (Multiple Beds), Isolation Ward, Post-operative Ward, ICU, ICCU and Nursery. The patients in all these wards should be kept according to the severity of the disease and/or patient's paying capacity.

While groups of rooms/wards should be set apart for the treatment of different types of diseases, the principle of progressive patient care should still be followed. For example, the post-operative ward and the intensive care ward should be organized in such a way that constant skilled attention is available to the patients in these wards. These areas have already been discussed in the chapters of 'Intensive Care Units' (Chap. 18) and 'OT Complex' (Chap. 19).

Let us now discuss some other room types:

21.6.1 Single Bed Occupancy

These rooms are also known as 'Private Ward' and have one patient bed with other amenities. They can be sub-categorized as follows:

1. Normal Private Room
2. Deluxe Room
3. Super Deluxe Room
4. Suites

21.6.2 Sharing Rooms

These are also known as 'Semi-Private Rooms' and usually have 2–4 patient beds shared in a single room.

21.6.3 General Wards

These are the wards having multiple beds, generally between 6 and 30 beds in a single hall.

21.6.4 Isolation Ward/Rooms

These are separately demarcated areas for housing infectious patients. Under this category as well, there can be Private Rooms, Semi-private Rooms and General Wards.

21.7 Infrastructure Details of the Indoor Patient Units

General Ward (Multiple beds)	Patient Beds
	Nurse Desk
	Nurses Duty Room
	Store
	Dirty Utility/Sluice Room
	Clean Supply Room
	Examination and Treatment Room
	Ward Pantry
	Resident Doctors and Student Duty Room
	Extra Rooms for Future expansion
	Public Utility for Staff
	Public Utility for Patients and Attendants
	Visitors Bay
Semi-private Ward (Twin Sharing)	Patient Beds (Twin Sharing) with Toilet
	Nurse Desk
	Store
	Dirty Utility/Sluice Room
	Clean Supply Room
	Examination and Treatment Room
	Ward Pantry
	Resident Doctors and Student Duty Room
	Nurses Duty Room
	Extra Rooms for Future expansion
	Public Utility for Staff
	Visitors Bay
Private Ward (Single Bed)	Patient Beds (Single Bed) with Toilet
	Nurse Desk
	Store
	Dirty Utility/Sluice Room
	Clean Supply Room
	Examination and Treatment Room
	Ward Pantry
	Resident Doctors and Student Duty Room
	Nurses Duty Room
	Extra Rooms for Future expansion
	Public Utility for Staff
	Visitors Bay
Deluxe Ward (Single Bed)	Patient Beds (Single Bed) with Toilet
	Nurse Desk
	Store
	Dirty Utility/Sluice Room
	Clean Supply Room
	Examination and Treatment Room
	Ward Pantry
	Resident Doctors and Student Duty Room
	Nurses Duty Room
	Extra Rooms for Future expansion
	Public Utility for Staff
	Visitors Bay
Family Suites (Single Bed)	Patient Beds (Single Bed) with Toilet
	Family Room
	Nurse Desk
	Store
	Dirty Utility/Sluice Room
	Clean Supply Room
	Examination and Treatment Room
	Ward Pantry
	Resident Doctors and Student Duty Room
	Nurses Duty Room
	Extra Rooms for Future expansion
	Public Utility for Staff
	Visitors Bay

21.8 Location of the Indoor Patient Areas

Zoning of the indoor hospital area has to be carefully planned. It has to be kept in mind that the indoor area is a *Limited movement zone*, and only the patient and family members are allowed to enter this area. Hence, it is advisable to plan this area on the upper floors of the building. As per the 12 storey building design explained earlier, the suggested indoor area can be planned between fourth and seventh floors.

As we have different categories of indoor rooms and wards to be located, two options for allocating space to each one of them across floors have been suggested below.

The first option is to plan all single room types in a cluster on a single floor. For example, all the single bedrooms (private/deluxe/suite) on one floor, all semi-private room on another floor etc.

The second option is that each floor shall have a mixture of all the wards/rooms. For example, a few private rooms, semi-private rooms and one or more general wards on each floor.

Both systems have their own pros and cons. However, opting for the first option is reasonably better as the rooms will ideally be of identical size; thus, the room design will be better placed for family lounges can be planned better, the nursing station can be at a better place, toilets can be planned wall to wall in the same length, movement of the staff and people can be better controlled etc.

Ideally, in a 12 storey building, all general wards can be placed on the fourth floor, semi-private rooms on the fifth floor and the sixth and seventh floors can be reserved for all private wards. Along with these, required attachments and spaces shall also be planned on the same floor.

21.9 Zoning of the Isolation Areas

One potential response is dedicating specific areas, either within hospitals where infectious patients are managed or in dedicated non-infectious facilities, where elective care may be delivered. Post-COVID-19 designs shall be such where the zoning of the indoor patient area shall be a necessity. A separate zone shall be provided for infected patients. All types of ward/rooms shall be created in this zone only. For example, the isolation zone shall have a separate set of the general ward, semi-private rooms, private rooms, deluxe rooms, suites etc. If needed, a separate Intensive Care Unit shall also be provided in this zone for infected patients. It is recommended that all the categories of isolated indoor units of a particular zone shall be in a cluster (maybe on the same floor/block/building or adjoining floors/blocks/buildings).

21.10 Single Patient Room (Private Room)

Multiple occupancy rooms are on their way out. Most of the patients nowadays prefer to have a single-occupancy room to ensure privacy, comfort and availability of family members nearby. Also, patients prefer to have better care and treatment, irrespective of the cost. Any patient, who can afford the costs, always prefers to choose a single-occupancy private room than multiple occupancies. This increases the revenue of the hospital because the charges of single occupancy rooms are more than other low category wards/rooms. Therefore, the hospital owners shall prefer to have a greater number of single bed units. This cannot be true for the charitable hospitals, as their motive is to provide treatment to the poor for free or at a negligible cost. Under this scenario, the concept of the general ward with multiple beds is better. Otherwise, single occupancy rooms considerably help in controlling the spread of infections such as COVID-19, methicillin-resistant *Staphylococcus aureus*, Gram-negative bacteraemia in burn patients, and respiratory and enteric infections requiring contact isolation in paediatric units.

A well-designed patient room has also been found to be a factor in improved patient care by providing better patient consultations, improved patient and clinician satisfaction, decreased length of stay and continuity of care during the hospital stay.

21.10.1 Room Layout

The single patient occupancy room shall be divided into three zones—a) staff zone located at the room entrance to allow efficiency in performing their tasks, b) patient zone where the patient's bed is placed and c) family zone for providing comfortable seating for visitors.

21.10.2 Size of the Room

A private single room shall have an area of about 23.22 sq.m including the family space and toilet.

While designing a single occupancy private patient room, the following points shall be considered:

21.10.3 Walls

The room shall be covered with walls on all the four sides except the area for windows and door. The wall thickness shall not be less than 120 mm with plaster on both sides of the wall. The walls can either be made out of clay bricks or hollow blocks, as per the design and technical civil construction details.

21.10.3.1 Headwall

The wall behind and the ceiling over the patient's head are the most important spaces for incorporating clinical care elements. Provisions for medical gases, power, information systems, monitoring and critical equipment storage are located here.

21.10.3.2 Footwall

It displays those items that the patient will directly view, such as television, clock and tackboard with different information. It is an ideal location for artwork. Most hospitals nowadays incorporate a flat screen television monitor with computer capabilities on the footwall.

21.10.4 Doors

The door of the room shall not be less than 1829 mm wide, unobstructed. A wide door is suggested for easy movement of the bed in and out of the room in case of emergency.

21.10.5 Windows

As natural lights help in early recovery and avoid disorientation and a sense of claustrophobia in patients, windows shall be preferred in the room; however, direct sunlight shall be avoided. Further, a window with an outside view such as gardens, trees, courtyard, or other natural settings, may help to relieve anxiety and stress, improve care, enhance patients' comfort and improve their orientation. The window shall be located on the front wall, or any sidewall (left/right) so that the patient can see outside the window even in lying position. The window may be openable or non-open able, depending on the design. However, the glass shall be tinted or curtains/blinds shall be provided. If cost is not a criterion, then electronic windows, which are transparent when switched off and turn opaque when switched on, can be fixed.

21.10.6 Toilets

A separate toilet and bathroom with a handwashing station shall be provided in all rooms. For single occupancy rooms, shared or common toilets are not allowed. As far as the location of the toilet is concerned, there are three models for it as suggested below:

21.10.6.1 Mid-board Toilet Model

Under this concept, toilets are located back to back between two patient rooms. i.e. the toilets of both the rooms are sandwiched between two rooms. This design allows the rooms to be of square or rectangular shape, the best shape for any acuity level. The full-width wall along the corridor allows maximum visibility at the patient, while the full-width window wall allows maximum space for family seating and outside viewing. The bed can also be nearer to the corridor door for easy staff access. The toilet door is on the foot side of the bed. The negative point of such a design is that each pair of rooms generate approximately 6 ft of additional corridor length (Fig. 21.1).

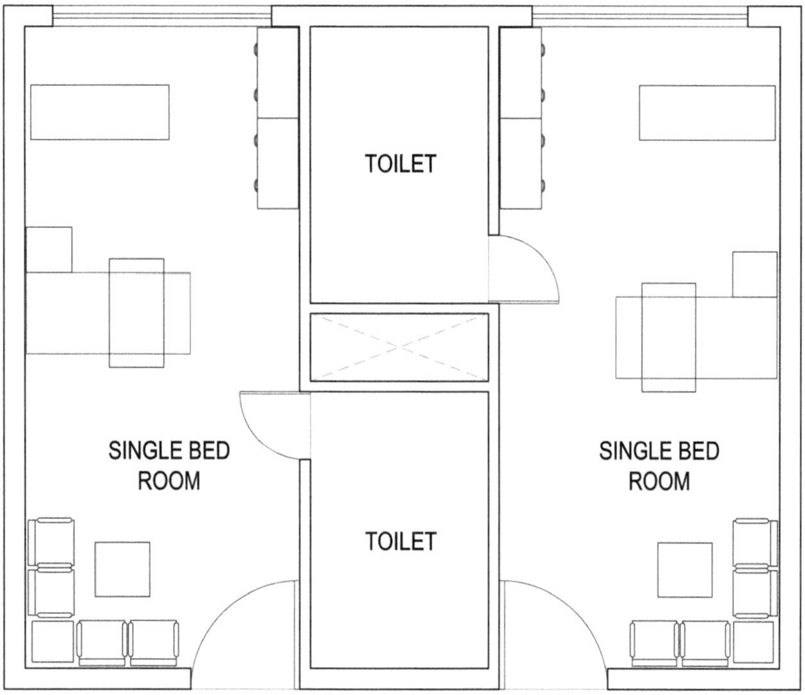

Fig. 21.1 Sample layout drawing of mid-board single occupancy room

21.10.6.2 Inboard Toilet Model

Under this concept, toilets are located on the corridor side, adjacent to the patient room door. This type of design allows the toilet to be more accessible to the patient and the housekeeping. It also allows the window wall to be open to its full width, maximizing natural light and views, and allows more space for a family. By placing the toilet inboard, there is more sound attenuation from corridor noise and more privacy. A drawback is a reduced visibility from the corridor and the distance of the patient's bed from the door makes this room type less ideal for patients. Another drawback is difficulty of moving the patient out of the room in case of emergency. The design shall be such where the staff moving in the corridor can have an easy look at the patient's condition and provide immediate help if needed (Fig. 21.2).

21.10.6.3 Outboard Toilet Model

Under this concept, toilets are placed on the back side of the patient room, on the outer wall. This allows maximum visibility of the patient from the corridor and reduces the distance between the bed and the corridor. However, the window and family area are a setback from the patient, reducing views and light, and making family interaction more difficult. The housekeeping must traverse the room to clean the toilet room (Fig. 21.3).

After comparing the advantages and disadvantages of all three concepts, it is recommended to opt for the Mid-board Toilet Model concept because:

1. It gives a proper rectangular shape to the room.
2. On the corridor side, a wide window can be provided to view and keep a watch on the patient's condition.
3. On the back wall, bigger windows can be provided for better natural light and outer views. This can relieve the patient from landing into claustrophobia.
4. Toilet being sandwiched between a pair of rooms, shall provide the space for water supply and drain line to be taken directly outside the building and terminate them in the service shafts provided for this purpose.

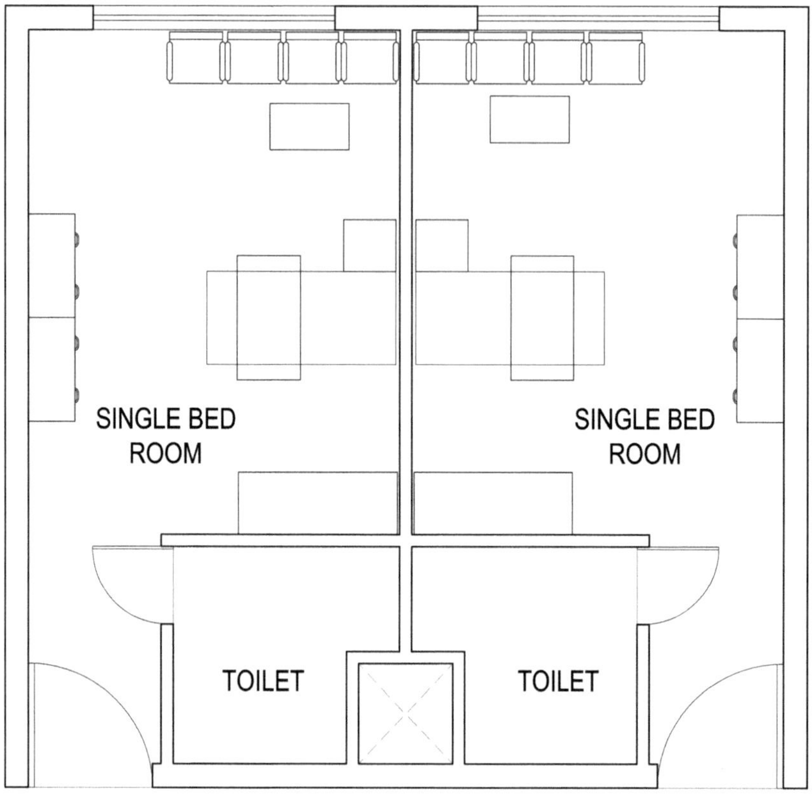

Fig. 21.2 Sample layout drawing of in-board single occupancy room

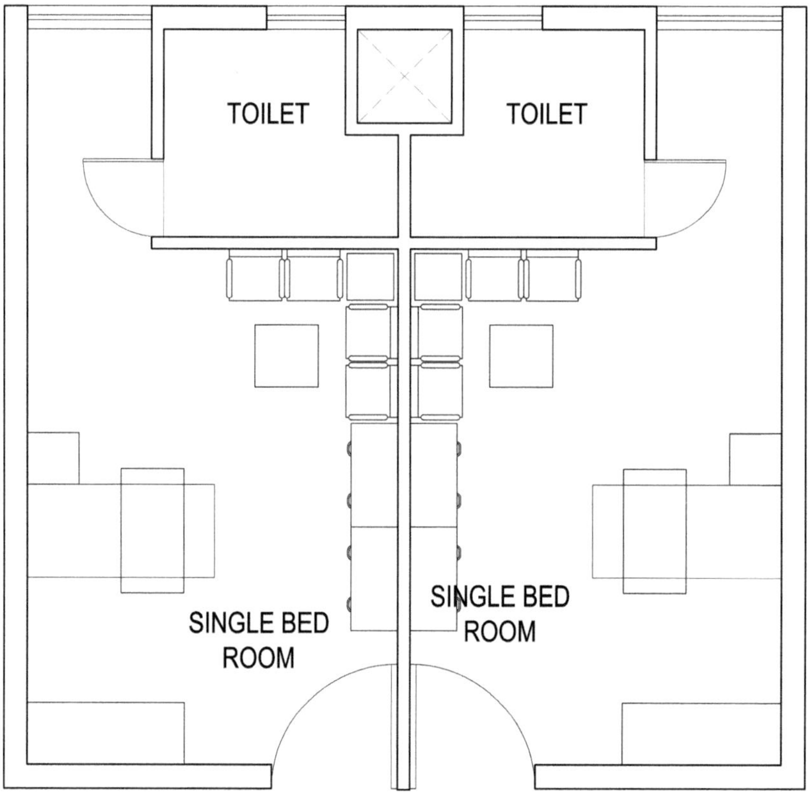

Fig. 21.3 Sample layout drawing of out-board single occupancy room

5. More length of the toilets can be achieved. Suppose the length of patient room is 4267 mm, we can have two toilets of 2134 mm length and the width can be 1524–1829 mm (as per requirement), allowing more spaces for sanitary fittings.
6. The toilets shall be designed considering the safety factors. For bariatric and handicapped patients, accessible toilets shall be provided with proper support, grab bars and hand rails.
7. The toilets shall have a proper and effective exhaust system of appropriate size.
8. The floor level of the toilet shall be at zero level compared to the floor level of the room, for easy movement of the wheelchair.
9. For bath, non-slippery pads shall be provided.
10. Indian type of WC shall not be provided in the toilets.
11. Non-slippery tiles shall be used for flooring of the toilet.
12. The toilets shall not have a bolt locking system from inside. So that in case of emergency, it can be opened with a key from the outside.
13. Provision of both hot and cold water shall be provided in the toilets.

21.10.7 Bed Layout in Patient Room

The bed in the patient room shall be laid out in such a way that it allows easy and smooth working all around the bed. The following points shall be kept in mind while laying down the bed in a room:

1. Head end of the bed shall be at least 610 mm away from the wall.
2. The head support panel of the bed shall be removable.
3. On the foot end, a clear space shall be about 1524 mm so that the stretcher trolley can easily be turned around and patient can be transferred from/to bed.
4. Distance of family couch/sitting from the patient bed shall not be less than 914 mm.

21.10.8 Furniture and Instruments in Patient Room

Patient Furniture

Patient Bed (preferable should be Multi-positional ICU Bed on lockable wheels with bed side safety rails or otherwise the fowler bed with bed side railing can be used)	
Bed Side Locker	IV Stand
Over Bed Table	IV Rod
Step Stool	Back Rest

Other Furniture

Pull-out bed or plain sofa set	Dining chairs
Attendant bed	Centre Table
Small dining table (if space is available)	Cupboard

Equipment

Multi-para Vital Sign Monitor (if required)	Air Mattress

Tools and Instruments

Walkers (if required)	Weighing Machine
Refrigerator	Other required instruments

21.10.9 Air Conditioning System of Patient Rooms

Patient rooms shall be fully air-conditioned, which allows control of temperature, humidity and air exchanges. Suitable and safe air quality must be maintained at all times. Following issues are important while designing the Air Conditioning System:

1. For air conditioning of patient rooms, either the Chilled Water Pipeline with Fan Coil Units (FCU) or the Ductable Split or VRV system can be opted.
2. Each room shall have individual return air provisions. The return air of any room shall not be mixed with other rooms/units/areas.

3. Air flow, direction and air exchanges have to be as per the industry norms.
4. Heating shall be done with water pipeline and FCUs having hot water generator instead of water chillers. Otherwise, room heaters can be opted; however, they are generally not recommended.
5. Temperature shall be between 21 and 24 °C.
6. Depending on the type of room/unit, the choice of positive or negative operating pressures shall be made. For isolation rooms, negative pressure shall be adopted.

   For full details on Air-conditioning, heating and air exchanges, please refer to the chapter of 'HVAC' (Chap. 38) in this book.

21.10.10 Central Piped Medical Gas Supply

In all the patient rooms, Piped Centralized Medical Supply shall be provided to handle any emergencies. Usually, the provision of mechanical ventilation is not provided in the patient room, as it is difficult to handle ventilated patients in the rooms. Therefore, such patients need to be transferred to the ICU for further management. The following gases are supplied:

Oxygen

Wall-mounted Suction

In patient rooms, the facility of supply of these lines shall be on every bed. In some hospitals, the outlets of these gases are fixed on the wall itself. Nowadays, the bedhead panel is used for this. It is a 1219-mm panel made of extruded sections of aluminium. This panel has a provision for fixing the gas outlets and the electrical points. Also, this panel has a service railing on which the IV rod, monitor tray and utility basket can be fixed. This panel is fixed at the height of 1524 mm above the floor level and goes up to 1829 mm. The panel is fixed on the head side wall of the patient.

21.10.11 Electrical Points in Patient Room

1. Main Switch board shall be at the entrance wall for controlling fans and lights of the hall along with one 6 Amp Switch/Socket.
2. Air Conditioning Control button with temperature adjustment.
3. On each of the Bedhead Panels, the electrical points are provided. There shall be at least three pairs of 6/16 Amp switches/sockets, i.e. six points. Half of these points shall be on UPS supply.
4. On the left and right sides of the patient, and at a distance of 1219 mm from the centre of the bed, one pair of 6/16 Amp. switches/sockets shall be provided at the height of 457 mm from the floor level, i.e. four points. Two pairs shall be on UPS supply.

21.10.12 Other Communication Points in Patient Room

1. Point for Nurse Call device
2. RJ 45 point for computer networking
3. RJ 11 for intercom and extension line
4. Point for reading light for patient

21.10.13 Curtain Partitions

The patient bed in the room shall be provided with hanging curtain partitions. Following points shall be considered for the same:

1. The bed shall have a curtain on all other three sides.
2. The ceiling suspended curtain track is fixed at 2134 mm above the floor level.
3. Curtains shall be hung on these tracks and shall be moveable and collapsible.
4. The bottom of the curtain shall have a clear area of about 457 mm from the floor to allow easy cleaning of the floor.

21.10.14 IV Track

The patient bed in the room shall be provided with a ceiling suspended IV track. Following points shall be considered for the same:

1. In the centre of the bed, the track shall be mounted length wise.

2. The track is mounted and screwed to the ceiling/false ceiling of the room.
3. The IV hanger shall be fixed in the track, which shall be moveable in the track.
4. The IV hanger can be with the provision of three, four or five hooks.

21.10.15 Psychiatric Patient Rooms

Psychiatric patients are normally in a disturbed state of mind and may have aggressive behaviour, resulting in incidents of violence and may cause psychological harm, and often physical injury, to themselves and staff. Therefore, while preparing the psychiatric patient rooms, special attention shall be paid to the following points:

1. The light fixtures, air vents, sprinkler heads and other appurtenances shall be tamper-resistant.
2. The bedrooms must have a private toilet with a non-lockable door that is capable of swinging outward, with a tamper-resistant ceiling and tamper-resistant light fixtures, air vents etc.
3. The room for psychiatry patients shall be separate and shall not be mixed with other patients. It is recommended that the psychiatry ward/rooms shall be located on the lower floors of the hospital building.
4. Avoid providing windows in the psychiatric patient rooms. If provided, the bottom height shall not be less than 6 ft from the floor level.
5. All the windows shall have a provision of grills.
6. The corridors leading to the psychiatry room shall be provided with the barriers or doors and shall be kept locked. These barriers or doors shall also be guarded.
7. Proper CCTV camera surveillance shall be provided.

21.11 Deluxe Single Patient Room (Deluxe Room)

The deluxe single bedroom is more or less the same as a single bed patient room, however, it has a few additional amenities like:

1. Size of the deluxe room shall be about 27.87 sq.m.
2. Size of the toilets can be bigger, and they can be designed to look more appealing by fixing patterns on the wall instead of pain tiles. The chinaware and the sanitary fittings shall be of better quality.
3. Bedhead panel can be 1524 mm long with more electrical points.
4. Ceiling finishes can be better.
5. The patient bed shall be a multi-positional ICU bed on lockable wheels, with bedside safety rails.
6. Other patient furnitures like over bed table and the bedside lockers shall be more elegant and of good quality.
7. A small kitchenette equipped with an electric kettle and a microwave shall be provided to make tea/coffee, snacks etc.
8. Size of the refrigerator can be bigger.
9. Good quality pull-out bed or sofa set shall be provided for visitors.
10. More space shall be provided for family and visitors.
11. The quality of dining table and chairs can be improved.
12. The cupboards can be bigger and designer.
13. Better quality artwork and sceneries can be provided.

All other details and requirements shall be the same as for a single patient room in this chapter.

21.12 Family Suite with Single Patient Room (Suite Room)

Family suite differs from other single bed patient rooms as one additional room for the family is provided, which is attached to the patient room. Apart from this, it has a few additional amenities like:

21.12.1 Patient Room of the Suite

1. Size of the deluxe room shall be about 27.87 sq.m.

2. Size of the toilets can be bigger, and they can be designed to look more appealing by fixing patterns on the wall instead of pain tiles. The chinaware and the sanitary fittings shall be of better quality.
3. Bedhead panel can be 1524 mm long with more electrical points.
4. Ceiling finishes can be better.
5. The floorings shall be better.
6. The patient bed shall be a multi-positional ICU bed on lockable wheels, with bedside safety rails.
7. Other patient furnitures like over bed table and the bedside lockers shall be more elegant and of good quality.
8. A small kitchenette equipped with an electric kettle and a microwave shall be provided to make tea/coffee, snacks etc.
9. Size of the refrigerator can be bigger.
10. Good quality pull-out bed or sofa set shall be provided for visitors.
11. More space shall be provided for family and visitors.
12. The quality of dining table and chairs can be improved.
13. The cupboards can be bigger and designer.
14. Better quality artwork and sceneries can be provided.

21.12.2 Family Room of the Suite

1. Size of the family room shall be about 18.58 sq.m.
2. The family room shall be attached to the patient room.
3. The family room can be separated from the patient room either by a solid wall or by a glass partition (Fig. 21.4).
4. The family room may or may not have a separate door. If only one door is provided for the suite, the family room shall be in the front and the patient room at the back.
5. Separate toilet in the family room shall be preferred.
6. A small kitchenette equipped with an electric kettle and a microwave shall be provided to make tea/coffee, snacks etc.
7. In the kitchenette, a working slab shall be provided along with a washing sink and drainboard.
8. Family room shall have a sofa set for seating 5–7 people, along with a centre table.
9. Dining table and chairs shall be provided in the family room.
10. One extra refrigerator shall be provided in the family room.

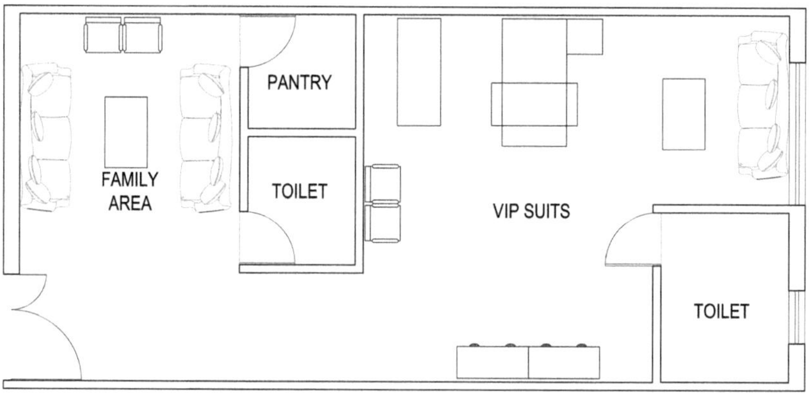

Fig. 21.4 Sample layout drawing of family suite

11. Separate cupboard shall be provided in the family room.
12. Painting of the family room shall be better.
13. Separate television shall be provided for the family.
14. Separate computer with Internet connection can be provided.
15. If required, a reading table with chair can be provided.

All other details and requirements shall be the same as for deluxe and single patient rooms mentioned in this chapter

21.13 Sharing Patient Room (Semi-private Room)

At times, due to financial issues, patients prefer a twin sharing room, by compromising on privacy. The occupancy in such rooms varies from two to four patients. Ideally, it is recommended that no more than two patients shall share a room, else it appears to be similar to the general ward. Based on the above recommendation, we suggest the following points to be taken care of while designing semi-private rooms (Fig. 21.5):

21.13.1 Room Layout

The room shall be divided into three zones—the first shall be a staff zone at the entrance of the room to allow staff to perform their tasks efficiently, second shall be the patient zone where patient beds are placed and the third shall be the family zone for seating visitors. Here, two family zones have to be provided, separate for each set of families of the patients.

21.13.2 Size of the Semi-private Sharing Room

The room shall have an area of about 32.52 sq.m including family spaces and toilets.

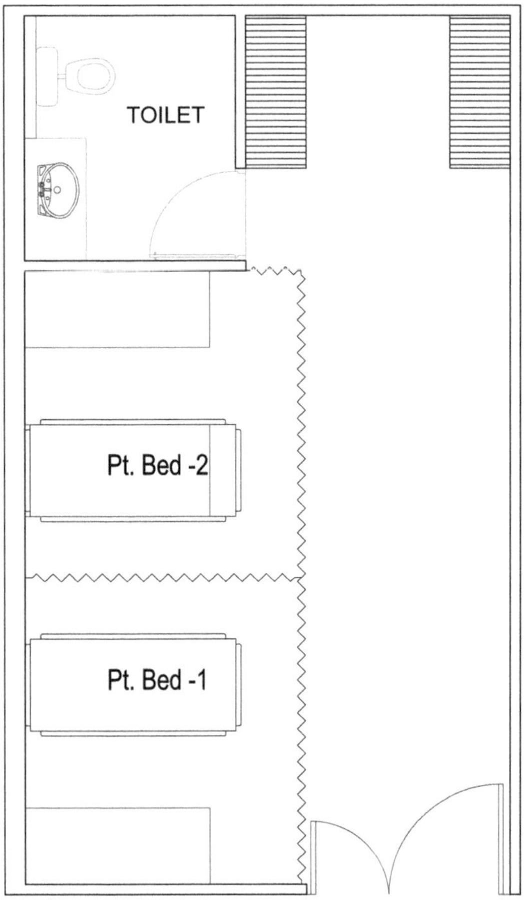

Fig. 21.5 Sample layout drawing of twin occupancy sharing room

21.13.3 Design of the Semi-private Sharing Room

21.13.3.1 Walls

The walls shall remain the same as those of a single occupancy patient room.

21.13.3.2 Doors

The door of the room shall not be less than 1829 mm wide, unobstructed. A wide door is suggested for easy movement of the bed in and out of the room, in case of emergency.

21.13.3.3 Windows

A window shall be preferred in the room, but direct sunlight shall be avoided. It shall be located on the outer wall, left or right side of the patient, opposite to the door side. The window may be openable or non-openable depending on the design. The glass can be tinted, or curtains/blinds shall be provided.

21.13.4 Toilets

A common toilet and bathroom with a handwashing station shall be provided for both the patients in the room. As mentioned earlier, the Mid-board concept for toilets shall be adopted. The toilets shall remain the same as those of a single occupancy patient room in all other aspects.

21.13.5 Bed Layout in Patient Room

Two patient beds shall be laid down in the room. For this, the centre of the room is marked, and a space of 610 mm is kept vacant on both sides of the centre marking. Then the beds are laid down on both sides. Hence, there is a distance of 1219 mm between two patient beds. This layout will permit easy and smooth working around the bed. Curtain partitions shall be provided between both the beds to maintain privacy.

21.13.6 Furniture and Instruments in Patient Room

Patient Furniture

Patient Bed (Fowler bed with bedside railing can be used)	
Bed Side Locker	IV Stand
Over Bed Table	IV Rod
Step Stool	Back Rest

Other Furnitures

Two numbers of Pull-out bed or plain sofa set (separate for families of each patient)	Two Attendant beds (if Pull-out bed is not provided)
Two Chairs (if space is available)	Two Cupboards (separate for each patient)

Equipment

Multipara Vital Sign Monitor (if required)	Air Mattress

21.13.7 Air Conditioning System of Patient Rooms

It shall remain the same as that of a single occupancy patient room.

21.13.8 Central Piped Medical Gas Supply

The Piped Centralized Medical Supply shall be provided on both the beds to handle any emergencies in the patient room. The arrangement shall remain the same as that of a single occupancy patient room.

21.13.9 Electrical Points in Patient Room

They shall remain the same as those of a single occupancy patient room, except that these points shall be provided for both the beds, separately. With the following pattern, the electrical points will be available on both sides of the patient:

1. On either side, at a distance of 610 mm from the bed, one pair of 6/16 Amp. switch/socket shall be provided on the wall at the height of 18 in. from the floor level.
2. Apart from this, between the centre of both the beds, a pair of 6/16 Amp. switches/sockets shall be provided on the wall at the height of 457 mm from the floor level.
3. Out of these, two pairs shall be on UPS supply.

21.13.10 Other Communication Points in Patient Room

They shall remain the same as those of a single occupancy patient room, but these points shall be provided on both the beds.

21.13.11 Curtain Partitions

They shall remain the same as those of a single occupancy patient room, but these curtains shall be provided on both the beds.

21.13.12 IV Track

It shall remain the same as those of a single occupancy patient room, but the tracks shall be provided on both the beds.

21.13.13 Lighting in the Patient Room

It shall remain the same as those of a single occupancy patient room.

21.14 General Ward (Multiple Beds Room)

In earlier days, multiple occupancy rooms were very popular, but slowly their demand decreased. Patients usually opt for this ward as the treatment cost is very low and they do not mind compromising on privacy. However, as the living standards and income of patients increased over the period of time, the demand for multiple bed wards reduced. Still some charitable hospitals and free hospitals prefer more number of multiple wards as compared to the paid wards. Patients with limited financial resources prefer to stay in a multiple bed general ward (Fig. 21.6).

There are a few issues with the multiple bed wards, such as:

1. Maximum chances of spread of infection in the wards.
2. Environmental conditions may be compromised, and wards can have a foul smell.
3. Proper hygiene is difficult to be maintained.
4. Toilets are shared among different patients.
5. Reduced privacy of the patients.
6. No proper entertainment source, as televisions cannot be provided in such wards.
7. Wards may be noisy, as a lot of people tend to be inside the ward at once.
8. Reduced inter-bed spaces.
9. No proper space for the family members to stay along with the patient.

Still some hospitals have a setup of multiple bed wards to cater to financially hampered patients. However, a well-designed multiple bed ward can curtail the above issues to some extent.

21.14.1 Location of the Multiple Bed Wards

All the multiple bed wards shall be located in a cluster, in a particular zone and a particular floor

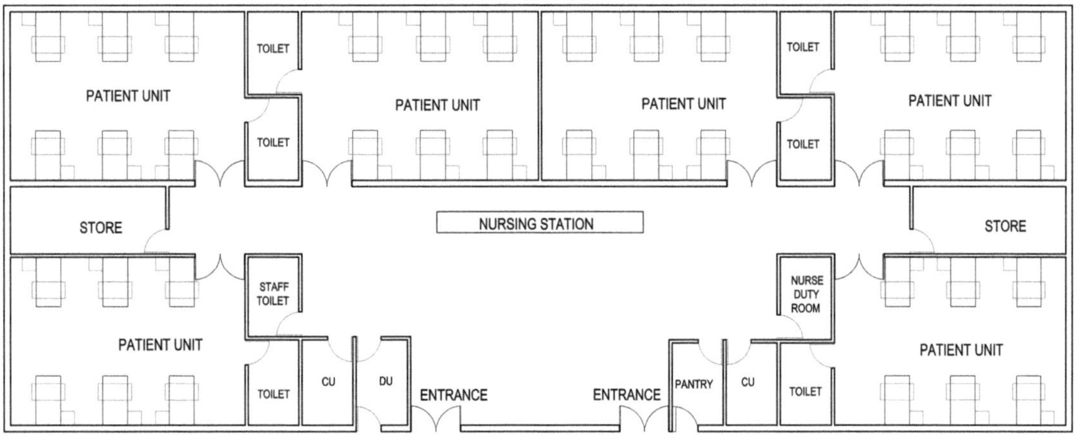

Fig. 21.6 Sample layout drawing of multiple bed general ward

of the hospital. Isolation ward shall be located in the isolation zone of the hospital.

21.14.2 Room Layout

The multiple bed wards shall have a patient area, nursing area and service area.

21.14.3 Number of Beds in the Multiple Bed Ward

There are no specific standards related to the number of beds to be placed in the multiple bed wards. Earlier it used to be 30–40 beds in a single ward. Nowadays, an arrangement of six beds per multiple bed ward is also seen. It depends on the designer and the management's requirement to decide on the number of beds to be laid in a particular ward.

Irrespective of the number of beds in the ward, after COVID-19, it is recommended that the entire ward shall be divided into cubicles with glass partitions and each cubicle shall not have more than four beds. In such a case, each cubicle shall have a separate supply and return of HVAC so that the exhausted air does not mix up with other cubicles or the space of the hospital. Also, more inter-bed space shall be provided.

It is also recommended that the multiple bed wards shall not have less than 6 or more than 30 beds in a single ward. Considering the COVID-19 and such future pandemics, it is highly recommended that the hospital shall opt for a design having about 30 beds in a ward, with separate cubicles of 4 beds each.

21.14.4 Size of the Multiple Bed Ward

The size of the ward shall depend on the number of beds to be laid in the ward. If we consider having four beds in a ward, the per bed space shall not be less than 11.15 sq.m, so the ward size shall be 6096 mm × 6096 mm. On the other hand, if we have 30 beds in a ward, the per bed space shall not be less than 9.29 sq.m, so the ward size shall be about 22,860 mm × 12,192 mm.

21.14.5 Design of the Multiple Bed Ward

21.14.5.1 Walls

The ward shall have walls on all four sides except the area for windows and door. The wall thickness shall not be less than 120 mm with plaster on both sides. They can either be made out of the clay bricks or hollow blocks, as per the design and technical civil construction details.

21.14.5.2 Doors

If the ward has 4–20 beds, a single door shall be provided. If the ward has more than 20 beds, two doors shall be provided. Door shall not be less than 1829 mm wide, unobstructed. A wide door is suggested for easy movement of the bed in and out of the room, in case of emergency.

21.14.5.3 Windows

They shall be provided on the outer wall of the ward. The size and number of windows shall depend on the outer elevation of the building and the designer's perceptions. The window may be openable or non-openable depending on the design. The glass can be tinted, or curtains/blinds shall be provided.

21.14.6 Toilets

For each such multiple bed Ward, a separate set of toilets including bathrooms and a handwashing station shall be provided. The toilets shall be separate for males and females. The number of WCs and bathrooms shall depend on the number of beds in the ward. As a thumb rule, at least one WC for four patients and one bathroom for eight patients shall be provided. This set of toilets shall be attached to the ward. If the concept of four bed cubicle is opted for, then each cubicle shall have a separate toilet attached to it. The design and facilities in the toilets shall remain the same as those of single occupancy patient rooms.

21.14.7 Bed Layout in Ward

The beds in the ward shall be laid out in such a manner that it allows easy and smooth working all around the bed. The following points shall be considered while laying down beds in the ward:

1. The beds shall be laid down along both the large-sized walls opposite to each other. Hence, leaving the free movement area in between.
2. Headend of the bed shall be at least 610 mm away from the wall.
3. On the foot end of both the beds, a clear space shall be about 1829 mm so that a stretcher trolley can easily be turned around and patient can be transferred from/to bed.
4. Inter-bed distance shall not be less than 914 mm.
5. If the width of the ward is more, say 12,192 mm, a low height wall can be provided in the centre of the hall and beds be laid down on both sides of the low height wall. It means there will be four rows of the bed in a ward. Two on each side of the low height wall and two on both the long walls of the hall.

21.14.8 Furniture and Instruments

Patient Furniture

Patient Bed (Semi-fowler bed with bedside railing can be used or otherwise plain patient bed can also be used)	
Bedside Locker	IV Stand
Over Bed Table	IV Rod
Step Stool	Back Rest

Other Furnitures

Stool or reclining chair for attendants	Cupboard (if possible)

21.14.9 Air Conditioning System

It shall remain the same as that of a single occupancy patient room, except that instead of FCU, AHU and ducting shall be used in the multiple bed wards.

21.14.10 Central Piped Medical Gas Supply

It shall remain the same as that of a single occupancy patient room and preferably it shall be provided on all the beds of the ward.

21.14.11 Electrical Points in Ward

1. Main switchboard shall be at the entrance wall for controlling fans and lights of the hall along with one 6 Amp. switch/socket.
2. Air Conditioning control button with temperature adjustment.
3. On each of the bed head panels, there shall be at least two pairs of 6/16 Amp. switch/socket, i.e. four points. Half of these points shall be on UPS supply.
4. Between two beds, in the centre, two pairs of 6/16 Amp. switches/sockets shall be provided on the wall at the height of 457 mm from the floor level. Out of these, one pair shall be on UPS supply.

21.14.12 Other Communication Points in Ward

1. Point for Nurse Call device.
2. Point for reading light for patient.

21.14.13 Curtain Partitions

They shall remain the same as those of a single occupancy patient room, but these curtains shall be provided for all the beds in the ward.

21.14.14 IV Track

It shall remain the same as those of a single occupancy patient room, but the tracks shall be provided for all the beds in the ward.

21.14.15 Lighting in the Patient Room

It shall remain the same as those of a single occupancy patient room.

21.15 Isolation Rooms/Wards

Controlling the spread of airborne infectious diseases in hospitals is a serious concern for the patients, staff and visitors. A recent example of this has been set by the COVID-19 virus. The world has experienced problems faced by hospitals due to limited availability of isolation beds.

To minimize the spread of airborne infections, certain rooms within a hospital shall be designed as airborne infection isolation rooms, with negative pressure, or protective environment rooms with a positive pressure.

As mentioned above, there shall be a separate zone in the hospital termed as the Isolation Zone. This area shall be located on any floor/unit of the building. It shall have a restricted access, proper barricading and be under the control of the security. Only authorized personnel shall be allowed to enter this area. At the entrance, air curtains shall be provided. The services in this area like pantry, gas supply and laundry shall be separate from other areas.

All types of isolation patient units like single occupancy rooms or sharing rooms/wards (which are generally not recommended) shall be separate and located in this dedicated isolation zone. These isolation wards/rooms shall not be spread at any other area of the hospital. If possible, the isolation ICU shall also be located in this zone.

While the isolation rooms/wards shall meet all general requirements of a standard room/ward as discussed earlier in this chapter, they also have the following specific requirements:

1. Patient isolation rooms shall have only one patient bed.
2. Space shall be provided for downing and doffing of the PPE kits and other personal safety devices.
3. Space shall be provided for storage of clean and soiled materials directly outside or inside the entry door.
4. Each room should be provided with a separate toilet with a handwashing sink.
5. Isolation room needs to be well-sealed to prevent excess air leakage into or out of the room.
6. Tighter the room is constructed, more efficiently the air pressure differential can be maintained.
7. Walls, floors and ceilings shall be sealed to prevent air leakage.
8. Self-closing doors shall be used.
9. Devices can be installed to monitor airflow.

21.15.1 Isolation in ICU

ICU is the area where patients are kept under intensive monitoring and those with life-threatening diseases are provided treatment and care. Out of all these patients, there may be some patients suffering from contagious diseases like Tuberculosis and COVID-19. These patients shall be placed separately from other non-infected patients to avoid the spread of disease. Therefore, along with normal beds, ICUs shall have the provision for a few beds for infected patients called Isolation cabin/unit/cubical.

It is recommended that a separate ICU shall be provided in the isolation zone. If this is not possible, about 25% of the beds in general ICUs shall be reserved for isolation bed/room/unit. This can be done using collapsible shutters around the bed or by fixing temporary acrylic partitions.

Isolation rooms/units shall have a separate entry other than the normal entry of the ICU. Isolation rooms should have a separate attached toilet. The isolation room/units shall be properly air-tightened and negatively pressurized. These shall not be mixed with other beds in the same hall, but shall be a separate zone with a barrier in between. Separate staff shall take care of the patients in isolation cabins.

21.15.2 Single Bed Isolation Rooms

These intend to prevent the spread of infectious agents by using pressure differentials to contain them, and are effective only if the room is tightly sealed. Thus, in terms of controlling infection in isolation rooms and other patient rooms, the greater risk may be associated with nurses not implementing evidence-based practices regarding handwashing and aseptic techniques to prevent infections.

21.15.3 Air and Pressure Monitoring System for Isolation Rooms

Each isolation room shall have a permanently installed visual device or mechanism to constantly monitor the air pressure differential of the room, when occupied by a patient, who requires isolation.

An electronic room pressure monitor can provide continuous confirmation of the required pressure differential across the room boundary. Most electronic monitors consist of two main components: a wall-mounted control panel and a sensor. The control panel shall be mounted on a corridor wall adjacent to the entrance of the isolation room and generally displays the pressure difference in inches of water column (WC). In addition to providing a continuous readout of pressure differential, the control panel should include both audible and visual alarms to warn staff when room pressurization is lost. For example, in a room designed to maintain a pressure differential of minus 0.03-in. WC, the alarm could be programmed to activate when the pressure differential falls to minus 0.01-in. WC. Monitors shall include an extra identical signal that allows the pressure differential and alarm signals to be displayed at a remote location. The common location for this remote alarm is either the nurses' station or the building's automation system.

21.15.4 Pressurization of the Isolation Rooms

The isolation rooms shall follow the standard norms of pressurization. The pressurization can either be negative or positive.

21.15.4.1 Negative Isolation Rooms

A negative-pressure room is designed to isolate a patient who is suspected of or has been diagnosed with an airborne infectious disease. The negative-pressure isolation room, therefore, is designed to help prevent the spread of a disease from an infected patient to others in the hospital.

Negative-pressure isolation rooms require a minimum of 12 air changes of exhaust per hour and must maintain a minimum 0.01-in. WC. Typically, a set point closer to minus 0.03-in. WC is used. The negative-pressure relationship to the corridor should be upheld; however, it is not required to be maintained at the minimum of minus 0.01-in. WC.

When an anteroom is provided, airflow should be from the corridor into the anteroom, and from the anteroom into the patient isolation room. To maintain the required pressure differential, the exhaust air quantity must always be higher than the supply airflow. Depending on factors such as the room size and the room's heating and cooling loads, more than 12 air changes per hour may be necessary. Typically, a minimum airflow difference of 150–200 cubic feet per minute (CFM) is adequate to maintain a pressure differential in a well-sealed room.

Exhaust from negative-pressure isolation rooms, associated anteroom and associated toilet rooms must be directly discharged outdoors, without mixing with exhaust from any other rooms. However, multiple isolation rooms may be connected to the same exhaust system. The exhaust ductwork serving negative isolation rooms should be permanently labelled as contaminated air.

Supply air outlet in the room is located in the ceiling at the foot end of the patient bed, with exhaust air taken from exhaust grills or registers located directly above the patient bed, on the ceiling, or on the wall near the head of the bed, lower than 7 ft above the floor.

21.15.4.2 Positive Isolation Rooms

A positive-pressure isolation room is designed to keep contagious diseases away from patients with compromised immune systems, such as those with cancer or transplants. These rooms require a minimum of 12 air changes per hour of supply air and must maintain a minimum 0.01-in.

WC positive-pressure differential, ensuring that the patient is protected from airborne contamination regardless of whether an anteroom is used. Typically, positive-pressure rooms are designed to maintain an even stricter set point of positive 0.03-in. WC. The positive-pressure relationship to the corridor should be preserved; however, it is not required to be maintained at the minimum of positive 0.01-in. WC.

When an anteroom is used, airflow must be from the patient room into the anteroom and from the anteroom out into the corridor. As with the AII negative room, typically a minimum airflow difference of 150–200 CFM is adequate to maintain a pressure differential in a well-sealed room. Positive-pressure rooms are required to be supplied with HEPA-filtered air, with the filters installed at the main air-handling unit or at the supply terminals in the room.

Supply air for the room must be located in the ceiling above the patient bed, with return air taken from the ceiling near the patient room door. The supplied diffuser shall be a non-aspirating, laminar-flow device and should be designed to limit the air velocity at the patient bed, to reduce the possibility of patient discomfort. Airflow to the PE isolation room shall be maintained at a constant volume to provide consistent ventilation in the room.

21.15.5 Air Conditioning of the Isolation Wards/Units

When designing the air-conditioning system for isolation rooms, the designer shall consider and calculate the airflow, temperature and pressure requirement to maintain the proper pressure differential and temperature. Instead of smaller standalone units, depending on the number and type of isolation rooms in the facility, a single larger system can be provided to serve multiple rooms. This practice is generally more economical.

The same air-handling system that serves other standard patient rooms may be used for isolation rooms. The only difference is in the filtration of the air and treatment of the return air. Air-handling unit (AHU) serving the isolation rooms shall have proper pre-filters, and high-efficiency particulate air (HEPA) final filters.

For detailed air conditioning system of the isolation rooms, please refer to the chapter 'HVAC' (Chap. 38) in this book.

21.16 Supporting Room/Units for Indoor Patient Service

Apart from the patient units/rooms/wards, there are a few other rooms and utilities that are required to serve patients and provide them with good care and treatment. Some of these are:

1. Nurse Station/Desk
2. Nurses duty rooms
3. Doctors duty rooms
4. Procedure and Treatment Room
5. Clean Utility
6. Dirty Utility/Sluice Room
7. Store for medicines, consumables and disposables
8. Medication Area
9. Equipment Park/Store
10. Trolley Park Area
11. Ward Pantry

21.17 Nursing Station

For efficient care and treatment, the location of a nursing station is very crucial. The location shall allow the nursing staff to keep a continuous watch on all patients in the unit. If we place the nursing station on one side or corner of the unit, the nurse may not be able to see the patient on the other end.

For general multiple bed ward, the nursing station shall be located in the centre of the hall, on the back wall of the ward. The counter shape can be straight or L-shaped.

For semi-private rooms, private rooms, deluxe rooms and suites, the nurse stations shall be outside the rooms. One nursing station shall be provided for a group of rooms put together, i.e. one nursing station for 8–10 such rooms shall be sufficient. It will be better if this nursing counter is placed somewhere in the centre of these rooms, so that the distance from all the rooms is as less as possible.

For general multiple bed wards, the nursing station shall be at some height so that the nurse can easily see the patients. For this, a platform of about 305 mm height can be provided on which the counter can be placed.

Nurse station design shall be such that the caregivers also maintain adequate distance. Normally, hospitals have a nurse counter, from where the patient/visitors interact with the nurse. This type of counter can be more prone to spreading infection because of no barrier in between. To overcome this issue, consider going away from open nurse stations and enclosing them in 'glass bubbles'. It is advised to make a proper 1829 mm high acrylic or glass partition at the top of the nurse counter so that the staff is always on the other side of the partition while interacting with the patient/visitor. We can also use technology like Audio-Video Controlled Nurse Call System.

Nursing station shall have sufficient storage facility for instruments, tools, patient files and stationery. Sufficient electrical and communications points shall be provided. A view box shall also be fixed on a wall near the nursing station. Each nursing station shall be provided with the following:

1. At least 5–7 numbers of 6 Amp. switches/sockets.
2. Point for Nurse Call Control Console.
3. RJ 45 point for Computer networking.
4. RJ 11 for Intercom and extension line.
5. HDMI point for computer display at other locations.

21.17.1 Hand Hygiene

For hand hygiene, in the indoor patient area, two-way scrub stations shall be used and placed near the nursing stations. Soap dispensers, paper towel dispenser and trash receptacle should be next to the scrub station. It should enable hands-free operation. The sensor-controlled and/or foot-operated scrub stations shall be used. It shall have the provision of both hot and cold water.

21.17.2 Alcohol Gel/Sanitizer Dispensers

Alcohol gel/sanitizer dispensers should be located in the patient room as well as at other staff locations around the unit. In the patient room, this can be hung with the help of a holder at the foot end of the bed.

21.18 Nurses Duty Rooms

These rooms allow the nurse to take rest/breaks and store their personal belongings, while on duty. Each nursing station shall have one nursing duty room. The following issues shall be considered while designing nurses duty rooms:

1. The room shall be of the size 3048 mm × 3048 mm.
2. It shall have an attached toilet.
3. It shall have one bed and a cupboard.
4. Apart from light and fan, the room shall have points for computer with Internet connection and Intercom facility.
5. It shall be air-conditioned and the control button with temperature adjustment shall be provided in the room.

21.19 Doctors Duty Rooms

It shall be provided with a group of patient rooms. As per experience, one such room shall be provided for 30–50 patients. This number can be increased or decreased as per the requirement. The following issues shall be considered while designing doctors duty rooms:

1. The room shall be of the size 4572 mm × 4267 mm.
2. It shall have an attached toilet.

3. It shall have one office table, chair, bed and a cupboard.
4. Apart from light and fan, the room shall have points for computer with Internet connection and Intercom facility.
5. It shall be air-conditioned and the control button with temperature adjustment shall be provided in the room.

21.20 Procedure and Treatment Room

At times, patients may require undergoing minor procedures like catheterization, suturing of small wounds, dressing and bandaging. However, it is difficult to do these procedures in the patient room, due to high chances of getting infected, the privacy of the patient, or the procedure requires anaesthesia. Therefore, a treatment room or procedure room shall be attached to each set of patient rooms. One such room shall be sufficient for 50 patients in the indoor area.

21.20.1 Location of Treatment/Procedure Room

These treatment rooms shall be near the patient rooms, preferably in the centre of the rooms. For example, the treatment room can be sandwiched between two general wards.

21.20.2 Size of Treatment/Procedure Room

The size of the Treatment/Procedure Room shall not be less than 4572 mm × 4572 mm.

21.20.3 Issues Related to Infrastructure of Treatment/Procedure Room

1. It shall be a sterilized room.
2. A single OT table shall be placed in the room.
3. It shall have a single-entry door.
4. A gowning and scrub station shall be attached to the treatment room.

21.20.4 Furniture in Treatment/Procedure Room

Patient Furniture

OT Table	Scrub Station
Stretcher Trolley	IV Stand
Dressing Trollies	IV Rod
Instrument Trollies	Crash Cart
Step Stool	Oxygen Cylinder Trolley

Equipment

Multi-para Vital Sign Monitor	Laryngoscope
Portable Operating Light Single Dome	Suction Machine
Infusion Pump	Oxygen Cylinders With Masks
Defibrillator	View Boxes

Tools and Instruments

Sterilizing Drums	Chetal Forceps
Extension Cord and Boxes	Forceps of all styles and sizes
Instrument Boxes	Needle Holders
Torches	Tray of all styles and sizes
Examination Light	Scissors of all styles and sizes
All other required instruments	General Operating Instruments

21.20.5 Doors

The door of the treatment/procedure room shall not be less than 1524 mm wide, unobstructed. The door shall be openable on both sides in and out.

21.20.6 Windows

These are not needed in the Treatment/Procedure Room.

21.20.7 Handwashing

For handwash, a single bay scrub station shall be provided, which shall be operational with sensors and foot.

21.20.8 Central Piped Medical Gas Supply

As surgical interventions have to be done in Treatment/Procedure Room, the following gas outlets shall be mounted on the ceiling suspended pendant:

1. two outlets for Oxygen
2. two outlets for Compressed Air
3. two outlets for Suction Oxygen

21.20.9 Electrical Points in Treatment/Procedure Room

1. The main switchboard shall be at the entrance wall for controlling fans and lights of the hall along with one 6 Amp. switch/socket.
2. Air Conditioning control button with temperature adjustment.
3. On hanging pendant, the electrical points are to be provided. There shall be at least three pairs of 6/16 Amp. switches/sockets on the back wall of the pendant. These points shall be on UPS supply.
4. On three walls of Treatment/Procedure room (leaving the wall on which door is provided) in the centre of each wall, a pair of two 6/16 Amp. switches/sockets is to be provided at the height of 457 mm from the floor level. Out of these two, one pair shall be on UPS.
5. The provision of lighting for patient examinations shall also be provided on the bedhead panel or the wall column.

21.20.10 Other Communication Points in Treatment/ Procedure Room

1. RJ 45 point for Computer networking.
2. RJ 11 for Intercom and extension line.
3. HDMI point for computer displays at other locations.

21.21 Clean Utility

A clean utility shall be attached to each nursing station of the indoor areas, which shall be used for the storage of clean linen. Sterilized material like a drum and drapes is also stored in this room.

Normally, the room shall not be less than 3658 mm × 3658 mm, but depending on the requirements, the size of the room can be changed. The room shall be provided with closed cabinets, drawers and racks. This room shall have only one door of about 3 ft.

21.22 Dirty Utility/Sluice Room

A dirty utility shall also be attached to each nursing station and shall be used for the storage of the soiled linen. From here the linen is moved for pre-wash before sending it to the laundry.

Normally, the room shall not be less than 3658 mm × 3658 mm, but depending on the requirements, the size of the room can be changed. The room shall be provided with covered linen collection hampers or containers to collect the dirty linen. This room shall have two doors of about 914 mm. One door opens in the ward/nursing station and the other in the corridor from where the laundry staff can collect the linen and he/she need not come to the ward/nursing station for collecting the linen. Air from this room shall be exhausted, hence exhaust fans are a must.

21.23 Store for Medicines, Consumables and Disposables

All nursing stations shall be provided with a general store to keep ample stock of required medicines, consumables and disposables. The room shall be at least 3048 mm × 3048 mm in size. Adequate lockable cupboards, racks and drawers shall be provided in the store. It shall also have a countertop. It shall be in charge of the Ward Supervisor.

21.24 Medication Areas

While designing the nursing station, an area shall be provided in the shape of the room, or a cupboard to keep patient medications in clear plastic boxes. These boxes are marked with the patient's name, and the room or bed number of the patient. A separate box shall be prepared for each patient. Depending on the requirement, the medicine is taken out of these boxes and given to the patient. The medication room or the cupboard shall be lockable. A refrigerator shall also be provided for this medication room.

21.25 Equipment Park/Store

Each nursing station shall be provided with an equipment storage area, where the less required equipment can be stored. For this, a small room with a size of not less than 2438 mm × 2438 mm shall be provided, attached to the nursing station. This area can be a closed room with a door or otherwise open area attached to the nursing station. The room shall have the provision of grounded electrical charging points for charging the unused medical equipment.

21.26 Trolley Park Area

Each nursing station shall be provided with a trolley park area for parking wheelchairs and stretches when not in use.

21.27 Ward Pantry

As the patients admitted in rooms/wards have to be served full-day diet, there shall be a space for storage of diet and further distribution. This space is called Ward Pantry. It is not necessary that the diet has to be cooked in the premises; the diet can be prepared in the kitchen and then sent to the ward pantry for further distribution. The diet is sent in bulk from the kitchen either packed for direct distribution or otherwise unpacked.

The size of the ward pantry shall be about 3658 mm × 3658 mm, with a single door opening outside in the corridor. The ward pantry shall have a countertop for packing food. Along with it, a sink with hot and cold water shall be available. A waste bin has to be kept in the ward pantry and a trolley for collecting the soiled utensils. A microwave oven may be useful.

Further Reading

Brown KK, Gallant D. Impacting Patient Outcomes Through Design: Acuity Adaptable Care/Universal Room Design. Crit Care Nurs Q. 2006 Dec;29(4):326–41.

Choi J-H, Beltran LO, Kim H-S. Impacts of indoor daylight environments on patient average length of stay (ALOS) in a healthcare facility. Build Environ. 2012 Apr 1;50:65–75.

Cullinan K, Wolf M. The Patient Room: what is the ideal solution? 60.

Design and Management of Negative Pressure Isolation Room for Infectious Disease-- 《Chinese Journal of Nosocomiology》 2007年12期 [Internet]. [cited 2021 Jun 22]. Available from: https://en.cnki.com.cn/Article_en/CJFDTotal-ZHYY200712041.htm

Design, Construction and Regulation of the Negative Pressure Isolation Room-- 《Chinese Medical Equipment Journal》 2004年01期 [Internet]. [cited 2021 Jun 22]. Available from: https://en.cnki.com.cn/Article_en/CJFDTotal-YNWS200401023.htm

Eijkelenboom A, Bluyssen PM. Comfort and health of patients and staff, related to the physical environment of different departments in hospitals: a literature review. Intell Build Int. 2019 May 18;0(0):1–19.

Griffin CH, Joint Commission, Joint Commission Resources, Inc, Joint Commission International, AIA Academy of Architecture for Health, editors. Planning, design, and construction of health care facilities: addressing Joint Commission and JCI standards and other considerations--from planning to commissioning. Third edition. Oak Brook, IL: Joint Commission Resources; 2015. 138 p.

Hendrich AL, Fay J, Sorrells AK. Effects of Acuity-Adaptable Rooms on Flow of Patients and Delivery of Care. Am J Crit Care. 2004 Jan 1;13(1):35–45.

Hyttinen M, Rautio A, Pasanen P, Reponen T, Earnest GS, Streifel A, et al. Airborne Infection Isolation Rooms – A Review of Experimental Studies. Indoor Built Environ. 2011 Dec 1;20(6):584–94.

Lee JK, Jeong HW. Rapid expansion of temporary, reliable airborne-infection isolation rooms with negative air machines for critical COVID-19 patients. Am J Infect Control. 2020 Jul 1;48(7):822–4.

New treatment room design model for future hospitals [Internet]. ScienceDaily. [cited 2021 Jun 22]. Available from: https://www.sciencedaily.com/releases/2016/05/160526092743.htm

Plate JDJ, Leenen LPH, Houwert M, Hietbrink F. Utilisation of Intermediate Care Units: A Systematic Review. Crit Care Res Pract. 2017;2017:8038460.

Smith TJ. Occupancy and patient care quality benefits of private room relative to multi-bed patient room designs for five different children's hospital intensive and intermediate care units. Work. 2016 Jan 1;54(4):853–72.

Stichler JF. The New Standard: Single Family Room Design. JONA J Nurs Adm. 2012 Oct;42(10):447–50.

Tsao T, Chang cheng-ping, Chuang C-Y, Juang Y-J, Lin S-J, Dai Y-T. The Effect of Doorway Size on the Negative Pressure in Airborne Infection Isolation Room The Effect of Doorway Size on the Negative Pressure in Airborne Infection Isolation Room. J Occup Saf Health. 2010 Sep 15;18:307–19.

Waydhas C, Herting E, Kluge S, Markewitz A, Marx G, Muhl E, et al. Intermediate care units : Recommendations on facilities and structure. Med Klin Intensivmed Notfallmedizin. 2017 Nov 7;113.

Weng C-L, Kau L-J. Planning and Design of a Full-Outer-Air-Intake Natural Air-Conditioning System for Medical Negative Pressure Isolation Wards. J Healthc Eng. 2021 Mar 26;2021:e8872167.

Zhang Y, Han O, Li A, Hou L, Olofsson T, Zhang L, et al. Adaptive wall-based attachment ventilation: A comparative study on its effectiveness in airborne infection isolation rooms with negative pressure. Engineering [Internet]. 2021 Jan 23 [cited 2021 Jun 22]; Available from: https://www.sciencedirect.com/science/article/pii/S2095809921000059

22 Radiology

Radiology is the department that uses medical imaging to diagnose and treat diseases. There are a variety of imaging techniques upon which imaging modalities are based:

1. X-Ray based
2. Ultrasound Waves based
3. Magnetic Fields based
4. Nuclear Medicine based

Imaging modalities based on these techniques are:

1. X-ray Radiography
2. Ultrasound Machines
3. Computed Tomography (CT)
4. Magnetic Resonance Imaging (MRI)
5. Mammography Imaging
6. Nuclear Positron Emission Computed Tomography (PET CT)
7. Nuclear Positron Emission Magnetic Resonance Imaging (PET MRI)
8. SPECT CT
9. Cyclotron/Radio Pharmacy
10. Densitometer, Bone
11. Digital Subtraction Angiography (DSA)

22.1 Diagnostic vs Therapeutic Radiology

Diagnostic Radiology is a science where a disease is diagnosed with the help of various imaging techniques, and the treatment part is left to the physicians. Here, diagnostic imaging helps physicians to accurately diagnose a disease.

Therapeutic Radiology is a science where in addition to diagnosis, the treatment part is also taken care of, for example peripheral shunting. Interventional radiology is a part of therapeutic radiology, which allows performing (usually minimally invasive) medical procedures with the guidance of imaging technologies.

22.2 Location of the Radiology Department

Radiology services are often used by:

1. OPD
2. Emergency
3. IPD
4. ICU
5. Operating Rooms

It is essential to understand that the department is at a place which is easy and convenient for patients to access. Importantly, it shall have adequate facilities to ensure protection from radiation exposure and does not interfere with the working of the other departments. Hence, it is better if the department is located on the ground floor. The second justification is, as the flow to this department is more, it has to be in a fast-moving zone. The radiology department shall be

A. Garg, A. Dewan, *Manual of Hospital Planning and Designing*,
https://doi.org/10.1007/978-981-16-8456-2_22

near the OPD complex, emergency department and Intensive Care Units.

As X-rays are hazardous, and most of the machines are based on X-Ray technology, adequate protection has to be given to the public. The protection has to be to an extent where the rays shall not penetrate out of the walls of the machine room. If we talk about CT Scans, PET CT, DSA and Radiotherapy, the radiation dose rate is much higher and harmful to the public. Thus, it is reasonable to locate radiology department in the basement, so that the outside radiation can be protected as beyond the outer wall there will only be soil, and any penetrating rays will be absorbed by it.

While designing the department of radiology, special care shall be taken about the size of the corridors. Corridor dimensions (clear width and height) should be sized to permit the movement and installation of all pieces of the equipment. If the size of the corridors and the corners are not well planned, it will create a big problem to transport the equipment to the respective point of installation. The route of transport of equipment shall be well planned at the time of designing the spaces. If need be, the sizes, weight and space required for transport, shall be checked from the manufacturers of the equipment.

22.3 Infrastructure on Centralized Radiology Department

The Department of Radiology consists of the following:

Utility Area	Reception and Enquiry
	Registration
	Record Room
	Reporting Room
	Store for unused films and Related material
	Store for used films
	Public Utility for Faculty
	Public Utility for Patients and Attendants
	Report Delivery Room
	Sub waiting
	Extra Rooms for Future expansion
X-ray	Radiography Rooms for DR or X-Ray Machine
	Radiography Room IITV System and Fluoroscopy
	Room for 60 mA Mobile X-Ray System
	Change Rooms
	Sub-waiting
	Patient Preparation Room
	CR Room
Ultrasound	Ultrasound Room
	Change Room
	Toilets
	Sub-waiting
CT Scan	Examination Room
	Control Room
	UPS room
	Change room
	Store
	Sub-waiting
MRI	Examination Room
	Control Room
	UPS room
	Machine Room
	Change room
	Store
	Sub-waiting
Mammography	Examination Room
	Change room
	Store
	Sub-waiting
DEXA Scan	Examination Room
	Sub-waiting
PET CT/MRI Scan/ SPECT CT	PET CT Room
	PET MRI Room
	SPECT CT Room
	Console Rooms for all machines
	UPS rooms
	Machine Panel Rooms
	Technologist Room
	Physician Consultation Room
	Post-drug Administration Holding cubicles
	Active Toilet
	Dose administration Room
	Hot Lab cum Radio Pharmacy Room
	Radioactive Store
	Medicine Preparation Room
	Radioactive waste Room
	Change room
	General Store
	Sub-waiting

Other new Investigation	Examination Room
	Control Room
	UPS room
	Machine Room
	Change room
	Store
	Sub-waiting
Support	Electric Panel room
	Reporting Room
	Seminar cum Library
Staff Accommodation	HOD with Toilet
	PA to HOD
	Doctors Rooms
	Senior Resident Room

22.4 Main Equipment in the Department of Radiology

Camera Scintillation (Gamma)	MRI Fibre optic pulse oximeter
Computed Tomography (CT)	Nuclear Computed Tomography (PET CT)
Cyclotron/Radio Pharmacy	Nuclear Magnetic Resonance Imaging System (PET MRI)
Densitometer, Bone	PACS
Digital Subtraction Angiography (DSA)	Portable X-Ray Machine DR
Laser Imager Camera	Pressure Die Injector
Lead Apron	Rebreathing Systems, Radionuclide
Lead Screen	Ultrasound Machine
Leakage Tester	Vascular Doppler
Magnetic Resonance Imaging (MRI) with Spectroscopy	X-Ray Machine DR systems 800/500/300 MA with Fluoroscopy
Mammographic Machine Digital	

22.5 Utility Area

This area is for the utility and comfort of the patients. We can also call it as the patient zone. This includes the spaces for registration, enquiry and reports delivery apart from the waiting area for patients, pre-procedure and post-procedure. The main design of this shall include the following:

22.5.1 Reception and Enquiry

This is the first point of contact for a patient arriving in the department. The reception provides all required information to the visitors/patients, book appointments, guide through the registration process, explain the collection of reports and guide them to the investigation room. Therefore, it shall be placed at the entry of the Radiology Department. The reception should be at such a place, where it is easily approachable. The length of the counter can be about 2438–3048 mm On the countertop, an acrylic sheet of about 914 mm height shall be provided as a precaution to protect the staff from infectious diseases.

22.5.2 Registration and Cash Counter

Near to the reception counter, the registration/cash counter shall be located. The Registration counter shall check the requisition form of investigation issued by the physician, register the patient for investigation, receive payment for investigation (if any), Issue Token number etc. and make the patient seated. The counter staff shall also guide the patient to the concerned room for investigation. The length of the counter can be about 2438–3048 mm in length. On the countertop, the acrylic sheet of about 914 mm height shall be provided as a precaution for the staff from infected diseases. It is also recommended that the cash counter shall be at a distance of about 1829 mm from the registration counter.

22.5.3 Waiting Lobby

After getting registered, patients need to wait for their turn to be investigated. The size of the waiting area shall be decided by the designer considering the patient load and the average time taken for the investigation. Waiting area shall be provided with comfortable chairs/sofa set, drinking water and toilets. A pre-COVID era concept allowed to create more and more spaces for waiting lobbies, to make it comfortable for patients and attendants to wait. Now post-COVID-19, the waiting areas will have to be planned carefully and designed to create a greater physical separation between people with appropriate queuing. Few suggestions for doing so are:

1. The foremost principle to be followed is that individual seats shall be provided to maintain social distancing.
2. *Sub-waiting lobbies*

   It is recommended that instead of a single large waiting lobby, sub-waiting lobbies shall be designed for each imaging modality. For example, MRI shall have a different sub-waiting area and CT scan shall have another sub-waiting area. However, such measures may not be practical in all situations, especially for small healthcare facilities, nursing homes, clinics etc. The number of people who can be allowed to wait in hospital lobbies may be limited to a certain maximum with a specific spacing between their seats. So, future waiting lobbies could be smaller in size and scattered across the department.
3. *Minimize Interaction with others*

   Trends like self-check-in and self-rooming will accelerate to minimize interactions with other people. The concept of a smaller enclave waiting space that separates the sick from other patients or visitors will be preferred. The seating has to be in clusters of small numbers of chairs, say 2–3 chairs per cluster. Further, each cluster shall be portioned from the other with a 1524-mm acrylic or glass partition to reduce exposure with other patients/visitors.
4. *Outside waiting*

   Patients and families shall be encouraged to wait outside or in their car, instead of waiting in the lobby.
5. *Adopting a Token system*

   To reduce the crowd in waiting lobbies, a token system shall be introduced. With this system, the patient or visitor is issued a token at the time of registration, so that they are well aware of their turn, and need not wait in the lobby near the service room, but can wait elsewhere. LCDs can be provided at various locations across the hospital, wherein a token holder can see the status of his/her token number. We can even use advanced technology like SMS service, which will be sent to the mobile number of the token holder as and when his/her token number arrives.

22.5.4 Reporting Room

Most of the hospitals have a central reporting room, where reporting of all the modalities is done. The size of the room will depend on the number of people to be accommodated in the room at a particular time, but ideally, it shall not be less than 6096 mm × 4572 mm. The room shall be provided with a required set of computers and printers, sufficient tables and comfortable chairs. Wall-mounted big-size view boxes (maybe up to four films) shall also be provided to examine the films. The room shall have space for a typist to sit.

Most importantly, all computers shall be connected to PACS (Picture Archiving and Communication System) through a secured network. PACS is a medical imaging software to communicate and transfer images either through a closed network or through the Internet. The images of all the modalities of radiology (except Ultrasound) are archived and stored in a separate server, called PACS server. When required, the images can be retrieved anywhere either for reporting by radiologists or for diagnosis by the physicians.

22.5.5 Stores for Unused Consumables and Films

The department has to be ready for investigation round the clock. Therefore, it is essential to always have ample stock of consumables and films, and for this, the department needs a store. This store shall be of the size of 3658 mm × 3658 mm, but depending on the number of items, the size may vary. The store needs to have a sufficient number of countertops, cupboards and drawers. It is highly recommended that for storage of films (as films are highly inflammable), a fireproof cabinet is provided. The light switch of such a store shall be given outside the room and a single light shall be provided, to avoid the chances of fire caused by sparks. The temperature of the room shall be between 17 and 21 °C, and it shall not have any window or other source of direct sunlight.

22.5.6 Stores for Used Films and General Items

At times the department needs to store exposed films, particularly those related to medico-legal cases or interesting cases for studies and references. Apart from this, waste films and other items like machine accessories also need to be stored. Thus, there shall be a dedicated space for storing such items. This store shall be of the size of 3658 mm × 3658 mm, but depending on the number of items, the size may vary. The store needs to have a sufficient number of countertops, cupboards and drawers. It is highly recommended that for storage of films (as films are highly inflammable), a fireproof cabinet is provided. The light switch of such a store shall be given outside the room and a single light shall be provided, to avoid the chances of fire caused by sparks. The temperature of the room shall be between 17 and 21 °C, and it shall not have any window or other source of direct sunlight.

22.5.7 Report Delivery Counter

Reports, along with films or CDs, can be delivered from any location as per the hospital policy. Some hospitals may like to deliver such reports directly from the radiology department, whereas others may want to deliver it from the main hospital reception. Whatever the case may be, a report delivery counter has to be provided. This counter can either be in the room or an open counter. We recommend an open counter, as it looks more elegant. The length of the counter can be about 2438–3048 mm. On the countertop, an acrylic sheet of about 914 mm height shall be provided to protect staff from infectious diseases. On the back wall of the counter, proper pre-numbered bins shall be provided to keep the reports ready for delivery.

22.6 X-Ray Zone

This zone of the radiology department is related to X-rays and X-ray-related investigations and/or procedures, including fluoroscopy. As X-rays are harmful, special care has to be taken while designing the investigation rooms. This zone includes the following:

22.6.1 Radiography Rooms

These are the actual rooms where the X-ray machine is installed, and the exposure of X-rays is given to the patient. As far as the number of radiography rooms is concerned, it depends on the number of machines required to be installed at once, and also on the plans of adding more machines. There are different varieties of machines starting from conventional X-ray machines to Digital Radiography (DR) machines. Further, the capacity of the machine may vary from 60 mA to 1000 mA. Also, X-ray tables are available in a wide variety starting from fixed tables to multi-positional motorized tables (Fig. 22.1).

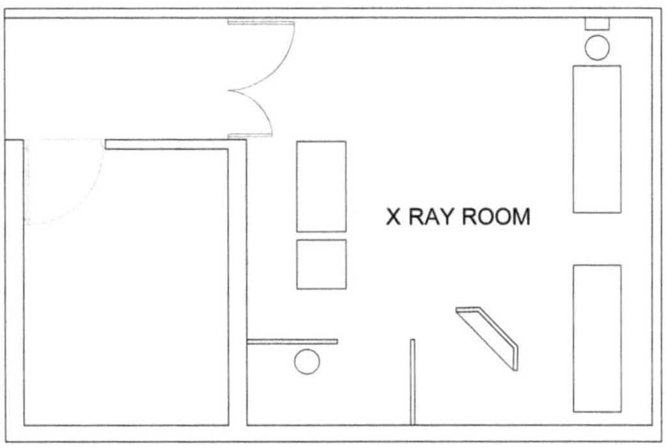

Fig. 22.1 Sample layout drawing of X-Ray Room

Some of the important points related to the designing of the radiography rooms are as follows:

1. *Before designing the radiography rooms, the guidelines and norms of the controlling authority of the country must be taken into account. e.g. in India, Baba Atomic Research Institute issues all such norms and guidelines.*
2. A separate room shall be provided for each machine.
3. Irrespective of the types of machines and tables, the size of the radiography rooms remains the same.
4. A rectangular room is suggested, and the size of the room shall not be less than 25 sq.m.
5. All the walls of the room shall be at least 229 mm thick, with plaster on both sides. The ideal thickness for the primary wall of an X-ray room is at least 250 mm solid baked clay bricks, and 150 mm mortar/concrete walls for plain radiography. Hollow bricks should be plastered with a thickness of 6 mm barium plaster and should be protected up to 2200 mm from the floor level.
6. No single wall dimension of the X-ray room shall be less than 4 m.
7. Flooring can be of tiles/marble/granite, but it shall not be slippery to avoid accidents and injury to the patient.
8. The room shall have a single door with a width of about 1524 mm, to ease the movement of trollies.
9. The door should be at least 1500 mm long and 2000 mm high. The door and its frame need to have a 2-mm thick lead lining. There shall be no leakage of the radiation from the door. Doors should overlap by a minimum of 100 mm on each side when closed. The overlap requirement applies to flap doors that make a single entrance door but close from a different side. Doors should have handles and locks, both on the inside and on the outside so that they are always closed during exposure and access can be controlled.
10. Windows are not allowed in the radiography room.
11. A warning light (red colour bulb) shall be provided outside the door. This light must be connected to the generator in a way that it illuminates only during the tube activation.
12. The chest stand or the chest frame can be fixed on the wall opposite to the entrance door and the control console.
13. A shielded barrier should be placed at the X-ray control console to protect the staff from radiation exposure.
14. Depending on the machine capacity, the power load required by the machine shall be calculated, and the main switch and cable shall be separately terminated in each radiography room.
15. If a Digitalized Radiography (DR) type of machine is planned, then a separate small control room, adjoining the DR room shall be provided. Between the two rooms, a lead glass shall be fixed in a wooden frame with a 2-mm lead lining.
16. Lighting shall be provided using normal LED, with sufficient lumen. No extra illumination is required in the room.
17. The temperature in the room shall range between 18 and 21 °C, and the humidity level shall not be more than 60%. Before finalizing the humidity level or temperature, environmental requirements shall be confirmed with the equipment supplier, as some machines may require varied environmental standards.
18. All machines shall have proper ground earthing provisions.
19. A stand with heavy-duty hangers shall be provided outside all rooms to hang the lead apron.
20. A cabinet shall be provided in each room to keep other radiation safety devices like lead gloves, lead goggles, groin guards and lead collar.

22.6.2 Room for Mobile X-Ray System

Usually, hospitals have mobile X-ray units for bedside X-ray of immobile patients. These machines are generally placed in the units where they are required, but in some hospitals, they are centrally located in the department of Radiology. Therefore, a store shall be provided in the department for storing these machines. Size-wise, the store can be 3658 mm × 3658 mm, but the size can be increased depending on the number of machines.

22.6.3 Change Rooms

Patients often need to change clothes before entering the X-Ray room as the clothes may have some metal parts which shall disturb the imaging. Hence, change rooms are provided in the department to enable the patient to remove all outside clothes and change to a hospital dress. The room shall be approximately 3048 mm × 3048 mm in size. It shall have an adequate provision of personal lockers to keep patient belongings. Also, hooks, hanger rod and hangers shall be provided to hang clothes. There shall be a cabinet to keep sterilized dresses.

22.6.4 Patient Preparation Room

A room shall be provided along with the radiography unit for preparing patients before specific imaging like barium sallow through. In such a case, the patient has to be given oral barium solution. The size of the room can be 3658 mm × 3658 mm with an examination couch and chair.

22.6.5 Computerized Radiography (CR) Room

X-ray exposure is taken on a special X-ray cassette. This cassette has a screen inside it on which the image is collected post-exposure. The cassette is then loaded in a machine called CR, where the screen inside the cassette comes out and the CR reads the image. After reading, the image on the screen is washed out by the CR and the cassette is ready for next use. The image captured by CR is then sent to a PC attached to it. Radiographer can then modify the image parameters, followed by printing the image on a film.

The size of the CR room shall be about 4267 mm × 3658 mm. The room shall have a countertop or table to keep the CR system or alternately it can be placed on a wooden table. Although a countertop is better as the unit can generate vibrations on a wooden table. For a PC, a table with chair is required. The camera can either be a tabletop model or a floor model. If it is a tabletop model, it can be placed on both the countertop and the table. But if it is a floor model, a small foundation shall be required. The temperature in the room shall be about 18–21 °C and the RH shall be 40–50%. Lighting shall be normal as in other rooms.

22.6.6 Sub-waiting for Radiography

Shall be the same as for the Utility area.

22.7 Ultrasound Zone

Ultrasound is an imaging technique which utilizes high-intensity sound waves, measured in MHz. In this technology, sound waves are induced in a specific part of the body with the help of the transduces. When these sound waves hit various body tissues at different time of milliseconds, they are reflected to the surface, where the transducer picks up the returned waves which have different intensities and different time periods. The machine reads these returned waves and forms an image. This zone includes the following:

22.7.1 Ultrasound Room

This is a room where the Ultrasound of the patient is performed. There are no specific requirements for the design of this room. It can either be a square or rectangular room of about 13.94–18.58 sq.m. On one side, a couch is placed next to the Ultrasound machine. Curtain partition shall be installed by hanging curtains from the curtain rails fixed on the ceiling. The temperature in the room shall be about 18–22 °C and the RH shall be 50%. The light of the room shall be dimmable.

22.7.2 Change Rooms

At times, a patient's cloth makes it difficult to perform an ultrasound. Hence, change rooms are provided in the department to enable the patient to remove all outside clothes and change to a hospital dress. The room shall be approximately 3048 mm × 3048 mm in size. It shall have an adequate provision of personal lockers to keep patient belongings. Also, hooks, hanger rod and hangers shall be provided to hang clothes. There shall be a cabinet to keep sterilized dresses.

22.7.3 Toilets

Each Ultrasound room shall have an attached toilet. This is required as some of the scans need to be done post void, particularly the ultrasound of the lower abdomen. The toilet shall have a WC, urinal and washbasin. Exhaust must be given in the toilet.

22.7.4 Sub-waiting for Ultrasound

Shall be the same as for Utility area.

22.8 CT Scan Zone

This zone of the radiology department is related to the Computerized Tomography. This machine is also X-ray based and very high doses of X-Rays are produced when exposure is given. Hence special care has to be taken while designing the CT Room. This zone includes the following:

22.8.1 CT Scan Machine Room

As far as the number of CT rooms is concerned, it depends on the number of machines required to be installed at once, and also on the future plans of adding more machines. The CT Scan machines are available in different configurations, but irrespective of it, the design and size of the room shall remain the same. The machine comes with a long slide table (Fig. 22.2).

Some of the important points related to the designing of the CT rooms are as follows:

1. *Before designing the CT Scan room, the guidelines and norms of the controlling authority of the country must be taken into account. e.g. in India, Baba Atomic Research Institute issues all such norms and guidelines.*
2. A separate room shall be provided for each machine.
3. If the machine is to be installed horizontally, a rectangular room shall be designed. If the machine is to be installed diagonally, a square room design would be better. However, we suggest installing the machine horizontally, in a rectangular room. In this case, the room space shall not be less than 42 sq.m, and the room size shall be 9144 mm × 4572 mm.
4. All the walls of the room shall be at least 229 mm thick, with plaster on both sides. The ideal thickness for the primary wall of an X-ray room is at least 250 mm solid baked clay bricks, and 150 mm mortar/concrete walls for plain radiography. Hollow bricks should be plastered with a thickness of 6 mm barium plaster and should be protected up to 2200 mm from the floor level.
5. Flooring can be of tiles/marble/granite, but it shall not be slippery to avoid accidents and injury to the patient.
6. It is advised to provide Air Interlocks by placing an additional door before the CT room door.
7. The CT room shall have a single door with a width of about 1524 mm, to ease the movement of trollies.
8. The door shall have to be with a proper 2 mm thick lead lining. The lining has to be done even on the door frame. There shall be no leakage of the radiation from any place in the door. Doors should overlap by a minimum of 100 mm on each side when closed. The door

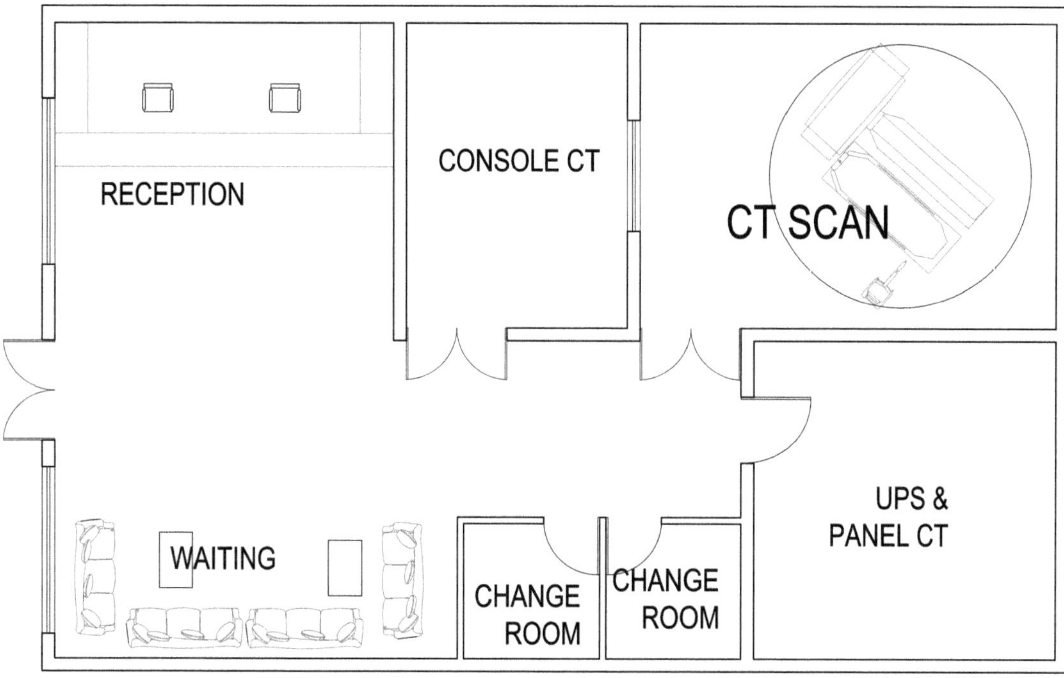

Fig. 22.2 Sample layout drawing of CT Scan Zone

should be at least 1500 mm long and 2000 mm high. The overlap requirement also applies to flap doors that make a single entrance door but closing from different sides of the door. The door should have handles and locks on the inside and the outside so that they may always be closed during exposures thus controlling access.

9. Windows are not allowed in the CT Scan room.
10. A warning light (red colour bulb) shall be provided outside the door. This light must be connected to the generator in a way that it illuminates only during the tube activation.
11. While installing the machine, care shall be taken to leave at least 1829 mm space behind the machine for the Gantry of the machine to tilt, and for easy maintenance of the machine. The machine shall be installed in the centre of the width of the room.
12. Depending on the machine capacity, the power load required by the machine shall be calculated, and the main switch and cable shall be separately terminated in each CT Scan room.
13. As the weight of the machine is more and the movement of the machine is very fast, it is advised to check the weight-bearing capacity of the floor. If needed, provide a foundation for the machine as per the suggestions of the machine manufacturer.
14. The equipment should be mounted on a base plate only with desired mounting anchor fasteners as specified by the manufacturer of the equipment.
15. Any shortcuts will result in vibrations of the unit during its operation and compression artefacts in the image, resulting in poor image quality, repetition in diagnostic tests and leading to eventual reinstallation of the unit.
16. Lighting shall be provided using normal LED, with sufficient lumen. No extra illumination is required in the room.

17. The temperature in the room shall range between 18 and 21 °C, and the humidity level shall not be more than 60%. Before finalizing the humidity level or temperature, environmental requirements shall be confirmed with the equipment supplier, as some machines may require varied environmental standards.
18. All machines shall have proper ground earthing provision.
19. Inside the CT Scan room, outlets for medical gas supply shall be given. There shall be one outlet for Oxygen, one for Vacuum and one for Air.
20. The proper two-way audio system shall be provided in the CT room, so that the patient can be directed by the technician sitting in the control room, without entering the CT room.
21. Position the gantry and couch in such a way that the patient is completely visible from the control console during scanning.
22. The entrance door to the gantry room, from the control console, shall have similar requirements as the patient entrance door.
23. A stand with heavy-duty hangers shall be provided outside all rooms to a hang the lead apron.
24. A cabinet shall be provided in each room to keep other radiation safety devices like lead gloves, lead goggles, groin guards and lead collar.

22.8.2 CT Control Room

Attached to the CT Scan room, a control room has to be provided. While the procedure is going on, no person shall be allowed to enter the machine room. All controls shall be done from the control room only. The size of this room shall be 3658 mm × 3658 mm. It shall be provided with a table to install the Control Unit of the machine. This table is usually supplied along with the machine. Apart from this, there shall be the provision of a secondary computer for transferring the CT images, for preparing reports. Some hospitals have a separate reporting room. In that case, the space for the secondary computer is not required in the control room. A lead glass (provided with the machine) of about 1200 mm × 1000 mm shall be fixed in a wooden frame with a 2-mm lead lining between the CT room and the control room to ensure no leakage of the radiation. A camera (printer) shall also be provided in the Control Room to print CT films.

22.8.3 UPS Room

As a CT Scan is an electronic machine, it requires a continuous power supply. If that is not provided, the machine will stop, increasing the chances of software corruption or even failure of different parts of the machine. To avoid this, mostly all users of the machine prefer to install an online UPS with the machine. As UPS is usually of high rating (above 100 kVA), a lot of batteries shall be required, and thus a separate room shall be provided for this. This room shall be attached to the CT Control Room or the machine room. Some hospitals install all UPSs used in the hospital at a commonplace, away from the machine. However, this is not recommended. The UPS shall be near the machine, as firstly the CT technician can keep a watch on the UPS, and secondly, in case of emergency, he/she can switch off the UPS immediately. Earthing of this UPS is essential.

The size of this room shall be about 3658 mm × 3658 mm with several racks to install batteries. Because of the acid in the batteries, sometimes fumes are formed in the room; thus, the UPS room shall have an exhaust. The UPS also generates a large amount of heat; thus, the room shall be air-conditioned and the temperature shall be about 17–20 °C with an RH of not more than 40%.

22.8.4 CT Panel Room

Apart from the gantry of the machine where the X-ray tube and detectors are fixed, other electronic parts are provided in the panels connected to the machine. These panels control the working of the machine but are not directly needed in the

CT Scan room. For better protection of these panels, it is advised to install these panels in a different room or enclosure, which is attached to the CT Scan room. Hence, such an area shall be designed after consulting the equipment manufacturer. The size and temperature etc. shall be confirmed by the manufacturer of the machine.

22.8.5 Change Rooms

Patients often need to change clothes before entering the CT room as the clothes may have some metal parts which shall disturb the imaging. Hence, change rooms are provided in the department to enable the patient to remove all outside clothes and change to a hospital dress. The room shall be approximately 3048 mm × 3048 mm in size. It shall have an adequate provision of personal lockers to keep patient belongings. Also, hooks, hanger rod and hangers shall be provided to hang clothes. There shall be a cabinet to keep sterilized dresses.

22.8.6 Sub-waiting for CT Scan

Shall be the same as for Utility area.

22.9 MRI Zone

This zone of the radiology department is related to Magnetic Resonance Imaging. As this machine has a strong magnetic field, special care has to be taken while designing the MRI rooms. This zone includes the following:

22.9.1 MRI Machine Room

As far as the number of MRI rooms is concerned, it depends on the number of machines required to be installed at once, and also on the future plans of adding more machines. The MRI machines are available in different configurations, and depending on the configuration of the machine, the design and size of the room shall change. For example, a room size of 0.25T MRI shall be small as compared to the 1.5T MRI, and it will be even more for a 3T MRI. The MRI machine comes with a long slide table (Fig. 22.3).

Some of the important points related to the designing of the MRI rooms are as follows:

1. A separate room shall be provided for each machine.
2. Magnetic field safety applies to MRI installations. Care should be taken to shield the magnet and procedure room from external magnetic interference, ensuring magnetic fields specified are not exceeded.
3. *RF Shielding*

   MRI systems are highly sensitive to radio frequencies. Therefore, the MRI machine is enclosed in an RF shield. It is essentially a six-sided copper-lined box around the room called 'Faraday Cage' which protects the MRI system from exterior radio frequencies for the clarity of scan. RF shielding can also be done with the galvanized steel and aluminium, but copper is considered to be the best. The footprint for the RF shield is set by the designer during the designing process. Also, the design of the RF shield has to be checked with the vendor, to establish where things like ductwork, conduits, plumbing and others, penetrate the shield.

   RF shields often require three partitions, including the parent wall, RF shield wall, and interior finishing wall. Parent wall means the brick or concrete wall already built. RF Shield is the actual metallic sheet, and the inner finishing is the artificial decorative interior. The inner interior can be done using wallpapers, wooden or PVC panels.

   The floor in MRI exam room often requires a structural subfloor, RF shielding, a protective layer and other finishing materials. Subfloor means the originally constructed floor, then the metallic cage, and then the protective layer. This layer can be made of wood, as it does not affect the magnetic field.

   An RF shield ceiling is often suspended from the structural deck overhead. Any ser-

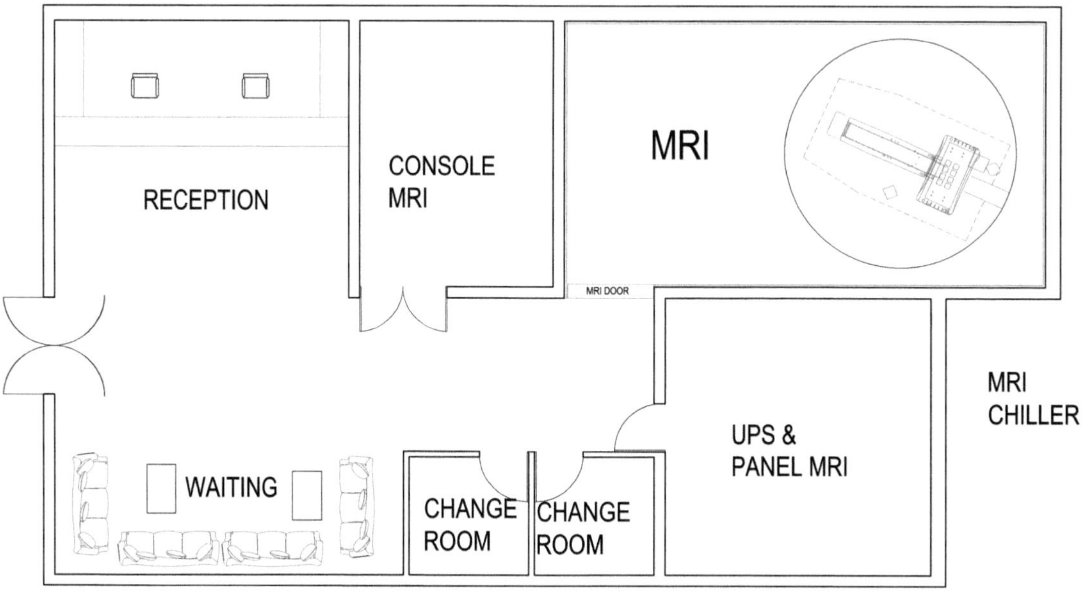

Fig. 22.3 Sample layout drawing of MRI Zone

vices that pass above the MRI scanner room (power, piping, cabling and ductwork) should do so in the plenum above the RF shield ceiling. Items that penetrate into the RF shield enclosure will require special fittings and materials to maintain the shield integrity. RF filters and waveguides are common materials used at the shielding feedthrough points. The bottom of the ceiling can be decorated with LED lights or 3D illuminated sceneries.

The window between the magnet room and control/console room usually requires RF shielding, which is often two layers of copper screens or perforated sheets.

4. The next thing a hospital needs to consider when designing an MRI suite is protecting the public from a high magnetic field. Designer shall work with MRI vendors to establish a precise location of the iso-centre of the magnet. From there, they design protective provisions to keep the public away from the most dangerous magnetic fields. Imagine an invisible shield radiating out from the magnet's iso-centre. This is called the Gauss Field. Distance from the iso-centre to the 5-gauss line is dangerous for anyone wearing ferrous metal, or for any metal objects. Anything metal within the 5-gauss line will essentially become a part of the magnet. To avoid this and keep everyone safe, designers intentionally design barriers to deter people from getting too close. Pacemakers, cell phones and credit cards are severely damaged when inside the 5-gauss line.
5. Maintain the desired minimum clearances from the objects, such as water-cooling systems, wheelchairs, carts, transformers, overhead power lines and vehicles including cars, as specified in the installation prerequisites supplied by the manufacturer to ensure trouble-free performance of the magnet. If accidentally it is taken near the magnet, the machine will pull it with a tremendous force, which can either damage the machine or cause injury to the patient.
6. In an event of such an emergency, the machine may have to be stopped by pushing the emergency stop button. If this is done, the magnet will quench, which means is the sud-

den loss of superconductivity in the magnet. A cryogen vent is required to be able to expel the super-cooled helium gas that the MRI uses. There is a huge expense behind reviving the machine in such cases.
7. It is advised to provide Interlocks before entering the MRI room. This can be done by providing another door before the MRI room door.
8. The size of an MRI room shall depend on the size of the RF cage. It is advised that while finalizing the configuration of the machine, a bigger-sized RF cage shall be taken if space allows. The designer shall take a specification of the room sizes from the vendor before planning the MRI room.
9. All the walls of the room shall be at least 229 mm thick, with a plaster on both sides.
10. The room shall have a single door, made from a material that does not interfere with the magnetic field, and it must be a sealed door. The size of the door shall be verified from the vendor of the machine.
11. Windows are not allowed in the MRI room.
12. While installing the machine, care shall be taken to leave at least 1829 mm space behind the machine for the MRI Table to move behind and for easy maintenance of the machine. The machine shall be installed in the centre of the width of the room.
13. As the weight of the machine is more, it is advised to check the weight-bearing capacity of the floor. If needed, provide a foundation for the machine as per the suggestions of the machine manufacturer.
14. The equipment should be mounted on a base plate only with desired mounting anchor fasteners as specified by the manufacturer of the equipment.
15. Any shortcuts will result in vibrations of the unit during its operation and compression art facts in an image, resulting in poor image quality, repetition in diagnostic tests, leading to eventual reinstallation of the unit.
16. Lighting shall be provided using normal LED, with sufficient lumen. However, ordinary light fittings are not allowed. There are special lights made of non-ferrous material for MRI room.
17. The temperature in the room shall range between 18 and 21 °C, and the humidity level shall not be more than 40%. Before finalizing the humidity level or temperature, environmental requirements shall be confirmed with the equipment supplier, as some machines may require varied environmental standards.
18. All machines shall have proper ground earthing provision.
19. Inside the room, a cabinet made of wood, Polycarbonate or other non-ferrous material has to be provided. This is required to store the MRI coils and any other non-ferrous material.
20. The MRI room needs the following outlets for medical gas supply: one outlet for Oxygen, one for Vacuum and one for Air. However, these outlets cannot be given directly in the room; instead, they are given in the RF cage, from where a rubber tube is provided inside the MRI room up to the patient table.
21. The proper two-way audio system shall be provided in the MRI room, so that the patient can be directed by the technician sitting in the control room, without entering the MRI room.

22.9.2 MRI Control Room

Attached to the MRI Scan room, a control room has to be provided. While the procedure is going on, no person shall be allowed to enter the machine room. All controls shall be done from the control room only. The size of this room shall be 3658 mm × 3658 mm. It shall be provided with a table to install the Control Unit of the machine. This table is usually supplied along with the machine. Apart from this, there shall be the provision of a secondary computer for transferring the MRI images, for preparing reports. Some hospitals have a separate reporting room. In that case, the space for a secondary computer is not required in the control room. A meshed glass (provided with the machine) of about 1200 mm × 1000 mm shall be fixed in a wooden frame with a 2-mm lead lining between the MRI room and the control room to ensure no leakage of the radiation. A camera (printer) shall also be provided in the Control Room to print MRI films.

22.9.3 UPS Room

As MRI is an electronic machine, it requires a continuous power supply. It is more essential, as the cold head of the machine shall always be on, failing which the Helium gas filled in the magnet will boil, and potentially lost. If that is not provided, the machine will stop, increasing the chances of software corruption or even failure of different parts of the machine. To avoid this, mostly all users of the machine prefer to install an online UPS with the machine. As UPS is usually of high rating (above 150 kVA), a lot of batteries shall be required, and thus a separate room shall be provided for this. This room shall be attached to the MRI Control Room or the machine room. Some hospitals install all UPSs used in the hospital at a commonplace, away from the machine. However, this is not recommended. The UPS shall be near the machine, as firstly the MRI technician can keep a watch on the UPS, and secondly, in case of emergency, he/she can switch off the UPS immediately. Earthing of this UPS is essential.

The size of this room shall be about 3658 mm × 3658 mm with several racks to install batteries. Because of the acid in the batteries, sometimes fumes are formed in the room; thus, the UPS room shall have an exhaust. The UPS also generates a large amount of heat; thus, the room shall be air-conditioned and the temperature shall be about 17–20 °C with an RH of not more than 40%.

22.9.4 MRI Panel Room

Apart from the gantry of the main MRI machine, other electronic parts are provided in the panels connected to the machine. These panels control the working of the machine but are not directly needed in the MRI room. For better protection of these panels, it is advised to install these panels in a different room or enclosure, which is attached to the MRI room. Hence, such an area shall be designed after consulting the equipment manufacturer. The size and temperature etc. shall be confirmed from the manufacturer of the machine.

22.9.5 Chiller

Along with the MRI, a water chiller is required to cool down the gradient coil and liquid helium compressor. The whole refrigeration part of MRI is composed of a chiller, a helium compressor and a cold head. Through their joint work, the temperature inside the magnet is controlled at −269 °C, to maintain the superconducting state of the coil. In order to maintain this temperature inside the magnet, the heat of the superconducting coil is taken away by the vaporization of liquid helium, which will cause the pressure inside the magnet to rise and thus the loss of liquid helium. If the MRI chiller fails, the entire refrigeration system will stop working; thus, it shall also be connected to the UPS for its continuous working.

The chiller is usually installed outside the hospital building to keep it cool. It is provided with a water tank, from where the chiller takes the water, cools it, and then sends it to the machine through a connected pipeline. This water cools the machine and returns to the chiller through a separate pipeline, and is cooled again.

22.9.6 Change Rooms

Patients often need to change clothes before entering the MRI room as the clothes may have some metal parts, which shall disturb the imaging. Hence, change rooms are provided in the department to enable the patient to remove all outside clothes and change to a hospital dress. The room shall be approximately 3048 mm × 3048 mm in size. It shall have an adequate provision of personal lockers to keep patient belongings. Also, hooks, hanger rod and hangers shall be provided to hang clothes. There shall be a cabinet to keep sterilized dresses.

22.9.7 Sub-waiting for MRI

Shall be the same as for Utility area.

22.10 Mammography Zone

This zone of the radiology department is related to the X-ray of breasts for females. As this is also an X-ray-based machine, hence care has to be taken while designing the mammography room. This zone includes the following:

22.10.1 Mammography Rooms

Mammography rooms are the actual room where the mammography machine is installed, and the exposure of X-rays is given to the patient. As far as the numbers of mammography rooms are concerned, generally one is sufficient, but the designer has to take into account the future plans as well.

Some of the important points related to the designing of the mammography rooms are as follows:

1. *Before designing the radiography rooms, the guidelines and norms of the controlling authority of the country must be taken into account. e.g. in India, Baba Atomic Research Institute issues all such norms and guidelines.*
2. A separate room shall be provided for each machine.
3. The room can either be a rectangular or square room as designed by the designer and the size of a room shall not be less than 10 sq.m.
4. All the walls of the room shall be at least 229 mm thick, with plaster on both sides. The ideal thickness for the primary wall of an mammography room is at least 250 mm solid baked clay bricks, and 150 mm mortar/concrete walls for plain radiography. Hollow bricks should be plastered with a thickness of 6 mm barium plaster and should be protected up to 2200 mm from the floor level.
5. No single wall dimension of the mammography room shall be less than 3000 mm.
6. Flooring can be of tiles/marble/granite, but it shall not be slippery to avoid accidents and injury to the patient.
7. The room shall have a single door with a width of about 1000 mm.
8. The door should be at least 1000 mm long and 2000 mm high. The door and its frame need to have a 2-mm thick lead lining. There shall be no leakage of the radiation from the door. Doors should overlap by a minimum of 100 mm on each side when closed. The overlap requirement applies to flap doors that make a single entrance door but closes from a different side. Doors should have handles and locks, both on the inside and on the outside so that they are always closed during exposure and access can be controlled.
9. Windows are not allowed in the mammography room.
10. A warning light (red colour bulb) shall be provided outside the door. This light must be connected to the generator in a way that it illuminates only during the tube activation
11. A shielded barrier should be placed at the mammography control console to protect the staff from radiation exposure.
12. Depending on the machine capacity, the power load required by the machine shall be calculated, and the main switch and cable shall be separately terminated in each mammography room.
13. Lighting shall be provided using normal LED, with sufficient lumen. No extra illumination is required in the room.

14. The temperature in the room shall range between 18 and 21 °C, and the humidity level shall not be more than 60%. Before finalizing the humidity level or temperature, environmental requirements shall be confirmed with the equipment supplier, as some machines may require varied environmental standards.
15. All machines shall have proper ground earthing provisions.
16. A stand with heavy-duty hangers shall be provided outside all rooms to a hang the lead apron.
17. A cabinet shall be provided in each room to keep other radiation safety devices like lead gloves, lead goggles, groin guards and lead collar.

22.10.2 Change Rooms

For mammography, generally, the upper body clothes have to be changed to a simple cotton gown. Hence, change rooms are provided in the department to enable the patient to remove all outside clothes and change to a hospital dress. The room shall be approximately 10 ft × 10 ft in size. It shall have an adequate provision of personal lockers to keep patient belongings. Also, hooks, hanger rod and hangers shall be provided to hang clothes. There shall be a cabinet to keep sterilized dresses.

22.10.3 Computerized Radiography (CR) Room

CR System of the main radiology department can be used for mammography. Just the cassette needs to be carried from the mammography room to the radiology CR room. Other processes will remain the same.

22.10.4 Sub-waiting for Mammography

Shall be the same as for Utility area.

22.11 DEXA Scan Zone

This zone of the radiology department is related to the high-precision type of X-ray that measures the bone mineral density and bone loss. If the bone density is lower than normal, it indicates a risk for osteoporosis and bone fractures. As this is an X-ray-based machine, hence care has to be taken while designing the DEXA Scan room. This zone includes the following:

22.11.1 DEXA Scan Machine Room

This is the area where the machine is installed and the exposure of X-rays is given to the patient. As far as the number of rooms is concerned, generally one is sufficient, but the designer has to take into account the future plans as well.

Some of the important points related to the designing of the radiography rooms are as follows:

1. *Before designing the radiography rooms, the guidelines and norms of the controlling authority of the country must be taken into account. e.g. in India, Baba Atomic Research Institute issues all such norms and guidelines.*
2. A separate room shall be provided for each machine.
3. The room can either be a rectangular or square room, as designed by the designer, and the size of the room shall not be less than 10 sq.m.
4. All the walls of the room shall be at least 9 in. thick, with plaster on both sides. The ideal thickness for the primary wall of an X-ray room is at least 250 mm solid baked clay bricks, and 150 mm mortar/concrete walls for plain radiography. Hollow bricks should be plastered with a thickness of 6 mm barium plaster and should be protected up to 2200 mm from the floor level.
5. Flooring can be of tiles/marble/granite, but it shall not be slippery to avoid accidents and injury to the patient.

6. The room shall have a single door with a width of about 1000 mm.
7. The door should be at least 1000 mm long and 2000 mm high. The door and its frame need to have a 2-mm thick lead lining. There shall be no leakage of the radiation from the door. Doors should overlap by a minimum of 100 mm on each side when closed. The overlap requirement applies to flap doors that make a single entrance door but closes from a different side. Doors should have handles and locks, both on the inside and on the outside so that they are always closed during exposure and access can be controlled.
8. Windows are not allowed in the DEXA scan room.
9. A warning light (red colour bulb) shall be provided outside the door. This light must be connected to the generator in a way that it illuminates only during the tube activation.
10. A shielded barrier should be placed at the DEXA scan control console to protect the staff from radiation exposure.
11. Depending on the machine capacity, the power load required by the machine shall be calculated and the main switch and cable shall be separately terminated in each DEXA scan room.
12. Lighting shall be provided using normal LED, with sufficient lumen. No extra illumination is required in the room.
13. The temperature in the room shall range between 18 and 21 °C, and the humidity level shall not be more than 60%. Before finalizing the humidity level or temperature, environmental requirements shall be confirmed with the equipment supplier, as some machines may require varied environmental standards.
14. All machines shall have proper ground earthing provisions.
15. A stand with heavy-duty hangers shall be provided outside all rooms to a hang the lead apron.
16. A cabinet shall be provided in each room to keep other radiation safety devices like lead gloves, lead goggles, groin guards and lead collar.

22.11.2 Sub-waiting for DEXA Scan

Shall be the same as for Utility area.

22.12 PET CT/MRI Zone

This zone of the radiology department is related to the Positron Emission Tomography (PET) scanners with the fusion of morphological imaging in the form of CT or MRI. This integrated system is called PET CT and PET MRI. Hence, we have to design the facility to incorporate the basic infrastructure of CT and MRI, and also the requirements and regulations of the PET Scanner, in which nuclear isotopes are used.

As the hot area consisting of the cyclotron and the radiopharmacy areas are the same, it is recommended that both the PET CT and PET MRI shall be installed in the same area. With such an arrangement, we can save a lot of space in the department.

As far as the number of PET CT and PET MRI is concerned, usually one machine each is installed, but the designer shall also take into account the future expansion plans of the hospital.

22.12.1 Location of the Zone in Hospital

As the PET area is a high positron emitter, it is essential to provide proper shielding and safety mechanisms like reinforced cement concrete (RCC) walls. Hence, it is advised to locate this zone in the basement, as the room will be surrounded by soil, which will reduce the risk of emission outside the zone.

The infrastructure of this zone includes (Fig. 22.4):

PET CT/PET MRI/ SPECT CT	PET CT Room
	PET MRI Room
	SPECT CT Room
	Console Rooms for all machines
	UPS rooms
	Machine Panel Rooms
	Technologist Room
	Physician Consultation Room
	Post-Drug Administration Holding cubicles
	Active Toilet
	Dose administration Room
	Hot Lab cum Radio-pharmacy Room
	Radioactive Store
	Medicine Preparation Room
	Radioactive waste Room
	Change room
	General Store
	Sub-waiting

22.12.2 PET CT Scan Machine Room

The infrastructure of the machine room shall be the same as a normal CT Scan machine room. The only difference is that the wall shall be made out of 300 mm thick RCC.

22.12.3 PET MRI Machine Room

The infrastructure of the machine room shall be the same as a normal MRI machine room. The only difference is that the wall shall be made out of 300 mm thick RCC.

All norms and specifications of other attached areas like console room, UPS room and machine panel room shall also be the same as CT Scan and MRI.

22.12.4 SPECT CT Machine Room

Earlier, a Nuclear Bone Scan was done with the help of a Gamma Camera. It was able to capture an image just like X-Ray, after inducing isotopes. As technology changed, SPECT came into the picture. It can capture images by cutting slices of the parts to be investigated. The infrastructure of the machine room shall be the same as a normal CT or PET CT machine room.

22.12.5 Operating Console Rooms

For each imaging modality, a separate console room shall be provided. Therefore, a wall separating the console room from the PET CT scanner, PET MRI and SPECT CT room shall be provided. This shall be a 300-mm-thick RCC wall with a 4-mm lead equivalent glass window.

Before planning the rooms for PET CT, PET MRI and SPECT CT, it is essential to meet the requirements and room specifications such as weight-bearing capacity, temperature stability, adequate power supply, as well as the issues concerning radiation safety, as advised by the machine manufacturer.

22.12.6 Low-Risk Areas or Cold Areas

22.12.6.1 Reception

It shall be located at the entrance of the zone, usually in the front. Also, a secretarial room shall be provided in the rear of the reception for administrative jobs like accounts. Roughly a space of about 15–20 sq.m shall be sufficient for both these utilities, but depending on the workload, the area may be increased or decreased. Other parameters like lighting, temperature and furniture shall be the same as in case of other reception areas and the administrative rooms.

22.12.6.2 Sub-waiting Room

Shall be the same as for Utility rooms.

22.12.6.3 Physicians Consulting Room

This room is for analyzing, interviewing and physically examining the patient before undertaking the patient for investigation. The patient is informed about the nature of the specific exami-

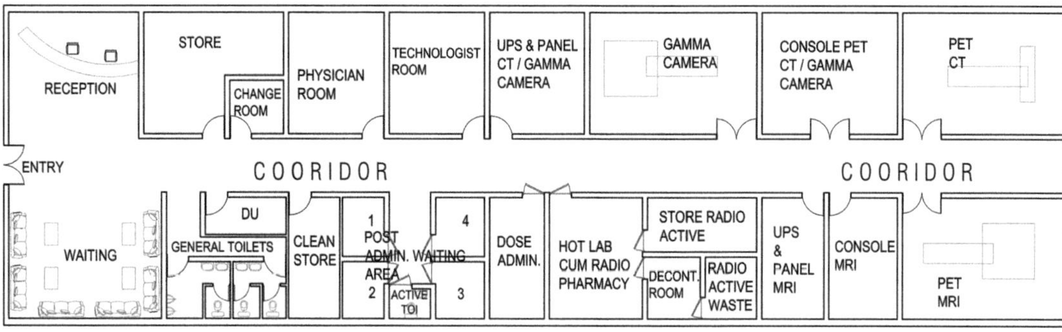

Fig. 22.4 Sample layout drawing of PET CT/PET MRI/Gamma Camera Zone

nation he/she is undergoing. This room shall be close to the waiting room and adequately equipped. The outlets for the supply of oxygen and vacuum shall be provided. The size of this room shall be about 4267 mm × 4572 mm.

22.12.6.4 Store

A small store of size 3658 mm × 3658 mm shall be provided to store the materials like QC phantoms, consumables and disposables. The room shall be provided with the worktops, cabinets and drawers for storage.

22.12.6.5 Technologist Room

A technologist room cum office shall be located near or opposite to the physician consultation room for planning the investigation and arranging resources for the department.

22.12.7 High-Risk Areas or Radiation Exposure Hot Areas

22.12.7.1 Hot Lab Cum Radiopharmacy Room

This room is required when the department has its own production unit (cyclotron and radiochemistry lab). This allows for mono-dose syringes to be delivered to each injecting room in lead containers. The walls of the room shall be 300 mm thick RCC.

22.12.7.2 Injection Room

An injection room is constructed with a 220-mm-thick RCC wall. An aperture is provided in this room which opens in the radiopharmacy. The patients are made to sit in the injection room and the staff prepares the injection in the adjoining radiopharmacy room. Through this aperture, the radiopharmaceutical is injected into the patient. This room shall roughly be 12–16 sq.m for each PET CT/PET MRI/SPECT CT installed. Patients after injection are a relatively intense source of radiation (of the order of 30–50 μSv/h per patient at 1000 mm just after the administration).

22.12.7.3 Post-dose Waiting Area

The injected patient is then made to wait in the post-dose waiting area, where he/she can rest comfortably during the uptake period. The walls of post-dose waiting area are made up of 300-mm-thick RCC, resulting in an exposure rate of about 1.22 uSv/h (for a patient injected with 300 MBq of ^{18}F radiopharmaceutical at a distance of about 1000 mm). The assembly of several patients in the uptake room area is a radiation protection problem that should not be overlooked; ensure proper positioning and shielding of the uptake rooms.

22.12.8 Toilet

After injection and an uptake period depending on the protocol, patients are asked to void their bladder before starting the actual PET scan procedure. Hence, a toilet must be located adjacent to the Post Dose Waiting Area. The discharge of this toilet is taken in a separate settlement tank where it is allowed to settle down and the effects of isotopes are neutralized before dropping the discharge in the main sewerage line.

22.12.9 Control and Scanning Room

This is the core of the facility. The scanning room must be easily reached from the preparation rooms and the toilet. The door is normally in front of the preparation block. Vendors' prerequisites and installation guidelines should be considered in the planning phase. Also, careful consideration should be given to the fact that PET/CT, PET MRI and SPECT CT scanners are somewhat demanding in terms of site prerequisites: the gantry of a multi-modality scanner could weigh more than 3000 kg. The corridors and angles should allow the biggest single package to be moved until its final position.

22.12.10 Post-examination Waiting Room

Patients should wait in the post-scan waiting room while their scans are checked. They will also need to change clothes if they are wearing a hospital gown. This allows for faster patient throughput. Patients are then released from the post-scan waiting room and leave the facility. It is advised to provide a separate exit gate so that these patients do not mix with others.

22.12.11 Waste Disposal Room

The materials used for dispensing FDG and anything which could be contaminated (clothes, linen etc.) should be stored in a dedicated area to let the radioactivity decay before being disposed of.

Further Reading

1.5T MRI Suite Size Requirements [Internet]. [cited 2021 Jun 22]. Available from: https://info.blockimaging.com/1.5t-mri-suite-size-requirements

CT Machine Site Plan Checklist | Amber Diagnostics [Internet]. 2021 [cited 2021 Jun 22]. Available from: https://www.amberusa.com/blog/ct-machine-site-plan-checklist/

Ct Scan Room Design Guidelines - ct scan machine [Internet]. Ct Scan Room Design Guidelines - ct scan machine. [cited 2021 Jun 22]. Available from: https://ctscanmachines.blogspot.com/2018/11/ct-scan-room-design-guidelines.html

CT Scan Room Layout | CT Scan Room Layout And Design [Internet]. Avanttec. 2019 [cited 2021 Jun 22]. Available from: http://www.avanttec.net/ct-scan-room-layout/

Design standards for imaging areas are changing [Internet]. [cited 2021 Jun 22]. Available from: https://www.hfmmagazine.com/articles/1426-design-standards-for-imaging-areas-are-changing

Designing MRI Suites: Navigating Structural Design Considerations for Success [Internet]. HGA. 2017 [cited 2021 Jun 22]. Available from: https://hga.com/designing-mri-suites-navigating-structural-design-considerations-for-success/

Dwiyanto A, Hardiman G, Budi WS. Human Safety Design Space In The Ct-Scan Service Unit A Case Study In An Indonesian Public Hospital. 2020;9(01):6.

Hawnaur J. Diagnostic radiology. BMJ. 1999 Jul 17;319(7203):168–71.

HealthManagement.org. Radiology Management, ICU Management, Healthcare IT, Cardiology Management, Executive Management [Internet]. HealthManagement. [cited 2021 Jun 22]. Available from: https://healthmanagement.org/c/imaging/issuearticle/safety-factors-in-planning-and-design-of-the-imaging-department

Jha AK, Singh AM, Mithun S, Shah S, Agrawal A, Purandare NC, et al. Designing of High-Volume PET/CT Facility with Optimal Reduction of Radiation Exposure to the Staff: Implementation and Optimization in a Tertiary Health Care Facility in India. World J Nucl Med. 2015;14(3):189–96.

Malone J. The Design of Diagnostic Medical Facilities where Ionising Radiation is used. 2009.

New Trends and Technology in Radiology [Internet]. Imaging Technology News. 2012 [cited 2021 Jun 22].

Available from: https://www.itnonline.com/article/new-trends-and-technology-radiology

Niu Y, Xian J, Lei Z, Liu X, Sun Q. Management of infection control and radiological protection in diagnostic radiology examination of COVID-19 cases. Radiat Med Prot. 2020 Jun 1;1(2):75–80.

Psm JL. Safety Guide for Radiation Protection in Nuclear Medicine. :111.

Radiology Room Requirements for Medical Imaging [Internet]. Everything Rad. 2017 [cited 2021 Jun 22]. Available from: https://www.carestream.com/blog/2017/02/14/radiology-room-requirements/

Skam J, Gloria I, Ibrahim Z, Zira D. Radiographic Room Design and Layout for Radiation Protection in Some Radio-Diagnostic Facilities in Katsina State, Nigeria. 2017 Nov 1;31:16–23.

Tandon P. Regulatory requirements for designing PET-CT facility in India. Indian J Nucl Med IJNM Off J Soc Nucl Med India. 2010;25(2):39–43.

White MJ, Thornton JS, Hawkes DJ, Hill DLG, Kitchen N, Mancini L, et al. Design, Operation, and Safety of Single-Room Interventional MRI Suites: Practical Experience From Two Centers. J Magn Reson Imaging. 2015;41(1):34–43.

23 Clinical Laboratories

A 'Clinical Laboratory' is a place where clinical pathology tests are carried out on clinical specimens to obtain information about the health of a patient to aid in diagnosis, treatment and prevention of disease.

The efficiency of the hospital to a large extent depends on the promptness and accuracy of the reports of pathological investigations. The clinical laboratory is one of the main investigative services of the hospital and should lend wholehearted support to the clinical services. In the hospitals it is also termed as the 'LAB'.

The laboratory provides the facilities to apply scientific techniques to the diagnosis and control of disease and for scientific investigations of clinical phenomena associated with a disease. Hence, this department should be well designed and supervised to assure it is being used to the greatest advantage. Pathology laboratory examinations are invaluable in supporting and supplementing clinical findings, but a diagnosis by the laboratory which deals with only selected functions of the human body must never be allowed to replace the clinical diagnosis based on a study of the individual as a whole.

The Clinical Laboratory of a hospital should have the following sections:

Clinical Pathology	Anatomical Pathology
	Clinical Pathology
	Cytopathology
	Derma Pathology
	Forensic Pathology
	Hematopathology
	Histopathology
	Molecular Pathology
	Neuropathology
	Oral and Maxillofacial Pathology
	Pulmonary Pathology
	Renal Pathology
	Surgical Pathology
	Toxicology
Biochemistry	Cell Biology
	Clinical Biochemistry
	Enzymology
	Genetics
	Immunology
	Metabolism
	Molecular Biochemistry

A. Garg, A. Dewan, *Manual of Hospital Planning and Designing*,
https://doi.org/10.1007/978-981-16-8456-2_23

Microbiology	Bacteriology
	Cellular Microbiology
	Generation Microbiology
	Immunology
	Microbial Cytology
	Microbial Ecology
	Microbial Genetics
	Microbial Physiology
	Microbial Systematics
	Microbial Taxonomy
	Molecular Microbiology
	Mycology
	Nano Microbiology
	Nematology
	Parasitology
	Phycology
	Phylogeny
	Protozoology
	Systems Microbiology
	Virology

23.1 Infrastructure of Clinical Lab

The following shall be the components of the lab.

Laboratories	Biochemistry
	Pathology
	Microbiology
Support Services	Autoclave
	Bulk storage room
	Biohazard/Trash/Recycle room
	Penta head/Deca Head Microscope room
	Record/File/Copy room
	RO water closet
	Gas storage closet
	Flammable storage
	Specimen storage/Recycle
	Block and slide storage
Utility Area	Doctors Room
	Laboratory Manager
	Technicians Room
Outpatient Phlebotomy	Phlebotomy room
	Fine-needle procedure room
	Toilet room
	Waiting
Employee Support	Staff lounge
	Lockers
	Male shower with water closet
	Female shower with water closet
	Unisex toilet

Planning and Designing of Laboratory
While designing the clinical lab there are many issues to be taken care of. Some of them are:

23.2 Size of the Lab

The size of the lab differs from hospital to hospital. The main factors while deciding the size of the lab are:

1. How much will be the patient load in the hospital, both OPD and IPD?
2. How many specimens are expected to be collected?
3. Once collected, how many tests will be performed on each?
4. What all investigations the hospitals want to start. In all the hospitals, all types of investigations are not carried out due to the low number of samples and a greater cost of infrastructures like spaces, equipment and reagents. These hospitals prefer to have an arrangement with outside labs for such investigations.
5. Nature and prime function of the hospital.
6. The presence or absence of specialized clinics.
7. The available financial support for investment in equipment and reagents etc.

23.3 Layout

Some common issues while planning the lab layout are:

1. All the sections of the lab shall be in different rooms and it is not advised to club the labs at a commonplace, e.g. the Biochemistry shall be in a different room, Pathology in a separate room and Microbiology in a separate room.
2. If the space is too less for a clinical lab, or the size of the lab is small, at the most Biochemistry and Pathology can be clubbed together, but the Microbiology has to be kept separate.

3. Collection counters shall be provided at different places, both in the wards and in the outpatient area.
4. Better to have a separate section for the emergency investigation to prevent delays in reporting.

23.4 Spaces

Laboratory requires space for:

1. Actually, carrying out tests
2. Collection of specimens
3. Dispatch of reports
4. Storeroom for equipment, glassware, chemical reagents etc.
5. Office space for reporting and administrative work

23.5 Location and Arrangement of Areas

As far as the location of the clinical labs is concerned, they can be located at any convenient place in the hospital, because the labs are generally not visited by the patients. The services to the patients like specimen collection and report delivery are carried out in the patient area like OPD.

23.6 Open Lab Designs

Till now the labs were designed in compartments. All the divisions of the laboratory were housed in separate walled rooms with the manual bench working system and the equipment relating to that particular division was installed in the room. As technology has advanced, more of the lab equipment is automated and moving away from the manual bench working system. The automated systems are compact systems without much manual interference; hence the concept of OPEN LAB designs is preferred.

With the open-plan or big room concept, a lab is built with no interior walls to allow the layout to be reconfigured as necessary. The equipment is installed in a row or other such fashion, as required. This system definitely gives the flexibility to add more equipment and modalities as may be required. In this type of open labs, the power, data and gas points are mounted overhead, rather than provided through the floor or walls. Modular furniture like cabinets with wheels is preferred. Sinks and floor drains, which cannot be moved without major construction, are placed in areas that are unlikely to change, like near to the walls.

23.7 Biosafety

Today, with increased concern about infectious disease following outbreaks of COVID-19, severe acute respiratory syndrome, swine flu, bird flu, Ebola and Middle East Respiratory Syndrome, as well as increased concern about bioterrorism, the hospitals are concerned about the safety of the workers. Therefore, the concept of BSL-3 labs shall be adopted, particularly for sections like Microbiology.

BSL-3 has to be designed carefully taking into consideration factors like multiplication of the pathogens. Proper partitions need to be given for handling the specimens safely. Hardened epoxy-coated or protected walls shall be given, plumbing and vacuum lines must be fitted with multiple vacuum breakers, all penetrations into the room must be sealed and working tops shall be of non-porous material like Stainless Steel. All these precautions shall decrease the chances of pathogen multiplication and infecting others.

23.8 Molecular Testing

Another recent medical advancement that is influencing the design of clinical labs is molecular testing. Molecular diagnostics has replaced traditional microbiology and is one of the fastest-growing areas of the clinical lab. With molecular testing, lab technicians can, for example directly test the blood of a patient with a suspected systemic blood infection. It is not necessary to incubate a specimen for a lengthy period. Directly testing a blood sample for DNA markers from specific organisms can produce results in an afternoon, rather than overnight or over several days. Based on specific genetic markers in the sample, technicians can determine what type of bacteria, virus or parasite is present and whether or not it's carrying, say, the genes for amoxicillin resistance.

23.9 Laboratories

All the laboratories, i.e. Biochemistry, Microbiology and Pathology (including the sub-divisions of these labs) have common norms for designing and construction except a few specifications which may differ from lab to lab. Once the size of the lab is finalized, the actual design shall be worked out (Fig. 23.1).

Some of the important issues relating to the design of the Clinical Laboratories are as follows:

1. *Before designing the Laboratory rooms, the guidelines and norms of the controlling authority of the country must be taken into account. Like NABL (a laboratory accreditation agency) prescribes the standards of clinical laboratories in India.*
2. We have seen the advantages of Open type laboratory design. There shall be no doubt that the open design is the best. But it is advised that for some particular divisions which deal with infectious or hazardous investigations, a close type of laboratory shall be designed. It means that the laboratory shall be designed considering both the options, i.e. open type laboratory and closed type laboratory.
3. If separate rooms are required for some particular division of the laboratories, it shall be planned accordingly. Before designing, the space required for equipment and movement of staff shall be considered.
4. At times even if the equipment is installed in an open hall, the manufacturers of that equipment prefer a separate enclosure for automated and sophisticated machines to maintain a better dust-free environment. Under such circumstances, partitions of glass or aluminium can be designed.
5. All the walls of the laboratory room shall be at least 9-in.-thick with plaster on both sides.
6. *Flooring*

   The floor must be non-porous and stain proof. It is recommended that floor tiles of large size, like 600 mm × 600 mm, shall be used. The only condition is that there shall be no spaces between the tiles, which means the tiles shall be joint less. Otherwise, optionally granite can be used as it is a hard stone. Marble is not recommended as it is porous and soft and gets stained easily. Some designers also prefer to use hot welded vinyl flooring or epoxy-coated concrete slab etc. The disadvantage with these floorings is that if the chemicals and contaminated water seep under the vinyl floorings, slowly complete flooring will be damaged and will come out.
7. *Doors*

   Preferably each laboratory shall have a single door with a width of about 1829 mm to ease control, like the movement of men and material, carrying the equipment in and out of the laboratory. The laboratory doors shall be automatically self-closing.
8. Windows shall be provided in the laboratory as per the design and elevation of the building.
9. The lightning in the room shall be normal LED lights with sufficient lumens. No extra illumination is required in the room.
10. The temperature in the room shall be between 18 and 22 °C and the humidity level shall not be more than 40%. Before finalizing the RH level or the temperature, the environment requirement shall also be confirmed from the equipment supplier as some machines may require varied standards of the environment.
11. All the machines shall have proper ground earthing provisions.

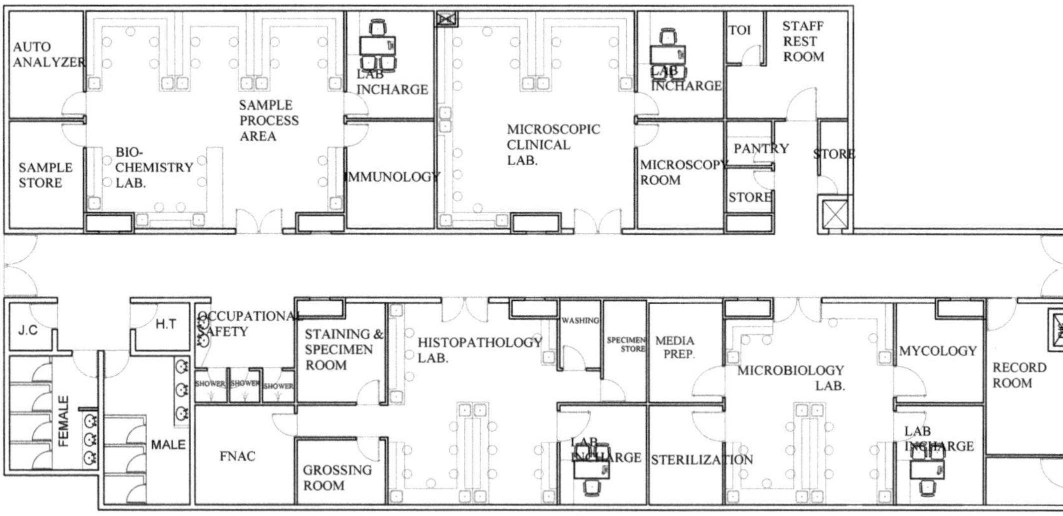

Fig. 23.1 Sample layout drawing of clinical laboratories

23.9.1 Working Slabs

For an efficient working in the laboratory, the role of working slabs shall not be underestimated. These working slabs are used for placing small tabletop machines, preparing the reagents and chemicals, preparing the slides or blocks etc. It means the working slabs are of multiple uses. If the open type of laboratory is designed, the working slabs shall be provided on the walls of the laboratory.

The top level of the working slab is normally 36–38 in. from the ground level. The width of the slab shall be about 762 mm, which can be reduced or increased depending on the requirement. On the top surface of the slab, granite stone can be fixed with round or half-round edges. Similarly, the vertical stone shall also be fixed on the wall starting from the top of the slab. The height of this vertical stone shall be between 305 mm and 610 mm. This vertical stone prevents the wall from getting damaged and stained.

Below the working slab, on the floor, a platform shall be provided. The thickness of the platform shall be about 183 mm. On the upper surface and throughout the thickness of the platform, stone or tiles shall be fixed.

Now between the upper surface of the platform and the lower surface of the slab, there will be vacant space. This space shall be used for providing cabinets. These cabinets are the most used spaces than any other spaces. This space can be used for storing reagents, chemicals, consumables, stationery etc. Even some shelves and drawers can be provided for more storage space and the safety of the material.

23.9.2 Sinks

Each laboratory must contain a sink for washing. Exposure to hazardous materials and/or pathogenic organisms can occur by hand-to-mouth transmission. It is extremely important that hands are washed before leaving the laboratory. Therefore, the sink should be located close to the egress.

The sinks shall be provided at appropriate places in the working slab itself. The sink shall be a deep laboratory sink and shall be about 610 mm long × 457 mm wide. The sink shall be of china clay as metal sinks are not recommended for laboratories. The sink shall be recessed in the working slab. The tap shall be about 305 mm in height from sink level and the drain shall be on the floor platform. Laboratory sinks shall have collars that protect sink drains from spills. Sink collars or brims should be ≥6 mm and designed to completely separate the lab bench from the sink drain.

23.9.3 Equipment Park/Store

Generally, in laboratories, there can be equipment that is not always in use but has to be ready all the time to be used whenever required. Hence, storage of these equipment shall be done at a separate place in the laboratories so that the floor space of the laboratory is not unnecessarily occupied with this equipment. Therefore, the equipment storage room/area is provided in the laboratories.

Normally, a room of size not less than 4267 mm × 4267 mm shall be provided attached to each laboratory. This area can be a closed room with a door or otherwise open area attached to a laboratory. The room shall have a provision of grounded and electrical charging points for charging the unused medical equipment.

23.9.4 Emergency Eyewash Station

Staff working in the laboratory are exposed to many hazardous fluids and chemicals. Despite universal precautions, splashes of chemicals/bodily fluids can occur. Therefore, an eyewash station shall be provided at a suitable place in each laboratory.

23.9.5 Clean Utility

The clean utility is a room attached to laboratories, which is used for storage of the clean material. Sterilized materials like drums and drapes are also stored in this room.

Normally, the room shall not be less than 3658 mm × 3658 mm but depending on the requirements; the size of the room can be changed. The room is provided with closed cabinets, drawers and racks. This room shall have only one door of about 914 mm.

23.9.6 Biohazard/Trash/Recycle Room

The Biohazard/Trash/Recycle room is attached to laboratories which are used for storage of the soiled material. Normally, the room shall not be less than 3658 mm × 3658 mm. But depending on the requirements, the size of the room can be changed. This room shall have two doors of about 914 mm. One door opens in the laboratory and the other in the corridor from where the staff can collect the material and he/she need not come to the laboratory for collection of material.

23.10 Pneumatic Tube Systems (PTS)

One station of the PTS shall be provided in each laboratory for receiving the specimens and requisition forms from different locations of the hospital. Similarly, it shall be used for sending the reports to the respective place.

23.11 Clear Floor Space

Clear floor space is the space that is not occupied by the fixed room furnishings and equipment. As a lot of medical equipment is being operated at a particular moment of time and a lot of technicians may be working at a particular moment of time, it is advisable to keep the maximum floor clear in the laboratories.

23.12 Electrical Points in Laboratories

As most of the equipment in the laboratories are electric driven and as the equipment is spread in the whole laboratory, careful designing has to be done for electrical points. The main issues to be considered while designing the electric points are as follows:

1. Main Switchboard shall be at the entrance wall for controlling fans and lights of the hall along with one or more 6 Amp Switch/Socket.
2. Air Conditioning Control button with temperature adjustments.
3. At least a pair of two 6/16/Amp switches/sockets shall be provided on the wall above the working slab. Such points shall be provided in series at a distance of 3048 mm from each other. Half of these should be on UPS supply.
4. 5 Amp switches/sockets shall be provided at a suitable place for refrigerators and deep freezers.
5. As the equipment will be scattered throughout the laboratory hall, they have to be provided with a power supply. First of all, the specification of the power requirement shall be taken from the manufacturer of the machine along with the dimensions of the machine. Then the location for placement of the machine has to be finalized. The required supply of the power shall be given through the floor. For this, the floor is chased and conduit is fixed in the chase. The wiring is done and the supply shall be given. These power points shall be on UPS supply. This electrical supply can also be given from the ceiling with a suspended conduit.
6. The power supply may also be required on the Office table for Microscopes. This can also be given through the floor supply.

23.13 Other Communication Points in Laboratories

Nowadays most of the laboratory equipment comes with the communication ports for interfacing with the Hospital Management Software so that the reports can be generated and the identification can be done by the machine through barcoding. Some of these machines may or may not have wireless connectivity. If there is no provision of wireless connectivity in the machine, a networking cable shall be provided to the machine. This can be provided through the floor as was done with the electrical point. The network cable can also be provided from the ceiling through the suspended conduit.

The following communication points shall be provided:

1. RJ 45 point for Computer networking
2. RJ 11 for Intercom and extension line

23.14 Air Conditioning System of Laboratories

Laboratories should be fully air-conditioned which allows control of temperature, humidity and air exchanges. Suitable and safe air quality must be maintained at all times. Following issues are important while designing the Air Conditioning System:

1. For Air Conditioning of laboratories, either Chilled Water Pipe Line with AHU's can be opted or the Ductable Split or VRV system can be opted. All the systems have their own advantages and disadvantages.
2. The return air of the laboratories shall be kept separate for all the laboratories. Under no circumstances the return air of any laboratory shall be mixed with another laboratory.
3. Air Flow, direction and air exchanges have to be as per the norms of the industry.
4. The temperature of the laboratories shall be between 18 and 22 °C, until and unless some machine requires varied temperature.

For full details on Air-conditioning, heating and air exchanges, please refer to the chapter 'HVAC' (Chap. 38) in this book.

23.15 Furniture in the Laboratories

Not much furniture is used in the laboratories. Only a few office tables, chairs, the laboratory stool etc. are provided in the laboratories. All work surfaces (e.g. benchtops and counters) must be impervious to the chemicals used.

23.16 Main Equipment in the Clinical Laboratories

Pathology	
Automated Platelet Counting	Laminar Air Flow Horizontal
Binocular Research Microscope	Lamps, Slide Warming
Cell Counter, Normal and Abnormal	Mass Spectrometer
Cell-Freezing Apparatus and Reagents	Micrometres, Microscope
Chromatography	Microscope Fluorescence/UV
Chromatography (GAS), Clinical Use	Microscope Inverted Stage, Tissue Culture
Chromatography For Bacterial Identification	Microscope Phase Contrast
Chromatography, Ion Exchange	Microtome
Chromatography, Thin Layer, Methadone	Multipurpose System In Vitro Coagulation Studies
Clinitek Status Analyzer	Platelet Aggregation Automated System
Coagulation, Automated	Platelet Aggregometer
Column Supports, Gas-Liquid Chromatography	Processor, Tissue Automated
Columns, Liquid Chromatography	Radioimmunoassay
Counter, Automated Cell	Rotary Microtome
Cytocentrifuge	Slide Stainer, Immersion Type
Cytospin	Spectrophotometer Digital
Enzyme Immunoassay	Stereoscopic Microscopes
Fibrometer	Suspension System, Cell Culture
Glass Ware	Trinocular Microscope with Phase Contrast attachment
Haematology Analyzer	Turbidity Meter
Haemoglobinometer	Vacuum Oven
Microbiology	
Automated Clinical Immunodiagnostic Systems	Laminar Air Flow
Bact Alert System	LIPA (Line Probe Assays)
Bio-Safety Cabinet	MGIT 960
BOD Incubator	Microscope Fluorescence/UV
BSL 3	QBC Microscope (Malaria)
CD4 Counter	Refrigerated Centrifuge
Cell Cultures for Isolation of Viruses	RT-PCR
Deep Freezer	T.B. Culture Bact/Alert 3D
Elisa Reader with Washer	Thermocycler
Gene Expert	Ultracentrifuge
High-Performance Liquid Chromatography (HPLC)	Vitek
Immunofluorescent Microscope	Vitek 2 Compact 60
Biochemistry	
Automated Clinical Chemistry Systems	Gamma Counter
Automated Urinalysis System	Gas, Oxygen Analyzer
Bichromatic Photometric Analyzer	Glass Ware
Carbon-Dioxide Analyzer	Microscope Fluorescence/UV
Card Reader Nyco II	Monochromator
Chemistry (Photometric, Discrete) Analyzer	Nephelometer
Chemistry (Sequential Multiple, Continuous Flow) Analyzer	Osmometers
Chemistry, Micro Analyzer	Pipetting Station
Colorimeter, Photometer, Spectrophotometer	Plasma Viscometer
Densitometric, Protein Fractionation	Radioimmunoassay
Freezer	Refractometer
Fully Auto. Analyzer (Immunoassay)	Semi-auto Analyzer

23.17 Support Services

These are the areas that support the laboratories at the back end to perform efficient working in the lab. Some of the areas are:

23.17.1 Autoclave

An autoclave room shall be provided with the microbiology lab to prepare the media and sterilize the glassware to be used in the laboratories. This room is located very near to the laboratory. The size of the room shall be about 3658 mm × 3658 mm. The room shall have a quick steam sterilizer and a hot air oven. The room shall have a proper supply of soft water to be used in the sterilizer and a required drain. The room shall have an adequate arrangement for exhaust and air exchanges. The room shall also be provided with the required electrical points to connect the machines.

23.17.2 Bulk Storage Room

This store is required for storing the reagents, chemicals, kits, glassware, consumables and disposables that are used in the laboratories. Depending on the quantum of material, a single room shall be provided but if the material to be stored is more, each laboratory can have a separate store. The room shall be at least 4572 mm × 4572 mm in size. The size of the room can also be increased or decreased as per the requirement. Adequate lockable cupboards, racks and drawers shall be provided in the store. The store shall also have a countertop to prepare the reagents if required. The storekeeper of the laboratories shall be in charge of this store.

23.17.3 Cold Storage Room

At times, some reagents or kits to be used in laboratories are temperature sensitive and cannot be stored at room temperature. Therefore, a cold room may be required. This cold room can be common for all the laboratories. It is also called the refrigerated room. The size of the room shall be about 3048 mm × 3048 mm. The walls and the ceiling of the room shall be made out of puff panel that acts as a thermal barrier. Inside the room, airconditioning is done and the temperature shall be between 5 and 12 °C and shall be adjustable as per requirement. The flooring is generally made out of wooden planks. The door of the room shall be lockable and shall not be less than 1200 mm and the door shall be made out of puff panel and shall be a hermetically sealed door. For storage, open racks made out of stainless steel shall be provided along the walls of the room.

23.17.4 RO Water Closet

Some of the machines like Auto biochemistry analyzer require the supply of RO water for its operation. Similarly, other machines may also require it. Therefore, a separate closet is provided in the laboratories area, where a RO plant is installed and from there through pipelines the water can be supplied to the machinery. Sizewise the room shall be about 3658 mm × 3658 mm with proper electrical points and a provision for the supply of water to the plant. Also, a treated water tank shall be provided (with a pump, if required) in the room for storage of the RO water.

23.17.5 Gas Storage Closet

Usually, cooking gas is required in the laboratories for burners. The best way is to supply the gas through pipelines instead of keeping gas cylinders at each point. Therefore, a small gas manifold room is provided at a convenient place in the laboratories to install the manifold. This area shall be open to the sky and shall not be a closed room. The manifold shall have a provision of fixing 2–5 cylinders at a time. From the manifold, a copper pipeline is laid down to the burner and at the end, a ball valve is provided. From here the burner is connected with a rubber pipe.

23.17.6 Record/File/Copy Room

This store is to be used for storing the records, files, requisition sheets, stationery etc. This store can be common for all the laboratories. But if more such space is required, a separate store may be provided to all the laboratories separately. The size of the room shall be 3658 mm × 3658 mm. There shall be no window in the room, no water outlet and no moisture. The room shall have an electric point for light and fan.

23.17.7 Flammable Storage

This store is used for storing flammable and hazardous materials like acids, spirit and alcohol. The room shall be located away from the general movement area. The room shall be of size 3658 mm × 3658 mm and the wall shall have glazed acid-proof tiles. Only one electric point for light shall be given in the room. The racks shall be of metal and not wood.

23.17.8 Specimen Storage/Recycle

This room is used for the storage of specimens that have been collected from the patients. Normally, the specimens are stored for a few days, because at times a repeat test may have to be performed. The specimens can be of blood, urine, stool, body fluids, semen etc. Each specimen may require a different environment and methods for storage. Therefore, adequate arrangements shall be made for refrigeration and humidity. Similarly, proper bins, racks, cabinets or racks shall be provided. The working top and the sinks shall also be provided in the room. The size of the room depends on the number of samples that have to be stored. Generally, a room with a size of 4267 mm × 3658 mm shall be sufficient.

23.17.9 Block and Slide Storage

This room is used for the storage of blocks and slides prepared for processing and investigation. As in the case of specimens, these blocks and slides are also stored for a few days, because at times a repeat test may have to be performed. Adequate arrangements shall be made for environment temperature and humidity. The room shall be provided with proper block storage cabinets for storage of blocks. Similarly, for storage of slides, slide storage cabinets shall be provided in the room. The working top and sinks shall also be provided in the room. The size of the room depends on the number of samples that have to be stored. Generally, a room with a size of 4267 mm × 3658 mm shall be sufficient.

23.17.10 Penta Head/Deca Head Microscope Room

This room is necessarily required in the teaching institutes, or in the hospital where more than one person has to examine the same slide. The Penta Head Microscope has five different binocular outlets connected through a pipe fitted with prisms and mirrors in between. Each head is focused on the common platform where the object is placed. Similarly, the deca head microscope has ten such outlets. Separate rooms shall be provided for both the microscopes. The room shall be square in shape. In the centre of the room, a table is placed which shall be sufficient to accommodate the microscope. On all the five or ten, as the case may be, laboratory stools are placed in front of the outlet from where they can sit and use the microscope. Proper electric points shall be given on the table where the microscope is placed.

23.18 Utility Area

This is the administrative area for controlling and coordinating the working of the laboratories. Some of the spaces are:

23.18.1 Doctors Room

This room is for the pathologists, biochemists and the microbiologists along with other doctors to carry out the official work of the laboratories. The size of this room shall be about 4572 mm × 4267 mm. The room shall have an arrangement for office tables, executive chair, visitor chairs, side rack etc. The room shall have an attached toilet. The room shall also have an attached P.A. room for the clerk to be seated. The room shall have proper arrangements for electrical points, intercom connection, IT network and air conditioning.

23.18.2 Laboratory Manager

This room is for the manager of the laboratories and shall be located on the laboratory premises. The size of this room shall be about 4572 mm × 4267 mm. The room shall have an arrangement for office tables, executive chair, visitor chairs, side rack etc. The room shall have an attached toilet. The room shall also have an attached P.A. room for the clerk to be seated. If required and long working hours are expected a small restroom can also be provided with this room. The room shall have proper arrangements for electrical points, intercom connection, IT network and air conditioning.

23.18.3 Technicians Room

This room is for the technicians working in the laboratories to carry out the official work of the laboratories. The size of this room shall be about 4572 mm × 4267 mm. The room shall have an arrangement for office tables, office chair, visitor chairs, side rack etc. The room shall have proper arrangements for electrical points, intercom connection, IT network and air conditioning.

23.19 Outpatient Phlebotomy

Phlebotomy is the collection of specimens of the patient for investigation. A person drawing the specimens is called the Phlebotomist. Normally the specimens are collected in the hospital at a number of locations like OPD, IPD, ICU, OR and Emergency. As far as the specimens from indoors are concerned, in some hospitals the phlebotomist is deputed, who at a fixed time collects the specimens of indoor patients. But at some places, the nurses and/or technicians have to draw the specimens. Normally, a phlebotomy room is planned in the OPD complex of the hospital. The following rooms are provided for phlebotomy in the OPD:

23.19.1 OPD Phlebotomy Room

Normally, a single or more than one such phlebotomy rooms are provided at a convenient place in the OPD complex. The Phlebotomist is placed in the room along with helpers to draw specimens. Size-wise the room shall be about 4572 mm × 4267 mm.

Attached to the phlebotomy room a separate space/room, called as Sample Collection Room/Space, shall be provided where the patient is seated or laid down and the specimens are drawn. This space shall be about 2438 mm × 2438 mm. Sample collection room/space contains one phlebotomy chair and one examination couch. There has to be a working top with the sink for keeping the drawn specimens. The couch shall have a curtain partition for the privacy of the patient. Sufficient stock of needles, vacutainer tubes, holders etc. shall be kept in this specimen collection room, hence proper cupboards, shelves and racks shall be provided.

As far as the phlebotomy room is concerned, the room shall be a normal room with a working top having sinks. Sufficient electrical points shall be provided on the working top. The provision of a refrigerator shall be provided. One office table, chairs, computer with printer and barcode printer shall be provided to complete the work like barcode fixing and taking consent. The specimens drawn are initially processed in the room and stored there to be sent to the laboratories in batches. The outlet point of the PTS shall be provided in the phlebotomy room so that the specimens along with the requisition forms can be sent to the laboratories without any delay.

23.19.2 Fine Needle Aspiration Room

This room is provided for drawing the specimens through fine needle aspiration. It can also be called the biopsy sample room. Normally, one such room is provided at a convenient place in the OPD complex. Size-wise the room shall be about 4572 mm × 4267 mm. As the collection of the specimen is through a fine needle, it is a kind of intervention. Therefore, the room has to be under sterile conditions. Attached to this room shall be a changing room for the patient and the staff. A scrub station shall be provided outside the room. A shoe rack has to be provided outside the room. Inside the room shall be the examination table covered with hanging curtain partitions. As it is an intervention procedure, the provision of the crash cart along with emergency medicines shall be kept in the room. One small storeroom shall also be provided attached to the room to maintain sufficient stock of needles, vacutainer tubes and holders etc.

23.19.3 Toilets

Some specimens like urine, stool and semen need to be taken in the toilet. Therefore, a toilet is provided attached to the phlebotomy room. If possible, separate toilets shall be provided for male and female. Toilet shall have a shelf with raised edges so that the patient can keep the sample while he/she prepares himself/herself to come out of the toilet.

23.19.4 Waiting Area

A waiting area near to the phlebotomy room shall be provided for the patients to wait till their turn comes to give the specimens. The hospital can introduce the token system so that the patient comes to know about their turn. Alternately, the waiting area shall be provided with speakers connected to a mike placed in the phlebotomy room. The phlebotomist can announce the name of the patient whose turn is to give the specimens.

23.20 Employee Support

The area for the facility of the staff. This area includes:

23.20.1 Staff Lounge

This lounge is given in the laboratory area for the staff to sit and relax in their spare time. The lounge shall be provided with an attached toilet and with the provision of tea/coffee which can be served from the pantry.

23.20.2 Lockers

Lockers shall be provided in the staff area for facilitating the staff to keep their personal belongings safely under lock and key. Each staff member shall be allotted a separate locker.

23.20.3 Shower with Water Closet

As the staff working in the laboratories is more prone to infection due to spillage of chemicals and reagents, a facility for taking showers shall be provided in the laboratories. Therefore, the staff area shall have a Shower room with a water closet for the staff, separately for the male and female.

Further Reading

Aulbach A, Provencher A, Tripathi N. Influence of Study Design Variables on Clinical Pathology Data. Toxicol Pathol. 2017 Feb 1;45(2):288–95.

Blanckaert N. Clinical pathology services: remapping our strategic itinerary. Clin Chem Lab Med. 2010 Jul 1;48(7):919–25.

Clinical Laboratory Design Concepts : March 2018 – MedicalLab Management Magazine [Internet]. [cited 2021 Jun 28]. Available from: https://www.medlabmag.com/article/1454/

Designing clinical labs [Internet]. [cited 2021 Jun 28]. Available from: https://www.hfmmagazine.com/articles/1703-designing-clinical-labs

Emerging Practices in Clinical Laboratory Design [Internet]. Clinical Lab Manager. [cited 2021 Jun 28]. Available from: https://www.clinicallabmanager.com/features/emerging-practices-in-clinical-laboratory-design-341

Medical laboratory safety management [Internet]. Medical Laboratory Observer. 2018 [cited 2021 Jun 28]. Available from: https://www.mlo-online.com/management/lab-safety/article/13017071/medical-laboratory-safety-management

Planning Premises And Design Considerations For Hospital Laboratory, GJRA - Global Journal For Research Analysis(GJRA), GJRA | World Wide Journals [Internet]. [cited 2021 Jun 28]. Available from: https://www.worldwidejournals.com/global-journal-for-research-analysis-GJRA/article/planning-premises-and-design-considerations-for-hospital-laboratory/MTA5MjQ=/?is=1

Race GJ, Tillery GW, Dysert PA. A history of pathology and laboratory medicine at Baylor University Medical Center. Proc Bayl Univ Med Cent. 2004 Jan;17(1):42–55.

Singh M. PLANNING PREMISES AND DESIGN CONSIDERATIONS FOR HOSPITAL LABORATORY. Glob J Health Sci. 2019 May 14;8:1–6.

Tan SS, Yan B, Saw S, Lee CK, Chong AT, Jureen R, et al. Practical laboratory considerations amidst the COVID-19 outbreak: early experience from Singapore. J Clin Pathol. 2021 Apr 1;74(4):257–60.

Technological Revolution in Hospital Design and Care Delivery Will Bring Changes for Clinical Pathologists and Medical Laboratories [Internet]. Dark Daily. 2017 [cited 2021 Jun 28]. Available from: https://www.darkdaily.com/2017/07/12/technological-revolution-in-hospital-design-and-care-delivery-will-bring-changes-for-clinical-pathologists-and-medical-laboratories/

Yoong NW. Transforming the 24/7 Clinical Laboratories - Design Considerations, Workflow and Relocation to New Diagnostics Building. [cited 2021 Jun 28]; Available from: https://clinmedjournals.org/articles/ijpcr/international-journal-of-pathology-and-clinical-research-ijpcr-2-024.php?jid=ijpcr

24 Blood Bank

Blood Bank is a place where blood is collected from donors, tested, separated into components, stored and prepared for transfusion to recipients.

24.1 Location of the Blood Bank in Hospital

The Blood Bank shall be located at the most easily accessible place in the hospital particularly in case of emergency. It shall be near to the Emergency, Operating Theatre Complex and Intensive Care Units. Preferably the blood bank shall be on the ground floor. The blood bank shall be a unitary complex and rooms of blood bank cannot be scattered into different areas.

24.2 Controlling Authority

Mostly in all the countries, the Blood Banks are controlled by some or the other controlling authority under a specified act, e.g. in India, it is controlled by the Drug Act. The norms, rules and regulations are prescribed by the controlling authorities.

As the Blood Bank is a regulated department in the hospital, it is advised to consider the rules, regulations and norms of the controlling authority of the respective country before planning and designing the blood bank.

24.3 Functions of Blood Bank

Blood banks have four major functions:

1. Receiving
2. Storage
3. Testing
4. Distribution

24.3.1 Receiving

Area designated for the collection of the blood from the donor and providing facilities to the donor after bleeding.

A. Garg, A. Dewan, *Manual of Hospital Planning and Designing*,
https://doi.org/10.1007/978-981-16-8456-2_24

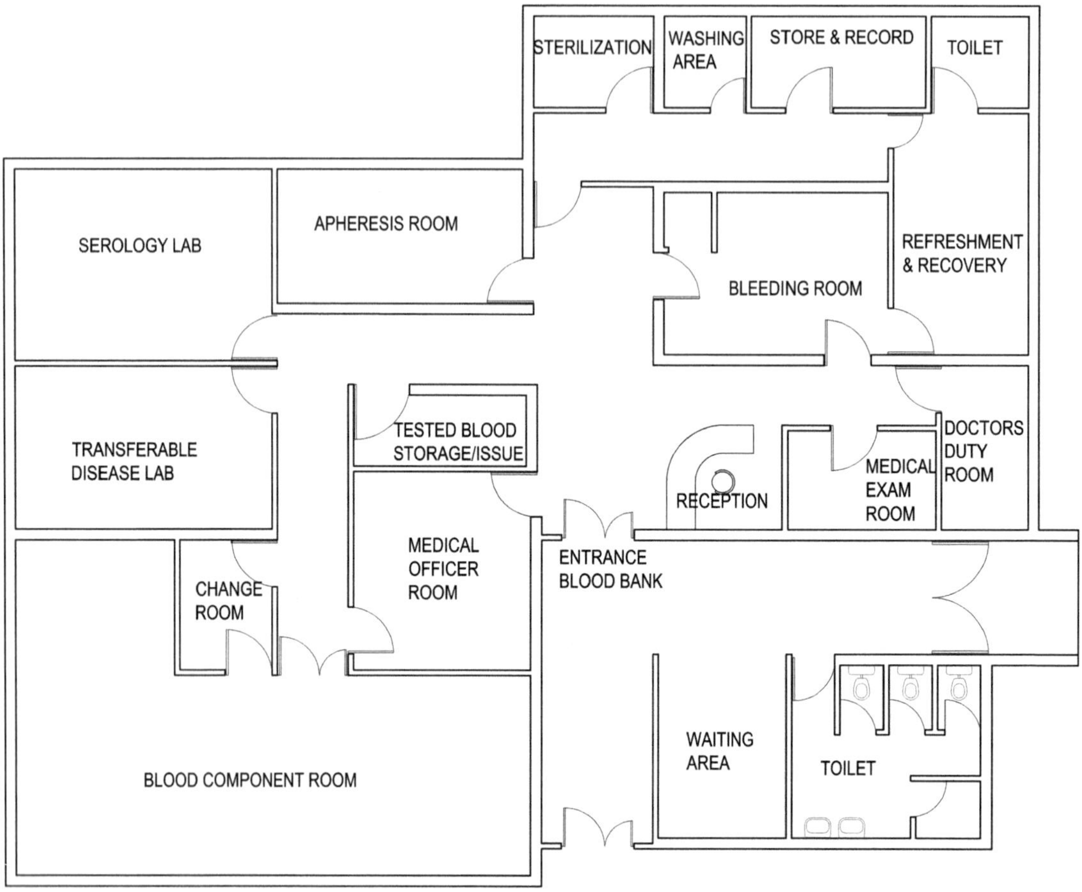

Fig. 24.1 Sample layout drawing of the blood bank

24.3.2 Storage

Storage is for storing the untested blood, tested blood and blood components.

24.3.3 Testing

Area designated for the screening of the donated blood for ruling out any infectious diseases in the blood.

24.3.4 Distribution

Area for distributing the blood for transfusion.

24.4 Infrastructure of the Blood Bank

Blood bank usually has the following infrastructure (Fig. 24.1):

Receiving	Entrance
	Reception
	Registration
	Waiting
	Medical Examination
	Bleeding
	Refreshment/Recovery/Rest Room
	Apheresis Room
Testing	Serology Lab
	Transferable Disease Lab

Storage and Processing	Blood Component Room
Distribution	Issue Counter
Utility Areas	Change Room
	Record
	Store
	Medical Officer Room
	Doctors Rest Room
	Sterilization room
	Washing Room
	Toilet

24.5 Area of Blood Bank

Generally, the area is specified in the norms issued by the controlling authority of the blood bank. So, while designing the blood bank, those area norms have to be adhered to, e.g. in India, the Drug Act prescribes the area as:

1. For Whole Blood—100 sq.m.
2. For Components—Additional 50 sq.m.
3. For Apheresis—Additional 15 sq.m.

Hence, the area shall not be less than 165 sq.m. After adding the movement area, the total area shall not be less than 200 sq.m.

24.6 Equipment in the Blood Bank

Normally, the following equipment is provided in the blood bank:

Apheresis Machine	Elisa Reader with Washer
Blood Bag Tube Sealer	HB Meter
Blood Bank Refrigerator	ID Centrifuge
Blood Collection Monitor	Mechanical Shaker
Blood Collection System, Vacuum-Assisted	Oven Universal
Blood Donor Couch (Mobile)	Plasma Extractor
Blood Mixing and Blood Weighing Device	Platelet Agitator
Cryo Bath Unit	Platelet Incubator
Deep Freezer −40 °C	Processing System for Frozen Blood
Deep Freezer −80 °C	Refrigerated Centrifuge
Dielectric Sealer	Thawing Bath
Double Pan Balance	Water Bath Serological

24.7 Receiving Area

This area pertains to the registration, examination and bleeding of the donor. This area shall also consist of spaces like a refreshment room and the Apheresis Room. The room wise details are:

24.7.1 Entrance

Entrance here means the main entrance to the blood bank. The entrance door of the blood bank shall be about 1219 mm wide so that the wheelchairs can easily enter the blood bank. Outside the entrance, a shoe rack is provided so that nobody enters the blood bank premises with outside shoes. Either there shall be a provision of shoe covers or otherwise, a separate set of slippers shall be provided. On the door of the blood bank, an air curtain can also be provided, but it is not necessary.

24.7.2 Reception

Reception shall be near the entrance of the blood bank. The reception shall be kept open. The Reception counter or the reception table can be provided with chairs for the receptionist. The reception counter shall have a provision for sufficient electric points, computer networking jacks, intercom points and an emergency telephone line. The reception shall have sufficient space for storage of stationery and other useful items. This storage can be provided in the cabinet or drawers on the counter. Otherwise, a side rack can be provided for storage. The area shall be 3658 mm × 3658 mm.

24.7.3 Registration

On the registration counter, the donor form is given and consent is taken from the donor. The registration counter can also be combined with the reception if required. An area of 2438 mm × 2438 mm shall be sufficient.

24.7.4 Waiting

Waiting area is for the waiting of donors till their turn comes or for the family members of the donor. It is also used for the family members who come to the blood bank for receiving the blood. The waiting area shall have a provision for seating of about 10–15 people. The area shall be about 4572 mm × 3048 mm.

24.7.5 Medical Examination

This room is used for examination of the donor pre-bleeding. The physician shall check the weight, height and examine the donor for any pre-existing diseases. Once the doctors feel that the donor is fit for donation, he/she is sent to the bleeding room. The size of this room shall be 3658 mm × 3658 mm. The medical examination room shall have a doctor table, chair, revolving stool and an examination couch. The provision shall be made for a view box on the wall near the doctor's chair. Electrical points shall be provided on the examination couch for fixing the examination lamp, above the doctors' table for view box, computer/printer etc. The communication points for intercom and networking shall also be provided. A height scale shall be fixed on the wall.

24.7.6 Bleeding Room

This room is used for bleeding the donor. Generally, a room of about 4572 mm × 4267 mm shall be sufficient. However, the room should be sufficient to accommodate two blood bank couches. If the donor load for bleeding is more and more bleeding couches are required to be placed, the size of the room can be increased. The room shall have two doors. One door from where the donor enters the bleeding room and the second door of the room shall open in the refreshment/recovery/restroom. Blood donor couches are placed adjoining the wall of the room. On the back side wall (on the back of the couch), an 488-mm wide working top shall be provided to place the blood collection monitor or the tube sealer. Emergency medicines can also be kept on that working top. On the front wall of the couch, a provision of Television shall be provided. Regarding the electrical points, two sets of 6/16 Amp switches/sockets shall be given below the working top to fulfil the requirement of supply to the couch. Each set shall have a pair of switch/sockets. On the wall above the working top, sufficient 6/16 Amp switch/sockets shall be provided at a distance of 1219 mm from each other to connect the medical equipment. An electrical point shall also be given for television. The room shall have a provision for emergency lights.

24.7.7 Refreshment/Recovery/ Rest Room

After the donation is over, the donor is asked to sit in this room for 15–30 min. This period is used for completing the records and also watching the donor for any untoward effect like oozing from the puncture site, dizziness or any other complaints. This room shall also have a provision for refreshment. The desirable area of the room shall be about 4572 mm × 3658 mm. Furniture wise, the room shall have a sofa set for the donor to relax, a couch for the donor to lay down and rest. There shall be a provision of refrigerator and tea/coffee vending machine for the refreshment of the donor. A television shall also be provided in the room in front of the sofa set. Electrical points shall be provided for the television, refrigerator and coffee vending machine.

24.7.8 Apheresis Room

This room is used to separate a particular component from the blood of the donor through apheresis. This is done with the help of the apheresis machine. The size of the room shall be about 4572 mm × 3658 mm. Furniture wise the apheresis chair is placed in the room adjoining the wall in the centre of the room. A television shall be provided in front of the couch. The Apheresis machine is placed on the right-hand side of the chair. A normal office chair shall also be provided for the technician to be seated there while the procedure is going on. Electrical points shall be given at the level of 457 mm from the floor level. Two such pairs of points shall be provided for the apheresis chair and the apheresis machine. These points shall have the supply through UPS. An electrical point shall be provided for television.

24.8 Testing Area

This area pertains to the screening of the donated blood. The laboratory is divided into two parts. One section is for blood group serology called the Serology Lab and another for screening the blood for HIV antibodies, hepatitis B antigen etc. called the TT Lab. The details of the structure of the Lab shall be as follows:

1. Two rooms, one for each lab shall be provided in the blood bank.
2. All the walls of the laboratory room shall be at least 229 mm thick with a plaster on both sides. As the blood bank is a clean area, therefore the laboratories shall also be designed as clean rooms. It is advised to make the wall with a puff panel with no corners and edges. The corners shall be rounded off with the help of the puff panel or the GI sheet. The walls and ceiling shall be finished with anti-bacterial and anti-fungal washable paints.
3. *Flooring*

   The floor must be non-pervious and stain proof. It is recommended that floor tiles of large sizes, like 600 mm × 600 mm, shall be used. The only condition is that there shall be no spaces between the tiles, which means the tiles shall be joint less. Otherwise, optionally granite can be used as it is a hard stone. Marble is not recommended as it is porous and a soft stone and easily gets stained. Some designers also prefer to use hot-welded vinyl flooring or epoxy coated concrete slab etc. The disadvantage with these floorings is that if the water or chemical seeps under the vinyl floorings, slowly and gradually complete flooring will be damaged and will come out.
4. *Doors*

   Preferably each laboratory shall have a single door with a width of about 1219 mm to ease the control, like the movement of men and material, carrying the equipment in and out of the laboratory. The laboratory doors shall be automatic and self-closing.
5. The lightning in the room shall be normal LED light with sufficient lumens. No extra illumination is required in the room.
6. The temperature in the room shall be between 18 and 22 °C and the humidity level shall not be more than 40%.
7. All the machines shall have proper ground earthing provisions.

24.8.1 Working Slabs

For efficient working in the laboratory, working slabs shall be provided to place small tabletop machines, preparing the reagents and chemicals, preparing slides or blocks etc. These working slabs shall be provided on the walls of the laboratory.

The top level of the working slab is normally 915 mm inches from the ground level. The width of the slab shall be about 762 mm, which can be increased or decreased depending on the requirement. On the top surface of the slab, granite stone can be fixed with round or half-round edges of granite stone. Similarly, the vertical stone shall also be fixed on the wall starting from the slab. The height of this vertical stone shall be between 305 mm and 610 mm. This vertical stone prevents the wall from getting damaged.

Below the working slab, on the floor, a platform shall be provided. The thickness of the platform shall be 152 mm. On the upper surface and throughout the thickness of the platform, stone or tiles shall be fixed.

Now, between the upper surface of the platform and the lower surface of the slab, there will be vacant space. This space shall be used for providing cabinets. These cabinets are the most used spaces than any other space. This space can be used for storing reagents, chemicals, consumables or stationery etc. Even shelves and doors shall be provided for more storage space and safety of the material.

24.8.2 Sinks

Each laboratory must contain a sink for washing. The sinks shall be provided at appropriate places in the working slab itself. The sink shall be a deep laboratory sink and shall be about 610 mm long × 457 mm wide. The sink shall be of China clay as metal sinks are not recommended for laboratories. The sink shall be recessed in the working slab. The tap shall be about 305 mm in height from sink level and the drain shall be on the floor platform.

24.8.3 Electrical Points in Laboratories

The main issues to be considered while designing the electric points are as follows:

1. Main Switchboard shall be at the entrance wall for controlling fans and lights of the hall along with one or more 6 Amp Switches/ Sockets.
2. Air Conditioning Control button with temperature adjustment.
3. At least a pair of two 6/16/Amp switches/ sockets shall be provided on the wall above the working slab. Such points shall be provided in series at a distance of 1524 mm from each other. Out of them, at least half shall be on UPS supply.
4. The power supply may also be required on the Office table for Microscopes. This can also be given through the floor supply.

24.8.4 Other Communication Points in Laboratories

The following communication points shall be provided:

1. RJ 45 point for Computer networking
2. RJ 11 for Intercom and extension line

24.8.5 Air Conditioning System of Laboratories

Laboratories should be fully air-conditioned which allows control of temperature, humidity and air exchanges. Suitable and safe air quality must be maintained at all times. Following issues are important while designing the Air Conditioning System:

1. For Air Conditioning of laboratories, either the Chilled Water Pipe Line with AHUs can be opted or otherwise the Ductable Split or VRV system can be opted. All the systems have their own advantages and disadvantages.
2. The return air of the laboratories shall be kept separate for each laboratory. Under no circumstances the return air of any laboratory shall be mixed with the other laboratory.
3. Air Flow, direction and air exchanges have to be as per the norms of the industry.
4. The temperature of the laboratories shall be between 18 and 22 °C, some machines require varied temperatures.

For full details on Air-conditioning, heating and air exchanges, please refer to the chapter 'HVAC' (Chap. 38) in this book.

24.8.6 Furniture in the Laboratories

Not much furniture is used in the laboratories. Only one office table, chair and the laboratory stool etc. are provided in the laboratories.

Use of wood in the blood bank is restricted. Therefore, all the items like tables, cabinets, racks and notice boards shall be made out of stainless steel.

No fittings like lights, fans, boards and stitches are allowed on the surface of the walls or the ceiling. Everything has to be recessed in the walls or the ceiling.

24.9 Storage and Processing Area

This area pertains to the storage of the blood pre- and post-screening. There are different storages of the blood. The blood is usually stored in the blood bank refrigerators, until and unless the quantity of the blood is huge and can be stored only in refrigerated rooms. This area is also for processing the blood to separate the components out of the blood.

1. The storage of untested blood (which has still to be screened) is generally kept either in the bleeding room or otherwise in a separate enclosure provided for this purpose. A blood bank refrigerator shall be provided in the bleeding room or the enclosure as the case may be. Wherever it may be, an electrical point shall be provided for connecting the blood bank refrigerator.
2. The storage of tested blood, ready for distribution, is done away from untested blood. This area is provided either in the delivery room or in a separate enclosure near to the delivery counter. A blood bank refrigerator shall be provided in the delivery room or the enclosure as the case may be. Wherever it may be, an electrical point shall be provided for connecting the blood bank refrigerator.
3. The numbers and capacity of blood bank refrigerators shall depend on the quantum of blood bags to be stored.

24.9.1 Blood Component Room

The component room is provided for the separation of the components from whole blood and for storage of the separated components. The size of the component room shall be about 7620 mm × 7620 mm.

1. All the walls of the component room shall be at least 229 mm thick with a plaster on both sides. As the component room is a clean area, it is advised to make the wall with a puff panel with no corners and edges. The corners shall be rounded off with the help of the puff panel or GI sheet. The walls and ceiling shall be finished with anti-bacterial and anti-fungal washable paints.
2. *Flooring*

   The floor must be non-pervious and stain proof. It is recommended that floor tiles of large size, like 600 mm × 600 mm shall be used. The only condition is that there shall be no spaces between the tiles it means the tiles shall be joint less. Otherwise, optionally granite can be used as it is a hard stone. Marble is not recommended as it is a porous and soft stone and easily gets stained. Some designers also prefer to use hot-welded vinyl flooring or epoxy coated concrete slab etc. The disadvantage with these floorings is that if the water or chemical seeps under the vinyl floorings, slowly and gradually complete flooring will be damaged and will come out.
3. *Doors*

   Preferably a component room shall have a single door with a width of about 1219 mm to ease the control, like the movement of men and material, carrying the equipment in and out of the component room. The door shall be automatic and self-closing.
4. The lightning in the room shall be normal LED light with sufficient lumens. No extra illumination is required in the room.
5. The temperature in the room shall be between 18 and 22 °C and the humidity level shall not be more than 40%.
6. All the machines shall have proper ground earthing provisions.

24.9.1.1 Furniture in the Component Room

Not much furniture needs to be provided in the component room. Only one office table, chair and the laboratory stool etc. are provided in the component room. Instead of the working tops, stainless steel tables are provided in the component room to keep the equipment or for other working. Lab sinks shall also be provided in these SS tables and there will be no need to provide extra sinks in the component room.

24.9.1.2 Electrical Points in the Component Room

The main issues to be considered while designing the electric points are as follows:

1. Main Switchboard shall be at the entrance wall for controlling fans and lights of the hall along with one or more 6 Amp Switches/ Sockets.
2. Air Conditioning Control button with temperature adjustment.
3. At least a pair of two 6/16/Amp switches/ sockets shall be provided on all the walls across the component room. These points shall be at the height of 18 in. from the floor level. Such points shall be in pairs and each pair shall be at a distance of 1524 mm from each other. Out of them, at least half shall be on UPS supply.

24.9.1.3 Other Communication Points in Laboratories

The following communication points shall be provided:

1. RJ 45 point for Computer networking
2. RJ 11 for Intercom and extension line

24.9.1.4 Air Conditioning System of Component Room

Component room should be fully air-conditioned which allows control of temperature, humidity and air exchanges. Suitable and safe air quality must be maintained at all times. The following issues are important while designing the Air Conditioning System:

1. For Air Conditioning, either the Chilled Water Pipe Line with AHUs can be opted, or otherwise, the Ductable Split or VRV system can be opted. All the systems have their own advantages and disadvantages.
2. The return air of the component room shall be kept separate from any other area.
3. Air Flow, Direction and air exchanges have to be as per the norms of the industry.
4. The temperature of the laboratories shall be between 18 and 22 °C, unless and until some machine requires varied temperature.

For full details on Air-conditioning, heating and air exchanges, please refer to the chapter 'HVAC' (Chap. 38) in this book.

Use of wood in the blood bank is restricted. Therefore, all the items like tables, cabinets, racks and notice boards shall be made out of stainless steel.

No fitting like lights, fans, boards and stitches are allowed on the surface of the walls or the ceiling. Everything has to be recessed in the walls or the ceiling.

24.10 Distribution Area

This area is to distribute the screened blood to be transfused to the patient. Usually, it is a room with a service window opening outside. The size of the room shall be about 3048 mm × 3048 mm and the window opening can be about 610 mm × 610 mm opening in the reception area. This room shall be located near the storage of screened blood. Alternatively, the screened blood can also be stored in this room. The issuing clerk shall check the cross-matching report and issue the blood. The room shall have a computer to enter issue details hence the necessary electrical and data points have to be provided in the room. Also, the communication port for intercom shall be provided.

24.10.1 Pneumatic Tube Systems

The distribution room shall have an outlet for Pneumatic Tube Systems (PTS). With PTS, it will be easy for the blood bank to receive the specimen of the blood of the patient along with the requisition form for cross-matching and also to send the blood bag to the required place.

24.11 Utility Area

These are the areas that support the functioning of the blood bank. Some of them are:

24.11.1 Change Room

Some areas like laboratories and the component room of the blood bank are basically clean areas and no person shall be allowed to enter these rooms without changing. Therefore, the staff must change into sterilized clothes by changing the outside dress. The following issues shall be considered regarding the Change room:

1. The room shall be of the size 2438 mm × 2438 mm.
2. Almirah shall be provided with the provision for hanging clothes.
3. In the change room, staff lockers shall also be provided where the staff can keep their personal belongings. Individual lockers shall be about 305 mm × 305 mm. Each locker shall be lockable separately. One such locker shall be allotted to one staff.
4. Handwashing and gowning facilities shall be provided in the change room.

24.11.2 Doctors Rest Rooms

Generally, a doctor is deputed in shifts who shall be available round the clock. Therefore, to facilitate the doctor on duty, a small doctor's restroom is provided in the blood bank.

1. The room shall be of the size 2438 mm × 3048 mm.
2. Furniture wise, the room shall have one office table, chair, bed and cupboard.
3. Apart from the light and fan, the room shall have points for a computer with Internet connection and Intercom point etc.
4. Also, the room shall be Air Conditioned and the Control button with temperature adjustment shall be provided in the room.

24.11.3 Store

Store shall be provided in the blood bank for equipment, supplies, consumable materials, medical disposables and other items in current use. The designer shall also consider future requirements while designing the storage space. The storage shall be lockable as far as possible and shall be free from humidity, should be termite proof and fire-resistant. Particular care shall be taken for storage of medicines and injectable etc. and shall be properly marked and under the strict control of an authorized person.

24.11.4 Record Room

Adequate storage space shall be allotted in the blood bank for storage of records. The size of the room shall be about 2438 mm × 2438 mm. The storage shall be lockable as far as possible and shall be free from humidity, should be termite proof and fire-resistant. The record room shall be provided with sufficient shelving, file cabinets and other storage for medical records. Donor record storage requirements will vary greatly according to local regulations. Typically current records (two to five years) will be held on-site. Archival donor record storage of up to 20 years will also be required.

24.11.5 Medical Officer Room

It is desirable to have a space for administrative control of the blood bank. As the in-charge of the blood bank is the Medical Officer, hence a Medical Officer Room shall be provided in the blood bank. The size of the room shall be about 4267 mm × 3658 mm. The room shall be provided with an office table, chairs, cupboard etc. Electrical points shall be provided near to the doctor's table for a view box and a computer. Communication ports shall be given for a computer and the intercom.

24.11.6 Sterilization Room Cum Washing Room

A small washing cum sterilization room shall be provided with the blood bank. The size of the room shall be about 3048 mm × 3048 mm. For washing, a countertop with deep sink shall be provided where the instruments can be washed. For sterilization, a single vertical autoclave with a capacity of two drums shall be provided. Necessary electric points shall be provided for the sterilizer.

24.11.7 Waste Management and Disposal

Blood banks generate a wide range of waste materials, including general waste, trade waste (i.e. chemical waste being discharged into the sewer), biological waste and waste radiation materials. The blood bank must review all its processes to identify the type and amount of each type of waste and develop policies and protocols for its handling, storage and disposal. Disposal of some waste materials may be carried out on-site while other materials may be collected and disposed of off-site by specialist contractors in accordance with local biomedical waste disposal regulations.

Further Reading

1. Health Services Department, Michael Okpara University of Agriculture, Umudike, Abia State, Nigeria. 2. Family Health International (FHI 360) Country Office, Garki Abuja Nigeria 3. Department of Medical Laboratory Science, Faculty of Health Sciences and Technology, Nnamdi Azikiwe University, Awka, Nigeria. Current concept of blood bank organisation and planning: A Review. Int J Curr Res Biol Med. 2016 Oct 21;1(7):19–26.

Choudhury N, Desai P. Blood bank regulations in India. Clin Lab Med. 2012 Jun;32(2):293–9.

Design guidelines for blood centres. Manila, Philippines: World Health Organization, Western Pacific Region; 2010. 104 p.

Drugs Control Media Services, Drugs Control, Regulatory, Pharma News, Research News, NPPA [Internet]. [cited 2021 Jul 7]. Available from: https://drugscontrol.org/blood-banks.php

Ltd TIS. JPAC - Transfusion Guidelines [Internet]. [cited 2021 Jul 7]. Available from: https://transfusionguidelines.org.uk/

Planning and Designing a Hospital Transfusion Service : September 2016 - MedicalLab Management Magazine [Internet]. [cited 2021 Jul 7]. Available from: https://www.medlabmag.com/article/1305

25 Other Investigations and Procedures

Apart from the Clinical Laboratories and Radiology, there are lots of other investigations, tests and procedures that are being carried out in the hospital. These investigations, tests and procedures may vary from one department to another.

All the special investigations, tests and procedures may or may not need special spaces in the hospital. Hence, it has to be planned well in advance as to which of these the hospital wants to set up immediately or maybe later in the future. The designer shall plan well in advance for providing spaces for them so that the hospital does not face problems in introducing them in future.

Most of these special investigations, tests and procedures may normally require some extra room with general facilities like adequate space, electrical outlet points and air-conditioning; but some of them may require specially designed rooms or complexes. The spaces which require special design have been described below:

25.1 Coronary Catheterization (Cath Lab)

The Cath lab, used for interventional cardiology, is an X-ray-based imaging machine and a very high dose of the rays are produced when exposure is given. Hence, it requires the design considering the norms of the regulatory authority. Proper designing has to be done to avoid radiation leakages. The main issues to be considered while designing the Cath Lab spaces are:

25.1.1 Location of the Cath Lab

Cath Lab shall be preferably located near the ICCU and shall be a sterilized and clean area.

25.1.2 Number of Cath Lab Procedure Rooms

The number of Cath Labs shall depend on the number of Cath Lab machines required to be installed as on date and also the future plans of the addition of more machines. The Cath Lab machine comes with a long slidable table.

Some of the important issues relating to Cath lab rooms are as follows:

Before designing the Cath Lab rooms, the guidelines and norms of the controlling authority of the country must be taken into account. In India the authority is Bhabha Atomic Research Institute.

A separate room shall be provided for each machine. More than one machine is not allowed in a single room.

For Cath Lab, if the machine is to be installed horizontally, a rectangular room shall be designed. If the machine is installed diagonally, a square room can also be considered. But the

A. Garg, A. Dewan, *Manual of Hospital Planning and Designing*,
https://doi.org/10.1007/978-981-16-8456-2_25

suggestion is to install horizontally in a rectangular room. The space of the room shall not be less than 42 sq. mtr. The approx. Size can be 9144 mm × 4572 mm.

All the walls of the room shall be at least 229 mm thick with a plaster on both sides. The ideal thickness for the primary wall of an X-ray room should be at least 250 mm solid baked clay bricks or 150 mm in case of mortar/concrete walls for plain radiography. Hollow bricks should be plastered with a thickness of 6 mm barium plaster and should be protected up to 2200 mm from the floor level.

The flooring shall be either tiles/marble/granite. But the flooring shall not be slippery to avoid the chances of an accident causing injury to the patient.

The room shall have a single door with a width of about 1829 mm, to ease the movement of trollies.

The door shall have to be with a proper 2000 mm thick lead lining. The lining has to be done even on the door frame. There shall be no leakage of the radiation from any place in the door. Doors should overlap by a minimum of 100 mm on each side when closed. The door should be at least 1800 mm long and 2000 mm high. The overlap requirement also applies to flap doors that make a single entrance door but close from different sides of the door. The door should have handles and locks on the inside and the outside so that they may always be closed during exposures thus controlling access.

It is advised to provide air interlock spaces by providing an additional door before the Cath Lab room door.

Windows are not allowed in the Cath Lab.

Outside the room, a Warning light shall be given by providing a Red colour bulb outside the door. The light must be connected to the generator in such a way that it will illuminate only during the activation of the tube.

While installing the machine, care shall be taken to leave at least 1829 mm space behind the machine for the movement of the C Arm of the machine to move. The machine shall be installed in the centre of the width of the room.

Depending on the capacity of the machine, the power load required by the machine shall be calculated and the main stitch and cable shall be terminated in each Cathlab room separately.

As the weight of the machine is more and the movement of the machine is very fast, it is advised to check the weight-bearing capacity of the floor. If needed to provide a foundation for the machine as per the suggestion of the machine manufacturer. If the machine is ceiling suspended model, care shall be taken to access the load-bearing capacity of the ceiling. If required proper treatment with the help of guarders of angle shall be done to increase the load-bearing capacity of the ceiling.

The lightning in the room shall be normal LED light with sufficient lumens. No extra illumination is required in the room.

The temperature in the room shall be between 17 and 21 °C and the humidity level shall not be more than 40%. Before finalizing the RH level or the temperature, the environment requirement shall also be confirmed from the equipment supplier as some machines may require varied standards of the environment.

All the machines shall have proper ground earthing provisions.

Inside the Cath Lab room, outlets for medical supply shall be given. The outlets shall be 1 of Oxygen, 1 for Vacuum and 1 for Air.

The proper two-way audio system is provided in the Cath Lab, from here the patient can be directed by the technician from the control room.

Position the gantry and couch such that the patient is completely visible from the control console during scanning.

Stand with heavy-duty hangers shall be provided outside the Cath Lab to hang the Lead apron.

Also, a cabinet shall be provided, for keeping other radiation safety devices like, lead gloves, lead goggles, groin guards and lead collars.

25.1.3 Cath Lab Console Room

Attached to the Cath Lab room a console room has to be provided. There shall be a provision of

Secondary Computer for transfer of images of the procedure which has been completed for starting the reporting. The size of the console room shall be a minimum 3658 mm × 3658 mm.

25.1.4 UPS Room

As the Cath Lab is an electronic machine, it requires a continuous power supply. If not, the machine will suddenly stop and the chances of corruption of software or the failure of the parts are high. To avoid this mostly all the users of the machine prefer to install an Online UPS with the machine. As the UPS is usually of high rating say above 100 KVA, a lot of batteries shall be required. Definitely, for this, a separate room will be required. This room shall be attached to the Control Room or the machine room. Some hospitals want to install all the UPS of the entire hospital at a common place away from the machine. This is not recommended. For Cath Lab type of machine, the UPS shall be near to the machine so that firstly the technician can keep a watch on the UPS, secondly, in case of emergency, he/she can switch off the UPS immediately. Earthing of the UPS is also desirable.

The size of the room shall be about 3658 mm × 3658 mm with a provision of racks to install the batteries. Because of the acid in the batteries, some fumes are formed in the room, so the UPS room shall have a provision of exhaust to remove these fumes out of the room from time to time. As the UPS also generates heat, the UPS shall be Air-conditioned and the temperature shall be about 17–20 °C with RH of not more than 40%.

25.1.5 Cath Lab Panel Room

Apart from the main machine where the tube and the detectors are fixed, other electronic parts are provided in the panels connected to the machine. These panels control the machine's working but are not directly needed in the Cath Lab room. For better protection of these panels, it is suggested to install them in a different room or enclosure attached to the Cath Lab room. Hence such an area shall be designed after consulting the equipment manufacturer. The size and temperature etc. shall be confirmed from the manufacturer of the machine.

25.1.6 Change Rooms for Patients

At times, with the patient's clothes which he/she is wearing it becomes difficult to perform the procedure. Hence the change rooms are provided near to the Cath Lab, to enable the patient to remove the outside clothes and change to the hospital dress. The size of this change room shall be 3658 mm × 3658 mm with a provision of a hanger rod and shelves for keeping the hospital dress.

25.1.7 Change Rooms for Staff

Some changing rooms are provided in the Cath Lab to enable the doctors and staff to remove the outside clothes and change to the sterilized hospital dress. Hospital dress is a pre-sterilized dress (normally Pyjama and Kurta) kept in the Change Rooms. The dresses of different sizes are stitched for different staff members. Different Change rooms are provided for different categories of staff members. Also, the change rooms for males are separate from Females. Following change rooms are generally provided in the Cath Lab.

1. Doctors Change Room—Males.
2. Doctors Change Room—Females.
3. Nurses/Technicians Change Room—Males.
4. Nurses/Technicians Change Room—Females.
5. Class IV Staff Change Room—Males.
6. Class IV Staff Change Room—Females.

Infrastructure wise:

1. The Room shall be of the size approximately 4267 mm × 4572 mm.
2. Along with the change room, an attached toilet with bath facility shall also be provided.
3. The room shall have the adequate provision of personal lockers to keep the personal belongings.

4. There shall be adequate hooks on the wall to hang the clothes.
5. Also, a hanger rod shall be provided with hangers to hang the clothes.
6. There shall be a cabinet to keep the sterilized dresses.
7. The hamper for dirty linen shall also be provided in the change room.

25.1.8 Waiting for Cath Lab

Cath Lab shall have a separate waiting area near the Lab for the family members of the patient whose procedure is being performed. The number of persons that can be allowed to wait in this lobby may be limited with proper spacing between their seats.

25.1.9 Stores for Unused Consumable

Cath Lab procedures require a lot of consumable materials like catheters, guide-wires and fluid. Hence ample stock of these consumables shall be available in the Lab. To stock these items, the department needs a store. This store shall be of the size of 3658 mm × 3658 mm. But depending on the quantity and number of items, the size may vary. The store needs to have sufficient countertops, cupboards and drawers. The Temperature of the room shall be between 17 and 21 °C.

25.1.10 Stores for Records and CDs

After the procedure, the images are generally transferred to a CD or DVD. These CDs/DVDs are marked with the patient ID and Name and are kept in the record along with other registers and reports. Hence, to stock these items, the department needs a store. This store shall be of the size of 3658 mm × 3658 mm. But depending on the quantity and number of items, the size may vary. The store needs to have sufficient countertops, cupboards and drawers. The Temperature of the room shall be between 17 and 21 °C.

25.1.11 Consultation Rooms

Family members and friends of the patient, being anxious to know the position and development in the condition of the patient need to meet the treating cardiologist and have an interaction with him. Therefore, Consultation Rooms are provided for this purpose. This room shall be about 4572 mm × 4267 mm with a provision of a doctor's table, chairs and sofa set. The cardiologist goes to that room, calls for the family members of the patient and has an interaction with them.

At times there can be hot discussions, for this, some security personnel shall be placed outside the room. Furthermore, this room shall be under CCTV surveillance from inside with audio-video recording (Fig. 25.1).

25.2 Thallium Scan

Thallium Scan is a high positron emitter, it is essential to provide the proper shielding and safety mechanisms like RCC walls. Hence it is advised that Thallium Scan areas shall be clubbed with the areas where PET CT/MRI machines are installed.

For details, please refer to the chapter 'Radiology' (Chap. 22).

25.3 Audiometry

Audiometry tests are to access the hearing functions. It tests both the intensity and the tone of sounds, balance issues and other issues related to the function of the inner ear. For the audiometry test, a specifically designed room is required.

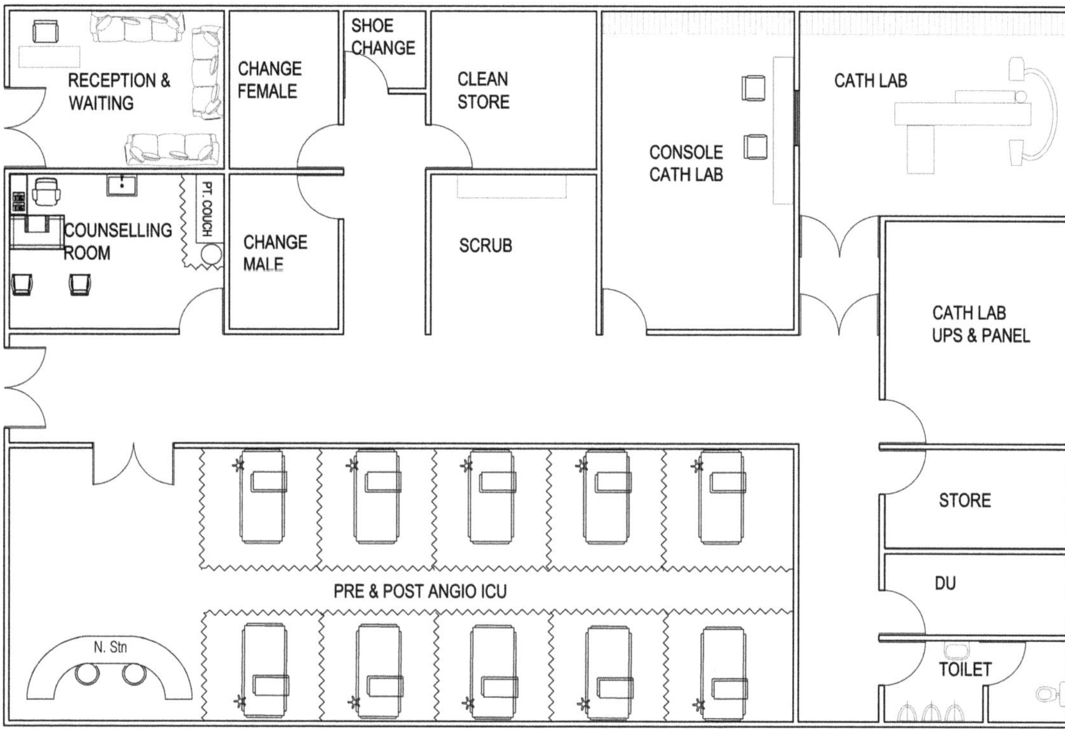

Fig. 25.1 Sample layout drawing of Cath Lab complex

25.3.1 Location of the Audiometry Room

This room shall be located near to the ENT OPD and in the general movement area. Clean and sterilized areas are not required for this.

25.3.2 Room Designing

The room of the audiometry shall be about 4267 mm × 4572 mm. This room shall have a glass partition in between. One shall be the patient room and the other the technician room. The patient room has to be completely soundproof and echo proof. For making the room soundproof and echo proof, acoustic treatment has to be done on the walls and ceiling. A wooden frame shall be fixed on the wall and ceiling, filling of glass wool shall be done. On the top fireproof cloth shall be fixed. Another alternative is to do wall panelling on the wall with specially designed sound and echo absorption panels. The flooring shall be done with wooden planks. The door of the room shall also be airtight so that no outer sound can enter the patient room.

The Technician room shall be a normal room with a glass window between the patient room and the technician room. This room shall have a working top below the glass window so that the technician can see the patient in the other room while the procedure is going on (Fig. 25.2).

25.4 Bronchoscopy

Bronchoscopy is used to assess reasons for persistent cough, infection or something unusual seen on a chest X-ray or other tests. Also used to obtain samples of mucus or tissue, to remove foreign bodies or other blockages from the airways of lungs, or to provide treatment for lung problems. Bronchoscopy is an invasive procedure where the bronchoscope is inserted into the trachea and the bronchi of the lung to see the picture of the lung and to find out any abnormality.

Usually, it is preferred to perform this procedure in the OT Complex. One particular OR is

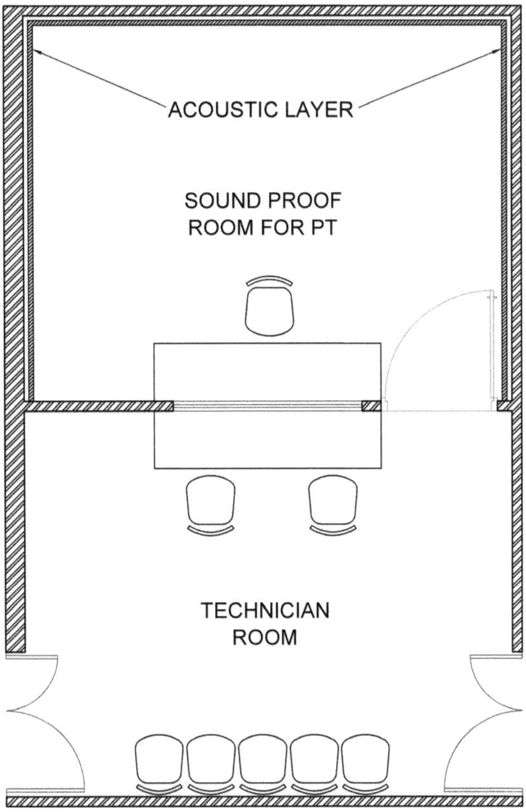

Fig. 25.2 Sample layout drawing of Audiometry Room

allotted for the bronchoscopy in the OT complex. If the procedure has to be done outside the OT complex, an OR type of setup has to be created at another place where the bronchoscopy has to be performed. The setup will require, sterilized bronchoscopy room, change rooms for staff, change room for the patient, store, bronchoscope wash area, patient recovery room etc.

The design of the rooms shall be exactly as described in the chapter 'OT Complex' (Chap. 19).

25.5 Capsule Endoscopy, Cholangioscopy, Colonoscopy, Duodenoscopy, Endoscopic Ultrasound, Upper Gastrointestinal Endoscopy etc.

All these procedures are basically invasive procedures performed by using the different types of endoscopes. Hence, they have to be done in a

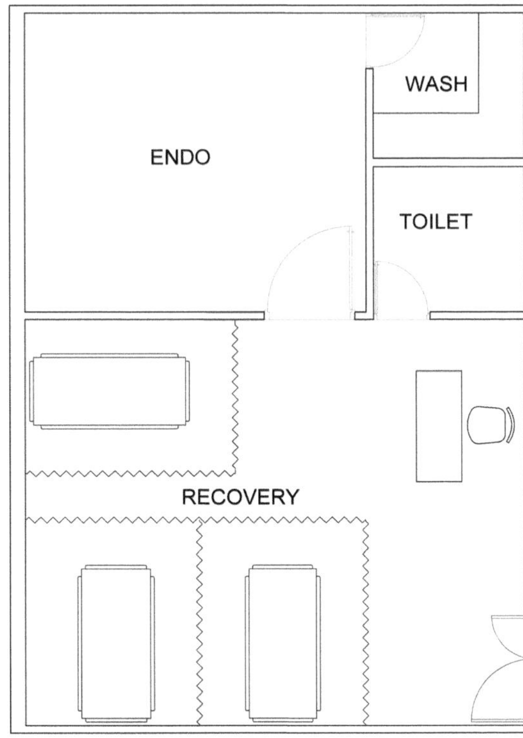

Fig. 25.3 Sample layout drawing of Endoscopy Room

sterilized and clean area. Therefore, it is preferred to get them done in the OT Complex (Fig. 25.3).

The details of the Endoscopy room have been described in the chapter 'OT Complex' (Chap. 19).

25.6 Neurology

Most of the neurological investigations like Electromyography (EMG), Neuropsychological Tests, NCV /EP Studies and Transcranial magnetic stimulation (TMS) are OPD-based investigation and space shall be provided in the OPD complex.

In the OPD Complex, a space called Neuro Lab shall be created and all such investigations shall be done in this lab. For convenience, a separate cabin for each investigation shall be provided to maintain the privacy of patients.

The size of the Lab shall depend on the number of such machines to be placed in the room and the number of cabins to be provided. Further, the size of the room shall also depend on the number of patients investigated at a particular moment of time. There shall also be ample space for movement of the staff in the Lab. It is advised that at least a space of 3658 mm × 3658 mm shall be provided for each machine to be installed in the lab.

Attached to the Neuro Lab a proper waiting area and a reception shall be provided for the convenience of the patients and family members. The facility of toilets shall also be provided for the patients and family members.

Regarding the temperature and the humidity in the Lab, normally it shall be between 18 and 22 °C and humidity of about 40–45%. But still, the equipment manufacturers shall be contacted for specific environmental conditions of the room.

Proper electric and communication points shall be provided for the machines.

25.7 Polysomnography (Sleep Lab)

Polysomnography, (sleep study) is a test used to diagnose sleep disorders. It records the brain waves, the oxygen level in the blood, heart rate and breathing, as well as eye and leg movements during the study. As this investigation is done while the patient is asleep, the room has to be in a silent space where there shall be no disturbance to the patient from outside sound and light.

25.7.1 Location of the Sleep Lab

This room shall be located near to the IPD area of the hospital. Clean and sterilized areas are not required for this.

25.7.2 Room Designing

The room of the sleep lab shall be about 4267 mm × 4572 mm. This room shall have a glass partition in between. One shall be the patient room and the other the technician room. The patient room has to be completely soundproof and with slight darkness to make the patient sleep comfortably. The door of the room shall also be airtight so that no outer sound can enter the patient room. The room shall have a bed for the patient.

As this machine is usually portable, some hospitals prefer to use a private single occupancy room to perform this procedure. This can also be done if preparing a separate room is not possible.

The Technician room shall be a normal room with a glass window between the patient room and the technician room. This room shall have a working top below the glass window so that the technician can see the patient in the other room while the procedure is going on. The machine is placed on the countertop and the technician records the findings of the patient while he/she is asleep.

Proper electric and communication points shall be provided for the machines.

25.8 Ophthalmology

In the department of Ophthalmology, separate specialized rooms are required for lasers. Lasers are very sophisticated machines and are highly sensitive to temperature and moisture. Therefore, special dust-proof rooms are required for lasers.

These rooms shall be located near to the Eye OPD and shall have a separate barricaded area with no general movement. The size of the room shall depend on the number and type of lasers to be installed in the room. Generally, each laser shall have an area of about 3658 mm × 3658 mm with an ample movement space.

The temperature in the room normally shall be between 18 and 22 °C and humidity of about 40–45%. But still, the equipment manufacturers shall be contacted for specific environmental conditions of the room.

Proper electric and communication points shall be provided for the machines.

25.9 ESW Lithotripter of Urology

Extracorporeal shock wave lithotripsy (ESWL) uses shock waves to break a kidney stone into small pieces that can more easily travel through the urinary tract and pass from the body.

For Lithotripter, a separate room shall be required. The size of the room shall be about 4572 mm × 4267 mm. In the centre of the room, the table (which comes along with the machine) is placed. On one side of the table shall be the lithotripter and the C-arm for focusing on the stone to be blasted.

The temperature in the room normally shall be between 18 and 22 °C and humidity of about 40–45%. But still, the equipment manufacturers shall be contacted for specific environmental conditions of the room.

Proper electric and communication points shall be provided for the machines. The Lithotripter and the table shall be properly earthed to absorb the leakage of the current.

25.10 Dialysis

Haemodialysis requires a separate area in the hospital. For dialysis, the following issues shall be kept in mind while designing the room:

25.10.1 Location of the Dialysis Room

Dialysis shall be preferably located near the department of Nephrology and shall be a sterilized and clean area.

25.10.2 Dialysis Procedure Room

The size of the Dialysis Room shall depend on the number of Dialysis machines required to be installed as on date and also the future plans for the addition of more machines.

Some of the important issues relating to Dialysis rooms are as follows:

A separate room shall be provided for the dialysis of the positive patients and shall not be mixed with the general patients under any circumstances. The machine shall also be separate for the positive patients.

The space for each dialysis machine shall not be less than 13.94 Sq. Mtr.

Sufficient power load as required by the machine shall be calculated and provided for each machine.

The bed or dialysis couch shall be placed at a distance of at least 1829 mm from each other so that there is ample space for keeping the machine on the right side of the patient (Fig. 25.4).

On the backside of each dialysis machine, the point for the supply of RO water shall be provided. Similarly, the drain points shall also be provided on the floor for each dialysis machine.

The lightning in the room shall be normal LED light with sufficient lumens. No extra illumination is required in the room.

The temperature in the room shall be from 17 to 21 °C and the humidity level shall not be more than 40%. Before finalizing the RH level or the temperature, the environment requirements shall also be confirmed from the equipment supplier as some machines may require varied standards of the environment.

All the machines shall have proper ground earthing provisions.

Each of the Dialysis bed/couch, the outlets for medical supply shall be given. The outlets shall be 1 for Oxygen, 1 for Vacuum and 1 for Air.

25.10.3 Washroom for Dialyzers

Attached to the Dialysis room shall be a dialyzer washroom, where the dialyzer washer is installed. On one of the walls, stainless steel bins shall be provided for keeping the washed dialyzers till they are dry. The size of the bins shall be 160 mm H × 150 mm W × 400 mm D. Provision shall be made for about 25–40 dialyzers.

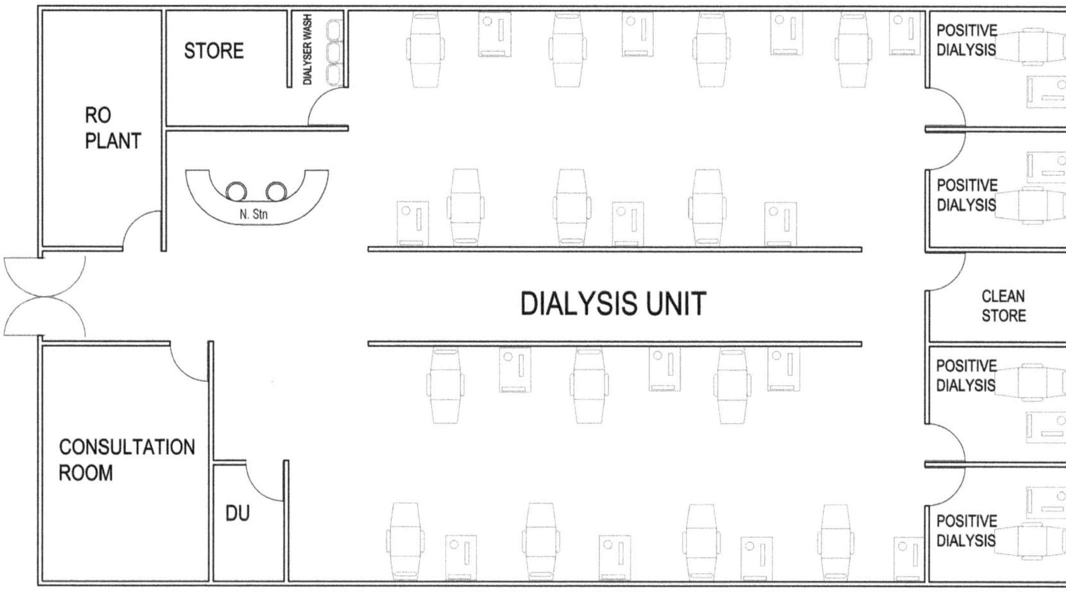

Fig. 25.4 Sample layout drawing of dialysis complex

25.10.4 Store

Dialysis procedure requires a lot of consumable materials like dialyzers and dialysis fluid Part A and Part B. Hence ample stock of these consumables shall be available in the dialysis. To stock these items, the department needs a store. This store shall be of the size of 4267 mm × 3658 mm. But depending on the quantity and number of items, the size may vary. The store needs to have sufficient countertops, cupboards and drawers. On one of the walls, lockable stainless steel bins shall be provided for keeping the used dialyzers for reuse. The size of the bins shall be 160 mm H × 150 mm W × 400 mm D. Provisions shall be made for about 40–60 dialyzers. The Temperature of the room shall be between 17 and 21 °C.

25.10.5 Change Rooms for Patients

Change rooms are provided near to the Dialysis, to enable the patient to remove the outside clothes and change to the hospital dress. The size of this change room shall be 3658 mm × 3658 mm with a provision of a hanger rod and shelves for keeping the hospital dress.

25.10.6 Change Rooms for Staff

The changing rooms are provided in the Dialysis to enable the doctors and staff to remove the outside clothes and change to the sterilized hospital dress. Hospital dress is a pre-sterilized dress (normally Pyjama and Kurta) kept in the Change Rooms. The dresses of different sizes are stitched for different staff members. Different Change rooms are provided for different categories of staff members. Also, the change rooms for males are separate from Females. Following change rooms are generally provided in the Dialysis.

1. Doctors Change Room—Males.
2. Doctors Change Room—Females.
3. Nurses/Technicians Change Room—Males.
4. Nurses/Technicians Change Room—Females.
5. Class IV Staff Change Room—Males.
6. Class IV Staff Change Room—Females.

Infrastructure wise:

1. The Room shall be of the size approximately 3658 mm × 3658 mm.
2. Rooms shall have adequate provision of personal lockers to keep their personal belongings.
3. There shall be adequate hooks on the wall to hang the clothes.
4. Also, a hanger rod shall be provided with hangers to hang the clothes.
5. There shall be a cabinet to keep the sterilized dresses.
6. The hamper for dirty linen shall also be provided in the change room.

25.10.7 Waiting for Dialysis

Dialysis shall have a separate waiting area near the dialysis room for the family members of the patient whose procedure is being performed. The number of persons that can be allowed to wait in this lobby may be limited with proper spacing between their seats.

For all other investigation/procedure rooms (which have not been specifically described in this chapter), shall be the normal rooms. Though the rooms are with the normal specification, as the machines are normally very sophisticated and highly sensitive, the following issues shall be kept in mind:

1. The rooms shall be dustproof and clean.
2. Proper electric and communication points shall be provided for the machines.
3. Proper environmental conditions shall be maintained as required by the equipment manufacturers.
4. Proper waiting spaces shall be provided.
5. The sizes of the rooms shall be decided individually and may vary depending on the number of machines, the number of patients etc.
6. All other requirements of infrastructure as required by the manufacturers of the machine shall be fulfilled.

Further Reading

Cardiac Catheterization Laboratory Facility Design and Equipment Selection [Internet]. HMP Global Learning Network. [cited 2021 Jul 7]. Available from: https://www.hmpgloballearningnetwork.com/site/cathlab/articles/Cardiac-Catheterization-Laboratory-Facility-Design-and-Equipment-Selection

Hendry C, Rashid R. Catheter Laboratory Design, Staffing and Training. In: Watson TJ, Ong PJ, Tcheng JE, editors. Primary angioplasty: A practical guide [internet]. Singapore: Springer; 2018 [cited 2021 Jul 7]. p. 69–81. Available from: https://doi.org/10.1007/978-981-13-1114-7_6

McGeary D. Catheterization Laboratories. Biomed Instrum Technol. 2008 Jan 1;42(1):49–52.

Pontoriero G, Tetta C, Wratten ML, Locatelli F. Design and Quality Assurance of New Dialysis Centers. Saudi J Kidney Dis Transplant. 2001 Jul 1;12(3):413.

Rajhans N, Sardar V, Sajgure A. Design of Wearable Dialysis Unit. In 2017.

Bower SB. Dialysis facility design—part I: Developing a strategic and financial plan. Dial Transplant. 2006;35(8):532–43.

Planning for the Ideal Cath Lab Requires the Multidisciplinary Approach [Internet]. [cited 2021 Jul 7]. Available from: https://www.cardiovascularbusiness.com/topics/coronary-intervention-surgery/planning-ideal-cath-lab-requires-multidisciplinary-approach

Predicting the Cath Lab of the Future [Internet]. DAIC. 2012 [cited 2021 Jul 7]. Available from: https://www.dicardiology.com/article/predicting-cath-lab-future

Setting up of hemodialysis unit. Indian J Nephrol. 2020 Jul 1;30(7):1.

26 Radiation Therapy

Radiation Therapy (RT) is a speciality of the Oncology Department and is used for the treatment of cancer through radioactive rays generated through Linear Accelerator (LINAC). Through radiation, specific malignant cells are damaged through external beams of radioactive waves. High-energy waves, such as X-rays, gamma rays, electron beams or protons, are accelerated in the LINAC to destroy or damage cancer cells.

In the Radiation Therapy Unit, the facilities and equipment for radiotherapy treatment are provided. The Radiation Oncology Unit contains spaces to support patient consultation, treatment simulation and planning, and the administration of treatment. The Radiation Oncology Unit generally contains both external and internal radiotherapy (brachytherapy) treatment areas.

26.1 Location of Radiotherapy Unit

The Radiotherapy department has two main machines. One is the LINAC and the other is the Brachytherapy. Because of the high radiation, it is mandatory to install these machines in the Bunkers. What is the Bunker? A bunker is made out of High-density RCC materials like concrete or steel. The wall thickness of the bunker is usually 2400 mm. Similarly, the roof is also 2400 mm thick. Another important issue is that the LINAC is a very heavy machine weighing about 8–9 tonnes. Hence, the flooring has to be very strong to bear such a weight. Usually, the bunker occupies 1.5 floors till the top of the bunker.

Taking into account the above factors, the Bunkers cannot be provided on any upper floors. It has to be on the ground floor. Still, it is preferable if the bunkers can be provided in the basement. The added advantage with the basement is that the wall thickness reduces because of the soil filled along the bunker walls. As the outer walls of bunkers are exposed to the outer surface, where the soil is backfilled, the thickness reduces, as the radiations penetrate the filled up soil.

Hence, the Radiotherapy department, particularly the bunkers shall be located either on the ground floor or in the basement. If basements are chosen, proper access and road connectivity shall be provided to transport the LINAC to the bunker site.

The Unit shall be provided with facilities for ready access for outpatients, including people with disabilities, people arriving by patient transfer services and ambulances, and for inpatients in wheelchairs and on beds or trolleys.

A. Garg, A. Dewan, *Manual of Hospital Planning and Designing*,
https://doi.org/10.1007/978-981-16-8456-2_26

26.2 Infrastructure of the Radiotherapy Department

The department shall have the following spaces:

Utility Area	Reception and Enquiry
	Registration
	Record Room
	Store
	Consultation Rooms
	Public Utility for Faculty
	Public Utility for Patients and Attendants
	Report Delivery Room
	Sub waiting
Treatment and Planning Area	Teletherapy Unit
	Intracavitary Treatment Room
	Interstitial, Endo-cavitory, Surface mould therapy room
	Planning room
	Metalling treatment planning equipment, Mould room
	Medical Physics Laboratory
	Radiation bunkers
	Control Room
	Brachytherapy bunker with a Control room
	Patient Holding Bay
	Patient Change Room
	Doctors Change
	Staff Change with Lockers
	Scrub
	Clean Supply Room
	Dirty Utility
	Toilet
	Store
Radiotherapy Ward	Patient Beds
	Nurses Duty Room
	Store
	Dirty Utility / Sluice Room
	Clean Supply Room
	Examination and Treatment Room
	Ward Pantry
	Resident Doctors and Student Duty Room
	Extra Rooms for Future expansion
	Public Utility for Staff
	Public Utility for Patients and Attendants

26.3 Utility Areas

The utility areas shall have:

26.3.1 Entrance to the department

1. The doors shall be at least 1829 mm wide with two doors openable on both sides.
2. For automation, sensor-operated glass doors can also be opted for.
3. An Airlock connecting external areas with internal areas shall be provided. This can be done by providing two doors at a distance of say 1829 mm from each other. The purpose is to decrease the infection rate and to maintain air-conditioning temperature and air pressurization from internal to external areas.
4. Prevent outside air contaminants such as dust entering the building by providing an air curtain.
5. There shall be a provision of thermal scanning of all the patients/attendants/visitors entering the Radiotherapy department.
6. The provision for providing masks, gloves and shoe covers shall be made at the entry gate.
7. The provision for sanitizations shall also be done at the gate.

26.3.2 Outside Entrance

These facilities shall be provided only if this department has a separate entrance other than the main entrance of the hospital.

1. The ambulance disembarkation area shall be provided near to entrance gate.
2. Preferably a Porch shall be provided at the entrance gate as a shelter from inclement weather.
3. The porch shall be wide enough to ease the pass of two vehicles at a time.
4. The height of the porch shall be at least 4572 mm from the road level.

5. The trolley bay shall be provided outside the lobby for parking of wheelchairs and stretcher trolley so that the patients dropping on the porch can use them.

26.3.3 Reception and Enquiry Counter

Immediately after the arrival of the patient in the department, this is the first area of contact. The Reception provides the required information to the visitors, guide the visitors to the required place, book an appointment or treatment schedule etc. Hence, the reception counter has to be placed just at the entry of the radiotherapy department. The reception shall be at such a place that it is easily approachable.

26.3.4 Registration Counter

Next to the reception counter, the registration counter has to be located. The Registration counter registers the patient for consultation or radiotherapy treatment. Prepare consultation form, receive payment for consultation, Issue token number etc. In some hospitals, the case records are stored in the registration department and patients are handed over a small card containing the registration number. Every time the patient visits the hospital the case record has to be taken out and sent to the physician for consultation. This job has to be done by the registration counter.

26.3.5 General Waiting

1. For Radiotherapy Treatment, usually with the patient, attendants also come to the hospital.
2. Each patient in a department shall be allowed only ONE accompanying attendant.
3. For the attendants, the waiting area shall be provided just at the entrance of the department. The attendants shall not be allowed inside the treatment area, because it is a high radiation area.
4. The waiting area shall not be very big, and distancing has to be followed.
5. The chairs shall be laid down at distancing.
6. There must be facilities available such as telephones, public address systems to call relatives of patients to inform them about the patient's condition etc.
7. Near to the waiting area shall be provided Toilets, both for males and for females separately. The provision of cold drinking water shall also be provided.
8. Mobile charging points shall also be provided in the waiting area.

26.3.6 Store

The department shall be provided with adequate storage for all equipment, supplies, consumable materials, medical disposables and other items in current use. Storage is also needed for personal items belonging to staff, patients and visitors. Equipment and supplies storage shall be designed to be stored as close as possible to point of use. The store shall be lockable as far as possible and shall be free from humidity, should be termite proof and fire-resistant. Particular care shall be taken for storage of medicines and injectable etc. and shall be properly marked and under the strict control of the authorized person.

26.3.7 Consultation Room

The required consultation rooms shall be provided in the radiotherapy department, where the patient can consult the doctors for their further treatments and protocols of treatment.

For other details of Consultation Rooms, Furniture, Equipment, Instruments and Tools, Doors, Windows, Central Medical Gas Supply, Electrical Points, Other Communication Points etc., please refer to the chapter 'Out-Patient Department' (Chap. 17) in this book.

26.4 Treatment and Planning Area

This area includes:

26.4.1 Mould Room

The mould is a kind of photon and electron shielding that is prepared to protect the patient from radiation exposure to other parts of the body except the area to be treated with radiation. The mould has to be prepared for each and every patient and the design and sizes vary from patient to patient. The mould room is to take the sizes and design of the mould to be prepared. The room shall be about 4267 mm × 3658 mm and shall be provided with the office table, chairs and the examination couch. The room shall also be provided with computer workstations connected to the hospital network. The connection to the PACS shall also be done.

26.4.2 Mould Workshop

Mould workshop is actually a place where the moulds are physically prepared. Mould Workshop shall have:

1. A special exhaust, as the mould is prepared out of molten metal, foam cutters, vacuum formers etc.
2. Proper acoustic treatment shall be done as there can be a lot of noise due to the use of the machinery like drills and cutters.
3. A separate store shall be provided to store the raw material of mould.
4. A store for storing the moulds that are presently being used for the treatment of the patient. Such moulds are stored during the entire duration of the treatment.

26.4.3 Medical Physics

Medical Physicists supervise the physical aspects of radiation treatment and radiation safety of staff, patients and visitors. They provide scientific support for all treatment machines like CT Simulators, LINAC, Brachytherapy, computer planning systems, and equipment as well as dosimetry, quality assurance and radiation safety. The spaces shall be provided for offices and workstations for physicists. The size of the room shall be about 4267 mm × 3658 mm. The room shall be provided with an office table, chairs and an examination couch. The room shall also be provided with computer workstations connected to the hospital network. Physics laboratory shall be provided to manufacture equipment not available commercially for patient treatment such as the installation of rigid attachments for patient hoists, calibration jigs for physics and mask creation appliances. Storage for Medical Physics equipment including bulky water tanks and phantoms.

26.4.4 CT Simulators

CT Simulator is utilized to set telegraphy fields and plan radiation treatment. Simulation is the process by which the radiation oncologists, physicians acquire images of the body in order to develop the appropriate treatment plan. Therefore, the treatment area shall also be provided with the CT simulator. The setup of the CT simulator is almost the same as that of the CT scan in the department of Radiology.

For other details about Furniture, Equipment, Instruments and Tools, Doors, Windows, Central Medical Gas Supply, Electrical Points, Other Communication Points etc. and CT Simulation, please refer to the chapter 'Radiology' (Chap. 22) in this book.

26.5 Radiation Therapy Treatment Area

The radiation treatment can be either the External Beam Radiation Therapy (LINAC) or the Internal Beam Radiation Therapy (Brachytherapy).

26.5.1 External Beam Radiation Therapy

For external beam radiation therapy, the LINAC is used. With LINAC, an electron beam is typically created which is used for killing cancer affected tissues by radiation while sparing the surrounding healthy tissue. Using these high-energy electrons (particle) beam accelerators, the patient's malignant cells and tumours of varying size and shape can be killed. While designing the External beam radiation unit, the following issues shall be considered:

1. The external beam radiation therapy LINAC is installed in the bunkers. Bunkers are made out of High-density RCC materials like concrete or steel.
2. The wall thickness of the bunker is usually 2400 mm. Similarly, the roof is also 2400 mm Thick.
3. The bunkers shall have a Maze type of design.
4. The size inside the bunkers shall be 7000 mm × 7000 mm with the iso-centre positioned approximately in the centre of the room.
5. The bunkers shall provide space for the structure of the LINAC unit and the maximum longitudinal extension of a typical patient treatment table.
6. The gantry and the patient treatment table shall be engineered to rotate around an iso-centre.
7. The width shall enable comfortable access around the gantry and the patient for all angles of rotation.
8. The plane of gantry rotation shall be parallel to the treatment control panel area.
9. While designing the orientation of the bunkers, the issues of high occupancy areas shall be taken into account.
10. The minimum structural room height shall be 4 m, including along the maze. This height is necessary for ease of access when equipment is delivered, to provide for the air conditioning, heating, exhaust and ventilation system design, and for installing additional electrical supply cabling.
11. A maze width of 2000–2200 mm shall be provided to ensure an adequate turning circle for equipment delivery.
12. LINAC is a very heavy machine weighing about 8–9 tonnes. Hence the flooring has to be very strong to bear such a weight.
13. While installing LINAC for the first time, provision for the base-frame shall be provided. This base frame shall be measured from the centre to the back and shall be 6000 mm × 2000 mm × 610 mm deep excavation.
14. Two or more bunkers shall be designed adjacent to each other to reduce costs by sharing the primary shielding structures.
15. The door shall be provided at the end of the maze, i.e. entry of the bunkers, just to avoid accidental entry in the bunkers, while the radiation is in progress. This door need not have the shielding as this door is not for protection from radiation, but to provide a physical barrier and restrict the entry in the bunkers.
16. Access during radiation shall be prevented with a combination of light sensors and/or push gates or barriers that are interlocked to the control panel.
17. Usually, the bunker occupies 1.5 floors till the top of the bunker. Access to the roof of the bunkers shall be restricted and cordoned off, with a security entrance, interlocked to the treatment machine.
18. However, the equipment like water chillier and the air-conditioning plants are placed on the roof, as these types of equipment require controlled access.
19. Linear accelerator bunkers require radiation protection that may include lead shielding and concrete walls, floors and ceilings to specified thicknesses, a neutron door may also be required depending on the type of linear accelerator used.
20. The radiation protection needs of the unit shall be assessed by a certified physicist or appropriate agency. This assessment is to

specify the type, location and amount of protection to be installed in accordance with the final approved department layout and equipment selection. The radiation protection requirements shall be incorporated into the final plans and specifications. Early consultation with the manufacturers of radiotherapy equipment is recommended.

21. For LINAC with a maximum energy of 10 MV, the neutron shielding is not required.
22. The lifespan of the facility and the need to upgrade technology should be considered when specifying the radiation shielding required. It is likely that the machines will be upgraded and newer machines may or may not emit stronger radiation. Therefore, it is sensible to allow for the highest energy machine and widest beam that is likely to be used in the future.
23. The bunker shall be provided with the plumbing and electrical provisions. The underground conduits for these lines shall not be straight but have to be angulated at an angle of 45 degrees.
24. The bunker shall be provided with the provision of power supply to the LINAC as per the requirement of the machine. Hence the manufacturer of the equipment shall be contacted beforehand while designing the bunkers.
25. Provisions for joints, ducting and sleeves should not follow the divergence of the primary beam, and this is easily achieved by placing these in the secondary shielding and using a curved path.
26. The issues relating to the mechanical, electrical and safety shall all be considered like, providing dimmable lights in the room, emergency switches and the provision of standby lighting.
27. Provision for ducting shall be provided in the bunker for connection between the gantry structure and the treatment control panel.
28. In addition, isolated ducts should be provided for dosimeter cables and connectivity to the chillier system.
29. After the installation of the machine, false ceilings shall be provided in the bunkers.
30. Each bunker shall be provided with Control Areas. These areas shall be located outside the maze of the bunker.
31. The bunkers shall be provided with a patient intercommunication device and at least two closed-circuit television monitors, to communicate with the patient while the therapy is in progress.
32. The working top in the control area shall be of adequate length to provide spaces for installation of all the monitors and other control equipment along with the patient information files, sheets and images to be used while therapy is in progress.
33. Electrical power points shall be provided along the whole length of the worktop to allow multiple devices to be powered, including additional emergency switches.
34. The X-ray viewing box with ambient lighting shall be provided in the control area.
35. Space shall be provided along with the control room area for networked imager or printer. This facility can also be shared with brachytherapy (Fig. 26.1).

26.5.2 Internal Beam Radiation Therapy

For internal beam radiation therapy, the Brachytherapy is used. Brachytherapy is a method of delivering radiation to tumours where radioactive sources are placed either within or immediately adjacent to tumour tissue. While designing the Brachytherapy Unit, the following issues shall be considered:

1. The Brachytherapy treatment room is used for delivery of a radiation source through a tube or applicator, implanted during surgery.
2. The Brachytherapy room is similar to that of the External Radiation therapy unit, i.e. for

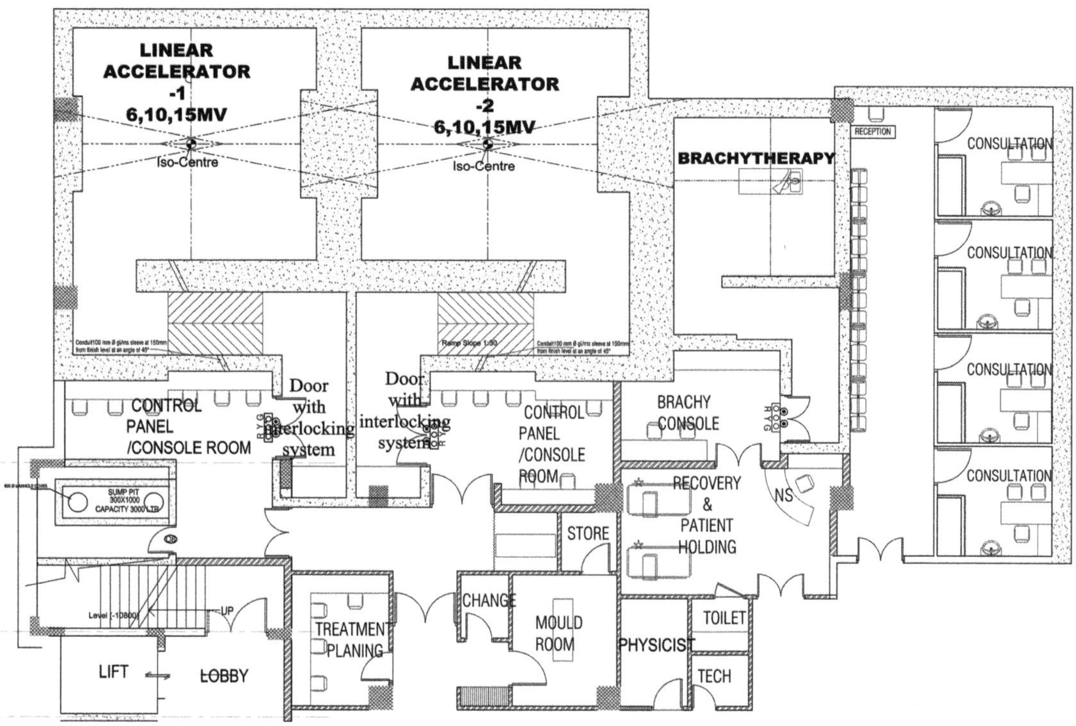

Fig. 26.1 Sample drawing of Radiation Department

brachytherapy, the bunker has to be provided. Hence all the issues relating to the bunkers as mentioned above in LINAC have to be taken care of.

3. Along with the Brachytherapy Unit, an equipped operating room along with other services like anaesthetic induction room, scrub area, patient recovery room and clean room shall be provided.
4. C-arm shall be provided in the Brachytherapy to be used for applicator placement and therefore will need to be installed in the appropriate room, either the procedure room or the treatment room depending on the local practice.
5. The brachytherapy bunker shall have wall and ceiling thicknesses of at least 1000 mm.
6. The maze shown is 1800 mm wide to allow for easy access in the event of an emergency and the design shown has no door.
7. The inside dimensions of the room shall be 4000 mm × 4000 mm × 3600 mm height (ceiling height of 3000 mm) in order for there to be enough space around the unit to manoeuvre a C-arm and a procedure trolley if the patient is prepared in the treatment room.
8. Because the source emits radiation isotopically, a shielded roof is required.
9. Except for the wall thickness and the dimensions of the Brachytherapy bunkers, all other issues of LINAC bunkers shall be taken care of while designing the bunkers for Brachytherapy.

26.6 Radiotherapy Ward

Though generally, a ward is not required in the radiotherapy department, but still some hospitals prefer to have a small setup of radiotherapy ward for any emergency. Hence a small ward with about 2 to 4 beds can be planned. The setup of the wards will be similar to any ward as mentioned in the chapter of Intermediate Care Area (Patient Rooms).

For other details about Radiotherapy Ward about construction details, Furniture, Equipment, Instruments and Tools, Doors, Windows, Central Medical Gas Supply, Electrical Points, Other Communication Points etc. please refer to the chapter 'Intermediate Care Area (Patient Rooms)' (Chap. 21) in this book.

26.7 Trolley Bay

For the convenience of the patient, the Radiation therapy shall be provided with an area reserved for the stretcher trolley and wheelchairs. The area shall be enough to park at least two stretcher trollies and two wheelchairs. The trolley park area shall be somewhere at the corner of the department so that it does not create hindrances in the routine working of the department.

26.8 Change Rooms

At times, with the patient's clothes which he/she is wearing it becomes difficult to perform the procedure, hence change rooms shall be provided in the department of Radiotherapy to enable the patient to remove the outside clothes and change to the hospital dress. The Room shall be of the size approximately 3048 mm × 3048 mm. Rooms shall have adequate provision of personal lockers to keep the belongings of the patient. There shall be adequate hooks on the wall to hang the clothes. Also, a hanger rod shall be provided with hangers to hang the clothes. There shall be a cabinet to keep the sterilized dresses.

26.9 Store

Small storeroom of at least 3658 mm × 3658 mm shall be provided near the treatment units for storing the major dosimetry equipment and all equipment, supplies, consumable materials, medical disposables and other items in current use. The designer shall also consider the future requirements while designing the storage space. Storage is needed for personal items belonging to staff, patients and visitors. Equipment and supplies storage shall be designed to be stored as close as possible to point of use. The storage shall be lockable as far as possible and shall be free from humidity, should be termite proof and fire-resistant. Particular care shall be taken for storage of medicines and injectable etc. and shall be properly marked and under the strict control of an authorized person.

26.10 Signage and Wayfinding

Proper Signage shall be provided in the department, which will make the visitors understand the layout of the department. Provide a simple and clear way finding solutions. This can be done with proper signage or with design and material solutions, such as colour-coordinating paths or accent lighting.

26.11 Sub-waiting Lobbies

It is recommended that instead of a large waiting lobby, sub-waiting lobbies shall be given for each modality of the department. The number of people who can be allowed to wait in Radiotherapy lobbies may be limited to a certain maximum with a specific minimum spacing between their seats.

26.12 Clean Utility

A clean utility room shall be provided in the department, which shall be used for storage of the clean linen. The room shall also be used for storing the sterilized material like drums, drapes etc. Normally, the room shall not be less than 3658 mm × 3658 mm. But depending on the requirements, the size of the room can be changed. The room is provided with closed cabinets, drawers and racks. This room shall have only one door of about 914 mm.

26.13 Dirty Utility/Sluice Room

The dirty utility shall be provided in the department which shall be used for storage of the soiled linen. From here the linen is moved for pre-wash before sending it to the laundry. Normally, the room shall not be less than 3658 mm × 3658 mm. But depending on the requirements, the size of the room can be changed. The room is provided with covered linen collection hampers or containers to collect the dirty linen. This room shall have two doors of about 914 mm. One door opens in the department and the other in the corridor from where the laundry staff can collect the linen. Air from this room shall be exhausted hence the exhaust fans are a must.

26.14 Handwashing

A Hand Basin shall be provided in Consult Rooms, Procedure Rooms and Imaging rooms, and shall be located conveniently to Simulator Rooms and Staff Stations or at other required places. The handwash basin shall have the facility of a soap dispenser and disposable paper towels.

26.15 Administration/Offices

Offices shall be provided for the Clinical Director of the unit, Radiation Oncologists and Radiation Therapy Managers. The size of these rooms shall be about 4572 mm × 4572 mm. The rooms shall have an arrangement for office tables, executive chair, visitor chairs, side rack etc. The rooms shall have an attached toilet. The rooms shall also have an attached P.A. room for a clerk to be seated. If required and long working hours are expected, a small restroom can also be provided with these rooms. The rooms shall have proper arrangements for electrical points, intercom connection, IT network and air conditioning.

Offices shall also be provided for Nursing Managers, Allied Health Professionals, Cancer Care Co-ordinators and Specialist Nurses. The size of these rooms shall be about 3658 mm × 3658 mm. The room shall have an arrangement for office tables, chairs, visitor chairs, side rack etc. The room shall have proper arrangements for electrical points, intercom connection, IT network and air conditioning.

26.16 Other Issues on Infrastructure of the Radiation Therapy Unit

26.16.1 Acoustics

Acoustic treatment shall be provided in all the examination rooms, consult rooms and offices to ensure privacy for discussions with patients, families and staff. Provide acoustic treatment for the control of noise associated with machinery in the appliance fabrication workshop areas.

26.16.2 Doors

All entry points, doors or openings requiring bed/trolley access including Radiation Therapy and Procedure Rooms shall be minimum of 1524 mm wide, unobstructed. Larger openings may be required for special equipment, to allow the manoeuvring of equipment without manual handling risks and risk of damage. Within workshop and appliance room areas, the number of doors should be kept to a size adequate to facilitate the movement of equipment; double doors should be provided to all workshop areas.

26.16.3 Finishes

All surface finishes shall be washable including walls and ceilings. Floor surfaces should be easy to clean, sealed and coved at the edges.

26.16.4 Other Communication Points in the Radiation Department

The following communication points shall be provided at all the required places in the department:

1. RJ 45 point for Computer networking.
2. RJ 11 for Intercom and extension line.
3. HDMI point for computer display at other locations.
4. Voice/data outlets and wireless networks.
5. Telephone and video conferencing capacity for meeting rooms.
6. PACS imaging system, electronic records and radiotherapy information management systems.

26.17 Heating Ventilation and Air conditioning

General air conditioning shall be provided in the whole department. The temperature of the unit should be maintained within a comfortable range between 18 and 24 °C and shall be comfortable for the patient.

The temperature of the treatment rooms shall be from 17 to 20 °C and the humidity level shall not be more than 40%. Before finalizing the RH level or the temperature, the environment requirement shall also be confirmed from the equipment supplier as some machines may require varied standards of the environment.

26.18 Central Piped Medical Gas Supply

Each of the treatment room, treatment planning room shall be provided with the Piped Centralised Medical Supply system. The gases supplied are:

- Oxygen.
- Compressed Air.
- Wall-mounted Suction.

26.19 Electrical Points in the Radiation Therapy Department

The following electrical points shall be provided in the consultation chamber, Administration rooms, Planning rooms and other areas except for the treatment rooms.

1. Main Switchboard shall be at the entrance wall (other than the wall on which door will open) for control of the fan and lights of the room along with one 6 A Switch/Socket.
2. Air Conditioning Control button with temperature adjustment.
3. Two 6 A Switches/Sockets above on the wall 1 ft. above the doctors/administrator table. Also, one 15 A Switch/Socket shall be provided adjoining to this.
4. Three 5 A Switches/Sockets above on the wall 305 mm above the doctor/administrator side rack for computer and printer. Also, one 15 A Switch/Socket shall be provided adjoining to this for equipment or heater.
5. Proper switch/sockets shall be provided in the treatment planning rooms for providing power to the required machinery.
6. Regarding the Power in the treatment rooms and the LINAC/Brachytherapy machines, the same shall be as per the requirement of the manufacturer of the machines. Therefore, before finalizing the electrical planning of these rooms, it shall be confirmed from the equipment supplier as some machines may have varied power requirements.

26.20 Power Backup

The power backup is very essential for the treatment rooms, where the machines are installed. These machines shall have their own power back up, which should start automatically in the event of a power failure. If possible the machine shall have a backup with the connected UPS. Also, the department shall have its own backup of an Auto

Start Diesel Generator. Also, the necessary provision for the regulation of voltage or power supplied to the department shall be made.

Further Reading

Baskar R, Lee KA, Yeo R, Yeoh K-W. Cancer and Radiation Therapy: Current Advances and Future Directions. Int J Med Sci. 2012;9(3):193–9.

Bonett J. Ceiling art in a radiation therapy department: its effect on patient treatment experience. J Med Radiat Sci. 2015;62(3):192–7.

Horton P, Eaton D. Design and Shielding of Radiotherapy Treatment Facilities: IPEM Report 75 second Edition: IPEM Report 75, second Edition [Internet]. IOP Publishing; 2017 [cited 2021 Jul 7]. Available from: https://iopscience.iop.org/book/978-0-7503-1440-4

Ashby D, Peterson F, Atterbury D. Designing chemotherapy and radiation therapy facilities. Health Care Strateg Manage. 1986 Oct;4(10):9–16.

Designing the New-age Oncology Radiation Therapy Department [Internet]. Healthcare Executive. [cited 2021 Jul 7]. Available from: https://www.healthcare-executive.in/blog/tdesigning-the-new-age-oncology-radiation-therapy-department

van der Merwe D. Planning a Radiotherapy Department. Clin Oncol. 2017 Feb 1;29(2):105–9.

Mc Morrow A. Radiation Shielding and Bunker Design. Biomed J Sci Tech Res [Internet]. 2019 May 17 [cited 2021 Jul 7];18(1). Available from: https://biomedres.us/fulltexts/BJSTR.MS.ID.003106.php

Wu S, Zheng D, Liu Y, Hu D, Wei W, Han G. Radiation Therapy Care During a Major Outbreak of COVID-19 in Wuhan. Adv Radiat Oncol. 2020 Jul 1;5(4):531–3.

Internationale Atomenergie-Organisation. Radiotherapy facilities: master planning and concept design considerations. Vienna: IAEA; 2014. 31 p. (IAEA human health reports).

Acosta R, Brick W, Hanna A, Holder A, Lara D, McQuilen G, et al. Radiotherapy optimAl Design: An Academic Radiotherapy Treatment Design System. Math Fac Res. 2009 Jan 1;47.

Mohan G, T P AH, A J J, K M SD, Narayanasamy A, Vellingiri B. Recent advances in radiotherapy and its associated side effects in cancer—a review. J Basic Appl Zool. 2019 Feb 27;80(1):14.

Spencer K, Jones CM, Girdler R, Roe C, Sharpe M, Lawton S, et al. The impact of the COVID-19 pandemic on radiotherapy services in England, UK: a population-based study. Lancet Oncol. 2021 Mar 1;22(3):309–20.

27 Rehabilitation and Allied Health Therapies

The Rehabilitation-Allied Health Unit provides a multidisciplinary rehabilitation service and therapies to improve the status of a patient suffering from an impairment, disability or is handicapped.

The Rehabilitation-Allied Health Therapies include (but is not limited to):

1. Physiotherapy including:
   (a) Gait Analysis.
   (b) Hydrotherapy.
   (c) Manual Therapy.
   (d) Electrotherapy.
   (e) Electromyography.
   (f) Laser Therapies.
2. Occupational Therapy.
3. Speech Therapy.
4. Podiatry.
5. Audiology.
6. Orthotics.

The department of Physiotherapy shall mainly be described here.

The facilities of these departments are utilized both by inpatients and outpatients. Apart from this, the services of the department are also utilized by long-term patients with a slow recovery rate. This is a department where the majority of patients attend on a daily basis. This department has to provide services to the patient both in the department or in the indoor patient wards/rooms also.

27.1 Location of Physiotherapy Department

As the patients suffer from various abnormalities, they may find it difficult to go to the upper floors of a building. Hence, the ground floor is the ideal location for this department. As the department has to serve both the outpatients and the inpatients, a location convenient to both areas would be preferable (Fig. 27.1).

27.2 Layout of the Physiotherapy Department

The Department of Physiotherapy shall include the following:

Physiotherapy	Entrance
	Reception and Enquiry
	Waiting Area
	Registration
	Examination room with Exam. cubicles
	Electrotherapy
	Thermotherapy
	Massage Therapy
	Laser Therapy
	Traction
	Gymnasium
	Administrative Rooms
	Store
	Public Utility for Faculty
	Public Utility for Patients and Attendants
	Trolley Bay

A. Garg, A. Dewan, *Manual of Hospital Planning and Designing*,
https://doi.org/10.1007/978-981-16-8456-2_27

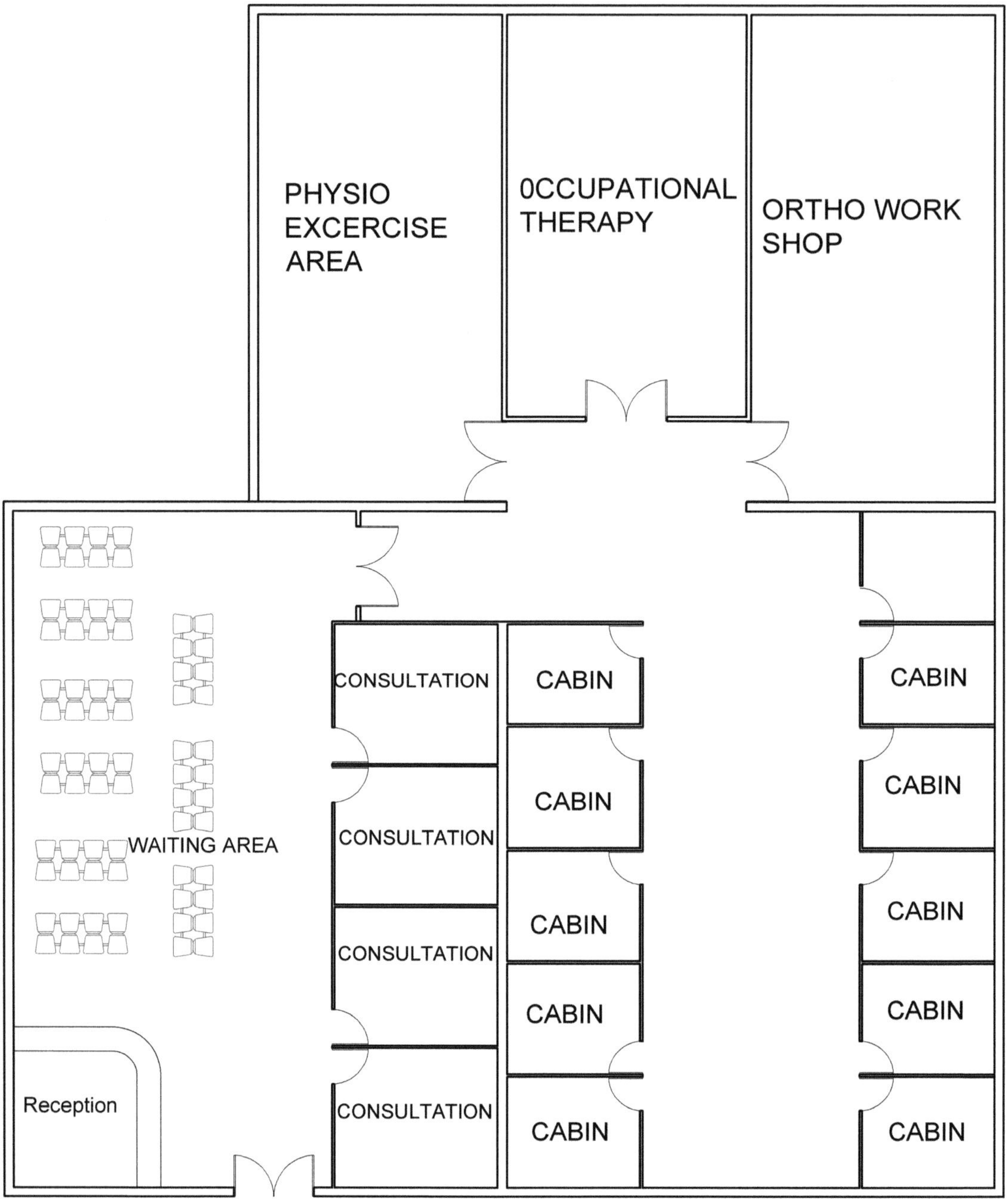

Fig. 27.1 Sample layout drawing of Department of Physiotherapy

27.3 Entrance/Entrance Lobby

If the department is located in a separate building, it shall have a separate entrance. The main issues relating to the reception shall be seen in the chapter of **'Entrance Lobby'** (Chap. 15) as given in this book.

27.4 Reception

The Reception of the department shall be at the entrance of the department. For details of the reception, please refer to the chapters **'Entrance lobby'** (Chap. 15) and **'Out-Patient Department'** (Chap. 17) given in this book.

27.5 Waiting Areas

The Waiting area shall be provided at the entrance lobby of the department. For details of the waiting area, please refer to the chapters **'Entrance lobby'** (Chap. 15) and **'Out-Patient Department'** (Chap. 17) given in this book.

27.6 Examination Room with Exam. Cubicles

The department shall be provided with an Examination room. For details of the examination rooms, please refer to the chapter **'Out-Patient Department'** (Chap. 17) given in this book.

27.7 Patient Therapy Areas

27.7.1 Physiotherapy

Physiotherapy area shall be provided with the following zones:

1. Physical Exercise Zone.
2. Electrotherapy.
3. Laser Therapy.
4. Thermotherapy.
5. Massage Therapy.
6. Traction Therapy.
7. Gymnasium.

First of all, the total physiotherapy shall be divided into the different zones as shown in the drawing below.

As the privacy of the patient shall be maintained, all these zones shall be provided with individual cabins for each modality. These cabins can either be made up of wall with civil work or by the partition of material like aluminium or board. As far as the exercise zone is concerned, it can be in one single hall and the cabins need not be provided. The following issues shall be considered while designing the cabins:

1. Each modality of service shall have a separate cabin, e.g. Traction to have a separate cabin, wax bath in a separate cabin, ultrasound therapy in a separate cabin and so on.
2. The size of the cabin shall be about 2743 mm × 1829 mm with a single door the width of which shall be 762 mm–914 mm.
3. The cabin shall be provided with a treatment couch sizing 1829 mm × 762 mm.
4. The required instrument trolley shall be provided in the cabin to place the machine.
5. The cabin shall be provided with sufficient electrical points for:
   (a) Light and fan of the cabin.
   (b) A pair of 6/16 A switches/sockets for providing power to the medical equipment. If required, more than one such pair of power supplies shall be provided.
6. The cabin shall be properly air-conditioned with a temperature between 18 and 23 °C.
7. One small cupboard shall be provided in the cabin, to store the accessories of the equipment and/or other items like linen.
8. For some modalities, instead of the couch, a chair or stool may be required. The same shall be provided.
9. If a mirror is required in the cabin to assist the patient, the same shall be provided.
10. For thera belts, required hooks shall be provided.
11. For ice pack therapy, the provision of the refrigerators shall be done in the cabin.
12. The cabins shall have outlets of Oxygen and Suction through the MGPS lines of the hospital. The outlets shall be fixed on the wall or in the bed head panel. If the distance of the building is more from the main hospital building, and the MGPS pipeline cannot be taken to the rehabilitation department, then a small manifold shall be created in the rehabilitation department itself. Similarly, for suction, a small suction pump shall be provided. For more details of MGPS please refer to the chapter **'MGPS'** (Chap. 30) given in this book.
13. In the cabins, the provision shall be given for monitor stands to install the Multi-parameter Monitor in case required. But a wall-mounted stand shall be provided in all the rooms.

14. **Nurse and Emergency Call Systems**
 Nurse call systems in all individual cabins including the Exercise area shall be provided.

For the Exercise zone, the following issues shall be kept in mind:

1. This zone can be accommodated in a single hall having sufficient spaces for installing all the equipment and modalities used in the exercise.
2. All the wall-mounted exercise modalities shall be properly screwed to the wall.
3. The required mirrors shall also be provided on the walls.

27.7.2 Occupational Therapy

The Occupational Therapy area shall be located adjacent to the Physiotherapy area, with ready access to waiting and amenities areas. The main issues related to occupational therapy are as follows:

1. The Occupational Therapy rooms and Workshop shall have larger spaces provided to enable a range of static and dynamic activities to take place.
2. The rooms shall be provided with spaces for installing tables for training the table based activities like sewing machine, woodwork and toys preparation.
3. The Rooms should be sized according to the number of patients to be accommodated, the activities to be undertaken etc.
4. Benches shall be fixed with sinks and shall be accessible by wheelchair.
5. Proper shelves, cupboards shall be provided for storage of equipment or tools.
6. Prefer the tables and chairs with adjustable height.
7. Handwashing basin with liquid soap and paper towel fittings shall be provided.
8. Provide Pinboard and whiteboard for displays.
9. A sufficient number of electrical outlets shall be provided for the tools and machinery to be used in the therapy.
10. Workshop areas shall have suitable air extraction and supply in the room. Air exchanges shall be preferred.

27.8 Administrative Area

The Rehabilitation department shall have the rooms to be used for general administrators, managers and clerical staff managing the department. The room shall be provided for:

27.9 In-Charge Rehabilitation Department

The room of the In-charge of the department shall be about 4572 mm × 4267 mm. The room shall have an adequate arrangement of cabinets, drawers and racks for smooth working. Some office tables and chairs shall also be provided. Preferably the room shall have an attached toilet. If required a separate store shall be attached to this room. The room shall also have proper arrangements for electrical points, intercom connection, IT network, CCTV surveillance and air conditioning.

27.10 Secretarial Staff

For a secretarial room, the room size shall be about 6096 mm × 4572 mm. The room shall have an adequate arrangement of cabinets, drawers, racks for smooth working. Some office tables and chairs shall also be provided. Preferably the room shall have an attached toilet. If required a separate store shall be attached to this room. The room shall also have proper arrangements for electrical points, intercom connection, IT network, CCTV surveillance and air conditioning.

27.11 Store

A store shall be provided in the rehabilitation department for storage of general items, stationery, old equipment not in use and other daily use items. The store shall be at least 3048 mm × 3048 mm in size, which may be increased or decreased according to the requirement. Adequate lockable cupboards, racks and drawers shall be provided in the store. The store shall also have a countertop.

27.12 Trolley Bay

The department shall be provided with the space for parking of the stretcher trollies and the wheelchairs. This area shall be provided near the entrance of the department. The parking area shall have power outlets for recharging electric wheelchairs and scooters when they are not in use.

27.13 Clean Utility

The clean utility is a room attached to the department that is used for storage of the clean linen. The sterilized material like drums and drapes are also stored in this room. Normally, the room shall not be less than 3048 mm × 3048 mm. But depending on the requirements, the size of the room can be changed. The room is provided with closed cabinets, drawers and racks. This room shall have only one door of about 3 ft.

27.14 Dirty Utility/Sluice Room

The dirty utility is a room attached to the department which is used for storage of the soiled linen. From here the linen is moved for pre-wash before sending it to the laundry. Normally, the room shall not be less than 3048 mm × 3048 mm. But depending on the requirements, the size of the room can be changed. The room is provided with covered linen collection hampers or containers to collect the dirty linen. This room shall have two doors of about 914 mm. One door opens in the department and the other in the corridor or outside the building from where the laundry staff can collect the linen and he/she need not come to the department for collection of linen. Air from this room shall be exhausted hence the exhaust fans are a must.

27.15 Change Rooms

At times, with the patient's clothes which he/she is wearing it becomes difficult to provide the therapy. Hence the change rooms are provided in the department to enable the patient to remove the outside clothes and change to the hospital dress. The room shall be of the size of approximately 3048 mm × 3048 mm. The room shall have adequate provision of personal lockers to keep the belongings of the patient. There shall be adequate hooks on the wall to hang clothes. Also, a hanger rod shall be provided with hangers to hang clothes. There shall be a cabinet to keep the sterilized dresses.

27.16 Other Issues About the Infrastructure of the Rehabilitation Department

While designing the department, the following issues shall be kept in mind:

1. The handwashing facilities shall be provided near each treatment space and shall have a provision of liquid soap and paper towel fittings.
2. The department shall be provided with the Resuscitation trollies with emergency tools and medicines in case of any emergency. The trollies shall be placed at a convenient place so that in an emergency, these can be easily and quickly wheeled to the required place.
3. Temperature, colour and lighting

   Care shall be about environmental factors such as temperature, humidity and ventilation. The air-conditioning shall be done in the department and the temperature shall be between 18 and 23 °C.

4. Natural Light/Lighting

   Wherever possible, the use of natural light shall be maximized for easy working of the staff.

5. Information Technology/Communications

   The department shall be provided with Intercom Lines at all the required places. Also, computer networking points shall be provided in the examination cubicles, reception and the cabins where the machines are required to be connected to the computers. At all the required places RJ45 jacks shall be provided in the department.

6. Electrical Services

   Apart from the electrical points, at all the required places the pair of 6/16 A switch/socket points shall be provided and all the computer points shall be backed up by UPS supply.

7. For the safety of the patients, handrails, grab bars and other support mechanisms shall be provided in the department.
8. The department shall be provided with wall guards and corner guards.

Further Reading

PRIME PubMed | Planning a new physiotherapy department--a personal experience [Internet]. [cited 2021 Jul 7]. Available from: https://www.unboundmedicine.com/medline/citation/7323205/Planning_a_new_physiotherapy_department__a_personal_experience_

28 Pharmacy Unit

In the hospital, the Pharmacy has an important role as it is the centre to disburse medicines, injectable, surgical disposables like catheters, cotton and bandage to all the inpatients and outpatients of the hospital.

Let us understand the working of the pharmacy department. In the hospital, there are two places where drugs have to be disbursed. One is for the inpatients and the second is for the outpatients.

Generally, for the inpatients, drugs are disbursed directly from the pharmacy store to the respective wards and there is no requirement of a separate drug distribution counter. Whereas in the case of Outdoor patients, a retail pharmacy counter needs to be provided.

The Pharmacy store or counter basically is a licensed facility and the Licence has to be taken for all the stores separately. A separate licence shall be required for outdoor pharmacy retail counter and the inpatient pharmacy. Both these licenses shall be for retail shops. If the hospital disburses drugs in wholesale, another license shall be required for wholesale pharmacy. Similarly, for dealing with the scheduled Narcotics drugs like Ketamine separate licenses will be required.

There are various combinations of providing Pharmacy services in the hospital. Those can be:

1. The hospital has a self-owned Pharmacy both for inpatients and for outpatients.
2. A Private Retail Pharmacy is provided both for inpatient and for outpatients.
3. Hospital has a self-owned pharmacy for inpatients and a Private Retail shop for outpatients.

Whatever the case may be, the hospital shall have two pharmacies, one for inpatients and the second for outpatients.

28.1 Location for the Pharmacy

For Outpatients, the pharmacy shall have a retail counter somewhere near the OPD block and shall be easily accessible to the patients. The best location can be at the exit point of the OPD block.

For inpatients, the pharmacy shall be provided at any place in the hospital where access is not common. It can either be in the basement or on the service floors.

28.2 Size of the Pharmacy

The size of the pharmacy shall depend on the number of patients to be served, numbers of formulations to be disbursed, the quantity of items to be stored etc. What is more important is that the size of the stores shall be large enough for storage of the drugs and disposables equal to the consumption of at least one month.

A. Garg, A. Dewan, *Manual of Hospital Planning and Designing*,
https://doi.org/10.1007/978-981-16-8456-2_28

28.3 Infrastructure of Pharmacy

The requirements of inpatient pharmacy and the outpatient pharmacy are more or less the same except for a few differences. Generally, the following are required in the pharmacy:

Pharmacy	Entrance
	Storage and Disbursing Hall
	Bulk Storage
	Cooled Storage
	Expiry Drug Room
	Costly Drug Room
	Drug Sorting Room
	Narcotics Drug Store
	Pharmacist Office
	Public Utilities for Staff

28.4 Pharmacy for Outpatients

The Outpatient Pharmacy of the hospital shall be centralized (all spaces in one complex) and shall be connected to key departments of the hospital like OPDs and emergency. The pharmacy shall have the following infrastructural facilities:

28.4.1 Entrance

There shall be one single entrance to the pharmacy unit. The entrance shall have a single door with a width of about 1829 mm. The door shall be openable on both sides. The door shall be guarded round the clock.

28.4.2 Drug Receiving Area

Within the Pharmacy, space or enclosure shall be provided where the drugs received from the suppliers shall be placed. After proper counting and quality verification, the drugs shall be moved to the respective store for shelving. This enclosure shall be about 3658 mm × 3658 mm. The area shall be provided with racks and shelves, an office table and chairs. The area or enclosure shall be lockable with restricted access of the staff. The receiving area shall be provided with a workstation for recording initial receiving/validation of medication orders.

28.4.3 Disbursing Hall

Disbursing hall is the main place where the routine drugs and disposables are stored and are disbursed to the patients. The following are the issues relating to designing of disbursing hall:

1. The size of the hall shall depend on the number of patients being served, the quantity and number of drug formularies to be disbursed.
2. The hall shall have the provision of racks divided into shelves for storage of the drugs. The racks shall either be made out of wood or stainless steel. The height of the racks shall not be more than 2134 mm the depth of the shelf shall be about 305 mm and the height from shelf to shelf shall be about 305 mm.
3. As an alternative to the racks, built-in cupboards can be provided on the walls of the hall which are divided into shelves.
4. The shelves shall be able to bear the load of the drugs stored in them.
5. For bulky material like cotton, pads, splints and walkers space can be provided above the rack above the height of 2134 mm. To operate this a double stand step ladder can be used.
6. For small and costly drugs lockable drawers and cabinets shall be provided.
7. On the front wall of the pharmacy, transaction/pass-through windows shall be provided. At least one such window shall be provided for every 50 patients being served during a day.
8. Below these transaction/pass-through windows, a working counter shall be provided for working of the staff. This counter shall be used for installing computers to be used for billing.
9. The counter shall have lockable drawers for keeping some collected cash.

10. Proper electrical points shall be provided on the working counter to supply power to the computers and printers.
11. Above the transaction or pass through windows, or on sides of such windows, a display case can be provided to display the general items being sold in the pharmacy.
12. An office table and chair shall be provided in the hall for the Pharmacist, who shall keep a watch on the working of pharmacy.
13. The pharmacist shall be provided with a computer system connected to the hospital network.
14. This area shall have restricted entry and shall be guarded.
15. Some refrigerators shall be provided in the room to store drugs requiring cold chains.

28.4.4 Bulk Storage

Usually, the pharmacies place orders in bulk for fast-moving items like fluids. Once the stock is received, it becomes difficult to store the entire lot in the disbursing hall and has to be stored at another place. Therefore, a bulk store shall be provided. This bulk store can either be located within the pharmacy complex or at any other convenient place. The size of the bulk store shall entirely depend on the requirements. This store shall have heavy-duty racks to store the cartons of the material. Accordingly, racks shall be designed. The room shall have a single door and the width of the door shall be about 1219 mm. The store shall be lockable and free from any kind of moisture. Special care shall be taken that the store is fire resistant, hence the electrical points shall be provided outside the store. In the store, only one or two light fittings shall be provided. Windows are not required in this store. Direct sunlight shall be avoided in the store.

28.4.5 Cold Store

A cold walk-in store shall be provided in the pharmacy for storing specific drugs which require a cold chain or are to be kept under cool temperatures. This cold room shall be located very near to the disbursement hall. It shall be better if the door of the cold room opens in the disbursement hall. This room is also called the refrigerated room. The size of the room shall be about 3048 mm × 3048 mm. The walls and the ceiling of the room shall be made out of a puff panel which acts as a thermal barrier. Inside the room, the air-conditioning is done and the temperature is kept between 5 and 12 °C and is adjustable as per requirement. The door of the room is also made out of the puff panel and is hermetically sealed. The flooring is generally made out of wooden planks. For storage, open racks are provided along the walls. The room shall be provided with a temperature monitoring system and connected to a centralized alarm/warning system. All access doors to this room shall be lockable.

28.4.6 Expiry Drug Room

Usually in any pharmacy, the expiry of the drugs is the main issue, and if not controlled properly, huge losses may occur. Efficient management always keeps a close track of the expiry of the drugs. As most of the drug manufacturers have a policy of replacing the near to expiry drugs, the pharmacist shall return the near expiry drugs well in time. To keep track of expired and near expiry drugs, most of the pharmacy software's have a provision of keeping track of the expiry dates and giving warning well in time. Once the pharmacist knows which drug is near expiry the same shall be removed from the shelf and kept in a separate place. This space shall be a separate room under lock and key. This place is termed as Expiry Drug Store. The store shall be about 3658 mm × 3658 mm. The room shall be provided with racks and shelves to store the drugs. This store shall be near to the disbursing hall. The room shall have a single door and the width of the door shall be about 1067 mm. The store shall be lockable and free from any kind of moisture. Special care shall be taken that the store is fire protected, hence the electrical points shall be provided outside the store. In the store, only one or two light fittings shall be provided. Windows are not required in this store. Direct sunlight shall be avoided in the store.

28.4.7 Costly Drug Room

Some drugs in any pharmacy are very costly, and there are a lot of chances of pilferage of such drugs, and if not controlled properly, huge losses may occur. Efficient management always keeps a close track of the costly drugs. Hence such drugs shall be stored in a separate room and shall always be under lock and key. Only authorized persons shall be allowed to enter the room. This room shall be termed as Costly Drug Room. The room shall be about 3048 mm × 3048 mm. The room shall be provided with racks and shelves to store the drugs. This room shall be attached to the disbursing hall. The room shall have a single door and the width of the door shall be about 1067 mm. The room shall be lockable and free from any kind of moisture. Special care shall be taken that the room is fire protected. Windows are not required in this room. Direct sunlight shall be avoided in the room.

28.4.8 Drug Sorting Room

While disbursing the stripped medicines in retail, at times it happens that the cut strips are left out. Secondly, due to the return of the medicines, these returned medicines have to be kept back on the shelf. Before placing these cut strips and returning drugs back on the shelves, they need to be sorted out. Therefore, a separate room shall be provided to sort out such drugs and strips. This room shall be termed as a Drug Sorting Room. The room shall be about 3048 mm × 3048 mm. The room shall be provided with racks and shelves to store the drugs. Also, the working counter along with the chairs shall be provided where the staff can sit and sort out the drugs. This room shall be attached to the disbursing hall. The room shall have a single door and the width of the door shall be about 1067 mm.

28.4.9 Narcotics and Controlled Drug Store

The pharmacy dealing with Narcotics and Controlled drugs shall always be alert to purchase, disburse and store these drugs. Hence such drugs shall be stored in a separate room and shall always be under lock and key. Only authorized persons shall be allowed to enter the room. This room shall be termed as Narcotic Drug Room. The room shall be about 3048 mm × 3048 mm. The room shall be provided with racks and shelves to store the drugs. This room shall be attached to the disbursing hall. The room shall have a single door and the width of the door shall be about 1067 mm. The room shall be lockable and free from any kind of moisture. Special care shall be taken that the room is fire protected. Windows are not required in this room. Direct sunlight shall be avoided in the room.

28.5 Pharmacy for Inpatients

The Inpatient Pharmacy of the hospital shall be centralized (all spaces in one complex) and shall be connected to key departments of the hospital like ICUs, Emergency, Operating Unit and IPD.

The pharmacy of inpatients shall have the same design, except that, in the disbursing hall the disbursing counters and windows are not required. Except this, all other areas/rooms, as mentioned above in outpatient pharmacy shall be provided.

28.6 Pneumatic Tube Systems

For a fast and efficient service of the pharmacy, the Pneumatic Tube Systems (PTS) systems shall be provided in the inpatient pharmacy.

The PTS is an air-operated system having the air pump attached to the control station. This system is used as a transport system of documents, material and medicines. This is the best, accurate and quickest mode of transport for documents, specimens, material and medicines.

In this system, at all the important points of the hospital (called stations) where the drugs have to be sent or from where the drugs have to be transported, the outlet of this system is installed along with the control unit. These areas can be ICUs, Emergency, Operating Room, Indoor wards etc. The carrier box (Capsule) carries the documents from the user department and supplies drugs to the user department.

It is very easy to operate. The user department has to just put the drug indent in the capsule and send it to the pharmacy. The pharmacy shall pack the drugs as required and send back the drugs to the same user. In seconds, the material or document is transported to the desired location.

28.7 Pharmacist Offices

Offices shall be provided for the Pharmacist near to or inside the pharmacy complex. These rooms shall be separate for inpatient pharmacy and outpatient pharmacy. The size of these rooms shall be about 4572 mm × 4267 mm. The rooms shall have an arrangement of office tables, executive chair, visitor chairs, side racks etc. The rooms shall have an attached Toilet. The rooms shall also have an attached P.A. room for the clerk to be seated. If required and long working hours are expected, a small restroom can also be provided with these rooms. The rooms shall have proper arrangements for electrical points, intercom connection, IT network and air conditioning.

28.8 Automation in the Pharmacy

The pharmacies are undergoing a lot of automation like using robots for filling up and disbursing the drugs and use of drug dispensing machines. The designer while designing the pharmacy shall consider all the requirements and issues relating to the automation. If need be the manufacturer of the automation equipment shall be contacted before planning.

Further Reading

ADVANCES IN HOSPITAL PHARMACY SERVICES: AN OVERVIEW [Internet]. PharmaTutor. [cited 2021 Jul 7]. Available from: https://www.pharmatutor.org/articles/advances-in-hospital-pharmacy-services-an-overview

Swensson ES. An Innovative Design in Hospital Pharmacy Facilities. Am J Hosp Pharm. 1971 Jun 1;28(6):440–6.

Taylor EN. Obesity, Weight Gain, and the Risk of Kidney Stones. JAMA. 2005;293(4):455.

Blum A, Merino GSAD, Merino EAD. Design strategies in hospital pharmacy department: Mapping a medication system. Strateg Des Res J. 2018 Jan 15;11(1):15–20.

Kay BG, Boyar RL, Raspante PS. Designing a modern hospital pharmacy. Am J Hosp Pharm. 1986 Feb 1;43(2):339–43.

Carroll N, Richardson I. Enablers and barriers for hospital pharmacy information systems. Health Informatics J. 2020 Mar 1;26(1):406–19.

Five pharmacy automation trends [Internet]. [cited 2021 Jul 7]. Available from: https://www.hfmmagazine.com/articles/2345-five-pharmacy-automation-trends

Gones V. HOSPITAL PHARMACY MANAGEMENT: AUSTRALIAN AND INDONESIAN PERSPECTIVES.: 196.

Pharmacy design can streamline patient care - Architecture [Internet]. Healthcare Facilities Today. [cited 2021 Jul 7]. Available from: https://www.healthcarefacilitiestoday.com/posts/Pharmacy-design-can-streamline-patient-care%2D%2D2720

Pharmacy Design, Design a Pharmacy [Internet]. [cited 2021 Jul 7]. Available from: https://www.pharmacydesign.org/Articles-PharmacyDesignTrends-0608.htm

Augusto V, Xie X. Redesigning pharmacy delivery processes of a health care complex. Health Care Manag Sci. 2009 Jun 1;12(2):166–78.

Sabzghabaee AM, Badri S, Ashari HE, Hosseini SM. The design and equipments of hospital pharmacies in Isfahan, Iran. J Res Med Sci Off J Isfahan Univ Med Sci. 2010;15(4):219–24.

Coblio NA. The Impact of Pharmacy Work Design on Pharmacist Productivity.: 176.

29 CSSD

The importance of sterilization cannot be overemphasized in any of the hospitals. Sterilization is a process through which the instruments, linen, O.T, Rooms and other parts of the hospital are made free from microorganisms and hence the prevention of infections in the hospital is made sure. The process of sterilization destroys all the microorganisms, whether disease producing or non-disease producing. In the hospital, while discharging its duties, one should safeguard human life, and that operative skill may be made as effective as possible. Hence it is necessary that adequate sterilization procedures be carried out.

The Central Sterile Services Department (CSSD) in the hospitals is an integrated place that performs sterilization of medical devices, instruments, linen and consumables. This is a support department for other hospital departments. The main operations of this department are cleaning, preparing, disinfecting, packing and sterilization of reusable medical devices, linen and surgical instruments.

A Central Sterile Supply Department (CSSD) should be established in the hospital to supply sterile dressings and sets to the wards and departments, including the operation theatre. The CSSD department should be a centralized department with all the modern equipment for effective sterilization.

The process of the sterilization can be broadly divided into the following categories:

1. Cleaning of the instruments and the linen before preparing for sterilization and Preparation for sterilization.
2. Pre-sterilization packing.
3. Sterilization.
4. Storing after sterilization.
5. Distribution of the sterilized material to the users.

Normally the following items are sterilized in the CSSD

1. Surgical Instruments.
2. Dressing drums.
3. Linen of O.T and Emergency.
4. Disposables.
5. Bedding.
6. Equipment.

29.1 Methods of Sterilization Processes

As the effectiveness of the sterilization depends upon the methods used for sterilization. Some of them being:

1. Dry Heat sterilization.
2. Steam sterilization.
3. Chemical sterilization.
4. Gas sterilization.

A. Garg, A. Dewan, *Manual of Hospital Planning and Designing*,
https://doi.org/10.1007/978-981-16-8456-2_29

5. Formaldehyde sterilization.
6. Fumigation.
7. Cidex sterilization.
8. Radiation sterilization.
9. Filtration sterilization.
10. Boiling sterilization.

29.2 Infrastructure of CSSD

The CSSD department shall have the following zones/room.

Central Sterile Supply	Staff Change
	Dirty Receipt
	Washing/Disinfection
	Assembly/Packing
	Sterilization
	Sterile Storage
	Delivery Room
	ETO Room
	CSSD Supervisor
	Staff Room
	Public Utility for Staff

29.3 Location

CSSD should be located as near as possible to the main user likes operation theatres, intensive care areas etc. Therefore, CSSD should be on the same floor or the floor immediately above or below the Intensive or operating floor.

At times, due to the limited availability of spaces, the CSSD cannot be provided near to the OT and may have to be located at some other location or floors. Under such cases, a dedicated sterile material elevator shall be provided, which shall open in the user's area like OT Complex and ICU Complex (Fig. 29.1).

29.4 Area Required for CSSD Department

Requirement of the area depends mainly on:

1. The workload of the department, which again is dependent on the number of OT's and ICU's.
2. Number of sterilization cycles that have to be run per day.
3. Operation hours of the CSSD (whether 24 h or for limited hours).
4. Number of sterilizers required in the department.
5. Type of sterilization to be done like Steam sterilization, ETO, Hot Air sterilization, Chemical Sterilization etc.
6. The equipment to be installed like instrument washer, ultrasonic cleaner etc.
7. Packing load of the department.
8. Number of sets of instruments prepared per day.

All these factors are important to decide the area that shall be required for the CSSD. Still, some standards have been worked out relating to the area required for CSSD. Minimum area requirement shall not be less than 1.39 Sq. Mtr. per bed (Minimum area of 27.87 Sq. Mtr. is required if the hospital is small).

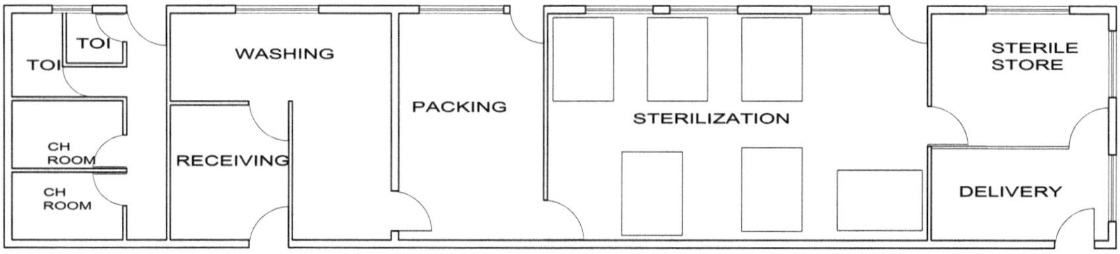

Fig. 29.1 Sample layout drawing of CSSD

29.5 Material Flows

While designing the CSSD, it is very important to keep in mind that the flow of material in the CSSD shall be unidirectional (one way), no backwards movement is allowed. It means the unsterile material shall enter from one end of the CSSD and shall be out after sterilization from the other end of the CSSD.

29.6 Functional Zones of CSSD

The CSSD shall have the following Zones:

1. Receiving Zone (Unclean Area).
2. Decontaminating, Washing and Disinfecting Zone.
3. Packing Zone.
4. Sterilization Zone.
5. Clean Storage Zone.
6. Clean Supply Zone.
7. Support Zone.

29.7 Receiving Zone (Unclean Area)

This area is demarked for receiving the material from various departments, which require sterilization. e.g. the surgical instruments are received from the OT Complex, Linen from the laundry etc. This can also be called the reception area of the CSSD.

The following issues shall be addressed to for the receiving zone

1. An area to act to receive the material coming in the CSSD.
2. Size of this Receiving area shall be about 3048 mm × 3048 mm.
3. Visual access shall be available from inside to main entrance door of the CSSD.
4. This room shall have proper working tops for unpacking and sorting.
5. The room shall be provided with racks and cupboards to stock the material till it is further processed.
6. All entrances should be secured to prevent access by unauthorized people.
7. The receiving room shall have either a window or a door to receive the material. A glass partition with lockable sliding hatch between this area and the corridor can also be provided.
8. Red-lines shall be applied at the receiving area to demarcate the movement of material and trolleys to enter the CSSD via this entrance.
9. The material is usually transported to this area with the help of trolleys. Hence the room shall have sufficient space for parking of the trolleys bringing the material in. A lockable hatch for trolleys shall be provided.
10. For the movement of such trolleys, it is better if dedicated material elevators are used.
11. The room shall have a provision for a computer connection to make the entry of material received in the department.
12. The room shall have a provision for Hand washing facilities with liquid soap dispenser and the paper towel dispenser.
13. The receiving area shall have.
    (a) Intercom outlets.
    (b) RJ 45 for data points.
    (c) Electrical outlets for computers and printers etc.

29.8 Decontaminating, Washing and Disinfecting Zone

The Decontamination area is where instruments are rinsed, ultrasonically cleaned (if required), washed/decontaminated and dried. Instruments may be tracked by using an instrument tracking system. Decontamination involves the use of automated and manual cleaning to remove harmful blood-borne pathogens on the surfaces of instruments. The contaminated articles are sorted, disassembled, pre-rinsed and cleaned in this decontamination/dirty area. Waste items are sorted into suitable containers for appropriate disposal. If items are heavily soiled, the automated cleaning process by instrument washer or ultrasonic disinfectors are used. The area shall be used for

1. Manual cleaning of instruments and Linen etc. not suitable for automated cleaning.
2. Disassembly and inspection of contaminated materials.
3. Rinsing of instruments and equipment.
4. Sorting and loading of medical instruments and equipment into trays/washer-disinfectors and other automated cleaning equipment.

This area shall have

1. Space for installation of the Automatic Instrument washer (Single door or double door) with a provision of the water supply line and required drain. The machine shall be mounted on the prescribed foundation. The required electrical outlets shall be provided. The earthing of the machine shall be done.
2. Similar arrangements shall also be done for the Ultrasonic cleaner.
3. The size of the decontamination and washing area shall be about 4267 mm × 3658 mm for both of them.
4. For manual cleaning, a double bay sink (one for cleaning and one for rinsing) along with the drain board fixed in the benches shall be provided. The sink shall be deep by at least 1 ft. and made out of 304-grade stainless steel. The size of the sink shall be about 457 mm × 610 mm. Proper arrangement for hot and cold water supply and drain shall be done. The benches shall also be made out of stainless steel.
5. The washing area shall also be provided with the outlet of compressed air (can be supplied from the piped medical pipeline) blowguns.
6. If need be, the pre-treatment area can be provided, where removal of pollutants is done with the help of an automatic cycle. This area shall be at "negative pressure" compared with the surrounding environment to reduce the risk of contaminating the other areas of treatment.
7. Handwashing facility with liquid soap dispenser and paper towel dispenser shall be provided.
8. The air-exhaust system shall be provided in this area.
9. Sufficient wall-mounted brackets for hanging cleaning chemicals and brushes shall be provided.
10. Space to park trolleys shall be provided.
11. Hatch window for the transfer of hand-washed items to the packing area and return of empty trays.
12. Deionized, distilled or reverse osmosis (RO) water for final rinsing is required.
13. Drying rack—workspace must be available for drying manually cleaned instruments.

29.9 Packaging Area

After decontaminating and washing the instruments, they are forwarded to the packing area for assembling them into pre-defined sets or trays. Instruments and other items that are prepared for sterilization must be packaged so that their sterility can be maintained to the point of use.

29.9.1 Location

Packing area shall be located between the Decontamination area and the Sterilization area, with a unidirectional workflow from contaminated to clean areas.

29.9.2 Role of the Packing Room

1. Inspecting, functionality testing, assembling and packing cleaned and disinfected medical devices and accessories, according to predetermined required standards, in preparation for sterilization.
2. Packs are checked, reassembled, double-wrapped, labelled, dated and signed on the checklist by the packer.
3. Delivering items to the sterilizer loading area.
4. Returning racks to the decontamination area.

29.9.3 Packing Room

Ideally, the size of the packing room shall be 4572 mm × 4267 mm. However, the size can be increased or decreased as per requirement.

1. The packing room shall be provided with packing tables of about 2438 mm × 1524 mm. The table is divided into two parts lengthwise. In the centre, a rack (914 mm height) with shelves is fixed. Hence four staff members can sit simultaneously for packing of the material. This table shall be made out of stainless steel.
2. One or more stainless steel countertops shall also be provided to pack the sets for cutting of the gauze of cotton rolls. Packing table(s) shall be about 2000 mm × 700 mm × 800 mm high, with a shelf below its surface and a basket rack above it.
3. The areas of the packing room shall be strictly marked for the purpose it is to be used. Like instrument preparation, linen folding and consumable packing etc.
4. A storage area for new surgical instruments may be created. These new instruments will serve as a backup of any devices that might arrive damaged.
5. The packing room shall be a sterile area that shall be positively pressurized. The pressurization shall be created just as it was created in the case or Operating Rooms. For details, please refer to the chapter of OR (Chap. 19).
6. Sealed windows can be provided in this room.
7. Sufficient wall-mounted brackets for equipment shall be provided.
8. The area must be divided by a hard barrier from the decontamination area, in order to prevent cross-contamination.
9. Packing tables require power connections for use with computers and instrument scanners.
10. A hand washing basin shall be provided at the perimeter of the room to avoid water contamination of wrapped instrument sets with a provision of the liquid soap dispenser and paper towel dispenser.
11. Equipment wise the room shall be provided with sealing machine, cloth cutters, heavy duty scissors and surgical trays, drums etc.
12. Hatch window or door shall be provided between the packing area and the sterilization room for transferring the material for sterilization.

29.10 Sterilization Area

Sterilization is an area where the actual processing is undertaken to make the packed materials like instruments, linen and consumables free from any kind of unwanted organisms which may harm the patient. Hence Sterilization is a defined process used to render a surface or product free from viable organisms, including bacterial spores. Depending on the product, this procedure could vary from steam sterilization, dry heat sterilization to low-temperature sterilization processes.

The sterilization area also is used for cooling the sterilized material before being sent to the clean storage room. The Sterilizing and Cooling Area provides accommodation for sterilizers and parking space for sterilizer and cooling trolleys. Following the unloading of the sterilizer, packs should not be handled until cool. Specialized sterilizers, such as ethylene oxide, require separate installation and accommodation. Low-temperature specialized sterilizers require separate installation according to manufacturer's recommendations.

29.10.1 Location and Relationships

The Sterilizing and Cooling area should be located between the Packing area and the Clean Storage area.

29.10.2 Main Activities of the Sterilization Process

The following activities are performed in the sterilization room;

1. Loading trolleys are parked.
2. Loading of the Sterilizers.
3. Unloading of the sterilizers.
4. Cooling of the sterilized packs.

29.10.3 Size of the Sterilization Room

The size will be dependent on the number and type of sterilizers installed and whether single or double-door. However, on average, the area per sterilizer shall not be less 9.29 Sq. Mtr.

29.10.4 Methods and Types of Sterilizers

Depending on the methods or load of the material to be sterilized, the type and size of the sterilizers are decided and provided. The sterilizers can be;

29.10.5 Steam Sterilizers

Steam under the pressure, greater than atmospheric, increases the temperature of steam for thermal destruction of microbial life. Death by moist heat in the form of steam under pressure is caused by the denaturation and coagulation of protein or the enzyme-protein system within the cells

1. Vertical Sterilizers.
   (a) Single drum.
   (b) Double Drum.
2. Horizontal Sterilizers.
   (a) Rectangular Sterilizers.
      - Single Door Sterilizers are available in different sizes and can be chosen as per the requirement.
      - Double door sterilizers are available in different sizes and can be chosen as per the requirement.

   (b) Cylindrical Sterilizers.
      - Single Door Sterilizers are available in different sizes and can be chosen as per the requirement.
      - Double door sterilizers are available in different sizes and can be chosen as per the requirement.

29.10.6 Ethylene Oxide Gas Sterilizer (ETO)

Ethylene oxide is used to sterilize items that are heat or moisture sensitive. Ethylene oxide (EO) is a chemical agent that kills microorganisms, including spores, by interfering with the normal metabolism of protein and reproductive processes (alkylation) resulting in the death of cells. Used in the gaseous state, EO gas must have direct contact with microorganisms on or in items to be sterilized.

29.10.7 Dry Heat Sterilizer

Dry heat in the form of hot air is used primarily to sterilize anhydrous oils, petroleum products, and bulk powders that steam and ethylene oxide gas cannot penetrate. Death of microbial life by dry heat is physical oxidation or slow-burning process of coagulating the protein in cells.

29.10.8 Hydrogen Peroxide Plasma Sterilizer

Hydrogen peroxide is activated to create a reactive plasma or vapour. It can be produced through the action of either a strong electric or magnetic field. Free radicals of the hydrogen peroxide in the space of the chamber of sterilizer, interact with the cell membranes, enzymes, or nucleic acids to disrupt the life functions of microorganisms.

29.10.9 Requirements for the Infrastructure of Steam Sterilizer

While setting up the steam sterilizers, the following issues shall be kept in mind. Depending on the type (Single Door or Double Door), the requirements may differ.

1. The single door sterilizer is installed adjoining the outer wall of the room.
2. An empty space of about 914 mm shall be kept between the sterilizer and the wall.
3. If the sterilizer is a double door unit, the unloading door shall open in the clean storage room. The common wall between the sterilization room and the clean storage shall be punctured, and then the sterilizer should be installed.
4. The sterilizer shall be installed on the foundation prepared for this purpose.
5. The sterilizer shall be securely bolted to the foundation with the help of fasteners.
6. An exhaust duct shall be connected to the sterilizer, which shall open outside the room by crossing the wall of the room.
7. Required electrical outlets shall be provided for supply to sterilizer.
8. Proper RO water line shall be provided.
9. Drain shall be provided on the floor below the sterilizer.
10. In the front side, free space of about 2438 mm shall be provided to load the sterilizer.
11. If more than one sterilizers are being installed, the distance between the two shall not be less than 1828 mm from each other.
12. Preferably sterilizers should be located in a restricted access area.
13. A hand washing basin shall be provided at the perimeter of the room with a provision of the liquid soap dispenser and paper towel dispenser.
14. The ventilation system should be designed so that air flows out of the sterilization area (via positive pressure).
15. Circulation space shall be adequate for the free and unhindered manoeuvring, loading and unloading of sterilizer trolleys.
16. If the vertical steam sterilizer is installed, nothing specific has to be done, but the sterilizer has to be placed on the floor. However, proper electrical points, water supply and drain shall be provided.

29.10.10 Requirements for the Infrastructure of ETO Sterilizer

While installing the ETO Sterilizer, the following issues shall be kept in mind.

1. The ETO sterilizer shall be installed in a separate room.
2. Depending on the size of the ETO sterilizer and model of the sterilizer (Tabletop or floor model), the size of the room shall be decided.
3. An empty space of about 914 mm shall be kept between the sterilizer and the wall.
4. An exhaust pipe for the drain of ethylene oxide gas shall be provided and shall be connected to the sterilizer, which shall open outside the room by crossing the wall of the room and shall terminate above the height of the building. A copper pipe or stainless steel is recommended for this purpose.
5. Required electrical outlets shall be provided for supply to sterilizer.
6. In the front side, free space of about 1524 mm shall be provided to load the sterilizer.
7. If more than one sterilizer is being installed, the distance between the two shall not be less than 1829 mm from each other.
8. Preferably sterilizers should be located in a restricted access area.
9. If the ETO cartage is being used, the proper waste disposal system shall be provided. However, if the ETO cylinders are used, the proper connection from the cylinder to the sterilizer shall be provided.

29.11 Clean Storage Area

After sterilization of items is complete, these have to be stored in the sterile area. Therefore, a room shall be provided for the storage of processed sterile material, including trays and drums etc.

29.11.1 Location of the Clean Storage Room

The sterile storage area should be located adjacent to the sterilization area, preferably in a separate, controlled, enclosed, limited-access area, the only function of which is to store sterile supplies.

29.11.2 Designing of the Storage Shelves

The storage room shall be provided with Stainless steel racks and/or alternately lockable cupboard made out of stainless steel. Some of these racks or the cupboards, as the case may be, shall be divided with the bins. Others can have open shelves. These racks shall be adjoining the walls of the storage room. The height of the racks can be about 1829 mm, and the width shall be according to space in the room. Better is if the width is kept to 914 mm each. Then multiple racks of 914 mm the width can be placed side by side. The shelves shall be 375 mm deep, easily cleaned and allow air to circulate around stored packs. Freestanding or mobile shelving provides a practical solution for handling the flow of products in and out of storage and cleaning. If the room size is bigger, the racks can be placed in the centre of the room to allow access from all sides of the racks. Open shelving is more commonly used as it allows dust to pass through making them easier to clean than solid shelves. For bins, the size of bins can be 305 mm × 305 mm × 305 mm each.

Packs should be stored away from direct sunlight and water and should not be stored next to or under sinks or on the floor where they are likely to get wet or damaged. Sterile packs should be stored at least 250 mm above the floor, and 450 mm below the ceiling or sprinkler heads and at least 50 mm from side walls to allow for air circulation in the room and to prevent contamination during cleaning.

The following issues shall be kept in mind while designing the clean storage room;

1. The size of the storage shall depend on the quantity of the material to be stored and also on the time period for which generally the material is held in the storage.
2. No window shall be provided in the room.
3. Direct sunlight shall be avoided in the room.
4. The entry to the storage should be restricted, and a person should be allowed to this area only after he has washed up and changed the clothes.
5. In this area, there shall be racks (as described earlier) of different sizes and the sterilized materials are kept in the racks for the use.
6. All the sets kept in the sterilized area should be marked for the date of sterilization so that if the set is not used within the sterilization life, it can be re-sterilized.
7. Ventilation, humidity and temperature control are required. The temperature of the room shall be between 18–22 degree and the RH around 40%.
8. The room shall be positively pressurized with filtration as in the case of OR's.
9. The storage shall be fitted with doors and shall be lockable.
10. This room shall be attached to the delivery counter. The material required to be delivered shall be moved from this room to the delivery counter.
11. The sterile area shall have arrangements for washing of the room and fumigation.

29.12 Delivery Counter

The delivery counter shall be at the extreme end of the CSSD from where the sterile material shall be delivered to the users. This area shall have a delivery counter to place the material to be immediately issued. Upon demand, the staff shall bring the required material from the sterile store, place it on the delivery counter, make the proper entries and deliver the material. The counter shall have a delivery window for the delivery of material. The size of the window can be 914 mm–1219 mm in length and 914 mm height.

Outside the delivery windows, sufficient space shall be provided for parking of the trolleys that arrive to collect the material. Here a computer station is provided for managing the delivery of materials and the transport documentation.

29.13 Support Areas

The support area to the CSSD are such areas that are not directly involved in the sterilization process, but directly or indirectly support the CSSD department. These are like;

29.13.1 Staff Changing Rooms

There are two different changing areas, one for the staff in the unclean area, another for the staff in the packaging and sterile areas. The details are.

29.13.1.1 Changing Rooms for the Unclean Area

Two pass-through changing rooms for males and females shall be provided in the unclean area. The change room maybe just at the entrance of the CSSD. Each changing room shall have an attached toilet.

29.13.1.2 Changing Rooms for Packaging and Sterile Area

If possible, a separate set of change rooms shall be provided at the entrance of the clean storage room, these change rooms shall be separate for males and females. Each changing room shall have an attached toilet.

While designing change rooms, the following needs to be considered;

1. Separate change rooms shall be provided, one for males and the second for females.
2. The room shall be of the size 3048 mm × 3048 mm.
3. The room shall have a provision of an attached toilet.
4. Furniture wise, the room shall have chairs and cupboard.
5. Almirah shall be provided with the provision for hanging the clothes.
6. Also, the room shall be Air Conditioned and the Control button with temperature adjustment shall be provided in the room.
7. In the change room, staff lockers shall also be provided where the staff can keep their personal belongings. Individual lockers shall be about 305 mm × 305 mm. These individual lockers can be combined and the locker almirah can be fabricated. Each locker shall be lockable separately. One such locker shall be allotted to one staff.

29.13.2 Administrative Area

The CSSD shall have room to be used for general administrator and clerical staff managing the CSSD. The size of this room shall be about 4572 mm × 4267 mm. But depending on the requirement and number of persons likely to sit, the size can be increased or decreased. The room shall have an adequate arrangement of cabinets, drawers, racks for a smooth working. The office tables and chairs shall also be provided. Preferably the room shall have an attached Toilet. If required a separate store shall be attached to this room. The room shall also have proper arrangements for electrical points, intercom connection, IT network, CCTV surveillance and air conditioning.

29.14 Finishing Details of the CSSD

29.14.1 Walls

1. Walls should be washable and painted with the anti-bacterial and anti-fungal paints. The vinyl-coated walls can also be used.

2. Walls should be adequately protected against damage by loose equipment and wheeled traffic by buffer rails and corner guards.

29.14.2 Ceilings

1. A ceiling height of shall be at least 2800 mm from the floor level.
2. Proper air vents shall be provided to control the temperature of the air.
3. Shall be washable, impermeable and non-porous.
4. Walls should be washable and painted with the anti-bacterial and anti-fungal paints.

29.14.3 Floors

1. Carpet or similar soft flooring should be avoided.
2. Impermeable, non-slip floor flooring shall be used. If tiles are used, there shall be no gaps in between and the tiles shall be joint less. PVC welded sheet vinyl coved up the wall can also be used.

29.14.4 Doors

1. Door shall be wide enough to allow trolley movement, and doors and corridors should be wide enough to accommodate trolley turning circles and protruding trolley fittings.
2. Door frames and door leaves should be designed and finished with protection cladding and bumper rails to withstand the inevitable bumps by trolleys.
3. Doors shall be adequately sized to allow clear passage of current as well as possible future equipment.
4. Automatic/semi-automatic doors make it easier for the collection and distribution of trolleys. If not automated doors should be self-closing. If the design allows it, doors shall open towards the higher pressure side where possible to overcome problems with weakening door closers, which may lead to lock-outs.
5. Vision panels shall be provided in the doors.

29.14.5 Sound/Noise

Noise must be controlled, and the threshold shall not exceed 60dBA (decibel). The walls and ceilings should be made of absorbent materials so that they do not reflect sound. Insulation of sterilizers and washer-disinfectors shall be thought off.

29.14.6 Natural Light

Natural lighting is highly desirable, especially in the work areas, and should be used wherever possible, especially in areas such as the cleaning and packing areas. However, direct sunlight on workspaces should be avoided.

29.14.7 Electrical Points

1. The sufficient number of 6/16 Amp electrical outlets shall be provided to supply power to all the appliances.
2. For higher load appliances, the connection shall be done with the help of the starters or directly with the proper rated MCB.

29.14.8 Lighting

1. Light fittings shall be fully recessed and selected to prevent dust and insects from entering.
2. LED type of light fittings shall be used and the light levels shall be not less than 400 lux.

29.14.9 Air Conditioning

The air conditioning and ventilation systems in the CSSD have an important role that can have an effect on air bacterial contamination. While during the design and implementation, particular attention shall be paid to the following issues;

1. The air conditioning of the areas such as changing rooms, administrative areas shall be without air recirculation and shall be designed as for other such areas of the hospital.

2. For clean areas like decontamination areas, packing areas, sterilization and clean storage areas, the provision shall be made for the required air exchanges. The design of such areas shall be the same as is done in the case of clean rooms.
3. To ensure proper air exchanges, a dedicated air-handling unit complete with primary air heating, cooling, humidification, dehumidification and filtration shall be used.
4. The temperature in the CSSD shall be between 18–22 °C and the Rh shall be about 40%.
5. Airflow should be designed so that air flows out of clean areas into dirty areas via positive pressure. Positive air pressure is required in the "clean" areas of the unit to reduce air movements into these areas from the "dirty" areas of the unit.

Acknowledgement I am grateful to Dr. Rohit Varshney for his great support in compiling this chapter. I wish to convey my thanks and gratitude to him for his time and efforts he has put in.

Further Reading

3 Design Considerations for Sterile Processing Departments [Internet]. HALYARD. [cited 2021 Jul 10]. Available from: https://www.halyardhealth.com/articles/sterilization/3-design-considerations-for-sterile-processing-departments/

Gonzalez P, Jacob MO. CENTRAL SERVICE: A systematic approach to design of efficient facilities layout. Hosp Top. 1969 Apr 1;47(4):119–26.

Hospaccx. Central Sterile Services Department Planning & Designing [Internet]. hospital and healthcare consultancy in india. 2019 [cited 2021 Jul 10]. Available from: https://hhbc.in/central-sterile-services-department-planning-designing/

Banu A. Central Sterile Supply Department – Need Of The Hour.:5.

Sen DJ, Saha DM. Central Sterile Supply Department: A Concept.:2.

CENTRAL STERILE SUPPLY DEPARTMENT: Planning Considerations | Healthcare Architecture [Internet]. [cited 2021 Jul 10]. Available from: https://healthcarearchitecture.in/central-sterile-supply-department-planning-considerations/

Swenson D. Designing and Developing a Central Sterile Supply Department. Biomed Instrum Technol. 2013 May 1;47(3):259–65.

Allison VD. Hospital Central Sterile Supply Departments. Br Med J. 1960;2(5201):772–8.

By JZ, Cao Y, Zhao H, Liran, Huang J, Zhu L, et al. MODERN CENTRAL STERILE SUPPLY DEPARTMENT ARCHITECTURAL DESIGN CONCEPT AND PRACTICE-NAVY GENERAL HOSPITAL CSSD DESIGN PRACTICE. Chin Hosp Archit Equip. 2014;(7):79–81.

Basu D, Bhattacharya S, Mahajan A, Ramanan VR, Chandy M. The Importance of the Central Sterile Supply Department in Infection Prevention and Control. Infect Control Hosp Epidemiol. 2014 Oct;35(10):1312–4.

The Leaflet Article [Internet]. [cited 2021 Jul 10]. Available from: https://www.hcarefacilities.com/newsletter/article.asp?id=1596

Piped Medical Gas Supply System (MGPS)

30

Medical gases are one of the main support services used in hospitals. Medical gases are specific gases that are separated from the air individually for various medical applications. Commonly used medical gases in hospitals are:

1. Oxygen (O_2).
2. Nitrous oxide (N_2O).
3. Medical air 400 KPa or 4 bar (MA 4).
4. Medical air 700 KPa or 7 bar (MA 7).
5. Carbon dioxide (CO_2).
6. Nitrogen (N_2).
7. Medical vacuum.

30.1 Oxygen (O_2)

Oxygen is the most important gas on the earth and the air of the planet contains about 21 percent of the Oxygen component. Apart from the respiration of human beings, it is also used to drive anaesthesia machines and ventilators in addition to other methods for manual ventilation like Ambu bags. Three sources are used for oxygen supply: Liquefied oxygen tank also called Vacuum-Insulated Evaporator (VIE), Gas Cylinders and Oxygen Concentrator (PSA) system. Further, oxygen is coded in white colour.

30.2 Nitrous Oxide (N_2O)

Nitrous oxide is a medical gas administered via an anaesthesia machine. It is mixed with oxygen and various anaesthetic agents. Therefore, operating rooms are the sole location where nitrous oxide gas is used. Usually, a manifold supply system is the source of nitrous oxide gas. Cylinders and the pipelines for Nitrous Oxide are coded with blue colour.

30.3 Compressed Medical Air 4 Bar

In general, medical air 4 is used for respiratory applications. The source of supply can be a centralized medical compressor plant. The colour code is black.

30.4 Compressed Medical Air 7 Bar

Medical air 7 is known as surgical air because it is used mainly to derive the surgical equipment like drills, tourniquet and bone saw etc. The supply source is similar to medical air through a compressor plant.

A. Garg, A. Dewan, *Manual of Hospital Planning and Designing*,
https://doi.org/10.1007/978-981-16-8456-2_30

30.5 Carbon Dioxide (CO_2)

Carbon dioxide is a medical gas used for insufflations purpose in the laparoscopy procedures. Usually, portable cylinders are the source of CO_2, which are coded with grey colour.

30.6 Nitrogen (N_2)

Nitrogen for surgical power tools is likely to be used only on the sites where there is availability for the production of synthetic air.

30.7 Medical Vacuum

The medical vacuum is provided by means of a vacuum central plant. The vacuum system shall always be used in conjunction with vacuum control units that include vacuum jars. In fact, it is not a gas, it is a negative pressure used for suctioning patients and for anaesthetic gas scavenging systems. Vacuum pipes are known for its yellow colour.

30.8 System Components

For supplying all these gases to the ultimate point of use, a set of components equipment is to be installed. This system starts right from the source of the gas till the outlet point on the patient bed. Combined all such system components are called MGPS systems. Each medical gas must be supplied through a separate system. Under no circumstances the gases can be mixed or cross-connected between systems.

30.9 Sources

Source is the system by which the gases are produced for flow through piping networks. There are different sources for medical gases, which vary from gas to gas. Each gas has a different source of production. These can be:

30.9.1 Bulky Systems

The bulk system may consist of specially insulated vessels, vaporizers etc. These systems can be constructed with cryogenic vessels or a high-pressure manifold, depending on the usage. Typically, oxygen, nitrous oxide and carbon dioxide are supplied to large hospitals in cryogenic tanks.

30.9.2 Manifold Systems

The manifold system is basically a set of gas cylinders connected in a series and forming a bank of cylinders. All the cylinders of the bank operate simultaneously. Generally, there are two such banks, out of which one bank is operational and the second is as a backup to be used when the first bank is empty and so on. For the operation of the bank, the control panel is installed which consists of primary and secondary regulators, pressure regulators and warning lamps.

30.9.3 Central Plants

Few gases like Medical air and the Vacuum supply are produced through the central plants. The central plant consists of the compressor pumps and the vacuum pumps. Generally, the pumps are installed in pairs, i.e. two compressors and two vacuum pumps. The pair of pumps operate one by one so that one pump is operational at a time and automatically switched to another pump at a set interval of time. These pumps are connected to the storage tanks. The storage tank is in turn connected to the pipeline. The pumps are automatically controlled by the Control Panel.

30.9.4 Generators

The oxygen is also produced by the Oxygen concentrators. These concentrators take air from the atmosphere, separate the oxygen component and fill up the tanks, from where it is supplied to the pipeline.

30.10 Piping Networks

All the Medical gases and vacuum are transported and distributed in the hospital through the copper pipeline distribution system to provide gas or vacuum at the end-point or terminal units. The pipes shall be made of high-quality copper, seamless type and non-arsenic. Moreover, it shall be protected against physical damage and corrosion and colour coded as per gas content.

The copper pipes are available in different sizes. The pipe size varies in Outer Diameter (OD), Inner Diameter (ID) and wall thickness. Some of the general pipe sizes are:

76 mm outer dia., 1.5 mm thick
54 mm outer dia., 1.5 mm thick
42 mm outer dia., 1.2 mm thick
28 mm outer dia., 0.9 mm thick
22 mm outer dia., 0.9 mm thick
15 mm outer dia., 0.9 mm thick
12 mm outer dia., 0.7 mm thick

30.10.1 Pipeline Installation

1. Material for pipes shall be phosphorus deoxidized, non-arsenical copper.
2. Other fittings for connection to copper pipes, for example valve and control panel fittings, may be of copper, brass, gunmetal or bronze to the appropriate standard.
3. All pipes must be cleaned and degreased for oxygen service and be free of particulate matter and toxic residues. They must be individually capped at both ends and delivered to the site identified as medical gas pipes.
4. All pipe jointing fittings and sub-assemblies of fittings for connection to pipes must be cleaned and degreased for oxygen service and be free of particulate matter and toxic residues. They must be individually sealed in bags or boxes and delivered to sites identified as medical gas fittings.
5. For jointing of the pipes and fittings, except for mechanical joints, copper-to-copper joints only will be permitted on site, made with brazing filler rods which can be used without flux and in the presence of oxygen-free nitrogen, which will be blown through the pipeline during brazing procedure to prevent the formation of oxides. Carbon dioxide shall not be used as the inert gas shield. This method eliminates the formation of oxide within the pipe, leaving a clean bore. Some slight burnishing may occasionally be observed on sectioned joints. Purging is still required to remove the internal shield gas and the other particulate matter not associated with the brazing operation.
6. Copper joints to brass or gunmetal fittings will require the use of flux, with subsequent cleaning to remove the flux residues and oxide deposits.
7. Heating of the joint for brazing shall be carried out with oxygen/acetylene or acetylene, hydrogen, liquid petroleum gas/ambient air torches. Additional heating may be required for some fittings, for example by means of a second torch.
8. In order to maintain the pipeline cleanliness and prevent the formation of verdigrises' after completion, it will be necessary to maintain the completed system charged with medical air until the installation is finally commissioned. On larger projects completed sections of the pipeline shall be similarly protected.
9. Mechanical (threaded or flanged) joints may be made where pipelines are connected to items such as valves and control equipment. For vacuum pipelines of 76 mm diameter and above, screwed or flanged compression fittings may be used. Mechanical joints shall not be used elsewhere for general pipework installation.
10. Allow joints to cool naturally to room temperature or at least to a temperature at which they can be handled. This is specifically for gunmetal fittings which, if cooled (or quenched) from the brazing temperature by dipping in cold water, could crack.
11. The pipeline shall be adequately supported at sufficient intervals to prevent sagging or distortion. For support, the PVC saddles shall be used. The saddles are fixed on the wall

with the help of screws and the pipe is supported on these saddles. Supports for surface mounted pipework shall provide clearance to permit painting of the surface.

12. For easy identification of the pipelines, the pipes shall be painted and with the prescribed colour and colour banding. Colour band identification shall be applied near to valves, junctions, walls etc. A band shall be 150 mm wide.

Oxygen	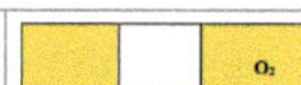
Nitrous Oxide	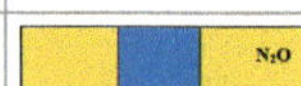
Oxygen/Nitrous Oxide Mixture	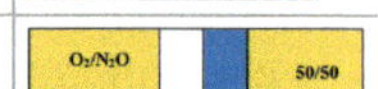
Medical Air	
Medical Vacuum	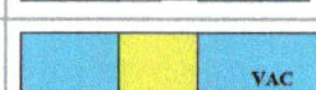

30.10.2 Valves

Valves are provided in the MGPS system to control the flow of the gases. Basically, two types of valves are provided in the system. Those are zone valves and service valves. Zone valves are used to isolate large areas of the system, like halls of floors. These valves are usually required to switch off the gases for maintenance or repair of the system. Whereas service valves are used to isolate small parts of the system like room for modification and/or repair.

Valve Boxes are available according to the number of gases for which it has to be used. Some are like:

5 Services
4 Services
3 Services
1 Services

30.10.3 Warning and Alarm Systems

The function of warning and alarm systems is to give alert in case of failure of the system or otherwise in case of inadequate pressures of gases. There are usually 2 types of alarms. One is the Master Alarm and second is the Area alarm. Master alarm monitors the main gas lines and sources conditions. Area alarms are used to monitor the conditions of specific smaller areas. For each gas service, there shall be pressure switches for high and low pressure. These conditions of pressure shall be clearly indicated on the alarm system with the facility to provide a common audio-visual alarm. All visual signal panels shall be permanently labelled having clear identification of the areas, rooms or departments served. Flashing visual signals shall have alternate periods on and off mode. When a warning or alarm signal occurs and the system condition subsequently reverts to normal, the corresponding visual and audible signals shall automatically reset to normal. The signal must re-sound after a nominal 15-minute period if the fault condition still exists.

Area Line Pressure Alarm Boxes are available according to the number of gases for which it has to be used. Some are like:

Area line Pressure Alarm up to 5 gases
Area line Pressure Alarm up to 4 gases
Area line Pressure Alarm up to 3 gases
Area line Pressure Alarm up to 2 gases

30.10.4 Gas Outlets

Outlets are the last endpoints of the MGPS from where the gases are delivered to the patients. The terminal units may be either wall- or pendant-mounted. The connectors are plugged in these outlets which in turn are connected to the delivery pipes through which the gases are delivered. Outlets shall be gas-specific and also colour coded as per standards.

30.10.5 Secondary Equipment

Other material, instruments required for MGPS systems are hoses, gas flow meters, gauges and vacuum regulators. Though these items are not part of the pipeline system, they contribute substantially to gas and vacuum consumption.

30.11 Designing the MGPS System

Before installation of the MGPS system, the most important factor is to design the system based on the present requirements as well as the future planning of increasing the outlets. There are a few issues to be considered before designing the system.

While designing the MGPS system certain norms, as issued by the competent authorities shall be followed. Usually, these norms are country specific. Hence while designing the MGPS system, these country-specific norms shall be taken into account and adhered to.

The factors to be considered are such as:

30.11.1 Analysis of the Area of the Hospital

First of all, the area where the outlets have to be provided shall be analyzed with respect to:

1. Numbers of beds in that area/hall/room.
2. Out of total beds, how many beds have to be provided by MGPS.
3. Location of those beds in the hall/area/room.
4. The purpose for which that area/hall/room has to be used. Whether it is an ICU or a normal patient room.
5. If ICU, what all medical equipment dependent on gas supplies are to be used, like Invasive Ventilators, Non-invasive ventilators and High Flow Nasal Cannula.
6. Depending on these uses and equipment decide the type of gases to be supplied, like Oxygen, Air or Vacuum.
7. Number of outlets to be provided on each bed.
8. What type of outlets shall be provided? Whether it will be push type or sliding type.
9. How the outlets shall be fixed. Whether these will be mounted on the wall directly or mounted in the bed head panel or in the ceiling hanging pendant.
10. Anticipate the expansion plans of the hospital relating to building, number of beds where the MGPS has to be supplied.
11. Location of the building expansion plans also has to be analyzed.
12. Determine the locations where the source of gases has to be installed. Like a manifold room, pump room and liquid oxygen tanks.
13. Check the availability of refilling of the Gas cylinder related to the number of empty cylinders available, the capacity of the supplier to supply filled cylinders and distance of the supplier from hospital etc.
14. The average stock of filled cylinders which the hospital wants to maintain at any particular time.
15. Check the estimated consumption of the gases, considering the type of patients that are expected in the hospital. Out of them how many are expected in the critical units.
16. Checks the estimated number of surgeries expected in the hospital.
17. After analysis, schematic drawings shall be prepared for piping layout locating zone valves, area valves, master alarms and area alarms.
18. Design of the technical details of the plant and machinery with their capacities shall be prepared. While designing, issues like estimated length of pipelines, the pressure at the delivery point shall be kept in mind.

30.12 Infrastructure for MGPS

The MGPS system shall have:

1. Liquid Oxygen Tank Area with Landing Bay (If Liquid Oxygen Tank is to be installed).
2. Manifold Room for Oxygen and Nitrous Oxide.
3. Plant room for Compressor, Vacuum units.
4. Medical Gases Control Room.
5. Public Utility for Staff (Fig. 30.1).

30.13 Manifold Room

The manifold room is provided to install the manifold for oxygen and Nitrous Oxide gases in the hospital. The manifold is basically a system

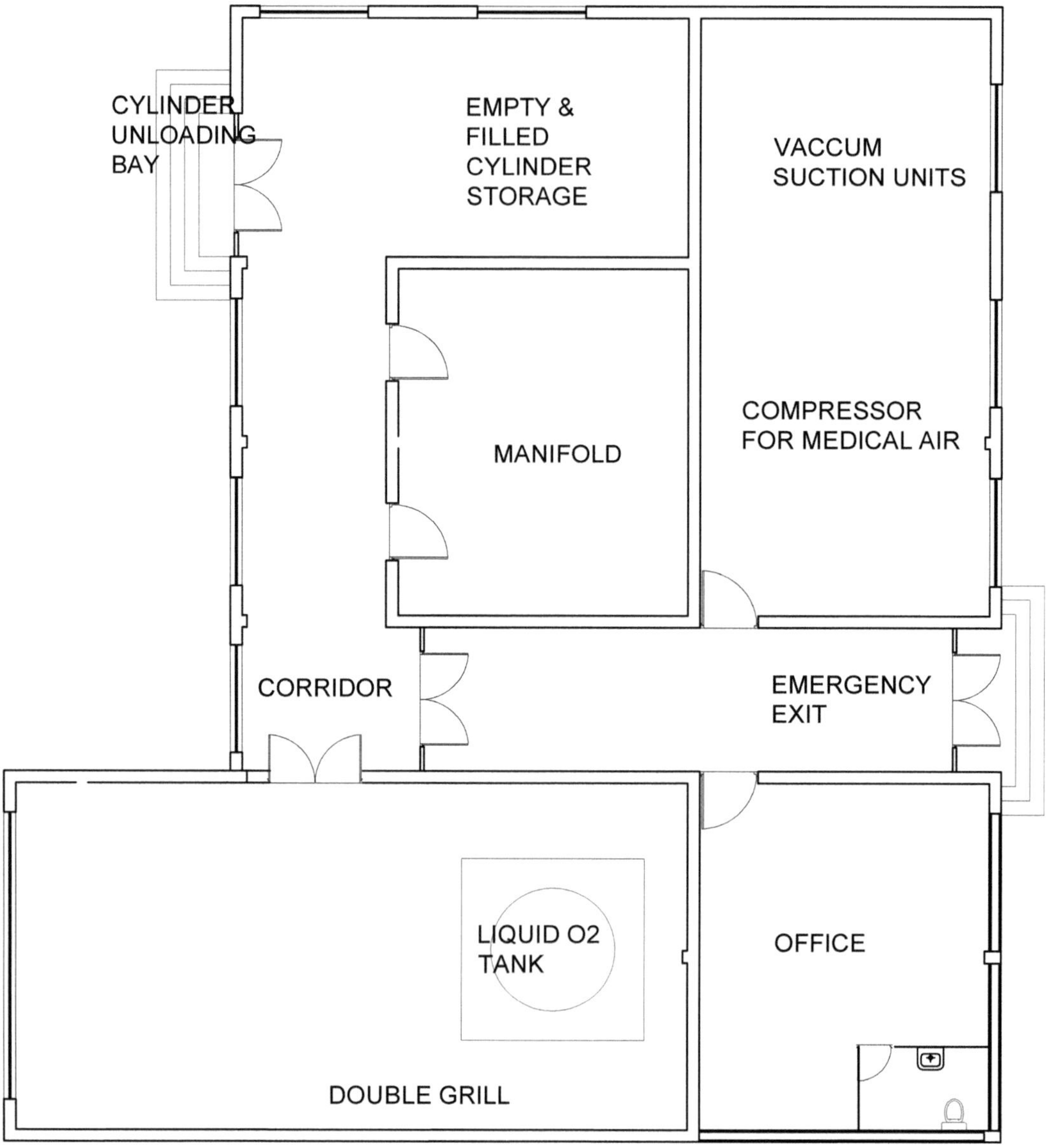

Fig. 30.1 Sample layout drawing of MGPS

where more than one cylinder is connected in series and then is connected to a common outlet. This set of cylinders connected in a series is called a BANK. Usually, 'D' type of jumbo cylinders are used for the manifolds.

A bank of cylinders may have 2 to 20 cylinders. The number of cylinders to be installed in each bank shall be decided as per the design that has been decided as mentioned above. Based on the number of cylinders to be installed in a bank, a common connecting copper pipe is fixed on the wall, and the outlet's sockets are provided on this common pipe at a distance of about 305 mm from each other. One socket shall be provided for each cylinder.

The total storage capacity of the manifolds is usually planned on the basis of one week's consumption of gases. Preference shall be that each bank of the manifold shall hold gases equivalent to at least two days' consumption. Similarly, the unconnected cylinders in stock shall have gases equivalent to at least three consumptions.

The copper tailpipe is attached to these sockets, which in turn are connected to the regulator of the cylinders. Each cylinder shall have a separate tailpipe and regulator. This regulator shall be fixed on the cylinders. Now the common connecting pipe, on which all the cylinders of the bank are attached, is connected to the control panel, which controls the flow of the gas.

The pig tail-pipe cylinder connector for oxygen, nitrous oxide/oxygen mixture (50% v/v) and medical air must be a pin-index yoke connector in accordance with laid down standards. Similarly, the connector for nitrous oxide shall be a side outlet valve connector in accordance with the standards.

It shall be kept in mind that, the temperature of the gas may fall as low as −30 °C as the gas passes through the regulator at maximum capacity, and the equipment shall be designed accordingly.

To complete the manifold, TWO such banks are installed and both are connected to the control panel. One bank is termed as 'Duty Bank' and the other as 'Standby Bank'. The control panel functions to control the flow of gases. As both the banks are connected to the control panel, this panel allows one bank to be operated at a time. As soon as the pressure of the current bank drops, the control panel automatically switches to the other bank. This job is done with the help of pressure regulating valves fitted on each bank. Once the empty bank is cut off, the cylinders of that bank are replaced with the filled cylinders and make ready for the next use.

The Control Panel can either be Automatic or Semi-auto type. The Automatic Control Panel automatically switches between 'Duty Bank' to 'Standby Bank' and visa-versa. Whereas in the case of Semi-auto panel, the warning is issued as soon as the bank pressure drops and the operator has to manually shift to the other bank.

The manifold headers shall be fitted with a non-return valve to allow removal and replacement of any cylinder and to prevent the discharge of a bank of cylinders in the event of pig tail-pipe rupture.

From the Control panel, the outlet is given which is connected with the copper pipe of the main supply line of the gas. The main supply line is the line that transports the gas to the hospital building.

To be on the safer side, it is anticipated that an emergency may arise at any time due to failure of the manifold system. To overcome such an emergency, an emergency manifold with two to four cylinders is also provided. The design of the emergency manifold shall be the same as that of the main manifold, with the difference that no control panel is provided on the emergency manifold.

The output of the emergency manifold is directly connected to the main supply line where the main manifold is already connected. In case of failure of the main manifold system, and as soon as the emergency manifold is switched on, the gas flow starts in the same main pipeline. A non-return valve and isolating valve shall be installed immediately upstream of the reserve manifold connection to the pipeline distribution system.

In the event of loss or failure of the primary source of supply, the emergency/reserve system shall be able to maintain (at least for a short time) the total system flow.

The manifold system is prepared for Oxygen Supply and Nitrous Oxide Supply. So for both the gases the main bank and the emergency supplies shall be provided (Fig. 30.2).

30.13.1 Purging of the System

The manifold shall have a facility of nitrogen purging, to purge any air introduced during cylinder changeover on each tailpipe. The purging system shall be provided with venting outside to allow purging with the working gas before the manifold is made ready for service. The pressure of the nitrogen supply used for purging needs to be set below the minimum operating pressure of the manifold, to prevent the supply of nitrogen to the patient and to prevent overriding of the alarm system.

Fig. 30.2 Sample layout drawing of Manifold

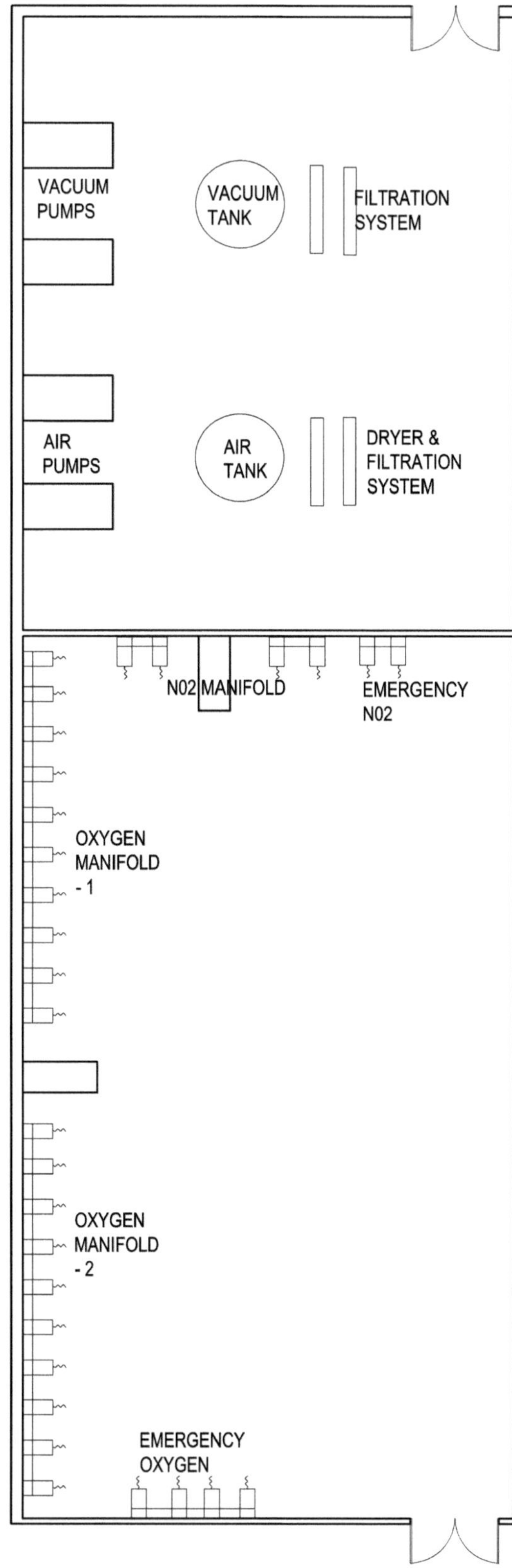

A system of manifolds shall be designed based on the number of outlet points and the requirement of gases. Based on the experience, it is recommended that the following patterns can be considered:

Number of Outlets	Cylinders (per bank) for Primary Supply	Cylinders (per bank) for Emergency Supply
For Oxygen		
Up to 50	4 + 4	1 + 1
50–100	6 + 6	2 + 2
100–200	10 + 10	3 + 3
200–500	15 + 15	4 + 4
Above 500	20 + 20	5 + 5
For Nitrous Oxide		
Up to 5	1 + 1	1
6–10	2 + 2	1 + 1
10–20	4 + 4	2 + 2
Above 20	6 + 6	3 + 3

30.13.2 Location of the Manifold

The manifolds shall be installed in the room/hall. The location of the manifold shall be outside the hospital building. Most important is that there shall be an approach road for the vehicles to reach up to the door of the manifold room. If not, it will be difficult to transport the jumbo cylinders to the manifold room.

Secondly, the room/hall shall be near to the shaft in the hospital building from where the rising main pipeline can be distributed in the hospital building.

At the cylinder unloading point, where the cylinders will fall from the vehicle, a thick wooden plank shall be inserted in the floor, so that the cylinders fall on the wooden plank, hence saving the floor from damage. The size of the wooden plank shall be about 1219 mm in length, 610 mm in width and at least 152 mm thick.

30.13.3 Size of the Manifold Room

The size of the manifold room shall entirely depend on the size of the manifold which in turn shall depend on the number of cylinders in the manifold system. Also, it will depend on the space required for storage of the filled cylinders and the empty cylinders. The movement area shall also be considered. Roughly, 0.28 Sq. Mtr. of area per cylinder shall be allotted.

30.13.4 Fixing the Manifold Systems in the Hall/Room

Three walls of the room/hall shall be used for fixing the manifold systems. One wall (of maximum Length) shall be used for Oxygen manifold. Opposite wall to this shall be used for Nitrous oxide and the third wall for emergency manifolds of both the gases. Depending on the size of the walls the arrangement can also be changed.

30.14 Compressed Medical Air

Medical air is used mainly for operating the Invasive Ventilators and the Nebulizers, as the compressed air is mixed with the oxygen in the ventilator and is provided to the patients. Secondly, it is also used to provide power to certain medical equipment for its operations. The equipment can be like Drill machines and Surgical Saws. Apart from this, it is also used to operate the dental chairs and also used for cleaning the instruments in the CSSD.

Medical air shall be provided at two different pressures: One is at a pressure of 400 kPa, required to drive ventilators and for other respiratory applications; Second is at a higher pressure of 700 kPa which is required to drive surgical tools.

30.14.1 Compressor Air Plant

The production of the medical air is done with the help of the compressor. The plant consists of the Electric Motors, Air Compressors, Air Reservoirs, Automatic/Semi-Automatic Control Panel, Bacteria Filter and the Air Dryer along with the required non-return valves, isolating valves, gauges and pressure switches, an operating and indicating system, an exhaust system and a test point.

First of all, the Electric Motor and the air compressor is mounted on the base frame, are fabricated for this purpose. The coupling of both is done with the help of V-Belts. This base frame (mounted with motor and compressor) is fixed on the pre-constructed foundation with the help of Fasteners. Please ensure to provide the anti-vibration pads while fixing the base frame as the unit creates a lot of vibration when operative. It has to be ensured that the compressors shall be Oil Free Compressors, failing which there are chances that the produced air may have traces of oil, which may be harmful to the patients or medical devices. The compressors shall either be air-cooled or water-cooled as the design may be. The plant shall have all-round access for maintenance purposes and allowance shall be made for changing major components.

The capacity of the compressors and motors shall depend on the air required and the number of outlets. It is measured in cfm.

There shall be a set of two such units as both will be operative reciprocally one after the other after a fixed interval of time.

The outlets of both the compressors are combined and connected to the Air Reservoir. The air reservoir is a tank made out of thick MS steel and is provided with the Air inlet, Air Outlet and the gate valve to drain the water (collected in the tank due to the moisture in the air). The tank's capacity is measured in litres. The capacity for each design varies as per requirement. It can be from 1000 Ltr. to 5000 Ltr. This tank is installed on the raised foundation (say by 152 mm to 305 mm).

From the Compressor, the air is stored in the reservoir. When required, the air comes out of the reservoir through the outlets and is passed through the Filters by increasing the pressure of the air.

30.14.2 Air Filtration

The air normally contains traces of impurities like carbon monoxide, carbon dioxide, sulphur dioxide, nitrogen monoxide and dioxide, moisture and oils. These contaminants can enter the compressed air system from three sources: the atmosphere, the compressor and the pipeline distribution system. Each potential source must be taken into account when specifying the type and location of air treatment equipment. Filtration equipment may include pre-filters, coalescing filters, carbon filters, particulate filters and any other additional filtration equipment necessary to provide the appropriate quality.

Similarly, the dirt particles in the environment cover a wide range of sizes, but approximately 80% are less than 0.2 μm and are therefore not removed by the intake filter to the compressor. Although particles smaller than 40 μm are unlikely to cause mechanical damage, a 5-μm intake filter is preferred, to avoid blockage of internal air/oil separators.

The filtration system can be in different stages depending on the type of filters. It can be from the single-stage filter to four-stage filter.

After passing through the filters the air passes to the Air Dryers. As the air contains moisture, it needs to be dried before sending it further to the user. If it is not dried, the wet air can be dangerous for the patients and also harmful for the medical equipment where it shall be used. The dryer system shall be a twin system so only one is operational at a time and the other is on standby. From time to time switching is done from one to another. There shall be separate power supplies for the 'duty' and 'standby' dryer assemblies taken from the same phase.

Thereafter, the air is connected to the main supply line of the Compressed Air.

The functioning of the air compressors is controlled by the Automatic / Semi-Automatic control panels. The electric connections to the motors are done through this control panel. The control panel switches from one set of compressor units to the other automatically at the pre-set interval of time. At any moment of time, both the compressors shall be in a working condition. If one unit goes out of order, the other unit of compressors shall be able to take the entire load of the air requirement.

30.14.3 Medical Air 400 kPa

The medical air with a pressure of 400 kPa, is mainly used for the operation of the Invasive Ventilators. Medical air is also directly inhaled by patients during ventilation and it may also be used to dilute oxygen before administration because of the potentially toxic effects of pure oxygen. Patient ventilators fall into two main categories—those used during anaesthesia and those used during intensive therapy. Pneumatically powered ventilators can use up to 80 l/min free air continuously. The exact flow requirements will depend on the design of the ventilator.

Medical air 400 kPa is also used for other equipment such as anaesthetic gas mixers, humidifiers and nebulizers. The flow rates normally required would not exceed 10 l/min, and this flow is always in excess of the actual volume respired.

The minimum pressure required at terminal units for respiratory use is 355 kPa at flows of 80 L/min in intensive therapy units and coronary care units; 40 L/min in special care units and operating suites and 20 L/min in ward areas.

While calculating the flow, the diversity shall also be taken into account considering that only 33% of the total points shall be operative at a time.

30.14.4 Surgical Air 700 kPa

The pressure requirements of surgical tools are between 600 and 700 kPa and flows may vary between 200 and 350 L/min. Most surgical tools are designed to operate within this pressure range. Higher pressures are likely to cause damage to tools.

The pipeline systems shall be designed to provide a flow of 350 L/min at 700 kPa at the terminal unit.

Surgical air 700 kPa is only required where surgical tools are to be used like orthopaedic, neurosurgery theatres and possibly plaster rooms. However, to facilitate maximum flexibility, surgical air shall be provided in all theatres. The diversified factor of 25% shall be considered while designing the system. The overall system shall be designed to provide a minimum of 700 kPa at the front of each terminal unit at a flow of 350 L/min.

30.15 Vacuum

The medical vacuum pipeline system provides suction facilities for medical needs, particularly in operation theatres and ICUs.

30.15.1 Vacuum Plant

The creation of the vacuum is done with the help of the vacuum pumps. The plant consists of the Electric Motors, Vacuum pumps, Vacuum Reservoir, Automatic/Semi-Automatic Control Panel and Bacteria Filter with drainage traps along with the required non-return valves, isolating valves, gauges and pressure switches, an operating and indicating system, an exhaust system and a test point.

First of all, the Electric Motor and the vacuum pumps are mounted on the base frame, fabricated for this purpose. The coupling of both is done with the help of V-Belts. This base frame (mounted with a motor and pump) is fixed on the pre-constructed foundation with the help of Fasteners. Please ensure to provide the anti-vibration pads while fixing the base frame as the unit creates a lot of vibration when operative. It has to be ensured that the vacuum pumps shall be Oil-Free. Water-sealed pumps shall not be used. It is desirable if the Rotary vane pumps are used instead of reciprocating vacuum pumps which are now obsolete. The plant shall have all-round access for maintenance purposes and allowance shall be made for changing major components.

The capacity of the pumps is measured in lpm. The exact capacity of the pumps to be installed shall depend on the requirement and number of vacuum outlets.

There shall be a set of two such units as both will be operative reciprocally one after the other at a fixed interval of time.

The outlets of both the vacuum pumps are combined and connected to the Vacuum

Reservoir. The vacuum reservoir is a tank made out of thick MS steel and is provided with the inlet connected to the vacuum pump, and an outlet connected to the filtration system. The tank's capacity is measured in litres. The capacity for each design varies as per requirement. It can be from 1000 Ltr. to 5000 Ltr. This tank is installed on a raised foundation (say by 152 mm to 305 mm).

30.15.2 Filtration System

The vacuum system is normally connected to the bacteria filters. The purpose is that any suction air coming towards the reservoir passes through the filtration system. Therefore, a Bacteria Filter station and secretion trap are provided in the system.

The filtration system can be in different stages depending on the type of filters. It can be from a single-stage filter to four-stage filter.

The functioning of the vacuum pumps is controlled by the Automatic/Semi-Automatic control panels. The electric connections to the motors are done through this control panel. The control panel switches from one set of pumps to the other automatically at a pre-set interval of time. At any moment of time, both the vacuum pump units shall be in a working condition. If one unit goes out of order, the other unit of the pump shall be able to take the entire load of the vacuum requirement.

The medical vacuum pipeline system shall be designed to maintain a vacuum of at least 300 mm Hg (40 kPa) at each terminal unit.

Where vacuum terminal units are provided in ward areas, it is unlikely that more than one terminal unit in any room (single or multi-bed) will be in use at any time. Therefore, the diversified flow shall be taken into account while designing the system.

At the terminal point, the outlet is connected to a Ward vacuum unit complete with regulator and collection bottles. The probe plugged in the vacuum outlet is connected to the ward vacuum unit with the help of the HP tube. HP tube is a High-Pressure rubber tube used for transportation of medical gases.

For Operating Rooms, instead of the ward vacuum units, theatre suction units are used.

30.16 Issues While Designing the Plant Room and the Manifold Room

The following issues shall be taken care of:

1. Two doors shall preferably be provided in the manifold room. One shall be large enough to facilitate cylinder handling and must be on an outside wall. This door must open outwards Second door shall be a normal 914 mm door and may open either outside or inside the manifold room. Exists must be free of all obstructions. All doors must normally be locked to prevent unauthorized access.
2. The internal walls, including any internal doors of the manifold room, shall be suitable non-combustible 2-hour fire-resistant material. Internal doors shall be avoided where practicable. Heat detectors shall be provided.
3. For ventilation louvres shall be provided at both high and low levels in the manifold room, to allow circulation of air.
4. In the plant room due to running of the motors and pumps, a lot of heat is generated. Further, these plants aspirate air from the atmosphere for its operation. Therefore, natural ventilation shall be provided. The ambient temperature of manifold rooms and plant rooms shall be between 18 and 30 °C.
5. In some cases, it may be necessary to provide mechanical ventilation for plant rooms, with supply air facing towards the compressors and pumps. Hence the direct air coolers shall be installed for this purpose.
6. **Noise control:** Plant rooms shall be designed and constructed to ensure the satisfactory control of noise emission. The effect of two vacuum pumps or compressors running together will increase the noise level in the plant room. Therefore, the plant rooms shall be provided with acoustic linings to reduce the noise levels.

30.17 Medical Gases Outlet Terminals

The gas outlets are the endpoint of the MGPS system. The pipelines carrying the gases terminate at this point and are connected to the gas outlets. For further supply of the gases to the user, the probe is plugged into the gas outlet and gases are provided to the patient.

The medical gases outlets are provided depending on the type of gasses like O_2, N_2O, Air and Vacuum. It means the outlets shall be separate and marked properly for each type of gas.

The Outlet shall be installed at the patient bed. Some hospitals prefer to affix the outlets of these gases directly on the wall itself. But nowadays, Bedhead panel is used for fixing the gas outlets. Bedhead panel is a 1524-mm panel made of extruded sections of aluminium. This panel has provisions for fixing the gas outlets and electrical points. Also, this panel has a service railing on which the IV rod, tray and utility basket can be fixed. This panel is fixed at the height of 1524 mm above the floor level and goes up to 1829 mm (Fig. 30.3).

Another option can be the Ceiling suspended pendant. This also has the same facilities as in the case of the Bedhead Panel. This panel is fixed on the ceiling and is suspended below so that the bottom of the pendant shall be a 1524-mm from the floor.

The Gas outlet points are fixed on the back wall of the pendant. On both, the side walls are electrical points and on the front wall shall be the utility tray for bedside multi-parameter vital sign monitor and also the utility basket can be fixed on the front wall. The pendant can revolve at 270 degrees. Further, the pendant can be a single arm or a dual-arm. The single-arm revolves at its own axis only, whereas the double arm pendant can

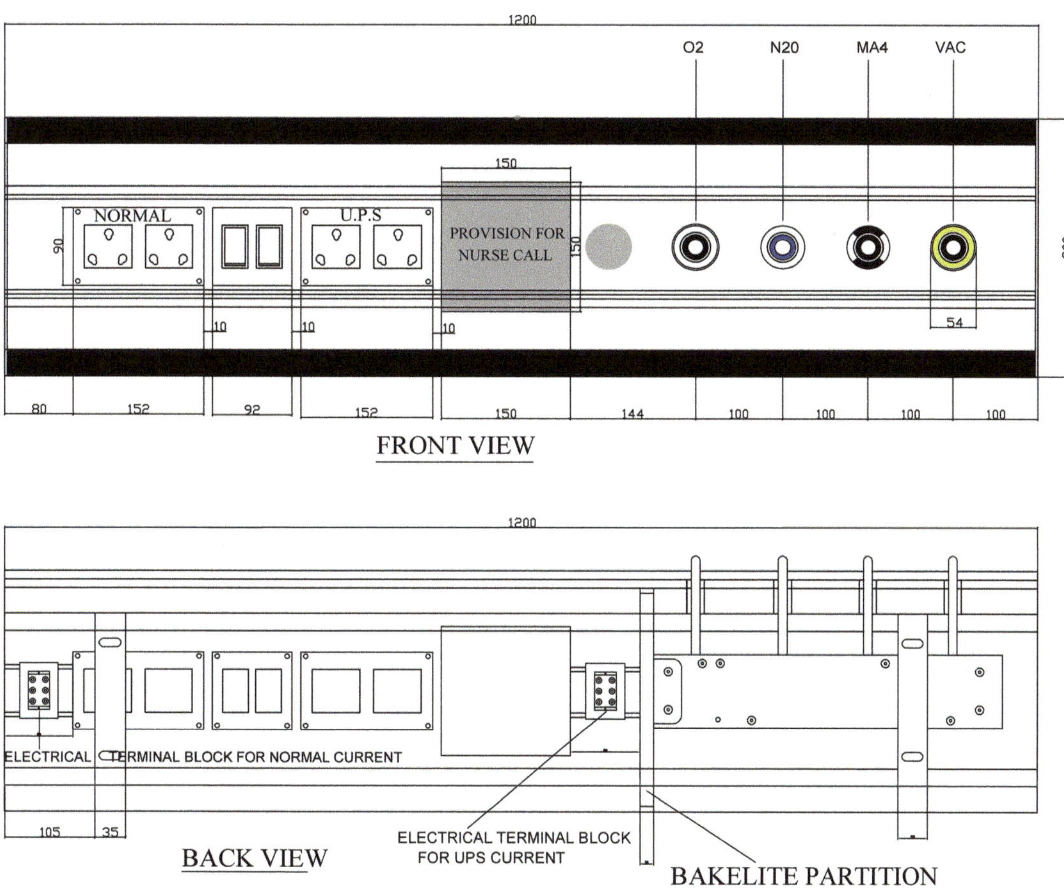

Fig. 30.3 Drawing of the Bedhead Panel for MGPS

revolve on both the arms hence covering more area around the bed.

30.18 Bulk Liquid Oxygen Gas System

In hospitals where the consumption of oxygen is quite high, it practically becomes difficult to handle the cylinders. Also, if the availability of the cylinders is not adequate, the hospital may face problems in fulfilling the demand of the oxygen required. Hence, the best option is to consider the installation of a bulk liquid oxygen tank.

This tank is used for the storage of any cryogenic liquid which can include oxygen, nitrogen and nitrous oxide. The tank is a cryogenic pressure vessel made of stainless steel supported within an outer vessel, similar to a vacuum flask.

The Liquid Oxygen plant consists of the Cryogenic tank, and the coils. The coils have a gas outlet, which is connected to the copper pipeline. Passing through the valves, pressure monitors and pressure controller, this pipeline is ultimately connected to the main oxygen supply line of the hospital. Working wise, the liquid oxygen in the vessel flows to the coils, where it is converted into the gaseous form. This gas then flows to the main pipeline for further supply to the endpoint.

30.18.1 Liquid Oxygen Vessel

The vessel, as mentioned, is a vacuum flask-type capsule made out of stainless steel. Vessels of various capacities are available varying from 500 litres to 20,000 litres. The vessel is installed on a pre-constructed foundation and is properly screwed to the foundation with the help of heavy-duty fasteners. The plant shall be located inside a fenced compound, which may also house the control panel and the standby manifold.

The plant has to be installed outside the hospital building in the open area only.

The area required for the vessel shall be about 18 m × 9 m. On the front side, the space of about 9 m × 9 m. Shall be left empty for parking the vehicle carrying the liquid oxygen to unload the liquid gas into the tank. On all other sides of the tank, a space of 3 m. Shall be left vacant before fixing the fencing. The Vessel area shall have fencing all around. The vessel area shall have a 6 m. Door in the front from where the vehicle will enter. Normally this door shall be locked and opened only when the vehicle arrives for unloading the gas. On the side, one small door shall be provided, which shall be used for regular monitoring of the plant. This door shall be about 914 mm wide.

The flooring of the vehicle parking area on the front side shall be made out of concrete, which shall be capable of bearing the load of the vehicle.

In the plant enclosure, a running water tap shall be provided, for melting the ice accumulated on the copper pipeline from time to time.

Before installing the plant, it may be necessary to comply with local authority planning constraints in some areas. Even before installations, the drawings have to be approved by the competent authority like the Explosive Department. Once completed, an inspection may be done by the department before issuing the licence to operate the plant (Fig. 30.4).

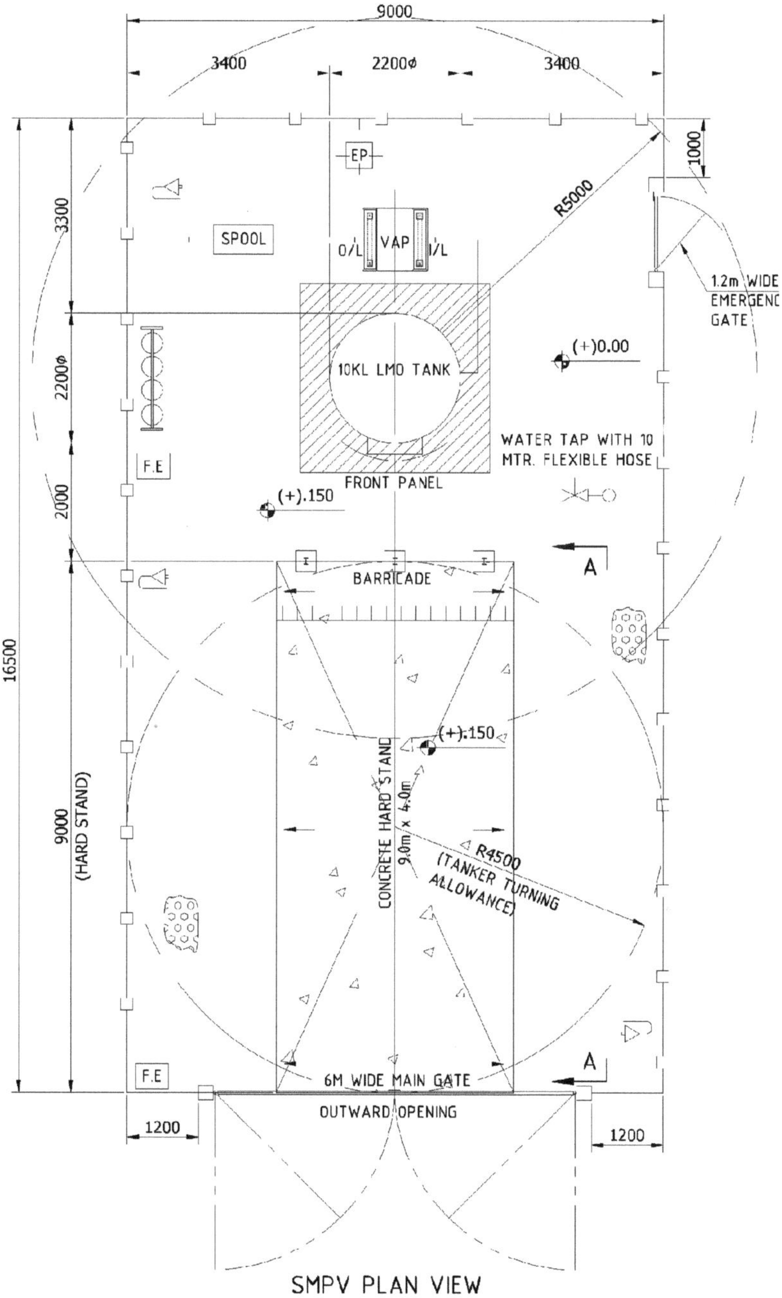

Fig. 30.4 Picture of the site layout of Liquid Oxygen plant

Further Reading

Ayman M. DESIGN OF MEDICAL GAS SYSTEM OF ASSIUT INJURES HOSPITAL`1. [cited 2021 Jul 10]; Available from: https://www.academia.edu/37965637/DESIGN_OF_MEDICAL_GAS_SYSTEM_OF_ASSIUT_INJURES_HOSPITAL1

Designing of medical gas pipeline system MGPS I HYDRO-GAZ-MED [Internet]. [cited 2021 Jul 10]. Available from: https://www.gazmed.pl/en/services/designing-medical-gas-pipeline-system/

General Procedure For The Design of MGPS I Chemical Engineering I Gases [Internet]. Scribd. [cited 2021 Jul 10]. Available from: https://www.scribd.com/document/481931877/GENERAL-PROCEDURE-FOR-THE-DESIGN-OF-MGPS-docx

14:00-17:00. ISO 7396-1:2007 [Internet]. ISO. [cited 2021 Jul 10]. Available from: https://www.iso.org/cms/render/live/en/sites/isoorg/contents/data/standard/04/04/40440.html

Group TM. Key Instrumentation Considerations in Medical Gas Delivery Systems [Internet]. [cited 2021 Jul 10]. Available from: https://www.medicaldesignbriefs.com/component/content/article/mdb/features/technology-leaders/20932

NHS Executive. Medical gas pipeline systems: design, installation, validation and verification. Stationery Office; 1997.

Medical Gases and Vacuum Systems in Hospitals - Healthcare Articles [Internet]. [cited 2021 Jul 10]. Available from: https://www.asianhhm.com/articles/medical-gases-and-vacuum-systems-in-hospitals

Great Britain, Department of Health. Medical gases: health technical memorandum 02–01: medical gas pipeline systems. Pt. A, Pt. A,. London: The Stationery Office; 2006.

VMEDO. NABH Standards for Medical gas pipeline system [Internet]. VMEDO. 2021 [cited 2021 Jul 10]. Available from: https://vmedo.com/blog/nabh-standards-for-medical-gas-pipeline-system/

Sarangi S, Babbar S, Taneja D. Safety of the medical gas pipeline system. J Anaesthesiol Clin Pharmacol. 2018;34(1):99–102.

31 Hospital Kitchen

Kitchen services is an important support in the hospital which is responsible for preparing and providing good-quality food to the patients in the hospital. Depending on the policy of the hospital, the Kitchen may also provide the food to the staff and visitors of the hospital.

The food service may also include catering for meetings and functions, such as board meetings, seminars, conferences and special occasions. Food must be familiar, tasty and appealing to patients from all age groups, religious, cultural and social backgrounds and those nutritionally vulnerable due to illness.

The hospital kitchen shall be designed and equipped in such a manner that it can fulfil the requirements variety of dietary needs. As the patients in the hospital are prescribed diets according to the disease, it is important that the kitchen shall be able to supply all such diets as prescribed.

31.1 Infrastructure of Hospital Kitchen

The Hospital Kitchen shall the following:

Hospital Kitchen	Entry of Staff
	Airlock Entry
	Change Rooms cum hand wash
	Receipt area for supplies
	Bulk Storage for tableware, linen, crockery and utensils
	Fruit/Vegetable storage
	Refrigerator/s, cool rooms and freezers
	Storage areas for dry ration/goods
	Pre Preparation
	Cooking/Baking
	Reheating facilities
	Packing/Plating areas
	Trolley parking area
	Loading/Distribution
	Trolley/cart washing area
	Pot Wash
	Dishwashing
	Waste Disposal area
	Manifold room and Cylinder Storage
	Staff Accommodation
	Kitchen Manager
	Dietician
	Dietetics Staff
	Public Utility for Staff

31.2 Location of Hospital Kitchen

The Kitchen (sometimes also known as Catering Unit) may be located on-site within the health facility or off-site, remote from the health facility. If it is On-site, the location of the hospital kitchen shall be away from the patient area or the clinical departments. Also, the Kitchen shall not

A. Garg, A. Dewan, *Manual of Hospital Planning and Designing*,
https://doi.org/10.1007/978-981-16-8456-2_31

be located on the floors, as the smell of the kitchen will be spread throughout the hospital. Hence, if the bylaws permit, the kitchen shall be located on the rooftop of the hospital building, otherwise, it shall be outside the hospital building. If proper ventilation is available and proper drainage of water supply is available, the kitchen can also be located in the basement. Also, the kitchen shall be located in a way that the noise does not cause any inconvenience to the other departments. At the same time, the location shall involve the shortest possible time in delivering food to the wards.

31.3 Size of the Kitchen

The size of the kitchen is dependent on the following;

1. How many beds are there in the hospital?
2. For how many people, the meals are cooked?
3. Is the Kitchen supplying meals to Visitors and Staff?
4. Is the kitchen supplying meals in the hospital cafeteria?

Leaving apart the dining area, the kitchen shall be approximately 0.28 m^2 per meal. I.e. if 500 meals have to be prepared per day, the area shall be about 140 m^2. This area shall again be subdivided into different utility areas. However, if the hospital set up is small, the area shall not be less than 50 m^2.

As far as the dining space is concerned, it shall also be about 0.28 m^2 per person.

A Well-Planned Kitchen Should Have:

1. Adequate storage for raw materials.
2. Adequate space for food being prepared.
3. Adequate space food awaiting service.
4. Adequate storage for equipment, utensils, crockery and cutlery.
5. Efficiency and effectivity in terms of movement of staff, equipment, materials and waste management system in place Food, Oil and Grease (F.O.G).
6. An area for checking in stock.
7. Janitorial store for kitchen, with janitorial sink in place and chemical store.

31.4 Entry

The Kitchen shall have one main entry and one emergency entry. The main shall be about 1524 mm wide and shall have a door opening on both sides. This entry door shall be provided with an Air Curtain to prevent insects inside the kitchen. Immediately after this door, an airlock shall be provided.

An Airlock Entry is required and to prevent external air, insects or contaminants such as dust entering the Catering unit and to control access to the Unit. The length of the airlock shall be about 1524–1829 mm. Immediately after the airlock, a second entry gate shall be provided. This door shall also be 1524 mm wide and openable on both the sides.

There shall also be an emergency exit near the cooking area for emergency evacuation out of the kitchen. This entry shall be about 1219 mm wide.

For materials, a separate entry door can be provided, which shall open in the storage area, so that the material can directly be sent to the storage without disturbing the main entry of the kitchen. This entry shall be about 1524–1829 mm wide.

31.5 Change Rooms cum Wash Areas

Immediately after the entry, a set of change rooms shall be provided for the staff change to remove outside clothes and wear kitchen dress. These change rooms shall be separate for males and females. While designing change rooms, the following needs to be considered;

1. Separate change rooms shall be provided, one for males and the second for females.
2. The room shall be of the size 3048 mm × 3048 mm.
3. Rooms shall have a provision of an attached toilet with a bath facility.

4. Furniture wise, the room shall have a cupboard.
5. Almirah shall be provided with the provision for hanging the clothes.
6. In the change room, staff lockers shall also be provided where the staff can keep their personal belongings. Individual lockers shall be about 305 mm × 305 mm. These individual lockers are combined, and the locker almirah can be fabricated. Each locker shall be lockable separately. One such locker shall be allotted to one staff.

Immediately at the exit of the change rooms, the handwashing area shall be provided. For hand washing, the sinks shall be provided with a provision of running hot and cold water. The drains shall be immediately below the wash sink. On average, one sink per 10 workers shall be provided.

31.6 Receipt Area for Supplies

This includes the receiving of purchased goods, ration and vegetables etc., which has to be used in the kitchen for cooking. This also includes the utensils and other such items like detergent powders, cooking gas etc. The receiving area shall have a separate entrance from the main entry and shall be near to the storage area. Here the materials/goods are received, handled, checked for quality/quantity. Entries are made in the stock registers, and then the material is sent to the concerned storage. Some of these functions may be combined or not, depending on the size of the kitchen. An area of 3658 mm × 3658 mm shall be sufficient. This area shall have two doors, one for entry of the materials/goods and the second for sending materials/goods to the respective storage.

31.7 Storage Area

There are different storage rooms depending on the properties of the item, like dairy products which may require a cold environment, vegetables which may require good ventilation etc. The following storages are generally required;

Bulk Storage	For storage of utensils, cooking accessories etc.
Fruit/vegetable storage	For storage of vegetables, fruits etc.
Refrigerator/s, cool rooms and freezers	For storage of milk and dairy products, meat and fish etc.
Storage areas for dry ration/goods	For storage of dry ration

As far as the sizes of the storage rooms are concerned, it shall depend on;

1. The size of the kitchen.
2. The volume of business.
3. Delivery frequency.
4. The length of storage.
5. The type of storage (frozen, refrigerated or dry).

31.7.1 Bulk Storage

This store is generally used for storage of the bulk items like cooking utensils, crockery, cutlery, glassware, linen, napkins, machinery which is not in use (like grinders, microwaves, toasters and gas stoves etc.), cleaning machines and cleaning agents and chemicals used in dish/pot washing equipment like detergents etc. Please note that these types of items shall not be mixed with any other storage where the eatables are stored. The store shall be at least 3658 mm × 3658 mm in size, which may be increased or decreased according to the requirement. Adequate lockable cupboards, racks and drawers shall be provided in the store. The store shall also have a countertop. The Kitchen Manager should be in charge of this store.

31.7.2 Fruit and Vegetable Store

This store is used for the storage of perishable food such as fruit and vegetables. The most important point for this storage is to control the temperature and humidity level so that the vegetables and fruits last long. The store shall have the capacity to store material sufficient for at least 4 days' consumption. The room shall be provided with bins or baskets made out of stainless steel wire mesh. These wire mesh baskets shall be placed on the racks. The racks shall be placed in such a fashion to make air circulation easy all around the racks. The baskets of wire mesh bins shall not be overloaded, and spaces shall be left for proper air circulation. The store shall be at least 3658 mm × 658 mm in size, which may be increased or decreased according to the requirement.

31.7.3 Refrigeration, Cool Rooms, Freezers

Cool rooms and freezers shall be used for the dairy products like milk, cheese, butter, cream, ice cream, meat, fish and frozen vegetables like peas, corn etc. It is also called the refrigerated room. The store shall be provided with the cold room with the temperature ranging from −20 to 2 °C, which shall be adjustable as per requirement. The size of the cold room shall be about 3048 mm × 3048 mm. The walls and the ceiling of the room shall be made out of a puff panel which acts as a thermal barrier. The flooring is generally made out of wooden planks. The door of the cold room shall also be made out of puff panel and shall be hermetically sealed. For storage, open racks are provided along the walls. The material is stored either on the shelves of the rack or otherwise in the baskets made of stainless steel wire mesh. Apart from this top-loading deep freezer may also be provided if required.

31.7.4 Storage Areas for Dry Ration/Goods

This storage is used to store the dry goods such as pulses, wheat, flour, spices, dry ingredients and cooking condiments etc. The store shall have the capacity for storing materials sufficient for at least 15 days' consumption. The room shall be provided with racks or bins/shelves/drawers etc. made out of the stainless steel. The racks shall be placed in such a fashion that the air circulation is easy all around the racks. The store shall be at least 3658 mm × 3658 mm in size, which may be increased or decreased according to the requirement. Proper care shall be taken for temperature and humidity levels. Also, precautions shall be taken for preventing the store from rodents, for this door brushes can be used.

Common to all the storage areas is that the food storage components shall be grouped for convenient access from receiving areas to the food preparation areas. All food shall be stored clear of the floor. The lowest shelf shall be not less than 305 mm above the floor or shall be closed in and sealed tight for ease of cleaning.

31.8 Preparation Areas

Food Preparation areas are for preparing the ingredient before starting the actual cooking process. The food preparation areas shall be separate from the cooking area. The processes normally done in the processing zones are like;

1. Peeling and cutting the vegetables
2. Grinding the condiments
3. Meshing the boiled vegetables
4. Mixing the items
5. Kneading the flour dome
6. Meat, Fish and Poultry preparation
7. Pastry/dessert preparation

Food preparation areas shall be located at such a place that it has ready access to vegetable/ration storage areas, refrigeration area for supplies. It shall also be near to the cooking areas, boiling water units and ice dispensing machines.

The preparation area shall be provided with the working counters (with granite stone on top), sinks, shelving and mobile trolleys for utensils. The equipment like food processors, slicers, mixers, grinders, cutters etc. shall be provided. For the operation of this equipment, the required electrical points shall be provided on the wall above the working top. For this, the 6/16 Amp switch/sockets shall be provided at a height of 305 mm from the top of the working counter. All equipment must be installed according to manufacturer's specifications. If possible a few important equipment shall be connected through the UPS in the event of power failure. Each preparation area shall have one single sink per station for washing of the food and ration. Hand basins shall also be provided in these areas with a provision of paper towels and soap dispensers. The peeling and cutting station shall be provided with a big-sized waste bin also.

Food preparation areas are provided as discrete areas for the separation of food types. Vegetarian, religious and cultural practices demand the preparation and serving of food with strict storage, preparation and serving requirements. Vegetarian and vegan food may need to be prepared, cooked and stored separately. Foods for particular health issues may include diabetes, food sensitivities or allergies such as lactose and glucose intolerance or nut, shellfish or egg protein allergies.

31.9 Cooking Areas

The cooking area is the most crucial area in the whole kitchen and shall be provided with the maximum area, as there are different means of cooking the food like boiling, frying, pan cooking etc. Different modes of cooking are used depending on the menu and may use convection or conduction heating. Cooking equipment must be of commercial quality and will require installation according to manufacturer's specifications, particularly with attention to services required, which may include power, gas, water or steam supply and drainage.

Cooking areas will be located in close proximity to food preparation areas and with convenient access to plating areas. Different sections in the cooking area have to be provided for different modes of cooking. Say for boiling, a separate space is required to install the boilers. For deep frying, a separate space for electric deep frying machine or a gas burner for deep frying, Gas stove area for preparing the vegetables etc. and a flat pan (Tawa) for making chapatis etc. Each section shall have proper low-height partitions to avoid mixing up and hampering the work of others. On the backside of these areas, the working tables (made out of stainless steel) shall be provided to keep the unprocessed material.

The gas stoves of other such cooking apparatus shall be kept at least 305 mm. away from the wall. Each such apparatus shall be provided with an area of at least 3.72 m^2.

Chapattis can either be made on the flat plate designed for this purpose or if the quantity of chapattis is huge, the automatic chapati making machine shall be installed.

Cooking areas must be properly ventilated, with an exhaust hood covering the entire area. Exhaust hoods must be designed and installed to prevent grease or condensation from collecting on walls, ceilings and from dripping into food or onto food-contact surfaces. The exhaust ducts of these hoods shall be opened out of the kitchen area.

The wall of the cooking areas shall have smooth and washable surfaces. Therefore, it is better to affix glazed tiles on the walls up to the height of 1524–2134 mm. Similarly, the floors of the cooking area shall not be slippery, particularly after the grease spills and washable. For this matt finish tiles can be used.

31.10 Reheating Areas

Reheating means again heating the cooked food before it is served in the dining areas. The heating can be done with the help of the gas burners or through devices like microwaves/induction plates/grills etc.

If it has to be done with the gas burners, the same burners can be used, which have been used for cooking. But if the other devices are used, a separate area shall be provided. This area shall have a working counter for the tabletop devices to be placed. For the operation of these devices, the required electrical points shall be provided on the wall above the working top. For this, the 6/16 Amp switch/sockets shall be provided at a height of 305 mm from the top of the working counter. All devices must be installed according to manufacturer's specifications. If possible few important devices shall be connected through the UPS in the event of a power failure.

If any of these devices are floor mounted, then adequate foundations and electrical points shall be provided. If required another working counter shall be provided opposite to such counter to keep the pre-heated and post-heated food items.

31.11 Packing/Plating

Once the meals are ready after cooking and heating, the next is to pack the meals or lay them on plates to be served to the patients, staff or visitors. In the hospitals, there are different types of diets to be supplied to the patients as prescribed by the physicians. Those can be the Normal Diet, Diabetic Diet, Salt-Free Diet, Oil-free diet, Semi-Solid Diet or Liquid diet etc.

Hence the packing or the plating has to be done accordingly with a clear marking on the plate. The Plate shall have a tag where the name, bed number, ward and type of diet are mentioned.

For such packing/plating, a separate area shall be provided in the kitchen. This area shall have a different working counter with granite top. The cooked food is brought in the packing rooms and the meals are filled up in the respective trays, plates or crockery. These plates/trays/crockery is properly covered with the silver foil or the wrapping slings.

The plating area equipment will be dependent on the number of meals to be plated and delivered to ensure meals are delivered at the correct time and a suitable temperature. In case the high number of plates have to be prepared, the Plating area may be provided with automated plating conveyor systems supported by food serving trolleys, tableware and utensil trolleys.

The tag is fixed on the tops of the plate and kept ready for loading in the service trolley to be served.

31.12 Meal Trolley/Cart Parking

The food is required to be distributed in the respective wards, room of the dining rooms. For this, the food has to be transported to the desired location with the help of the trolleys. And as the food has to be loaded from the packing/plating area, the trolley/cart parking area is required. Therefore, Trolley/Cart parking space shall be provided adjoining the plating/packing area for temporarily parking the meal trolley that shall carry the food to the respective location.

The packed food is then loaded in the trolleys/cart. Service windows shall be provided between the plating/packing area to pass on the plates/trays to the trolley parking area to be loaded in the trolleys.

If the number of trays to be loaded is more, an automatic loading conveyor can be used for quick loading the trolleys.

The size of the area will be dependent on the number of trolleys to be accommodated.

There can be trolleys that keep the food warm, and also there can be refrigerated trolleys to keep the food cold to be used for desserts. Therefore, to keep the trolleys/carts hot and cold, power is required. So the trolley/cart parking area shall be provided with the electrical PowerPoint for plugging in the trolleys/carts so that they are ready at the time of loading.

The trolley shall also be provided with chains of other mechanisms like hooks etc., to hold the trolleys at a place so that these trolleys/carts do not unnecessarily move.

31.13 Food Distribution

After loading the trays/plates in the trolleys/carts, the trolleys/carts are unhooked and moved to the respective wards/rooms or dining areas. The distribution service must ensure food is delivered to the patient hot or cold as required.

The trolleys/cart are wheeled to the respective ward/room/dining rooms and the trays/plates/ crockery are unloaded at the respective place.

Once the meals are over and the plates/trays/crockery is free, these plates/trays/crockery is reloaded in the trolleys/cart and is wheeled back to the trolley wash area in the kitchen.

31.14 Trolley Return/Stripping

The trolleys/carts returning from the wards/rooms/dining areas after serving food and filled up with the unwashed utensils, shall be brought to the Trolley Return area. Trolleys will then be taken into the trolley stripping area where the dishes, trays, plates, crockery and waste shall be removed, and the trolley is thus sent to the Trolley/Cart Washing area.

The Trolley Return/Stripping area shall be located adjacent to the Dishwashing and the Trolley/Cart Washing area. There shall also be convenient access to the Waste Disposal area.

The Trolley Return/Stripping area shall have a provision of proper wall guards and corner guards to prevent edges of the walls being damaged due to the impact of the trolleys hitting the walls.

The provision of handwashing shall also be given in the trolley stripping area.

31.15 Trolley/Cart Wash

After unloading the trolleys/cart, they shall be moved to the trolley washing area. This area shall be provided for washing/disinfecting and drying of trolleys and carts making them ready for the next use and sending them to the parking area for loading. There must be a clear flow from dirty to clean to prevent cross-flow of dirty with clean items.

The Trolley Wash area shall be located remotely from the food preparation and storage areas with convenient access from the Trolley Return/Stripping area. The Trolley Return/Stripping area shall have a provision of proper wall guards and corner guards to prevent edges of the walls being damaged due to the impact of the trolleys hitting the walls.

The trolley wash area shall have the provision of running hot and cold water. Also, a compressor system shall be provided to pressure clean the trolleys and to remove dirt or greasy components on the trolley. Similarly, the area shall have a provision for trolley drying area, may with the hot air blowing system. If the trolleys to be washed is more, an automated trolley/cart washing equipment may be provided.

31.16 Dishwashing

The trays/plates/crockery/cutlery received back after use have to be washed. Therefore, a dishwashing area shall be provided in the kitchen. This area shall be located near the trolley stripping area.

For washing, separate stainless steel sinks and drainers shall be provided, which shall be fixed on the working counter. The sinks shall be deep, long and wide enough to wash the utensils. Along with the sink, a drain board shall also be provided to drain out the excess water. The sinks shall have the provision of running hot and cold water with a flexible hose spray. Also, a provision shall be made on the wall for detergent dispensers and sponge holders.

After washing and drainage, space shall be provided for sorting the utensils. Once sorted, there shall be a space for stacking the utensils. For stacking, a wooden stripped cupboard can be fixed on the wall or alternately racks can be provided. The stacking can either be done in the dishwashing area or otherwise in the packing/plating area. If the number of utensils to be washed is more, automatic dishwashers may be used.

Crockery, utensil and cutlery washing facilities shall be located as far as possible from the food preparation and serving area. Washing facilities shall be designed to prevent contamination of clean wares with soiled wares through cross-traffic. The clean wares shall be transferred for storage or used in plating, serving or dining areas without having to pass through food preparation areas.

31.17 Pot Washing

The kitchen shall also have a pot washing area for washing and cleaning the pots and big utensils used for cooking the food. For this, a separate enclosure shall be provided near to the cooking area.

In this area, low-level taps are provided at the height of about 610–914 mm from the floor level giving enough space to move and rotate the pots below the taps. The taps shall have a provision of running hot and cold water. If required, an arrangement for pressure cleaning can also be provided.

On the backside, a stripped stainless steel rack shall be provided which shall work as a drain board to drain out the excess water from the pots. Once the pots are dry, they are sent back to the cooking area.

If the number of pots is more and manual cleaning is not possible, an automatic pot washing machine can also be provided.

31.18 Waste Disposal

In the kitchen, a lot of waste is generated from the cutting/peeling areas and the leftover waste in the utensils. The waste can be either wet or dry. Hence a proper provision shall be made for regular removal and disposal of such waste in accordance with the Waste Management guidelines and policies.

For handling and disposal of such waste, a separate waste disposal area shall be provided near and adjoining the kitchen. This room shall be about 3048 mm × 3048 mm and shall have a door that shall open outside the kitchen. The room shall contain big-sized waste bins with a disposable biodegradable polythene bag. In the kitchen side, a window shall be provided from where the waste can be thrown in the bin placed in the waste disposal room.

All garbage, and in particular wet waste, shall be stored in sealed bins. A provision shall be made for the removal and cleaning of these waste bins from time to time. Inside the room, space shall also be provided to wash the bins before the next use. For this, a tap shall be provided in the waste disposal area.

31.19 Gas Storage Closet

Usually, the cooking gas is required in the kitchen. The best way to supply the gas to these burners is through pipelines instead of keeping gas cylinders at each point. Therefore, a gas manifold room shall be provided at a convenient place outside the kitchen. This area shall be open to the sky and shall not be a closed room. The manifold shall have a provision of fixing 6 to 10 cylinders at a time. From the manifold, the copper pipeline is laid down on the wall from which it is then connected to the burner by the flexible gas pipe. But now a days, the cooking gas is provided through the piped gas lines (PNG). If so, the cylinders are not required and the burners can be directly connected to the gas pipeline with the help of the flexible pipe.

For storage of the stock of filled cylinders and the empty cylinders, a separate enclosure shall be provided near the manifold room. Both these areas, the manifold room and the gas store shall be enclosed with the help of wire mesh structure. No wall shall be constructed for these areas. Be very careful while designing these areas and that it shall be fully protected from any chances of fire nearby.

The size of the manifold shall depend on the number of cylinders. But on average, for a manifold of 10 cylinders, the room size shall be about 3658 mm × 3658 mm. Similarly, the size of the gas store shall also be 3658 mm × 3658 mm.

31.20 Staff and Support Areas

There shall be a small administrative area to control and monitor the functioning of the kitchen. Hence the following rooms shall be provided in the kitchen.

Offices shall be provided for

1. Kitchen Manager
2. Dietician
3. Dietetics Staff

These rooms are for the general administrators and clerical staff managing the kitchen. The staff can be like Managers, Dieticians, Asstt. Dieticians etc. The size of these rooms shall be about 4572 mm × 3658 mm. But depending on the requirement and number of persons likely to sit, the size can be increased or decreased. The room shall have an adequate arrangement of cabinets, drawers and racks for a smooth working. The office tables and chairs shall also be provided. Preferably the room shall have an attached Toilet. If required a separate room for the staff shall be provided. The room shall also have proper arrangements for electrical points, inter-

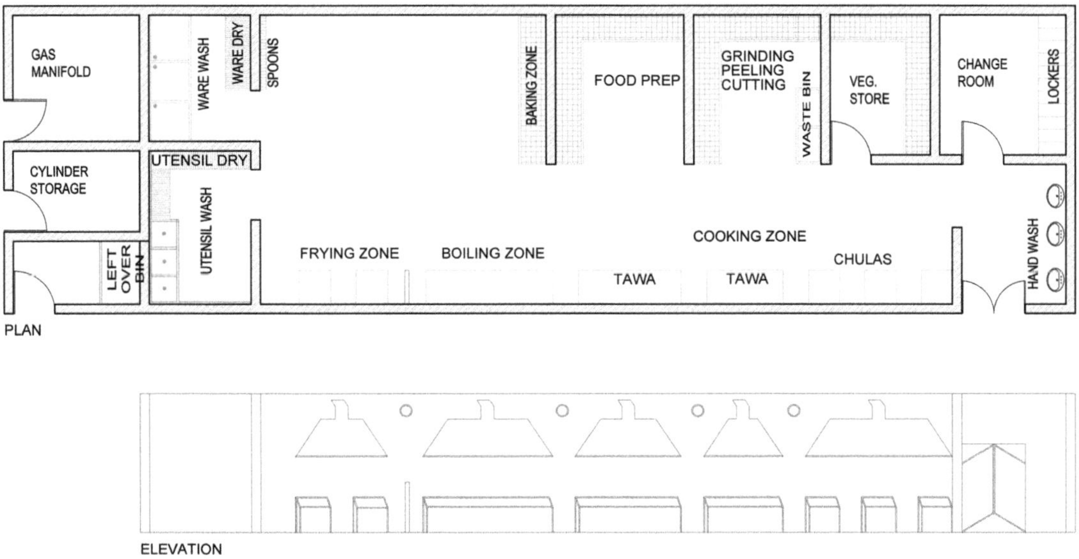

Fig. 31.1 Pic of layout of kitchen

com connection, IT network, CCTV surveillance and air-conditioning (Fig. 31.1).

31.21 General Issues About Infrastructure Requirements

1. *Doors*

   Doors shall be adequately sized for ease of passage of food distribution trolleys/carts. The doors can be either automatic/semi-automatic or otherwise manual doors.
2. Benches, storage shelves, sinks and preparation areas shall be of suitable working heights. Adjustable height equipment shall be used if possible.
3. For lifting and handling heavy equipment or supplies, the provision of lifting devices shall be provided.
4. *Safety*

   All electrical equipment shall have an emergency shut-off switches to prevent overheating.
5. Mobile food trolleys and catering equipment on casters must have locking brakes.
6. *Security*

   Unauthorized entry to the kitchen shall be restricted.
7. *Finishes*

   All tables, benches and other surfaces on which food is prepared or handled shall be covered in a smooth impervious material. Preferably the entire furniture, tables, benches etc. shall be made out of 304-grade stainless steel.
8. *Ceiling*

   Ceiling in food preparation or food storage areas shall be finished to ensure they are easily cleanable. In food preparation, any dust fallout would pose a potential problem.
9. *Floors and Walls*

   In the kitchen area, the floors shall be non-slippery, water-resistant and greaseproof. Floor finish must be easily cleanable with no crevices.
10. Floor and wall finishes shall be free of gaps/spaces that can harbour rodents and insects.
11. Wall finishes shall be smooth, impervious to moisture, easily cleanable and able to withstand repeated washing. Therefore, glazed tiles are recommended to be used in the kitchen up to the height of 1524 mm–2134 mm from the floor level.
12. *Communications*

    The following IT/Communications systems shall be provided in the kitchen:

(a) Voice and data points for telephones and computers with internet access.
(b) Wireless internet provision for Offices, Meeting rooms.
(c) Data provision for management and quality systems as required.

13. *Hand Basins*

Sufficient number of Handwashing basins shall be provided in all clean-up, preparation, cooking, serving areas of the Unit. Staff in food preparation and serving areas shall not be more than 6000 mm from a hand washing basin. Basins shall be hands-free operation with a paper towel and soap dispensers. Mirrors shall not be installed over basins in food preparation areas where contamination from touching hair may occur.

14. *Grease Traps*

Grease traps shall be provided in the kitchen area to prevent Food, oil and grease from entering the drainage system. These grease tanks shall have odour tight lids/air-tight to stop airborne bacteria from contaminating preparation/cooking surfaces.

31.22 Fixtures, Fittings and Equipment

Some of the equipment, devices and cookware required for the kitchen are

Blenders	Induction stove
Boilers	Juicer
Burners	Kettles
Chapati maker	Kitchen knives
Cookers and steamers	Ladles
Cooking ranges	Microwave ovens
Cooking utensils	Mixers
Deep freezers	Nutcracker
Dish warmer	Ovens
Dish washer	Pans and cooking spoons
Fire extinguisher	Refrigerators
Flat cooking pan	Rubber floor mats
Fryer	Shredders
Glass washer	Spatulas
Griddles	Stainless steel tables, benches
Grill	Vegetable cutters/choppers
Grinders	Waste bins large size

Further Reading

JK B. Cafeteria Design Guide | Architectural Design [Internet]. Architecture Student Chronicles. 2012 [cited 2021 Jul 10]. Available from: http://www.architecture-student.com/design-guide/cafeteria-design-guide-architectural-design/

Andersen BM. Hospital Kitchen. In: Andersen BM, editor. Prevention and Control of Infections in Hospitals: Practice and Theory [Internet]. Cham: Springer International Publishing; 2019 [cited 2021 Jul 10]. p. 995–9. Available from: https://doi.org/10.1007/978-3-319-99921-0_77

Hospital kitchen design - Hospital kitchen layout | Food Strategy [Internet]. Commercial Kitchen Designers Brisbane | Food Strategy Australia. [cited 2021 Jul 10]. Available from: https://www.foodstrategy.com.au/projects/hospital-kitchen-design-ideas/

Hospital Kitchen Design For Optimal Foodservice | LaBel [Internet]. LaBel Foodservice Equipment & Design. [cited 2021 Jul 10]. Available from: https://labelfoodservice.com/blog/hospital-kitchen-design-planning

Hospitals take a fresh look on cafeteria design [Internet]. [cited 2021 Jul 10]. Available from: https://www.hfmmagazine.com/articles/3181-hospitals-take-a-fresh-look-on-cafeteria-design

Moatari Kazerouni A, Chinniah Y, Agard B. Integration of occupational health and safety in the facility layout planning, part II: Design of the kitchen of a hospital. Int J Prod Res. 2014 Oct 27;53:1–15.

Kitchen Design: Intermountain Hospital's Efficient Kitchen and Bistro [Internet]. Foodservice Equipment Reports, Articles & News | FER Magazine. 2019 [cited 2021 Jul 10]. Available from: https://www.fermag.com/articles/9541-kitchen-design-intermountain-hospitals-efficient-kitchen-and-bistro/

Principles of Commercial Kitchen Design [Internet]. WebstaurantStore. [cited 2021 Jul 10]. Available from: https://www.webstaurantstore.com/article/6/commercial-kitchen-design.html

32 Laundry

Laundry service is responsible for providing an adequate, clean, sterilized and constant supply of linen to all users. Their basic tasks include sorting, washing, extracting, drying, ironing, folding, mending and delivery. The main purpose of this department is to provide clean material to the patients and ensure that hygiene is maintained in the process.

Hospitals can set up laundry in three ways: First, the hospital can purchase laundry equipment and employ workers to operate the laundry inside the hospital premises. Second, the hospital can provide space for laundry and hire a contractor for setting up the equipment and operate laundry. Third, the hospital can enter into a contract with a local laundry service, in which case the contractor carries dirty linen to the off-site/local laundry and brings it back after washing and processing.

32.1 Facilities and Space Requirements

Laundry infrastructure has the following setup:

Hospital Laundry	Central Storage Area
	Dirty Receipt
	Mending and Tailoring
	Sorting/Weighing
	Washing
	Ironing
	Packing
	Clean Storage
	General Storage
	Public Utility for Staff

Laundry shall have the facilities for the following areas;

1. Central storage space for collecting linen from interim storage.
2. Space for installation of equipment like washing machine, extractor, dryer etc.
3. Provision for an adequate supply of hot and cold water.
4. Provision for power supply.
5. Place for installing the boilers (if required).
6. Storage place for cleaning agents and detergents.
7. Space for sorting the soiled linen.
8. Clothesline to dry washed linen in the sun.
9. Place for sewing and mending area.
10. Place for ironing.
11. Office space for the management of the laundry.

A. Garg, A. Dewan, *Manual of Hospital Planning and Designing*,
https://doi.org/10.1007/978-981-16-8456-2_32

32.2 Location of the Laundry

The Laundry shall be located in the service area of the hospital, with close access to the clean and dirty loading dock areas. The surrounding area should have ample daylight and natural ventilation. Ideally, it should be on the ground floor of an isolated building connected or adjacent to the water and power plant.

32.3 Size of the Unit

The size of the Laundry area will depend on the size of the hospital, the total load of the linen to be washed per day, and the number and type of laundry equipment to be installed. The size shall also depend on factors like the amount of storage required for standard conditions, allowance for reserve clean linen and dirty holding in emergencies, and the frequency and reliability of linen supply and collection services.

32.4 Dirty and Soiled Linen Generation

During routine hospital operations, soiled linen is generated from various departments like Indoor patient wards/rooms, Operation Theatre Complex, OPDs etc. This soiled linen has to be replaced by washed and sterilized linen for the next use.

Following are the various types of linen that are normally used and washed in the hospital laundry:

Bedsheets	Doctors OT dress and Gowns
Draw Sheets	Theatre drapes
Blankets	Napkins
Towels	Kitchen Cloths
Patient dress	Curtains
Patient gowns	Uniform of the staff
Pillow Covers	Screens Cloths
Doctors Apron	Staff Apron

Infrastructure of Laundry
(Figure 32.1)

32.5 Dirty and Soiled Linen Interim Storage

The sorting of dirty and soiled linen starts right from the point of use of linen. As mentioned at various places in this book, Dirty Utility has to be provided at different location of the hospital, which contains a hamper to collect all dirty linen. It is also a place where contaminated linen is initially separated, which shall be put in the colour-coded plastic bags. From here, the linen is collected using a trolley and carried to the Central Storage Area.

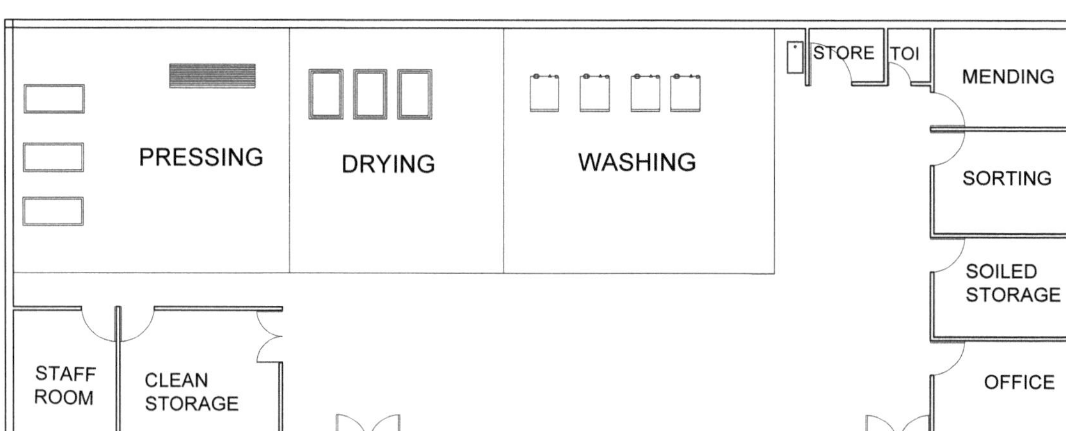

Fig. 32.1 Sample layout drawing laundry

32.6 Central Storage Area

This is an area where soiled linen is exchanged with the washed linen.

As linen is stored in the central storage area for a short time before it is taken to the hospital laundry, one portion of the central storage area is demarcated for the soiled linen, collected from various interim storages of the hospital. This area can be provided at a convenient place either inside or outside the hospital building. The size of the room shall depend on the quantity of the linen received daily and the frequency of transporting the soiled linen to the laundry. The room shall be provided with racks to store the sorted and packed linen. The room shall also possess transport trolleys for transporting the soiled linen to the laundry. Adequate trolley parking bay shall also be provided with this room.

This Central Storage area shall also have a separate room which shall be used only for the storage of clean linen. Please ensure there shall be no mixing of clean and soiled linen, else it may lead to cross-contamination. The entrance to this room shall be totally separate and managed by separate staff. The size of the room shall depend on the quantity of washed linen received daily from the laundry and the frequency of issue of washed linen to the departments. The most important thing to consider is that as per the hospital policy, how many day's stocks the management desires to keep for emergency situations. The room shall be provided with racks to store washed linen. The room shall also possess transport trolleys for transporting linen to the user department. Adequate trolley parking bay shall also be provided. Please ensure that trolleys for the supply of washed linen shall be separate from the trolleys used for soiled linen. It is better if closed trolleys are used for this purpose.

32.7 Dirty Receipt

This area receives the soiled/dirty linen from the Central Storage of the hospital under a receipt. This room shall be located just at the entrance of the laundry, with a separate entry. The size of the room shall depend on the quantity of the linen received daily and the average time for which the dirty linen stays in this room. However, a room of 3658 mm × 4267 mm shall be sufficient. The room shall have two doors, one from where the linen shall be received and the second that opens in the sorting and weighing area. As the linen is delivered through the trolleys, there shall be sufficient space outside the room for parking the trolleys. If required, racks or shelves shall be provided to store the linen. This linen is then transferred to the sorting and weighing room for further processing.

32.8 Sorting and Weighing

As mentioned earlier, the initial sorting of the soiled linen is done in the central storing area of the hospital. Further, different items requiring different washing conditions such as temperature, detergent, and length of wash cycle are sorted here. The received linen is divided into two basic loads: a load that will require drying after washer-extracting and a load that will require ironing.

Items that need mending or stain removal will be separated so that they can be dealt with accordingly. Depending on the size and type of facility, soiled linen should be pre-sluiced, either in a suitable sluicing machine or in stainless steel tubs, which must be provided in this area.

The linen is also sorted according to the type of fabric, item, colour, degree and type of soiling, and load sizes to suit the washer-extractors capacity. For this, the room shall be provided with stainless steel tables. After sorting, items should be placed in trolleys compatible with the loads allowed in the washer-extractors.

The size of the room shall depend on the quantity of the linen. However, a room of 3658 mm × 4267 mm shall be sufficient. The room shall have two doors, one attached to the receiving room and the second opening in the washing area.

32.9 Washing Area

It is the main area in the infrastructure of laundry, where linen is washed and kept ready for delivery.

This area also includes processes like extraction, drying, and ironing. The main areas required for the working of different machines are:

32.9.1 Loading and Washing

Once the linen has been sorted, weighed, and has arrived in the washing area, it shall be loaded into the washers. The washers are generally front-opening washing machine. Machines are available different in capacities and shall be chosen according to the requirement.

Washers are installed on a pre-constructed foundation and shall be screwed using fasteners. Also, vibrations occur during the operative of the washer; thus, appropriate anti-vibration pads shall be provided to protect the machine. The washer shall be connected to separate hot and cold water supply. There are different options available for heating the water required for washing, like steam heating, gas-fired burners or electric heaters. If steam is to be used, the washer shall be connected to the boiler, if gas-fired burners are to be used, the connection is done with the gas supply system, and if the electric heater is to be used, adequate power supply shall be provided to the washer. Washer-extractors are normally arranged against the perimeter of the laundry wall, and the drain-off is discharged into a floor drain channel, which is covered by a gate. The washers shall be installed at a distance of about 610 mm from the wall for better cleaning of the laundry. A common drain pipe of about 6 inches' diameter shall be provided on the back of the washers to which all drain pipes shall be connected. In front of the washer, a clear space of 1829 mm shall be provided for easy loading and unloading of the linen.

Usually, at least two such washers shall be provided in the laundry. But depending on the linen load and the future expansion plans, space for more than two washers shall be planned well in advance.

32.9.2 Extractors

After washing, excessive water has to be drained out of the linen. This is done with the help of the extractor. Earlier, hydro extractors were used as a separate machine, in which linen was taken out of the washer and loaded in the extractor for draining water. But nowadays, most washers have an inbuilt extractor. However, if separate extractors are used, they shall be installed on a pre-constructed foundation and shall be screwed using fasteners. Also, vibrations occur during the operative of the washer; thus, appropriate anti-vibration pads shall be provided to protect the machine. As balancing and levelling is an important thing to consider while installing an extractor, the alignment of the extractor must be accurate. For operating the extractor, adequate power supply shall be provided. For draining the water from the extractor, drain pipes shall be provided which shall terminate in a common drain. Like washers, extractors are also installed at a distance of about 610 mm from the wall for better cleaning of the laundry. A common drain pipe of about 152 mm diameter shall be provided on the back of the washers to which all drain pipes shall be connected. In front of the washer, a clear space of 1829 mm shall be provided for easy loading and unloading of the linen.

Usually, at least two such extractors shall be provided in the laundry. But depending on the linen load and the future expansion plans, space for more than two washers shall be planned well in advance.

32.9.3 Tumble Drying

This process entails reducing the moisture content of the washed linen, for making it suitable for ironing. Tumbler dryer is loaded from the front, with the linen, which has been processed in the extractor and is then dried in the dryer through heat. Dryers operate and heat with gas, steam, or electricity. They are installed on the pre-constructed foundation and shall be screwed using fasteners. Like washers, dryers are also installed at a distance of about 610 mm from the wall for better cleaning of the laundry. In the front of the dryer, a clear space of 1829 mm shall be provided for easy loading and unloading of the linen.

Dryers must be vented directly outside of the building, and these should preferably be located next to an external wall. They can be placed side by side or in a separate room that is well ventilated at the back. Dryers generate the most heat of all the equipment in the laundry, and all hot air should be relayed outside.

Usually, at least two such dryers shall be provided in the laundry. But depending on the linen load and the future expansion plans, space for more than two washers shall be planned well in advance.

32.9.4 Ironing

This is the last stage of the washing process, and a separate area shall be provided in the laundry for ironing. In this zone, various types of ironing machines are installed, which depends on the type of linen to be ironed. Some examples of ironing machines are:

32.9.4.1 Pressing Machines

This is used to iron clothes like shirts, pants, uniforms, curtains etc. This machine is available with either single or double heated bucks and may use electricity or steam for heating the bucks. Compressed air is used to rotate and lift the bucks, as well as for the pressing operation; thus a compressed air point shall be provided in the laundry near the pressing machine. These machines are usually operated manually or by foot in conjunction with a pneumatic system for the pressing operation.

The pressing machine is a floor mounting model and is screwed to the floor using the help of fasteners. It shall be installed at a distance of about 610 mm from the wall for better cleaning of the laundry. In the front of the machine, a clear space of 1829 mm shall be provided for easy working of the personnel. Usually, one machine is enough in the laundry. But depending on the linen load and the future expansion plans, space for more than two pressing machines shall be planned well in advance.

32.9.4.2 Calendar Dryer Irons

The calendar ironing machine is basically used for ironing bed sheets. Flatwork irons usually have a single large diameter heated roller, and the linen comes into contact with approximately 300° of its circumference. The linen is fed into the iron by a series of belts that span across the bed and the contact surface of the roller.

The machines have a return-feed but can be set up for through-feed. With a return-feed ironer, a single person can operate the machine, which can be positioned against a wall to conserve space. The temperature of the roller and the degree of contact of linen with the roller ensures adequate ironing and drying process. An automatic folding process can also be fitted.

Another type of calendar machine is the bed and chest heating calendar, in which instead of rollers, the bed and chest of the machine are heated. These irons can have up to four large diameter rollers. The bed is lined with 'clothing' to transfer the heat from the bed to the linen and ensure a clean and smooth passage of the flatwork through the machine. Most of these machines are through-feed machines. The linen has approximately 180° contact with the rollers. In the end, the linen can be folded manually or automatically.

Dry irons with a return-feed mechanism are usually placed near the perimeter wall, but the multi-roller heated-bed irons are free-standing and require considerably more space. In the front, a clear space of 1829 mm shall be provided for easy working of the personnel. Usually, one machine is enough in the laundry. But depending on the linen load and the future expansion plans, space for more than two washers shall be planned well in advance.

32.9.4.3 Flat Irons

This is the normal domestic iron and is used for the small cloths and dresses of the hospital (which are not possible to be done on the pressing machine). This iron requires electric power point and a wooden table of size 1219 mm × 914 mm and can be installed at any convenient place in the ironing area adjoining the wall.

32.10 Inspection and Repairing

An important function carried out by the laundry department is the mending and repairing of torn linen. As said earlier, the linen requiring repairs or mending are is sorted separately. Mending is done after washing the linen, as handling soiled linen involves a high risk of infection. Please note that the linen to be mended is washed separately and not mixed with the other linen. A separate mending room is provided in the laundry which is equipped with a stainless steel working counter, foot-operated sewing machine, and patching machine. The size of the mending room shall be about 4267 mm × 3658 mm, and adequate electric points shall be provided to operate sewing machines or cutters. Storage supplies such as threads, needles, repair fabrics and other haberdashery requirements shall be provided.

32.11 Packaging and Storage

This area is used to pack the linen which shall be wrapped in fluid-resistant, securely sealed plastic bags or placed unwrapped into fluid-resistant covered carts or hampers. The packing area can either be in an open hall or a specially dedicated room; it is recommended that a separate room measuring 4267 mm × 3658 mm shall be sufficient for packing. This area should be provided with sorting racks, shelves, bins etc. along with packing tables or working tops.

After wrapping, linen shall be stored in the clean storage room. The size of the room depends on the quantity of the linen to be stored and the number of days for which the linen has to be stored. On average, the room size of 6096 mm × 4572 mm shall be sufficient. The room shall be provided with stainless steel racks, shelves or bins for storage. The storage room shall have two sealable doors, one shall open in the packing room from where the linen is brought in and the other shall open in the dispatch room.

It is also recommended that the clean storage room shall be positively pressurized with proper air exchanges to maintain the hygiene of the linen.

32.12 Dispatch Room

The laundry shall also be provided with a dispatch room from where the linen will be dispatched either to the user department or the central storage provided in the hospital. This room shall be about 3658 mm × 3658 mm in size, provided with a dispatch counter or an office table with chair for administrative work. It shall have two doors, one shall open in the clean storage room, and the other shall open outside the dispatch room from where the linen will be dispatched. As linen is delivered through trolleys, there shall be sufficient space for parking the trolleys outside the room.

32.13 Trolley Washing

Trolleys carrying soiled linen have high chances of getting contaminated and must be washed before being re-used. This area shall be provided for manual washing/disinfecting and drying of trolleys and carts, making it ready for the next use. This area shall be located remotely from the clean storage room with convenient access from the linen receiving area. The trolley wash area shall have a provision of proper wall guards and corner guards to prevent edges of the walls from getting damaged when trolleys hit the walls. This area shall have the provision of running hot and cold water. Also, a compressor system shall be provided to pressure clean the trolleys and remove any dirt, stains, blood, pathogens or grease. Similarly, the area shall have a provision for trolley drying using hot air blowing system.

32.14 Store

This store is generally used for the storage of chemicals, detergents, and solution preparation. Storage space for at least 1 month's supply should be provided in the storeroom. It shall be near the washer-extractor area. The store shall be at least 3658 mm × 3658 mm in size, which may be increased or decreased according to the requirement. Adequate lockable cupboards, racks, drawers and a countertop shall be provided in the store. Environmental conditions in this store must be dry. As dry washing materials are contained in heavy bags or containers, they shall preferrable be stored on pallets. If required, a solution preparation and storage area might be requested.

32.15 Staff and Support Areas

The laundry shall be provided with an administrative room to control and monitor the functioning of the laundry. The size of the rooms shall be about 4572 mm × 3658 mm, but depending on the requirement and number of persons likely to sit, the size can be increased or decreased. The room shall have an adequate arrangement of cabinets, drawers, and racks for a smooth working. Office tables and chairs shall also be provided in the room. The room shall have an attached toilet. If required, a separate room for the staff shall be provided. The room shall also have proper arrangements for electrical points, intercom connection, IT network, CCTV surveillance, and air conditioning.

32.16 Other Issues Relating to the Infrastructure of Laundry

The following issues shall be considered while designing the laundry:

32.16.1 Infection Control

Laundry shall be provided with sufficient hand washing stations in the clean linen storage room, soiled linen receiving room, sorting room etc. Also, the following points shall be taken care of

1. Restricted/controlled access in the laundry
2. Uni-directional workflow, progressing from dirty to clean areas
3. Controlled airflow with positive air pressure from clean to dirty areas
4. Selection of suitable building materials and finishes
5. Adequate facilities for cleaning and waste management

32.16.2 Airflow

Positive airflow in the laundry shall be from clean to dirty areas, venting directly to the outside. This barrier will ensure that microbe-laden lint and other particle contaminants cannot enter the clean linen processing area and settle on the shelves, carts, or clean linen that is packed and delivered.

32.16.3 Floors

Floors of the entire laundry shall be impervious, non-slip in wet areas, easily cleaned, and robust to allow equipment to be moved over them without lifting or cracking. In the washing area and areas where the release of water may be occasionally unavoidable, floors should be adequately drained.

32.16.4 Walls

Wall surfaces should be easily washable and shall be provided with wall guards and corner protection guards to prevent trolley damage.

32.16.5 Natural Lighting

Natural lighting is the best and should be used wherever possible, especially in cleaning and packing areas. Direct sunlight and solar glare in workspaces should be avoided.

32.16.6 Mechanical Ventilation

As laundry is warm due to the hot working environment of tumble -drying, ironing etc. it becomes more important to provide relatively cool and comfortable working conditions. Adequate ventilation, by removal of stale air at a high level with an inflow of fresh air at a low level, shall be provided. For exhaust of the air, high-speed exhausts or centrifugal fans shall be used. Similarly, for the supply of air, blower fans shall be used.

32.16.7 Hot-Air Extraction

If possible and as per the recommendations of the manufacturers of the equipment, hot air should be extracted directly from the heat-emitting equipment and disposed of in the atmosphere through the ducts which shall be terminated outside the wall of the laundry. These include tumble-drying, where dryers should ideally be accommodated in a separate section.

32.16.8 Compressors

Certain washer-extractors in the laundry require compressed air for their operation. A separate compressed air supply should be used for this purpose instead of medical compressed air. Compressed air needs to dry, as required by the equipment suppliers. Moisture-trapping arrangements must be provided in the system design.

32.16.9 Steam

Adequate system shall be provided in the laundry for the supply of steam. If required, a boiler shall be installed outside the laundry premises to generate steam. Depending on the type of boiler, a provision of gas/coal/wood/electricity shall be provided near the boiler.

32.16.10 Water Supply, Heating and Water Treatment Equipment

Water shall be provided in the laundry at the pressure specified by the manufacturers. For this, booster pumps and water storage tanks shall be provided. Hot water should be generated and stored in sufficient quantity to ensure that the correct temperature can be achieved in the washer-extractors without compromising on the machine output. The use of air-to-water heat pumps coupled with large-volume hot-water storage tanks shall be considered. Hard water may pose serious problems in the laundry, thus, if required, a water-softening plant shall be provided.

32.16.11 Fire Prevention and Detection

Fire can probably be the biggest threat to a laundry. Therefore, proper fire protection devices such as a sprinkler system, hydrant supply, smoke detectors and fire extinguishers shall be installed in the laundry.

32.16.12 Communications

The following IT/Communications systems may be provided within the Linen Handling Unit:

1. Telephones in linen holding areas, linen inspection and mending rooms, offices and workstations.
2. Data outlets for computers/internet access to offices, workstations and delivery rooms.
3. Scanning systems for registering received supplies or dispatch.

Further Reading

Kumar MS, Goud BR, Joseph B. A study of occupational health and safety measures in the Laundry Department of a private tertiary care teaching hospital, Bengaluru. Indian J Occup Environ Med. 2014 Jan 1;18(1):13.

Lopes C, Scavarda A, Nunes M, Carvalho M, Vaccaro G, Korzenowski A. Analysis of Sustainability in Hospital Laundry: The Social, Environmental, and Economic (Cost) Risks. Resources. 2019 Feb 13;8.

Woodson S. Design and Construction of a Healthcare Laundry. 5(3):6.

Sehulster LM. Healthcare Laundry and Textiles in the United States: Review and Commentary on Contemporary Infection Prevention Issues. Infect Control Hosp Epidemiol. 2015 Sep;36(9):1073–88.

Beggs B. HSHS Shared Laundry Services consolidates laundry for 10 hospitals.:10.

National Health Services Estates, editor. Laundry. London: HMSO Publications Centre; 1994. 118 p. (Health building note).

OPL 101: Designing an On-Premises Laundry Room [Internet]. American Laundry News. 2013 [cited 2021 Jul 10]. Available from: https://americanlaundrynews.com/articles/opl-101-designing-premises-laundry-room

Planning, Designing And Maintaining Hospital Laundry To Reduce Carbon Foot Prints And To Make It Energy Efficient And Cost Competitive., IJSR - International Journal of Scientific Research (IJSR), IJSR | World Wide Journals [Internet]. [cited 2021 Jul 10]. Available from: https://www.worldwidejournals.com/international-journal-of-scientific-research-(IJSR)/article/planning-designing-and-maintaining-hospital-laundry-to-reduce-carbon-foot-prints-and-to-make-it-energy-efficient-and-cost-competitive/MTA3ODE=/?is=1

Quality Assurance Hospital Linen and Laundry Services. 2015;6(3):4.

Time to relook at infection control practices for hospital laundry [Internet]. Clean India Journal. 2020 [cited 2021 Jul 10]. Available from: https://www.cleanindiajournal.com/time-to-relook-at-infection-control-practices-for-hospital-linen/

33 Medical Record Department (MRD)

Medical Record is the systematic documentation of a patient's medical history and current treatment and care given to the patient. It serves as a basis for planning future patient care, documenting communication between the hospital and any other health professionals contributing to the patient care, and assisting in protecting the legal interest of the patient and the hospital responsible for patient care.

It also serves as a document to educate medical students and resident physicians, to provide data for internal hospital auditing and quality assurance, and to provide data for medical research.

In earlier days, most of the medical records used to be in hard copies and were to be stored. Now with the development of the information technology, most of the records are being shifted to electronic and digital modes. But still, 100% record cannot be maintained digitally, and some of the records have to be maintained in hard copies. Therefore, the MRD shall have an excellent set up of information technology for the effective preservation of the medical records.

33.1 Electronic Medical Records (EMR)

It is a computerized recording system that tracks and keeps details of the patients admitted in the hospital and their attendants. The EMR also enables to enter patient data at the point of care and allows authorized clinicians to access patient's records from any online location, at any time, for assessments and further treatment of the patient. An EMR system also requires scanning of miscellaneous paper records that may be sourced from outside the facility or brought in by the patient.

33.2 Location of MRD

As several departments may have to refer or visit the MRD frequently, it shall be located within the hospital building, in a low activity area. The location necessarily need not be in direct access to the patient. If the hospital has a basement, the MRD can be located in there, or otherwise on floors that are not a fast movement zone. Sometimes, due to shortage of space, the department can be located in another building but in close vicinity to the hospital building. MRD shall be located within easy walking distance from the admitting or outpatient department to ensure that the staff can easily refer files and retrieve records on an emergency basis.

A. Garg, A. Dewan, *Manual of Hospital Planning and Designing*,
https://doi.org/10.1007/978-981-16-8456-2_33

33.3 Layout

The MRD must have the following areas:

1. Entry and Reception
2. Receipt
3. Compilation Desk/Sorting Room
4. Indexing/Coding
5. Statistical Analysis
6. Computer Lab
7. Storage for Files/Register
8. Dictation Room/Cubicles
9. Transcription Room
10. Photocopy/Printing Room
11. Record Scanning Room
12. Binding Room
13. Waste Holding Area
14. Store
15. Administrative area including:
    (a) Staff Accommodation for Manager, Coders etc.
    (b) Medical Record Officer
    (c) Secretarial Staff
    (d) Public Utility for Staff

33.4 Entry and Reception

Reception shall be provided at the entrance of the MRD. If required, a small waiting area shall be provided near the reception. It shall have a reception counter, chair, and a computer, along with necessary electrical outlets. Entrance doors shall have a key card or electronic access for authorized staff only. Non-authorized visitors shall never be allowed in the MRD and sent back from the reception counter.

33.5 Medical Record Receipt Room

It shall be located at the entrance of the MRD. This is the room where medical records from IPD, OPD, emergency, diagnostic departments etc. are received for recording purposes. The size of the receipt room shall be about 3658 mm × 3658 mm. The room shall have one door, which shall open in the MRD. The outside wall shall have an openable window to receive the records, the size of which shall be about 914 mm × 914 mm.

Inside the room, a receipt counter made out of either wood, stainless steel or fixed counter with granite top shall be provided. On the backside, closed racks shall be provided to temporarily store the received records. A high-raised chair shall also be provided in the room.The room shall have a computer with a printer connected to the computer network of the hospital. The record received at the counter shall be entered immediately in the computer, and if the receipt is to be provided to the respective department, it can be printed and given to the person carrying the records.

33.6 Compilation Desk

The records received at the receipt counter are sent to the compilation desk for further sorting and compilation. While compiling, all the documents of the records are checked for correctness and completion. Main documents checked and verified at this stage are:

Name of patient	Operative ntes
Parents name	Investigation reports
Address	X-ray/CT/MRI films etc.
Contact details	Progress sheet
Unique IPD number and OPD number	Vital chart
Admission date	Medication sheet
Discharge date	Intake-output chart
Diagnosis	Temperature chart
Discharge card/summary	

For sorting and compilation of the medical records, a separate room shall be provided in the MRD. This room shall be located adjoining the receipt room so that the record can be easily transferred to the compilation room. The size of this room shall be about 4267 mm × 3658 mm. The room shall have one door, which shall open in the MRD.

The room shall be provided with the compilation and sorting desk, the size of which shall be about 1829 mm × 1219 mm, made out of either wood or stainless steel, and chairs. A filing rack shall be provided for temporarily storing the records until they are sent for further processing.

The room shall have a computer with a printer connected to the computer network of the hospital. The record-keeper shall check the record and confirm it with the checklist provided in the system.

The sorting and compilation room shall have a proper partition for storing the sorted and unsorted files separately. This room shall have access to the dictation room and photocopy and scanning room.

33.7 Indexing and Coding

This desk may be used for medical records, coding forms, coding books, and compiling disease and operative indexes manually. As most of the indexing and coding work is done on a computer, the room shall have a computer with a printer connected to the computer network of the hospital. After sorting and compilation, the record is indexed and coded as per the ICD codes.

For indexing and coding, a separate room shall be provided in the MRD. This room shall be located adjoining the compilation room so that the record can be easily transferred from there. The size of the room shall be about 4267 mm × 3658 mm. The room shall have one door, which shall open in the MRD. The room shall be provided with office tables and chairs. A filing rack shall be provided for temporarily storing the records until they are sent for further processing.

33.8 Statistical Analysis

A room shall be provided in the MRD for statistical analysis of the data relating to the medical records. As maximum records are on electronic digital media, the analysis is done on and from the workstations. Hence, a separate room of about 3658 mm × 3658 mm, with an office table and chairs, shall be provided. The room shall also be provided with workstations connected to the hospital network. The room shall have a storage cupboard to temporarily store the files that are being used for the statistical analysis.

33.9 Computer Lab

As maximum records are on electronic digital media, the data in the medical records have to be fed in the workstations. Hence, a separate room of about 4572 mm × 3658 mm shall be provided to be used as a computer lab. The room shall be provided with working tops for installing workstations connected to the hospital network to carry out the work of data feeding and retrieval. The number of workstations shall depend on the requirement and workload of the MRD. The sufficient number of chairs to sit and storage cupboards shall also be provided in the room to temporarily store the files that are being used for the data feeding or the retrieval of the data.

33.10 Medical Record Storage Room

Depending on the country's local statutory requirements/guidelines, medical records have to be stored for a long time which can anywhere between 7 and 15 years after last attendance, whereas the Medico-Legal Records may have to be stored for a longer period. Thus, records must be stored in a fire-rated construction as indicated in the local building bylaws. Active medical records in constant use shall be stored in open metal shelving units to provide easy access. The size of the storage room shall depend on the load of the patients and the beds in the hospital. However, the recommended size is about 93 m^2 for a 300-bed hospital.

For storing medical records, compact slidable units may be used. Storage cabinets shall be lockable, and storage of records in the open shelves or racks shall not be allowed. The systems shall have 7 shelves. On an average, if the shelf is 1219 mm long and proper adjustable partitions are given, it can accommodate about 1000 records files. If there are 7 such shelves, it can house about 7000 record files. The highest shelf should not exceed 2134 mm and be reachable by staff using a library step stool. The highest shelf for staff reach, without a step stool, should not be higher than 1829 mm. Aisle between bays of shelving should have a minimum width of 762 mm, however, 914 mm is recommended to allow space for records trolleys, library stools, and staff transit.

If the management of the hospital does not want to use the compacted slidable system, the open file rack system shall be opted for; however, the adequate arrangement shall be done to prevent the record from fire, termite, and pilferage.

The storage area shall have a properly air-conditioned room of about 3048 mm × 3048 mm for storage of CDs/DVDs and hard disks on which the data backup of electronic digital records has been taken. The room shall be provided with a properly sealed, fireproof cabinet to keep these items.

The room shall also be provided with step stools, chairs and working tops made out of stainless steel. The doors of the room shall be properly sealed and provided with the door brushes to prevent rodents from entering the room. All electric cables shall be properly covered to prevent any short-circuiting. Fire sprinklers shall not be installed in the storage area. Records storage areas must be temperature and humidity controlled for the preservation of records.

33.11 Dictation Room/Cubicles

This area is used by the medical staff and others to view and research medical records, as well as dictating and completing the discharge summaries. The cubicles should be located on the perimeter of the unit, adjacent to, but inside the reception area. The number of cubicles will depend on usage. The auditory separation of personnel is preferred, as extraneous noise will be distracting to the person dictating. The required power and data provisions shall be provided.

33.12 Transcription Room

A room in the MRD shall be provided for the transcription of medical records. The room shall be of size 4267 mm × 3658 mm and shall be noise and echo proof, so that the staff can listen to the transcription machines. This room should be located between the entry area and the sorting room. The room shall be provided with an office table, chair, computer and transcription machine. The required power and data provisions shall be provided.

33.13 Photocopying/Printing Room

A room for photocopying and printing shall be provided in the MRD. The room shall be about 3658 mm × 3658 mm with a photocopy machine, computer workstation, office table, and chairs. This space may also be used for generating bar code labels and stationary storage. The room shall also be provided with cupboards for storing stationery to be used in the MRD.

33.14 Scanning Room

At times, some of the documents, particularly the documents brought from outside by the patients or the paper documents created in the hospital, need to be scanned to record them in the electronic digital records. Therefore, a scanning room shall be provided in the MRD. This room shall be about 3658 mm × 3658 mm with a provision of the office table, chairs, workstation, and a good quality multi-sheet high-resolution scanner.

33.15 Binding Room

As medical records have to be stored for a long period, they shall be properly indexed and bound before storage. Therefore, a binding room shall be provided in the MRD. The room shall be about 3658 mm × 3658 mm with a provision of at least one office table, chair, and working top for binding of the records. Binding shall be done for paper-based medical records. For electronic digital record, hard disks, CD's or DVD's shall be packed in the binding room and kept ready for the storage. The room shall also have a storage cupboard to temporarily store the files, registers or any other paper-based records that have to be bound.

33.16 Waste Holding Room

The documents discarded in the MRD shall be destroyed in this room by shredding. The room shall be about 3658 mm × 3658 mm with a provision of the office table, chairs, a high capacity shredding machine and waste holding bins.

33.17 Store

A store shall be provided in the MRD for storage of general items, stationery, unused old equipment, and other daily used items. The store size shall be 3048 mm × 3048 mm, which may be increased or decreased according to the requirement. Adequate lockable cupboards, racks, drawers and countertops shall be provided in the store.

33.18 Administrative Area

The MRD shall have separate rooms to be used for general administrators, managers and clerical staff managing the MRD. The rooms shall be provided for:

1. In-charge MRD
2. Medical Record Officer
3. Coders
4. Data Analyst
5. Secretarial staff

The size of the room shall depend on the designation of the staff. The rooms of the In-charge and Medical Record Officer shall be about 4572 mm × 4267 mm. The room shall have an adequate arrangement of cabinets, drawers, racks, office tables, and chairs for a smooth working. The room shall have an attached toilet. If required, a separate store shall be attached to this room. The room shall also have proper arrangements for electrical points, intercom connection, IT network, CCTV surveillance, and air conditioning.

For other staff members, smaller rooms of size 3658 mm × 3658 mm shall be provided. The room shall have an adequate arrangement of cabinets, drawers, racks, office tables, and chairs for a smooth working. The room shall also have proper arrangements for electrical points, intercom connection, IT network, CCTV surveillance, and air conditioning.

The secretarial room shall be about 6096 mm × 4572 mm in size. The room shall have an adequate arrangement of cabinets, drawers, racks, office tables, and chairs for a smooth working. The room shall have an attached toilet. If required, a separate store shall be attached to this room. The room shall also have proper arrangements for electrical points, intercom connection, IT network, CCTV surveillance, and air conditioning.

33.19 Other Issues About the Infrastructure of MRD

1. *Temperature, Colour and Lighting*

   Care shall be taken about environmental factors such as temperature, humidity, and ventilation. These factors have a direct effect on the records stored in the MRD.
2. *Protection from Fire*

   The entire MRD, especially the filing area of records and X-rays, should be fire protected by installing fire extinguishers and smoke detector. Important documents like medico-legal cases should be preserved in fire-proof cabinets. All electrical lines should be covered to avoid short-circuiting.
3. *Protection from Rodents and Termite*

   The MRD section shall be designed to make it free from vermin, silverfish and other insects likely to attack and destroy the records. Provision shall be made for proper wire mesh or door brushes. Also, MRD shall have a sealed ceiling with no air gaps or leakage.

Regular pest control treatment must be carried out in thein MRD.

4. *Natural Light/Lighting*

   Wherever possible, use of natural light shall be maximized for easy working of the staff. However, storage areas shall not be provided with natural light as it may enhance the deterioration of paper records.

5. *Safety and Security*

   Records in the MRD are confidential, thus, to prevent their loss or damage, the security of the MRD must be carefully considered. Entry and exit points of MRD shall be limited and fitted with access control—manual or electronic.

6. *Information Technology/Communications*

   MRD section shall be provided with intercom lines, computer networking points connected to the central server of the hospital, and RJ45 jack at all the required places.

7. *Electrical Services*

   A pair of 6/16 Amp switch/socket shall be provided at all the required places in the MRD, and all computer points shall be backed up by the UPS supply.

8. *Pneumatic Tube Systems (PTS)*

   It is an air-operated system having an air pump attached to the control station. This is the best, accurate, and quickest mode of transportation for documents, specimens, materials and medicines. One station of the PTS shall be provided in the MRD for receiving documents and records from different locations of the hospital.

Further Reading

Moghaddasi H, Hosseini A, Sheikhtaheri A. A New Model for the Organizational Structure of Medical Record Departments in Hospitals in Iran. Perspect Health Inf Manag AHIMA Am Health Inf Manag Assoc. 2006 May 23;3:4.

Vlayen A, Marquet K, Schrooten W, Vleugels A, Hellings J, De Troy E, et al. Design of a medical record review study on the incidence and preventability of adverse events requiring a higher level of care in Belgian hospitals. BMC Res Notes. 2012 Aug 29;5:468.

Wadhwa M. Electronic Health Records in India.:23.

Dugar D. Future of Electronic Medical Records 2021 | EMR Trends [Internet]. 2021 [cited 2021 Jul 10]. Available from: https://www.selecthub.com/medical-software/emr/electronic-medical-records-future-emr-trends/

Publication I. MEDICAL RECORD DEPARTMENT: AN ANALYTICAL STUDY. [cited 2021 Jul 10]; Available from: https://www.academia.edu/19864782/MEDICAL_RECORD_DEPARTMENT_AN_ANALYTICAL_STUDY

He X, Cai L, Huang S, Ma X, Zhou X. The design of electronic medical records for patients of continuous care. J Infect Public Health. 2021 Jan 1;14(1):117–22.

34 Mortuary

Hospital Mortuary is the place where dead bodies are temporarily kept, under the specified climatic conditions, until either post mortem is carried out or it is handed over to the police or family, or it is finally disposed of. Thus, hospital mortuary can be either used only for storage and disposal of bodies or as a post mortem facility with adequate provisions.

Mortuary
It is primarily used for the storage of bodies and includes a refrigerated body storage facility and may include a body viewing and preparation room.

Autopsy Unit
It is a facility attached to the mortuary which is used to investigate the cause of death. It comprises an autopsy room, change room and observation area. Additional autopsy functions may be provided at large hospitals or as per the country's guidelines.

The size of the mortuary shall depend on the number of cabinets/body storage spaces required and the death rate in the hospital. As a general rule, space for four bodies per 300 beds is workable, excluding isolation storage.

34.1 Location of the Mortuary

The hospital Mortuary/Autopsy Unit shall be located away from the main clinical areas. It can either be the same building or some annexure building to the main hospital. Also, the mortuary shall have a separate route that is not generally used by the patients or staff. The best solution is to have a separate back door from the hospital building, from where the bodies can be moved to the mortuary.

The mortuary shall ideally be located on the ground floor or basement of the hospital for easy and discrete access for ambulances, police, and funeral vehicles to deliver and/or remove bodies through an exit door.

34.2 Infrastructure of Mortuary

The following areas shall be incorporated in a mortuary which operates with post mortem facility:

Mortuary	Entry Lobby
	Body Wash
	Body Holding Area
	Waiting/Viewing Area
	Administration
	Exit Lobby
	Staff Area

If post mortem is to be conducted in a mortuary, it shall have the following facilities in a separate autopsy area:

A. Garg, A. Dewan, *Manual of Hospital Planning and Designing*,
https://doi.org/10.1007/978-981-16-8456-2_34

Autopsy Area	Staff Change Rooms
	Pre Autopsy Room
	Autopsy Room Indoor
	Autopsy Room Outdoor
	Post Autopsy Room
	Autopsy surgeon's room
	Instrument Wash Room
	Viscera Preparation Room
	Viscera Store
	Staff Toilet

34.3 Mortuary (Fig. 34.1)

34.3.1 Entrance Lobby

The Mortuary shall have an entry gate and a small entrance lobby. In the lobby, a small counter shall be provided to receive the body and identify and tag the received body. At this place, records related to receiving and disposal of the bodies

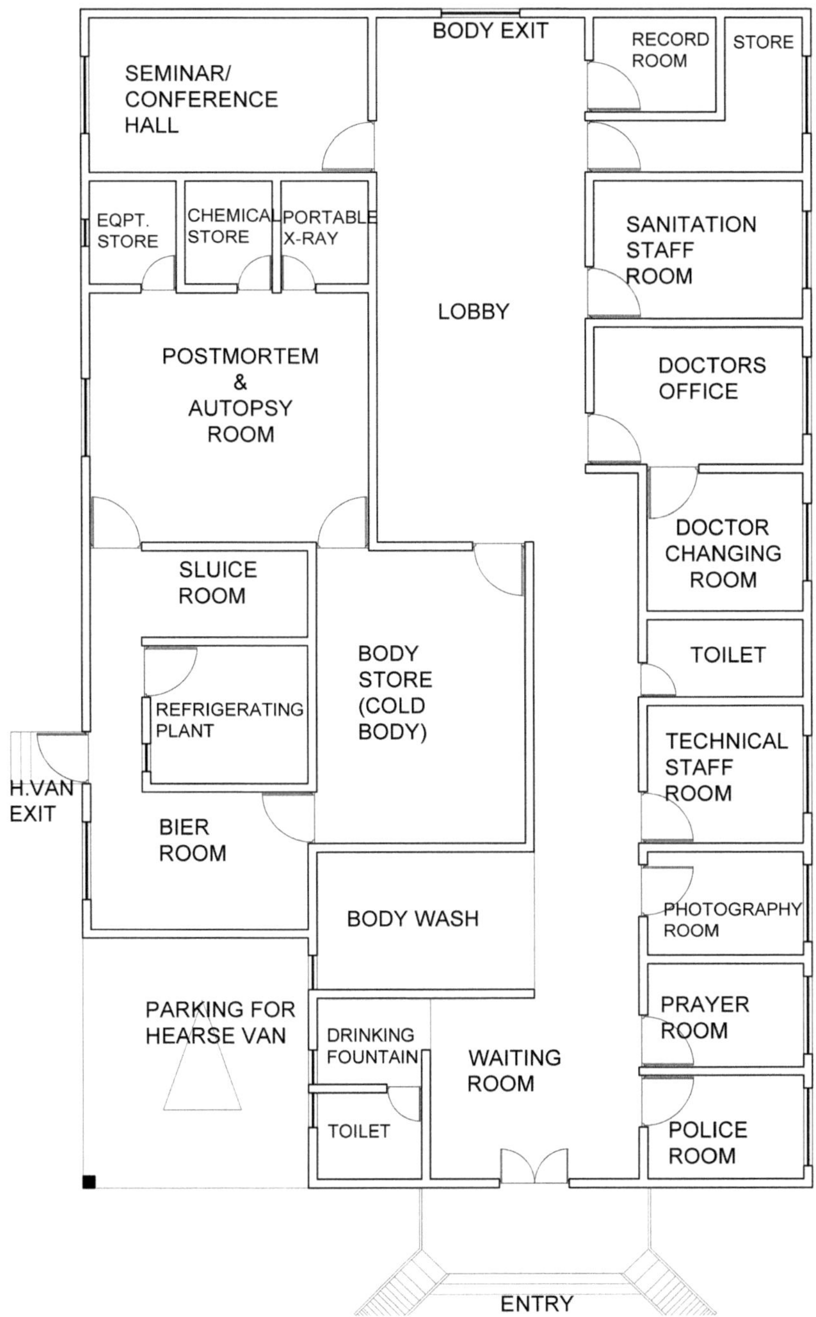

Fig. 34.1 Sample layout drawing of mortuary

shall be maintained. The main gate of the mortuary shall be at least 1829 mm wide, openable both sides. The size of the reception/waiting hall shall be about 6096 mm × 4267 mm.

It shall have direct access to the Body Wash and Body Holding Area. The lobby shall be provided with a hand wash basin with the soap dispensers and towel.

Outside the entrance, adequate space shall be provided for parking ambulances and trolleys bringing the body to the mortuary. A trolley bay shall also be provided, where stretcher trolleys can be placed to unload bodies from the ambulances.

34.3.2 Body Wash

At times it may happen that the bodies are dirty or soiled due to roadside accident, death due to stabbing etc. Under such cases, the body shall be thoroughly washed before taking it in the body holding area. The body wash area shall have a platform with a size 2134 mm (L) × 914 mm (W) × 914 mm (H). The top of the platform shall be slightly curved. The platform shall also have the proper drain, to drain out the water after the wash. On the entire platform, glazed tiles shall be provided for an easy drain of water and proper cleaning of the platform.

For washing the bodies, showers shall be provided on top of the platform. Also, a tap with hose pipe shall be provided in the body wash area. If required, the body can be packed in the body bag here.

34.3.3 Body Holding Area

This is the area where a refrigerated space is provided for the temporary storage of bodies. For this, the following options are available:

1. Provide a walk-in Cool Room for individual trolleys.
2. Install refrigerated cabinets

34.3.3.1 Walk-in Cool Room

In this concept, a chamber is built where the walls and ceiling are made of insulated panels, and wooden flooring is used for thermal control. The door of the chamber is also insulated and sealed, so that outside air shall not enter the chamber. The size of the chamber shall depend on the expected number of bodies to be placed at once and the average holding time of bodies. Generally, 3 m^2 space is required for a body placed on a loose tray or trolley in a cool room. The temperature of the chambers shall be maintained between 2 and 4 °C.

34.3.3.2 Refrigerated Cabinets

In this system, refrigerated body storage cabinets are provided, which have inbuilt slidable drawers to place the body. Generally, a cabinet has two such drawers in one row, i.e. one above the other, and the multiple numbers of such cabinets can be installed. If more than two are provided, it becomes difficult to lift the bodies at height. Still, if cabinets have to be stacked vertically to optimize the use of space, provision of suitable lifting equipment and consideration of equipment turning circles shall be provided. However, this method of storage is not appropriate for bariatric (obese) bodies. Manoeuvring space shall be provided in front of refrigerated cabinets to pull and push the drawers. The temperature of the cabinets shall be maintained between 2 and 4 °C. Please note, separate spaces/cabinets shall be allocated for isolation bodies, and consideration shall be given to storage and handling of a bariatric body.

The body holding area shall be about 6096 mm × 4877 mm in size. However, depending on the requirement, the area can be increased or decreased. The area shall be provided with a power backup system, either by a separate self-start generator or UPS.

34.3.4 Waiting/Viewing Area

The mortuary and autopsy room shall be provided with a waiting area for police and relatives of the deceased. This area shall be just at the entrance of the mortuary and shall have the capacity to accommodate 20–30 people. However, the capacity can be increased or decreased depending on the requirement. An accessible toilet shall also be provided near the waiting area.

As mortuary and autopsy rooms do not have access for the public, the waiting area shall be provided with a viewing area, which shall have a window/partition that it is revealed when a curtain is drawn.

34.3.5 Storage

A store shall be provided in the mortuary and the autopsy room to store clean linen, gowns, aprons, gumboots, towels, cleaning materials, plastic body bags, etc. Also, a lockable storage area shall be provided for storing the deceased's belongings. The size of this store shall be about 3658 mm × 3048 mm. An area shall also be provided in the mortuary for the collection of the used linen and gowns.

34.3.6 Administration Area

Staff area shall be provided depending on the size of the mortuary. This area may include an office, workstations, toilet and any other required amenities. The area should be used by pathologists, mortuary staff, and police for a variety of administrative tasks and confidential telephone calls. At least 2–3 such rooms shall be provided; one for the manager of the size 3658 mm × 3658 mm, one for class IV staff of size 3048 mm × 3048 mm, and one for police officials of size 3048 mm × 3048 mm.

34.3.7 Exit Lobby

The mortuary shall have an exit lobby and exit door. When the body has to be delivered to the relatives or police, it shall be moved out from this door. The door shall be at least 1829 mm wide, openable both sides. The exit lobby shall have direct access to the Body Holding Area. It shall be provided with a hand wash basin with soap dispensers and towel. Outside the exit lobby, adequate space shall be provided for parking ambulances and vehicles taking the body.

34.4 Autopsy Area

34.4.1 Pre Autopsy Room

This room is required for storing bodies before post mortem begins. This can be a walking cool room or refrigerated cabinets can be provided, however, this space shall be separate from that used in the mortuary. As soon as the police bring the body to the mortuary, it should be kept in this room with complete identity. The size of the pre autopsy room shall be about 4267 mm × 3658 mm. Temperature of the room or cabinet shall be between 4 and 6.5 °C.

34.4.2 Autopsy Room (Indoor)

The size of the room shall be about 6096 mm × 6096 mm. The room shall be provided with two dissection tables, preferably made out of 304-grade stainless steel, with arrangements for free drainage of constant water flow from top to bottom. Proper ventilation and the ducting system shall be installed for the exit of foul smell and gases out of the room. Provision shall also be given for inlet of fresh air and air exchanges. The room shall have big-sized windows to allow maximum sunlight in the room.

The flooring of the room shall either be of washable tiles or granite, with an adequate slope to the drain side for easy washing. The walls of the room shall be washable, thus, either tiles can be fixed to up to the height of 2134 mm or washable epoxy paints can be applied.

X-ray view boxes, portable X-ray machines and necessary electric points shall be provided in the room for the operation of the X-ray machine. Also, an electrical point shall be provided near the autopsy table for a portable OT light. A provision of photography shall also be provided in the room.

34.4.3 Autopsy Room (Outdoor)

This room is required for the post mortem of infected or decomposed bodies, which cannot be handled in the main autopsy room. The room shall have all the facilities as in an indoor autopsy room, except the roof, which is generally covered with net.

34.4.4 Post Autopsy Room

This room is required for shifting bodies after completing the post mortem. The body is kept here until it is handed over to the investigating officer, who subsequently handovers the body to the relatives for final disposal. The size of the room shall be about 4267 mm × 4572 mm, and it shall have a platform of about 914 mm × 2134 mm to lay down the bodies.

34.4.5 Autopsy Surgeon's Room

This room shall be provided where the autopsy surgeon/medical officer can discuss details of the case with police and relatives and write reports. The size of the room shall be about 3658 mm × 4267 mm. But depending on the requirement and number of persons likely to sit, the size can be increased or decreased. The room shall have an adequate arrangement of the office table, chairs, cabinets, drawers and racks for a smooth working. It shall also have an attached toilet. If required, a separate store shall be attached to this room. The room shall also have proper arrangements for electrical points, intercom connection, IT network, CCTV surveillance and air-conditioning. Along with the surgeon's room, a small room shall be provided as a staff office to the surgeon. The size of this room shall be about 3658 mm × 3048 mm.

34.4.6 Instrument Wash Room

After every post mortem, the used instruments need to be washed thoroughly before the next use. Hence, an instrument washroom is required for this purpose. The size of the room shall be about 2438 mm × 3048 mm. The room shall be provided with a large-size sink with drain board and countertop for drying up the instruments.

34.4.7 Viscera Preparation Room

This room is required for the preparation of viscera taken after the post mortem. The size of this room shall be about 3658 mm × 3048 mm. The room shall be provided with a countertop, handwash basin, soap dispenser, and towel hanger.

34.4.8 Viscera Stores

The viscera store shall be a lockable room of the size 3658 mm × 3048 mm. This is used for the storage and preservation of the viscera and viscera packing material. The store needs to have sufficient countertops, cupboards, and drawers. The temperature of the room shall be between 17 and 21 °C. The store shall not have any window, and direct sunlight shall be avoided.

34.4.9 Surgeon Change Room

Along with the autopsy room, separate change rooms shall be provided for males and females. The rooms shall be of the size 3048 mm × 3658 mm, and provided with cupboards and cloth hangers. It shall also have staff lockers to store personal belongings.

34.5 Other Infrastructural Issues Relating to the Mortuary/Autopsy Room

While designing the mortuary/autopsy room, the following issues shall be considered:

1. The hot and cold water supply shall be provided in all handwash basins.
2. The entire complex shall be air-conditioned with a separate system for the autopsy rooms to prevent foul air permeating the rest of the area.

No air should be re-circulated in the mortuary in order to ensure a clean air environment.

3. The complex should have the adequate arrangement for fire detection and firefighting, including fire sprinkler, smoke/thermal detector in all rooms and a fire alarm system.
4. The mortuary complex should have all adequate arrangement for the disposal of different types of waste products according to the country's waste disposal rules and regulations.

Further Reading

Hospital Mortuary / Autopsy Unit. Part B. 2015;29.

Brassil KE, Zillman MA. Design for a hospital mortuary. Pathology (Phila). 1993 Oct;25(4):333–7.

Malik AR, Rizvi IH, Ibrahim S. Design and Layout of Standard Autopsy Suite. Ann King Edw Med Univ [Internet]. 2019 Oct 12 [cited 2021 Jul 12];25(3). Available from: https://annalskemu.org/journal/index.php/annals/article/view/3042

Sirohiwal BL, Pk P, Sharma L, Chawla H. Design and Layout of Mortuary Complex for a Medical College and Peripheral Hospitals. 2011;2(6):4.

Chawla H, Sirohiwal B, PK P, Sharma L. Design and Layout of Mortuary Complex for a Medical College and Peripheral Hospitals. J Forensic Res. 2011 Jul 21;2:4.

3 ways to maximize postmortem spaces in medical facilities [Internet]. [cited 2021 Jul 12]. Available from: https://www.hfmmagazine.com/articles/2114-3-ways-to-maximize-postmortem-spaces-in-medical-facilities

35 Administration Area

In any organization, there is a set of people who manage the day to day affairs of the hospital. This set of people is jointly named as the 'administrative team', who reports to the management or the owners of the organization.

As this team has to look after the daily activities of the hospital, their daily presence is required in the hospital. Hence, space has to be allotted in the hospital for accommodating their offices. This space together is known as the 'Administrative Area'.

This area provides spaces for offices, workspaces, and associated facilities for supporting the management of the hospital and includes both clinical and non-clinical support staff.

The size, number, and level of offices will depend on the size of the hospital.

Director's Office	Office
	Toilet
	P.A Room
	Secretarial Staff
	Waiting Area For Visitors
Medical Superintendent's Office	Office
	Toilet
	P.A room
	Secretarial staff
	Waiting area for visitors
Dy. Medical Superintendent's Office	Office
	Toilet
	P.A Room
	Secretarial staff
	Waiting area for visitors

Nursing Administration

Nursing Superintendent's Office	Office
	Toilet
	P.A Room
	Secretarial Staff
	Waiting Area For Visitors
Dy. Nursing Superintendent's Office	Office
	Toilet

General Administration

Personnel Office	Personnel Manager
	Training and Skill Development Manager
	Attendance Management
	Leaves record
	Clerks
	Toilet
Accounts Office	Finance manager
	Chief cashier
	Accounts officers
	Clerks
	Stores
	Sub-waiting
	Public utility for staff

A. Garg, A. Dewan, *Manual of Hospital Planning and Designing*,
https://doi.org/10.1007/978-981-16-8456-2_35

Marketing Office	Marketing manager
	Marketing staff
	Design room
	Meeting room
	Stores
	Sub-waiting
	Public utility for staff
Purchase Office	Purchase manager
	Purchase officer
	Stores
	Sub-waiting
	Public utility for staff
Hospital Information	IT manager
	IT control room
	Server room
	Public utility for staff

35.1 Levels of Administrative Staff

There are various people responsible for the management of the hospital. These people can be at different staff positions, including Senior Management, Senior Executive Level Management, Executive Level Management, Junior level Management etc. We can categorize the staff as follows:

Senior Level Management	Directors
	Chief Executive Officer (CEO) or (COO)
	Medical Superintendent
	Dy. Medical Superintendent
	Nursing Superintendent
Senior executive level management	Dy. Medical superintendent
	Dy. Nursing superintendent
	Personnel manager
	Training and skill development manager
	Finance manager
	Marketing manager
	Purchase manager
	HVAC engineer
	Civil engineer
	Electrical engineer
	Biomedical manager
	IT manager
	Stores manager
Executive level management	Chief cashier
	Accounts officers
	Design officer
	Marketing executives
	Purchase officer
	Store officers
	IT officers
Junior level management	Personal assistants
	Accounts clerks
	Store keepers
	Electrical line man
	Purchasers
	BioMedical assistants

The above list is not exhaustive but just an example. The actual grading shall depend on hospital policies.

35.2 Infrastructure of the Administrative Area

The administration unit may include the following spaces:

1. Main Reception and Enquiries.
2. Offices for Senior Management and their support staff.
3. Offices for Senior Executive Management and support staff.
4. Offices for Executive Management.
5. Nursing Office.
6. Human Resources and Payroll Office.
7. Finance and Accounting Office.
8. Facility Management Office.
9. Public Relations Office.
10. Legal Services Office.
11. Quality Management Office.
12. Training, Education and Research, this may be a separate area in large healthcare facilities.

35.3 Location of the Administrative Area

The administrative area shall either be located in the hospital building or in a separate annexure building to the main hospital. If it is in the main hospital building, it shall be located away from the clinical departments. However, it shall be easily approachable as a lot of visitors and hospital staff needs the services of this department on a day-to-day basis.

35.4 Reception

This is the place where visitors and staff contact before entering the administration office and shall also act as an Enquiry Counter.

35.5 Infrastructure of Reception

1. The reception counter shall be just near the entrance of the administrative area.
2. The waiting area shall be in front of reception but at a distance to maintain social distancing.
3. Reception should be clearly visible and reachable without blocking human traffic.
4. Depending on the size and volume of the visitors in the administrative area, the size of the reception shall be decided.
5. A record room shall be provided with the reception to keep the necessary records and files.
6. *Furniture*

   The following furniture shall be placed in the reception:

(a) Reception Counter
(b) Reception Chair

35.6 Waiting Lobby

After arriving at the reception, visitors need to wait for their turn to meet the concerned person in the administrative area. In the pre-COVID era, waiting lobbies were designed to create a more comfortable space and accommodate a large number of chairs for seating. However, post COVID-19, all public spaces, like waiting areas, shall be carefully planned and designed to create a greater physical separation between people with appropriate queuing. Few suggestions to ensure such social distancing are:

1. Provide individual seats/chairs than clustered.
2. *Sub-Waiting lobbies*

   It is recommended that instead of a large waiting lobby, hospitals shall design small sub-waiting lobbies. For example instead of providing a large lobby at the reception, a separate sub-waiting lobby shall be created for different administrative offices. However, such measures may not be practical in all situations, especially for small healthcare facilities, nursing homes, clinics, etc. In such settings, the number of people allowed to wait in hospital lobbies may be limited to a certain maximum, with a specific minimum spacing between their seats. Thus, future waiting lobbies could be smaller but in scattered clusters.
3. Minimize Interaction with Others

   Trends like self-check-in minimize interaction between people. The concept of a smaller enclave waiting space that separates the visitors shall be preferred. The seating shall be in clusters of small numbers of chairs, say 2–3 chairs per cluster. Further, each cluster shall be portioned from the other with at least 1524 mm acrylic or glass partition to reduce exposure.
4. VIP Waiting Areas

   For important visitors, a VIP waiting area shall be created with a seating of about 8–10 persons. Instead of waiting chairs, the room shall be provided with a sofa set and centre table. The room shall also be provided with a television, drinking water, and an attached toilet. Even a small pantry can be attached to serve tea/coffee to the visitors.

35.7 Offices of the Senior Management

Each and every senior officer of the management shall be provided a separate room as his/her office. The size of this room shall be about 6096 mm × 6096 mm. But depending on the designation, the size of the room can be increased or decreased. The room shall have an adequate arrangement of cabinets, drawers and racks for a smooth working. Preferably the room shall have and attached toilet. If required, a separate store shall be attached to this room. The senior management room shall also be provided with a small personal conference room. If required and long working hours are expected, a small restroom can also be provided with this room. The room shall have proper arrangements for:

35.7.1 Electrical Points

1. Main switchboard at the entrance wall (other than the wall on which door will open) for control of fan and lights of the room along with one 5 Amp Switch/Socket.
2. Air-Conditioning Control button with temperature adjustment.
3. Three 6/16 Amp Switch/Sockets on the wall adjoining the office table. If the table is placed in the centre of the room, an underground cable shall be carried to the table, and electrical points shall be provided on the table.
4. Two 5 Amp Switch/Socket on the wall 305 mm above the office table. Also, one 15 Amp Switch/Socket shall be provided adjoining this.
5. USB charging points shall be provided on the table and near the sofa set placed in the room.

35.7.2 Other Communication Points in the Room

These points can be provided in the office at any convenient place/wall

1. RJ 45 point for Computer networking.
2. RJ 11 for Intercom and extension line.
3. HDMI point for computer display at other locations.
4. Connection to the CCTV surveillance system.

35.7.3 Lighting in the Offices

Lighting for general illumination and specific tasks has to be carefully planned. The following points shall be considered while finalizing the light plan in the offices:

1. Lights shall not be too bright or too dull. Proper lumens have to be planned as per the standards.
2. Use of LED lights is always recommended because of their long life and lower energy consumption.
3. Lights shall be equally distributed in the unit/room.
4. Ceiling flush-mounted lights shall be used instead of surface-exposed lights.
5. Avoid wall lights as they are not effective.
6. Fancy lights can be used.
7. To prevent burns, incandescent and halogen light sources should be avoided.
8. Flexible arms, if used with this light source, must be mechanically controlled to prevent the lamp from contacting linen.
9. Emergency battery-operated light shall be provided in the corridors and offices.
10. It will be better if light controls are done through variable-control dimmers at the user end.

35.7.4 Doors

Preferably the door of the offices shall be made out of wood, or flush doors shall be used. The width of the doors shall not be less than 1219 mm wide, unobstructed. The door shall be provided with a door closer and stopper. The door shall have a provision of being locked both from inside and outside.

35.7.5 Windows

The window shall be as wide as possible and fitted with tinted glass, maybe with a double vacuum glass. The windows shall be covered either with curtains or vanishing blinds.

35.7.6 Flooring

Flooring of the office shall look aesthetic, give a clean appearance, and shall provide a positive and welcoming atmosphere. The flooring of the offices can be either laid with Italian marble or some other stone. Carpet can also be used in the executive rooms.

35.7.7 Air-Conditioning

The office shall be provided with air-conditioners. The system shall be connected to the central HVAC system, with separate AHU's for the administrative area. Ducts can be provided in the rooms which shall be connected to the AHU. Alternatively, Fan Coil Units can be provided in the room individually. The temperature in the offices shall be between 18 and 24 °C and RH of about 45–50%.

35.7.8 Room Décor

Pleasant aesthetic surroundings and increased comfort result in better work output. Hence, the following points shall be considered:

1. Good colour schemes affect mood and stress levels. Thus, use light green and blue colour tone on the walls.
2. Wall furnishings shall be excellent with waterproof washable paints.
3. Pictures, paintings, murals and artwork shall be placed appropriately.

35.7.9 Furniture in the Executive Offices

The following furniture shall be provided:

1. Offices
   (a) Executive Office Table
   (b) Side Rack
   (c) Back Rack
   (d) Executive Chair
   (e) Executive Visitors Chair
   (f) Sofa Set
   (g) Centre Table
   (h) Coat Hanger
   (i) Refrigerator
   (j) Television
2. Conference room
   (a) Conference Table
   (b) Conference Chairs
   (c) Projector
   (d) Projector Screen or Multi-Media Television
3. Rest Room
   (a) Resting Bed
   (b) Study Table
   (c) Chair

35.7.10 Acoustics

Acoustic treatment shall be done in the meeting and conference rooms to reduce the noise between rooms, particularly those used for teleconferencing, video-conferencing, and large meetings. Acoustic separation should be provided between offices, meeting rooms, interview rooms, and adjacent corridors to reduce the transfer of noise between rooms, particularly for private conversations which should not be audible outside the room.

35.7.11 Privacy

Visual privacy shall be considered while designing places where confidential conversations are likely to take place in offices, meeting and conference rooms.

35.8 Offices of the Senior Executive Level Management

Each and every senior executive shall be provided a separate room as his/her office. The size of this room shall be about 4572 mm × 4267 mm, but depending on the designation; the size of the room can be increased or decreased. The room shall have an adequate arrangement of cabinets, drawers and racks for a smooth working. Preferably the room shall have an attached Toilet. The room shall have proper arrangements for:

35.8.1 Electrical Points

1. Main switch board at the entrance wall (other than the wall on which door will open) for control of fan and lights of the room along with one 5 Amp Switch/Socket.
2. Air-Conditioning Control button with temperature adjustment.
3. Three 6/16 Amp Switch/Sockets on the wall adjoining the office table. If the table is placed in the centre of the room, an underground cable shall be carried to the table, and electrical points shall be provided on the table.
4. Two 5 Amp Switch/Socket on the wall 305 mm above the office table. Also, one 15 Amp Switch/Socket shall be provided adjoining this.
5. USB charging points shall be provided on the table.

35.8.2 Other Communication Points in the Room

Can be provided in the executive office at any convenient place/wall

1. RJ 45 point for Computer networking.
2. RJ 11 for Intercom and extension line.
3. HDMI point for computer display at other locations.

35.8.3 Lighting in the Offices

Lighting for general illumination and specific tasks has to be carefully planned. The following points shall be considered while finalizing the light plan in the offices:

1. Lights shall not be too bright or too dull. Proper lumens have to be planned as per the standards.
2. Use of LED lights is always recommended because of their long life and lower energy consumption.
3. Lights shall be equally distributed in the unit/room.
4. Ceiling flush-mounted lights shall be used instead of surface-exposed lights.
5. Avoid wall lights as they are not effective.
6. Fancy lights can be used.
7. To prevent burns, incandescent and halogen light sources should be avoided.
8. Flexible arms, if used with this light source, must be mechanically controlled to prevent the lamp from contacting linen.
9. Emergency battery-operated light shall be provided in the corridors and offices.
10. It will be better if light controls are done through variable-control dimmers at the user end.

35.8.4 Doors

Preferably the door of the offices shall be made out of wood, or flush doors shall be used. The width of the doors shall not be less than 1219 mm wide, unobstructed. The door shall be provided with a door closer and stopper. The door shall have a provision of being locked both from inside and outside.

35.8.5 Windows

The window shall be as wide as possible and fitted with tinted glass, maybe with a double vacuum glass. The windows shall be covered either with curtains or vanishing blinds.

35.8.6 Flooring

Flooring of the office shall look aesthetic, give a clean appearance, and shall provide a positive and welcoming atmosphere. The flooring of the offices can be either laid with Italian marble or some other stone. Carpet can also be used in the executive rooms.

35.8.7 Air-Conditioning

The office shall be provided with air-conditioners. The system shall be connected to the central HVAC system, with separate AHUs for the administrative area. Ducts can be provided in the rooms which shall be connected to the AHU. Alternatively, Fan Coil Units can be provided in the room individually. The temperature in the offices shall be between 18 and 24 °C and RH of about 45–50%.

35.8.8 Furniture in the Executive Offices

The following furniture shall be provided in the offices:

1. Offices
   (a) Office Table
   (b) Side Rack
   (c) Officer Chair
   (d) Visitors Chair
   (e) Television

35.8.9 Acoustics

Acoustic treatment shall be done in the rooms. Acoustic separation should be provided between offices, meeting rooms, and adjacent corridors to reduce the transfer of noise between rooms, particularly for private conversations which should not be audible outside the room.

35.9 Offices of the Executive Level Management

One or more than one (Better if not more than two) executives shall be provided with a room as their office. If two persons are to be placed in one room, the size of this room shall be about 4572 mm × 4267 mm. If Single person is to be placed, the size shall be about 3658 mm × 3658 mm. But depending on the designation the size of the room can be increased or decreased. The room shall adequate arrangement of cabinets, drawers, racks for a smooth working. The room shall have proper arrangements for.

35.9.1 Electrical Points

1. Main switch board at the entrance wall (other than the wall on which door will open) for control of fan and lights of the room along with one 5 Amp Switch/Socket.
2. Air-Conditioning Control button with temperature adjustment.
3. Three 6/16 Amp Switch/Sockets on the wall adjoining the office tables.
4. Two 5 Amp Switch/Socket above on the wall 305 mm above the office table. Also, one 15 Amp Switch/Socket shall be provided adjoining this.

35.9.2 Other Communication Points in the Room

Can be provided in the office at any convenient place/wall

1. RJ 45 point for Computer networking
2. RJ 11 for Intercom and extension line
3. HDMI point for computer display at other locations

35.9.3 Lighting in the Offices

LED ceiling-mounted lights shall be provided in the rooms.

35.9.4 Doors

Preferably the Door of the offices shall be made out of wood or flush doors shall be used. The width of the doors shall not be less than 1067 mm wide, unobstructed. The door shall be provided with a door closer and stopper. The door shall have a provision of being locked both from inside and outside.

35.9.5 Windows

The window shall be as wide as possible and fitted with tinted glass, maybe with a double vacuum glass.

35.9.6 Flooring

The flooring of the offices can be either laid with simple marble or some other stone.

35.9.7 Air-Conditioning

The office shall be provided with air-conditioners. The system shall be connected to the central HVAC system, with separate AHU's for the administrative area. Ducts can be provided in the rooms which shall be connected to the AHU. Alternatively, Fan Coil Units can be provided in the room individually. The temperature in the offices shall be between 18 and 24 °C and RH of about 45–50%.

35.9.8 Furniture in the Executive Offices

The following furniture shall be provided in the offices:

1. Offices
   (a) Office Table
   (b) Officer Chair
   (c) Visitors Chair

35.10 Offices of the Junior Level Management

For junior level, rooms are not required, but they shall be provided with a hall where multiple desks/workstations are installed. Each workstation shall have an adequate arrangement of cabinets, drawers and racks for a smooth working. The size of the hall shall depend on the number of persons to be seated in the hall.

Each administrative department of the hospital shall be provided with separate halls fitted with multi desk workstations, where their staff can be accommodated. For example, one hall each shall be given for the purchase department, HR department, accounts etc.

The room shall have proper arrangements for.

35.10.1 Electrical Points

1. Main switch board at the entrance wall (other than the wall on which door will open) for control of fan and lights of the room along with one 5 Amp Switch/Socket
2. Air-Conditioning Control button with temperature adjustment
3. Each workstation shall have Two 6/16 Amp Switch/Sockets on the modular wall of the desk

35.10.2 Other Communication Points

The following communication points shall be provided on each workstation

1. RJ 45 point for Computer networking
2. RJ 11 for Intercom and extension line
3. HDMI point for computer display at other locations

35.10.3 Lighting in the Offices

LED ceiling-mounted lights shall be provided in the rooms.

35.10.4 Doors

Preferably the Door of the offices shall be made out of wood or flush doors shall be used. The width of the doors shall not be less than 1067 mm wide, unobstructed. The door shall have a provision of being locked both from inside and outside.

35.10.5 Windows

The window shall be as wide as possible and fitted with tinted glass, maybe with a double vacuum glass.

35.10.6 Flooring

The flooring of the offices can be either laid with simple marble or some other similar stone or tiles.

35.10.7 Air-Conditioning

The office shall be provided with air-conditioners. The system shall be connected to the central HVAC system, with separate AHU's for the administrative area. Ducts can be provided in the rooms which shall be connected to the AHU. Alternatively, Fan Coil Units can be provided in the room individually. The temperature in the offices shall be between 18 and 24 °C and RH of about 45–50%.

35.11 Support Room/Facilities

The following support rooms/facilities are generally required in the administration area:

35.11.1 Senior Management's PA Room

For the senior management personnel, a PA room shall be provided. This room shall either be attached to or in close vicinity to the officer's room. The size of this room shall be about 3658 mm × 3658 mm, but depending on the requirement, the size of the room can be increased or decreased. The room shall have adequate an arrangement of cabinets, drawers and racks for a smooth working. The room shall have an extra door which shall open in the officer's room. The room shall also have proper electricity, communication points and air-conditioning arrangement.

35.11.2 Secretarial Staff

Separate rooms are not required for the secretarial staff, but they shall be provided with a hall where multiple desks/workstations are installed. Each workstation shall have an adequate arrangement of cabinets, drawers and racks for a smooth working. Each workstation shall be provided with electricity and communication points, and air-conditioning shall be common in the hall.

35.11.3 Kitchen

A small kitchenette shall be provided in the administrative area for preparing tea/coffee for the guests and the staff. This kitchenette shall also have the provision for warming food which the staff brings from home as lunch. The size of the kitchenette shall be about 3658 mm × 4267 mm. It shall be provided with a working top for cooking and installing kitchen gadgets. The countertop shall have a deep stainless steel sink with a drainboard for washing utensils. A gas burner shall also be provided within a connection to a gas cylinder. The kitchenette shall have a refrigerator, microwave oven, induction heating pad, OTG, utensils, and other required items like a mixer, juicer etc.

35.11.4 Dining Area

Close to the kitchenette shall be a dining room with a dining table and chair to accommodate 10–15 people. The size of the room shall be about 4572 mm × 3658 mm. It shall be provided with a handwashing facility with soap dispenser and paper towel.

35.11.5 Staff Toilets

They shall be separate for males and females. The toilets shall have WC's, urinals, and washbasin. If required, the bathing facility can also be provided.

35.11.6 Store

Stores shall be located at a conveniently accessible place for storing all required files and stationery. It shall be 3658 mm × 3658 mm in size, but the size may vary depending on the quantity and number of items to be stored. The store needs to have a sufficient number of countertops, cupboards, and drawers. The temperature of the room shall be between 17 and 21 °C. It shall be lockable and secure to keep confidential administration, finance, and human resources records.

35.11.7 Notice Boards

A notice board shall be planned near the reception so that it is visible to all those arriving in the administrative area. The board shall be made out cork to allow easy use of board pins. If possible, a light shall be provided above the notice board to make it more readable.

35.12 Meeting Rooms

A single large meeting room or multiple small meeting rooms shall be provided in the administrative area. Before designing these rooms, the designer shall consider the requirements of different administrative departments of the hospital. Small meeting room shall be designed to accommodate 10 people, and the size of the room shall be about 6096 mm × 4572 mm. If a large meeting/conference room is planned, the size of the room shall be about 15,240 mm × 6096 mm, and it shall have seating arrangement for 50 people.

In either case, the following points shall be considered:

1. The meeting room shall be provided with teleconference or video-conference facilities.
2. At all seats, conference audio system shall be provided.
3. Speakers connected to the audio system shall be installed in the ceiling.
4. A projector and projector screen shall be provided in the room.
5. If possible, a smart board shall be provided.
6. A stage or podium with audio system connection shall be provided.

35.12.1 Electrical Points

1. Main switch board at the entrance wall (other than the wall on which door will open) for control of fan and lights of the room along with one 6 Amp Switch/Socket.
2. Air-Conditioning Control button with temperature adjustment.
3. On the conference table, a module of electrical points shall be provided. The module shall have, three 6/16 Amp Switch/Sockets, 1 USB charging point, RJ 45 point and 1 HDMI point.
4. 1 electrical point for projector shall be provided at the podium.
5. If a smartboard is used, the required electrical outlet shall be provided near the board.

35.12.2 Other Communication Points in the Room

The following communication points shall be provided in the room at any convenient place/wall:

1. RJ 45 point for Computer networking.
2. RJ 11 for Intercom and extension line.
3. Connection to the CCTV surveillance system.

35.12.3 Lighting

Lighting for general illumination and specific tasks has to be carefully planned. The following points shall be considered while finalizing the lighting of meeting rooms:

1. Lights shall not be too bright or too dull. Proper lumens have to be planned as per the standards.
2. Use of LED lights is always recommended because of their long life and lower energy consumption.
3. Lights shall be equally distributed in the room.
4. Ceiling flush-mounted lights shall be used instead of surface-exposed lights.
5. Avoid wall lights as they are not effective.
6. To prevent burns, incandescent and halogen light sources should be avoided.
7. Emergency battery-operated light shall be provided in the room.
8. It will be better if light controls are done through variable-control dimmers at the user end.

35.12.4 Doors

Preferably the door of the meeting room shall be made out of wood or flush doors shall be used. The width of the doors shall not be less than 1829 mm wide, unobstructed. The door shall be provided with a door closer and stopper. The door shall have the provision of being locked both from inside and outside.

35.12.5 Windows

The window shall be as wide as possible and fitted with tinted glass, maybe with a double vacuum glass. The windows shall be covered either with the blackout curtains or vanishing blinds.

35.12.6 Flooring

Flooring of the room shall look aesthetic, give a clean appearance, and shall provide a positive and welcoming atmosphere. The flooring of the meeting room can be either laid with Italian marble or some other stone. Carpet can also be used in the meeting rooms.

35.12.7 Air-Conditioning

The office shall be provided with air-conditioners. The system shall be connected to the central HVAC system, with separate AHU's for meeting rooms. Ducts can be provided in the rooms which shall be connected to the AHU. Alternatively, Fan Coil Units can be provided in the room individually. The temperature in the offices shall be between 18 and 24 °C and RH of about 45–50%.

35.12.8 Room Decor

Pleasant and aesthetic surroundings shall be designed, and the following issues shall be addressed while designing the room:

1. The good colour scheme shall be used on the walls, particularly light green and blue colours.
2. Wall furnishings shall be excellent with waterproof washable paints.
3. Pictures, paintings, murals and artwork shall be appropriately provided.

35.12.9 Furniture in the Meeting Room

The following furniture shall be provided in the meeting rooms:

1. Conference Table
2. Conference Chairs

3. Projector
4. Projector Screen or Multi-Media Television
5. Smart Board

35.12.10 Acoustics

Acoustic treatment shall be done in the meeting and conference rooms to reduce noise between rooms, particularly if used for tele-conferencing, video-conferencing, and large meetings.

35.12.11 Privacy

Visual privacy shall be considered while designing spaces where confidential conversations are likely to take place in the meeting and conference rooms.

Further Reading

Lakshmi EV, Kumar PD. Planning, Analysis And Design Of An Administrative Building At N.B.K.R.I.S.T. 2019;7(1):5.

GmbH E. Lighting for offices and administrative buildings | ERCO [Internet]. [cited 2021 Jul 12]. Available from: https://www.erco.com/en/designing-with-light/work/work-6443/

Mohammad K, Ranjan R, Singh A, Siddharth V, Sharma D. Hospital Administration Control Room- An Effective Concept for Managing Hospital Operation Issues: A Study in Tertiary Care Public Sector Hospital. International Journal of Research Foundation of Hospital and Healthcare Administration. 2018 Dec 1;6:82–90.

Dani Jose, Donna Rajan, Jitha K. R, Praveen Mathew, Treesa Varghese M, M A College of Engineering. Functional Planning of An Administrative Building. Int J Eng Res. 2015 Mar 27;V4(03):IJERTV4IS030897.

Stores in the Hospital

36

The stores are a vital part of all industrial undertakings, including the hospitals. It is the centre of activities from where materials used in the hospital are controlled.

The main objectives of the store are:

1. Availability of a balanced and timely flow of all materials like consumables, medical disposables, spare parts and components, tools and equipment and other general supplies.
2. Receive, inspect and issue the above supplies/stores to the hospital.
3. Accept, store and arrange disposal of scrap and unwanted supplies/stores.

36.1 Functions of Stores

The following functions need to be performed by the stores:

1. *Identification* is the process of codifying and describing all items required to be stocked.
2. *Receipt* is the process of receiving the materials ordered by the purchase department after verification and inspection of quality and quantity of all materials received in the stores.
3. *Inspection* is checking of all incoming materials for quality and quantity.
4. *Storage* is the process of storing the materials in warehouse, stockyards etc.
5. *Stock control* is the process of provisioning which means continuously arranging recoupment, receipts and issues of stocks to ensure required service is consistent with the economy. The store has to keep the materials in safe custody.
6. *Issues and dispatch* is the process of receiving demand from different hospital departments and issuing the demanded materials without losing time.
7. *Stock records* have to be maintained, showing day-to-day position of receipt issues and stock balances.
8. *Stores accounting* is entering each receipt and issue a voucher in a manner so that the balance material in-store can be worked out and also know the funds spent on each department of the hospital. This also includes passing the bills of the received materials.
9. *Stocktaking* is the process of physically verifying the quantities of materials and their condition in the stock at specified intervals and to compare it with the quantities shown in stock records.
10. *Raising demand* to the purchase department for materials to be procured.

A. Garg, A. Dewan, *Manual of Hospital Planning and Designing*,
https://doi.org/10.1007/978-981-16-8456-2_36

36.2 Types of Hospital Stores

The hospital stores can be divided into two broad categories:

1. *Non-Consu mable Stores*
   These stores include the items which are not used so frequently like surgical instruments, patient furniture, general furniture, rubber goods, enamelware, electrical items etc. or otherwise for the capital items.
2. *Consumable Stores*
   These stores include items that are used more frequently or are used repeatedly, like cotton, bandages, catheters, linen, stationery, lab reagents, chemicals etc.

36.3 Planning of Hospital Stores

Hospitals have a different type of stores, depending on the nature of the items dealt with. Generally, hospitals have the following stores:

1. *Medical and Drug Stores*
   This store deals with medicines, formulary, emergency drugs, general drugs, special drugs, medical gases, chemicals etc.
2. *Surgical Stores*
   This store deals with items like bandages, gauzes, sutures, instruments, equipment, rubber goods, glass items, cotton and general surgical items.
3. *General Stores*
   This store deals with cleaning materials like soaps and detergents, enamel wares, ward/ general furniture, small electrical items etc.
4. *Equipment Stores*
   This store deals with medical equipment like machines, spares of the equipment, and consumables to be used in the equipment.
5. *Linen Stores*
   This store deals with textiles, synthetic fabric, woolen articles, patient dress, doctors dress, staff dress, ward linen, blankets, pillows, bedsheets, curtains and furnishings.
6. *Stationery Stores*
   This store deals with medical forms, papers for medical documentation, registers, office stationery etc.
7. *Dietary Stores*
   This store is usually attached to the kitchens and deals with items like vegetables, fruits, tinned item and dry ration.
8. *Engineering and Maintenance*
   This store deals with the items required for maintenance of the hospital, such as civil maintenance, electrical maintenance, HVAC maintenance, plumbing maintenance, wooden and steel maintenance, IT maintenance, mechanical and electronic maintenance, etc. Depending on the material load, a single store can be provided for all maintenance departments or separate store can be provided for each department.
9. *Condemnation Store*
   This store deals with the acquisition and disposal of condemned items of the hospital.

36.4 Location of the Stores

Stores shall be located at a place that is away from the general movement or clinical areas of the hospital. This space shall be restricted to unauthorized persons.

The areas like the basement, which is otherwise unusable for clinical departments can be used for stores.

If the main hospital building does not have enough space for stores, they can be taken in the annexure building of the main hospital.

While deciding the location of the store, the safety of material form unnecessary pilferage, theft and the fire must be ensured.

The location shall allow easy shifting of materials and easy approachability of small vehicles. Vertical lifts shall be provided in the stores.

The store building should be close to the area where materials are required. While selecting a suitable site for a store, consideration should be given to temperature, humidity, and lighting arrangements, along with future expansion plans.

36.5 Infrastructure of Stores

The following points shall be considered while designing the stores:

36.5.1 Store

Depending on the number of stores, nature of the material to be handled, workload, number of items to be dealt with, and the cost of material to be handled, the size of the store shall be worked out. There is no fixed size, but it depends on the user to decide the size of the store. The following store size recommendations are given based on experience:

Store type	Size of the store room
Medical and drug stores	9144 mm × 9144 mm
Surgical stores	9144 mm × 9144 mm
General stores	12,192 mm × 9144 mm
Equipment stores	12,192 mm × 12,192 mm
Linen stores	9144 mm × 9144 mm
Stationery stores	6096 mm × 9144 mm
Engineering and maintenance	30,480 mm × 15,240 mm
Condemnation store	30,480 mm × 15,240 mm

36.5.2 Storekeeper Room

A separate room shall be provided for the storekeeper. This room shall either be attached to the store premises or shall be in close vicinity to the store. Depending on the requirements, there can be one or more rooms for different storekeepers. Some hospitals prefer to have a separate room for each type of store. The size of this room shall be about 4267 mm × 3658 mm, but depending on the requirement the size of the room can be increased or decreased. The room shall adequate arrangement of cabinets, drawers, and racks for a smooth working. The room shall also have proper arrangements for electricity, communication points and air-conditioning.

36.5.3 Store Secretarial Staff

For secretarial staff, rooms are not required, but they shall be provided with a hall where multiple desks/workstations are installed. Each workstation shall have an adequate arrangement of cabinets, drawers, and racks for a smooth working. Each workstation shall have proper arrangements for electricity and communication points, with air-conditioning being common to the hall.

36.5.4 Kitchen

A small kitchenette shall be provided near the stores for preparing tea/coffee for the guests and the staff. This kitchenette shall also have the provision for warming food which the staff brings from home as lunch. The size of the kitchenette shall be about 3658 mm × 3658 mm. It shall be provided with a working top for cooking and installing kitchen gadgets. The countertop shall have a deep stainless steel sink with a drain board for washing utensils. A gas burner shall also be provided within a connection to a gas cylinder.

36.5.5 Staff Toilets

Toilets shall be separate for males and females. The toilets shall have WC's, urinals, and washbasin. If required, the bathing facility can also be provided.

36.5.6 Special Store Room

Special locked room shall be provided within the stores for storing expensive items and confidential store documents. This storeroom shall be located at a conveniently accessible place but shall be directly visible from the storekeeper room. The store shall be 3658 mm × 3658 mm in size, but the size may vary depending on the quantity and number of items to be stored. The store needs to have sufficient countertops, cupboards, and drawers. The temperature of the room shall be between 17 and 21 °C.

36.5.7 Cold Room

A cold walk-in store/refrigerated room shall be provided in the medical and drug store for storing specific drugs which require a cold chain or are to be kept under cool temperature. The size of the room shall be about 3048 mm × 3048 mm. The walls and ceiling of the room shall be made out of puff panel, which acts as a thermal barrier. The door of the room shall also be made out of puff panel and shall be hermetically sealed. The flooring is generally made out of wooden planks. For storage, open racks shall be provided along the walls. Inside the room, air-conditioning shall be done, and the temperature shall be kept between 5 and 12 °C, which might be adjusted as needed. The room shall be provided with a temperature monitoring system and shall be connected to a centralized alarm/warning system. All access doors to this room shall be lockable.

36.5.8 Issue Counter

The store shall have an issue counter near the entrance door. The user shall remain at the issue counter while the material is being taken out and issued to the user. Sufficient space shall be provided outside the issue counter for the user to be seated, and there shall be adequate space for parking trolleys carrying material.

36.5.9 Receiving Area

The store shall have a separate enclosure for keeping the material received from outside, either from a vendor or from within the hospital. This area is required for keeping material till its quality and quantity validation is complete. Once completed, the material is shifted to the store, and this area is vacated.

36.6 Other Infrastructure Issues

While designing stores, the following shall be considered:

36.6.1 Electrical Points

1. Main switch board at the entrance wall (other than the wall on which door will open) for control of fan and lights of the room along with one 6 Amp Switch/Socket.
2. Air-Conditioning Control button with temperature adjustment.
3. The suitable electrical point with 6 Amp Switch/Sockets shall be provided on the vacant walls of the stores to help testing of items, charging of machinery, or otherwise for miscellaneous use. If required, 16 Amp switch/sockets can also be provided.

36.6.2 Other Communication Points in the Room

The following communication points shall be provided near the office table of the storekeeper:

1. RJ 45 point for Computer networking.
2. RJ 11 for Intercom and extension line.
3. Connection to the CCTV surveillance system.

36.6.3 Lighting in the Stores

Lighting for general illumination and specific tasks has to be carefully planned. The following points shall be considered while finalizing the light plan in the stores

1. Lights shall not be too bright or too dull. Proper lumens have to be planned as per the standards.
2. Use of LED lights is always recommended because of their long life and lower energy consumption.
3. Lights shall be equally distributed in the store.
4. If the store has been provided with a false ceiling, ceiling flush-mounted lights shall be used; however, if the false ceiling is not provided, then surface mounted ceiling lights can be used.
5. Avoid wall lights as they are not effective.
6. To prevent burns, incandescent and halogen light sources should be avoided.
7. Emergency battery-operated light shall be provided in the stores.

36.6.4 Doors

Preferably the door of the stores shall be made out of wood, or flush doors shall be used. Aluminium doors can also be used as an alternative. However, MS steel doors are not recommended as they rust and give a poor appearance. The width of the doors shall not be less than 1829 mm wide, unobstructed. The door shall be provided with a door closer and stopper. The door shall have a provision of being locked both from inside and outside.

36.6.5 Windows

The window shall be as wide as possible and fitted with tinted glass, maybe with a double vacuum glass. The windows shall be covered either with curtains or vanishing blinds.

36.6.6 Flooring

Flooring of the store shall be steady to tolerate a heavy load of material. On the other hand, it shall look aesthetic, give a clean appearance, and shall provide a positive and welcoming atmosphere. The flooring of the offices can be either laid with marble, Kota stone, or tiles.

36.6.7 Air-Conditioning

If required, stores shall be provided with air-conditioners. The system shall be connected to the central HVAC system, with separate AHUs for storage area. Ducts can be provided in the stores which shall be connected to the AHU. The temperature in the stores shall be between 18 and 24 °C and RH of about 45–50%.

36.6.8 Furniture in the Stores

The following furniture shall be provided in the storerooms:

1. Slotted angle racks.
2. Heavy-duty racks made out of Stainless Steel or Mild Steel with proper shelves. The shelves shall be of different heights to accommodate all type of materials. It can be 229 mm to 610 mm high, depending on the requirement.
3. Bins for storing small items like bolts, sanitary items like elbows, tees, plugs, electrical materials like connectors, switches, PVC tape and plugs etc. The size of the bins shall be as per the requirement. It can range from as low as 152 mm × 152 mm to as large as 305 mm × 305 mm.
4. Wall fixed cupboard with locking facility.
5. Office table for storekeeper.
6. Office Chairs.
7. Visitor Chair.
8. Plastic or wooden pallets for stocking material on the floor.
9. Twin leg stairs for climbing to the rack height.
10. Material handling fork lifters, if required.

36.6.9 Notice Boards

A notice board shall be planned near the storekeeper so that it is visible to all those arriving in the store. The board shall be made out cork to allow easy use of board pins. If possible, a light shall be provided above the notice board to make it more readable.

Further Reading

What works for storeroom, warehouse design [Internet]. Healthcare Purchasing News. 2017 [cited 2021 Jul 12]. Available from: https://www.hpnonline.com/sourcing-logistics/article/13000939/what-works-for-storeroom-warehouse-design

Kent AM, Kirby AE. The design of the store environment and its implications for retail image. Int Rev. Retail Distrib Consum Res. 2009 Sep 1;19(4):457–68.

Supply Chain: Health care reform [Internet]. [cited 2021 Jul 12]. Available from: https://www.mmh.com/article/supply_chain_health_care_reform

Material Handling and Storage Safety Topics [Internet]. SafetyInfo. [cited 2021 Jul 12]. Available from: https://www.safetyinfo.com/material-handling-and-storage-safety-index/

Material Handling [Internet]. [cited 2021 Jul 12]. Available from: https://www.mhi.org/fundamentals/material-handling
Facility Layout and Material Management in the Healthcare Industry | Thought Leadership [Internet]. HMC Architects. 2019 [cited 2021 Jul 12]. Available from: https://hmcarchitects.com/news/facility-layout-and-material-management-in-the-healthcare-industry-2019-09-13/

37 Engineering and Maintenance Unit

It is a universal fact that whatever asset you create, requires repairs and maintenance. In hospitals also, all medical equipment and buildings require repairs and maintenance. This can either be outsourced or in-house repair and maintenance facilities can be developed. Outsourcing, however, elevates the cost of repair and maintenance cost and often, it takes longer time repair an asset. Hence it is recommended to develop in-house repair and maintenance facilities in a hospital.

Type of Repair and Maintenance Required in Hospital:

1. Medical Equipment
2. Electrical Services
3. Plumbing Services
4. HVAC Services
5. MGPS Services
6. IT/CCTV/Low Voltage Services
7. Firefighting Services
8. Mechanical Equipment
9. Building including
   (a) Civil Repairs
   (b) Painting
   (c) Wooden Works
   (d) Steel Works
   (e) Aluminium Works
10. Landscape works
11. Automobile Workshop

37.1 Worksshops

To carry out the above repairs and maintenance work, several workshops are required. Different workshops are designed and planned depending on a load of work or frequency of repairs and maintenance. There are some which shall necessarily be provided, however, others can be clubbed together if the workload of a single workshop is not high. Following are some workshop that shall necessarily be provided:

37.2 Biomedical Workshop

This is used for repair and maintenance of the biomedical equipment in the hospital like X-Ray, Ventilators, Vital Monitor, Defibrillator, Lab instruments, Ultrasound and other medical equipment.

37.3 Electrical Workshop

This is used for repair and maintenance of the electrical supply, switches, sockets, electric motors, MCB and DB boxes, UPS and other electrical items. This workshop is also provided to help the biomedical workshop in repairing and maintaining electrical parts of the biomedical equipment.

A. Garg, A. Dewan, *Manual of Hospital Planning and Designing*,
https://doi.org/10.1007/978-981-16-8456-2_37

37.4 HVAC Workshop

This is used for repair and maintenance of the hospital air-conditioning and cold rooms in the hospital, including the mortuary cabinet, refrigerators and deep freezers.

37.5 MGPS Workshop

This is used for repair and maintenance of the medical gases supplied in the hospital, including the manifold room, pump room and liquid oxygen plant.

37.6 Low Voltage Workshop

This is used for repair and maintenance of the low voltage services in the building like CCTV, IT network, computer systems, Audio-Visual systems, and the internet and Wi-Fi services.

37.7 Building Maintenance

This is used for repair and maintenance of the civil works, plumbing works, painting jobs, wooden works, steel and aluminium works, welding works and mild steel works. Depending on the workload and size of the building, either a common building workshop can be designed, or separate workshops can be created. If one workshop is planned, then separate divisions can be designed for each service, as mentioned above.

37.8 Mechanical Workshop

This is used for repair and maintenance of mechanical machinery like lifts, generators, pumps, and mechanical medical equipment.

37.9 Firefighting Workshop

This is used for repair and maintenance of the firefighting services of the hospital. Depending on the size of the hospital building, either a separate workshop can be designed, or this can be clubbed with the building maintenance workshop.

37.10 Automobile Workshop

If the hospital owns a fleet of vehicles, then an in-house automobile workshop can be designed.

37.11 Location of the Workshops

Workshops shall be located at a place that is away from the general movement or clinical areas of the hospital. This space shall be restricted for unauthorized persons.

The areas like the basement, which is otherwise unusable for clinical departments, can be used for workshops.

The location shall allow easy shifting of materials and easy approachability of small vehicles. Vertical lifts shall be provided in the workshops.

Usually, except for the Biomedical Workshop and Low Voltage workshop, all other workshops can be located outside the main hospital building. This can either be created in a temporary structured building or can be taken in the annexure building of the main hospital.

37.12 Infrastructure of Workshops

The following points shall be considered while designing the workshop:

37.12.1 Workshop

Depending on the number of the workshop, nature of service rendered, and the workload, the size of the workshop shall be worked out. There is no fixed size, but it depends on the user to decide the size of the workshop. The following store size recommendations are given based on experience:

Workshop type	Size of the workshop room
Biomedical workshop	9144 mm × 6096 mm
Electrical workshop	6096 mm × 6096 mm
HVAC workshop	9144 mm × 6096 mm
MGPS workshop	6096 mm × 4572 mm
Low voltage workshop	6096 mm × 4572 mm
Building maintenance	30,480 mm × 15,240 mm
Mechanical workshop	12,192 mm × 6096 mm
Firefighting workshop	6096 mm × 4572 mm
Automobile workshop	30,480 mm × 15,240 mm with service duct

37.12.2 Workshop In-charge Room

A separate room shall be provided for the workshop-in-charge. This room shall either be attached to the workshop premises or shall be in close vicinity to the workshop. Depending on the requirements, there can be one or more rooms for different workshop-in-charge. Some hospitals prefer to have a separate room for each type of workshop. The size of this room shall be about 4267 mm × 3658 mm, but depending on the requirement, the size of the room can be increased or decreased. The room shall adequate arrangement of cabinets, drawers, and racks for a smooth working. The room shall also have proper arrangements for electricity, communication points and air-conditioning.

37.12.3 Workshop Engineers

For engineers and assistant engineers, rooms are not required, but they shall be provided with a hall where multiple desks/workstations are installed. Each workstation shall have an adequate arrangement of cabinets, drawers, and racks for a smooth working. Each workstation shall have proper arrangements for electricity and communication points, with air-conditioning being common to the hall.

37.12.4 Staff Toilets

Toilets shall be separate for males and females. The toilets shall have WCs, urinals, and washbasin. If required, a bathing facility can also be provided.

37.12.5 Receiving/Issue Counter

The workshop shall have a receiving and issue counter near the entrance door of the workshop. The user shall submit the item to be repaired at this counter, and after repairs, the same shall be handed over to the user at the same counter. Sufficient space shall be provided outside the counter for the user to be seated, and there shall be adequate space for parking trolleys carrying material.

37.13 Other Infrastructure Issues

While designing the workshops, the following shall be considered:

37.13.1 Electrical Points

1. Main switchboard at the entrance wall (other than the wall on which door will open) for control of fan and lights of the room along with one 5 Amp Switch/Socket.
2. Air-Conditioning Control button with temperature adjustment.
3. The suitable electrical point with 6 Amp Switch Sockets shall be provided on walls above the working counter of the workshops to help testing of items, charging of machinery, or otherwise for miscellaneous use. If required, 16 Amp switch/sockets can also be provided.

37.13.2 Other Communication Points in the Room

The following communication points shall be provided near the office table of the workshop in-charge:

1. RJ 45 point for Computer networking.
2. RJ 11 for Intercom and extension line.
3. Connection to the CCTV surveillance system.

37.13.3 Lighting in the Workshops

Lighting for general illumination and specific tasks has to be carefully planned. The following points shall be considered while finalizing the light plan in the workshops:

1. Lights shall not be too bright or too dull. Proper lumens have to be planned as per the standards.
2. The use of LED lights is always recommended because of their long life and lower energy consumption.
3. Lights shall be equally distributed in the hall and particularly the working countertop.
4. If the workshop has been provided with a false ceiling, ceiling flush-mounted lights shall be used; however, if the false ceiling has not been provided, then surface mounted ceiling lights can be used.
5. Avoid wall lights as they are not effective.
6. To prevent burns, incandescent and halogen light sources should be avoided.
7. Emergency battery-operated light shall be provided in the workshop.

37.13.4 Doors

Preferably the door of the workshop shall be made out of wood, or flush doors shall be used. Aluminium doors can also be used as an alternative. However, MS steel doors are not recommended as they rust and give a poor appearance. The width of the doors shall not be less than 1829 mm wide, unobstructed. The door shall be provided with a door closer and stopper. The door shall have a provision of being locked both from inside and outside.

37.13.5 Windows

The window shall be as wide as possible and fitted with tinted glass, maybe with a double vacuum glass. The windows shall be covered either with curtains or vanishing blinds.

37.13.6 Flooring

Flooring of the workshop shall be steady to tolerate a heavy load of material. On the other hand, it shall look aesthetic, give a clean appearance, and shall provide a positive and welcoming atmosphere. The flooring of the offices can be either laid with marble, Kota stone, or tiles.

37.13.7 Air-Conditioning

If required, workshops shall be provided with air-conditioners. The system shall be connected to the central HVAC system, with separate AHUs for workshops area. Ducts can be provided in the stores which shall be connected to the AHU. The temperature in the workshops shall be between 18 and 24 °C and RH of about 45–50%.

37.13.8 Furniture in the Workshop

The following furniture shall be provided in the workshop rooms:

1. Slotted angle racks.
2. Heavy-duty racks made out of Stainless Steel or Mild Steel with proper shelves. The shelves shall be of different heights to accommodate all type of materials. It can be 229 mm to 610 mm high, depending on the requirement.
3. Wall fixed cupboard with locking facility.
4. High-raised chairs for countertop working.
5. Office table for workshop keeper.
6. Office Chairs.
7. Visitor Chair.

37.13.9 Notice Boards

A notice board shall be planned near the workshop-in-charge so that it is visible to all those arriving in the workshop. The board shall be made out cork to allow easy use of board pins. If possible, a light shall be provided above the notice board to make it more readable.

Further Reading

WBDG | WBDG - Whole Building Design Guide [Internet]. [cited 2021 Jul 12]. Available from: https://www.wbdg.org/

Singh M, Patnaik S, Srivastava P, Satia H, Singh M. Planning and Designing of Clinical Engineering Department in a Hospital. Int J Res Found Hosp Healthc Adm. 2015 Dec 1;3:129–34.

Olanrewaju A, Fang WW, Tan SY. Hospital Building Maintenance Management Model. Int J Eng Technol. 2018 May 22;7(2.29):747–53.

Bronzino JD, editor. CHAPTER 6 - FACILITIES MANAGEMENT AND DESIGN. In: Management of Medical Technology [Internet]. Butterworth-Heinemann; 1992 [cited 2021 Jul 12]. p. 187–242. Available from: https://www.sciencedirect.com/science/article/pii/B9780750692526500138

Part V

MEP Planning & Designing

38 HVAC (Air-Conditioning) System

HVAC (Heating, ventilation, air-conditioning), in a hospital, is one of the most complicated systems, as compared to any other commercial building. It involves a lot of functionalities when used in a hospital setting than commercial settings, where it is used just for thermal comfort.

HVAC systems in hospitals involve providing comfortable climatic conditions for patients and employees while also providing a germ-free and clean environment to prevent the spread of disease. Further, medical equipment in hospitals is highly sensitive and their performance might be affected due to the uncontrolled temperature and humidity levels. Therefore, perfect air control is essential to make the equipment work accurately. Therefore, the designer needs to pay special attention to these issues while designing the HVAC systems for the hospitals.

Additionally, different rooms in the hospital have different uses, which add to the complexity of the HVAC system design. First of all, it becomes necessary to clearly define different zones and spaces and their uses. For example certain patient rooms may be required to isolate patients exposed to infectious-contagious diseases, and some shall be required for patients who may be immune-compromised. Hospitals have a high concentration of microorganisms and pathogen accumulation compared to any other commercial building, and some of these organisms and pathogens may travel with the air current. There are certain spaces in the hospital (such as ICUs, neonatal unit, OR etc.) where it is necessary to restrict the arrival and growth of pathogens. Hence, air-conditioning system has to be highly sensitive to accumulate and filter such pathogens. This can be achieved with a perfectly designed HVAC system, so that the patients, staff and visitors of the hospital are protected from exposure to such microorganisms and pathogens.

It is also important that the system shall have the provision of an exhaustive level of air filtration, particularly external air supply, which is inducted into the system for fresh air and air exchanges. This exercise prevents the growth, spreading and accumulation of micro-particles/pathogens.

Following are some designing factors that may help in reducing the spread of airborne infection:

- Proper Air Change Rates can reduce the time the air particles stay in the space.
- Microbes can be filtered and removed from the air using proper filters.
- The use of Ultraviolet Germicidal Lights can inactivate microorganisms in the space and prevent their growth.
- Proper control of temperature and humidity.

A. Garg, A. Dewan, *Manual of Hospital Planning and Designing*,
https://doi.org/10.1007/978-981-16-8456-2_38

- Hundred per cent air shall be exhausted from the high-risk areas to remove infected foreign particles.
- Proper distribution of air in the air-conditioned space can reduce the accumulation of such particles on the surfaces and provide a clear path for air to exit.

There are two options for HVAC system in the hospitals:

1. *Central Water Chilled Plant*
2. *DX (Direct Expansion) Chilling*

38.1 Central Water Chilled Plant

If the hospital project is large, it is advisable to select a Chilled Water Central Plant to install the HVAC system. This type of system reduces the initial capital cost and increases the overall efficiency of the system.

Under this type of system, water is chilled by central chillers, which then travel to the coils of Air Handling Units (AHU) through insulated pipelines. In AHU, the air is blown by fans placed behind the coils. The blown air gets cooled, and the same travel through the ducts to the terminal point, which is thrown in the spaces via diffusers.

The chilled water central plant's capacity shall be calculated based on the size of the spaces and the air-conditioning requirements of the particular area. The designer shall also consider the simultaneous peak load and not only the total of the individual system loads. In addition to this, diversity factors such as head load of the machinery in the spaces, number of people in the spaces, heat load of the lighting, thermal loss due to sunlight in the room etc. shall also be considered while calculating the capacity of the central cooling plant.

38.1.1 Chillers

Chillers are that part of the system which cools the water to be sent to the AHUs. The chilled water plant shall have multiple or a minimum of two chillers, as a single chiller will be overloaded due to continuous operation. Also, if there are two chillers, one can act as a standby.

While chilling the water, the chillers heat up and need to be cooled. Chillers can either be cooled with water (known as water-cooled chillers) or air (known as air-cooled chillers).

To provide heating in the building, hot water is transported to the AHU. As a result, warm air is supplied by the AHU instead of cool air. All other processes remain the same.

38.1.1.1 Water-Cooled Chillers

There are different types of water-cooled chillers and they can be either centrifugal/screw chillers or absorption chillers. However, centrifugal chillers, either with a single compressor or dual compressors, are most commonly used for water-cooled chiller plants. The number of compressors shall depend on the total tonnage of the chillers.

38.1.1.2 Air-Cooled Chillers

Where the tonnage of the chillier plant is over and above 100 tons, the screw-type air-cooled chillers can be used. If the installations are smaller, scroll-type chillers can be used. However, reciprocating types of chillers are not recommended for HVAC system in hospitals.

38.1.2 Cooling Towers

1. While the chillers are operative, they produce lot of heat and the body of the chillers also heat up. Therefore, before re-circulating the water in the chillers, it has to be cooled. This is done using cooling towers.
2. Only factory fabricated and tested cooling towers shall be used and they shall be induced draft-type with counter-flow.
3. The structure and basin of the cooling tower shall be made out of stainless steel 304 grade, with FRP removable louvers.
4. Basin cleaning system shall be provided with the cooling towers.

38.1.3 Air Handling Systems

38.1.3.1 Air Handling Units (AHU)

AHU is a box-type structure, which takes in the air, cools/warms the air to the desired temperature, and sends it to the diffuser for throwing it in the designated spaces. The AHU shall have provisions for:

1. Taking fresh air from the atmosphere. The quantity of the air to be taken can be controlled by the damper fitted in the AHU.
2. AHU shall also be connected to the return air duct, or a return air vent shall be provided in the AHU to collect the returning air from the spaces.
3. Fresh air and return air should not get mixed in the AHU.
4. A blower fan shall be provided in the AHU to throw the exhaust air out from the unit.
5. Chilled water circulates in the coils provided in the front of the AHU. When the air blown by the fan passes between these coils, it gets cooled and moves out from the AHU to the supply duct.
6. Each cooling coil of AHU shall have maximum of six rows and ten fins per inch (FPI). In case the cooling requirement is more, AHU shall be designed with twin coil sets of six rows instead of increasing the rows and fins in a single coil. Care shall be taken that the chilled water supply line is piping through both the coils and is in series with an access section of 1067 mm between two equal-sized coils.
7. Discharge face velocity of the cooling coil and heating coil shall not be more than 450 fpm and 800 fpm, respectively.
8. If cooling and heating are required simultaneously, AHU can use a two-coil system, where there are two separate coils, one for cold water and other for hot water. This system is used for specific areas like Operating Rooms, where controlling humidity is an important factor.
9. AHU also contains filters such as Pre Filter and Micro V filters fitted in the return pathway of the air to filter it air before it is sent out.
10. The provision of Ultraviolet Light can also be provided in the AHU for disinfecting the air.
11. The design of the AHU shall depend on the CFM and air-conditioning requirement in the spaces (in Tonne).
12. The capacity of a single AHU shall not be more than 50,000 m^3/hour.
13. To avoid cross-contamination, separate AHUs shall be provided at places like Operating Rooms, Mortuary/Autopsy Room, Clean Room, Lab and component rooms of Blood Bank and isolation areas.
14. Each AHU shall be installed as a stand-alone unit and it shall have no interface with another AHU. Vertical stacking of AHUs is not recommended.
15. The return air fan for each AHU shall be separate and shall not be combined with the return air fan of other AHU.
16. Use of Variable Frequency Drives (VFD) shall be encouraged for AHUs. VFDs shall be designed and configured in a way that in case one VFD fails, it shall not disable the entire unit. For this, a bypass switch can also be used.
17. Service access doors shall always open inside the AHU, i.e. on the positive side of the door. The opening shall not be blocked by internal parts of the AHU.
18. These doors shall be provided with the micro switches or safety switch interlocks to protect maintenance personnel from possible injuries.

38.1.3.2 Fan Coil Units

1. For smaller area or for a particular area like private patient room, instead of AHU, a Fan Coils Units (FCU) can be used. Both have the same working system; however, the only difference is that AHU supplies air in large quantity to a larger area, whereas FCU supplies less air in small area.
2. FCU is suitable for spaces like single patient rooms, computer rooms, communication rooms, offices, machine rooms of lifts/elevators, IT Rooms, electrical rooms, EPABX rooms, pharmacy, stores, restrooms, OPD, administration areas etc.

3. FCU shall not be used where an adequate space is available for distribution ductwork or where distribution ductwork is essential.

38.1.4 Variable Air Volume (VAV) Ventilation

1. In frequent part-load conditions of the ventilation equipment, VAV/DCV systems can give a better performance.
2. DCV automatically adjusts ventilation considering the occupancy in the room.
3. VAV system allows variable airflow but on the controls can also be manual.
4. Along with energy saving, VAV system can provide a better control on temperature and humidity. The life of the air-conditioning equipment also increases because of the less frequent switching on/off.
5. VAV systems depend on two main factors:
   (a) Dampers in VAV boxes that adjust the airflow of individual zones.
   (b) Controls of the fan speed. Variable Frequency Drives (VFD) are generally used for fan motors with a rating of above 1 hp, whereas Electronically Commutated Motors (ECM) provide a built-in speed controller.
6. In response to the air temperature of the space, VAV boxes open or close the air damper automatically.
7. VAV systems can save more than 30% energy as compared to CAV systems in buildings where ventilation load is variable.

38.1.5 Diffusers, Registers and Grills

38.1.5.1 Grills

The grill's primary function is to cover and allow the air to pass in and out through it. Grills are the only option out of the three, that are suitable for both air intake and air exhaust outlets from indoor spaces. Considering grills do not involve any moving components or dampers, it is also one of the easiest to maintain. But it is not suitable if there is a need to adjust the airflow direction or the amount of air flowing in and out.

38.1.5.2 Registers

Air register is almost the same as a grill but with adjustable dampers in it. Unlike grills, which are used for both intake and release of air in a room, a register only releases the air. An air register is used with air supply outlets feeding air into indoor spaces. The dampers help to control the airflow direction or shut off the flow.

38.1.5.3 Diffusers

Diffuser differs the airflow direction variability. A diffuser and its dampers are designed facing all-round rather than a register's single air direction. Many diffusers are found on ceilings, often covering an air-con or air release outlet. Most diffusers come in square or circular shape with vents designed to match the diffuser's shape, facing different directions.

38.1.6 Ductwork

1. Ducts are required to carry cool air to the terminal point. At the time the ducts are also used to carry return air back to the AHUs.
2. The supply duct is on one side connected to the AHU, terminating at the VAV or the grills/dampers/diffusers. Similarly, the return duct is connected to the grills and terminates by connecting to the AHU.
3. The clinical areas of the hospital shall have a fully ducted system.
4. The shape of the duct can either be rectangular, square or round, depending on the design and availability of the spaces below the ceiling.
5. The duct is generally made out of galvanized steel. For some specific areas like Operating Rooms, the duct is made out of Aluminium.
6. Air handling duct systems shall be accessible, which can be achieved by providing access panels in the ducts.
7. Anti-microbial coating shall be done on the internal surface of the duct.
8. Insulation shall be done on the ducts, preferably with nitrile sheet applied using adhesive.

38.1.7 Air Intake and Exhaust

1. Positioning of the air intake and exhaust louvers or vents in the hospital shall be planned carefully and ensured that there is no chance of undesired recirculation of air.
2. Adequate distances for separation between intake and exhaust shall be maintained.
3. In case of harsh climatic conditions, special attention shall be paid to air intake louvers. At least, the intake of outside air shall be drawn into the system through sand trap louvers.
4. Washable aluminium filters shall be installed at the rear end of the sand trap louver. Care shall be taken to provide access to clean these filters. If there are restrictions in providing access, the system shall allow for removing the filters without the need to shut down the AHU. If the filters are not cleaned, it may result in clogging the air stream and higher pressure may drop, in turn reducing the air volume.

38.1.8 Filtration

1. First stage filtration of not less than MERV 8/ ePM10 60% rating shall be provided with all AHUs. Similarly, the final filter of not less than MERV 14/ePM1 70% rating shall be provided downstream of all wet-air cooling coils and supply fan.
2. Ultraviolet (UV-C) shall also be used as a disinfection method to inactivate the microorganisms. The use of UV-C is recommended for cooling coil surfaces to avoid fungal amplification. Use of upper air UV for patient rooms in critical care or isolation rooms shall be provided to reduce the virus spread.
3. Filters like Pre-Filters, Sand Filters, Micro V filters and HEPA filters shall be used in the HVAC system wherever the design recommends.

38.2 Installation of Central Chilled Water Plant

38.2.1 Chillers (Fig. 38.1)

1. Adequate spaces shall be provided in the hospital building for installation of chillers. This space shall be away from the clinical or patient areas. It can be the basements, rooftop, or outside the building (in main or annexure building).
2. Before finalizing the location of the chiller, the weights of chillers and other allied equipment, it shall be ensured that the structure of the building is capable of handling the load of the HVAC equipment.
3. As a standard, a set of two chillers shall always be provided so that both of them can work alternately. It will also give a buffer in case of failure of one chiller. Though initially only two chillers are installed but considering the future expansion of air-conditioning plants, spaces shall be provided for installing more such chillers at the same location in the future.
4. The size of the chiller may vary with its capacity.
5. Spaces for chiller pumps and supply pumps shall be allotted near the chiller.
6. Space shall also be provided for pipeline of the chiller water supply and the pipelines for transportation of chilled water to AHUs.
7. Spaces shall be provided for equipment removal and maintenance.
8. For air-cooled chillers, sufficient open space shall be provided for fresh air to cool the chillers.
9. Space shall be allotted for installation of Hot Water Generator for warm air.
10. Emergency chilled water pipeline system covered with blind flanges and isolation valves shall be provided to be used in future or in case the additional chillers need to be installed.
11. Proper raw water pipelines shall be provided to connect the raw water supply line to chillers and cooling towers.
12. Higher delta T shall be used to save energy by lowering the cost of pumping.
13. For additional energy saving, equipment driven with VFD shall be considered for pump consuming over 7.5 kW.
14. A space shall be provided for the make up tank of water, which makes up the level of water to be used for cooling the chillers and also for chilling the water to be transported to the AHUs.

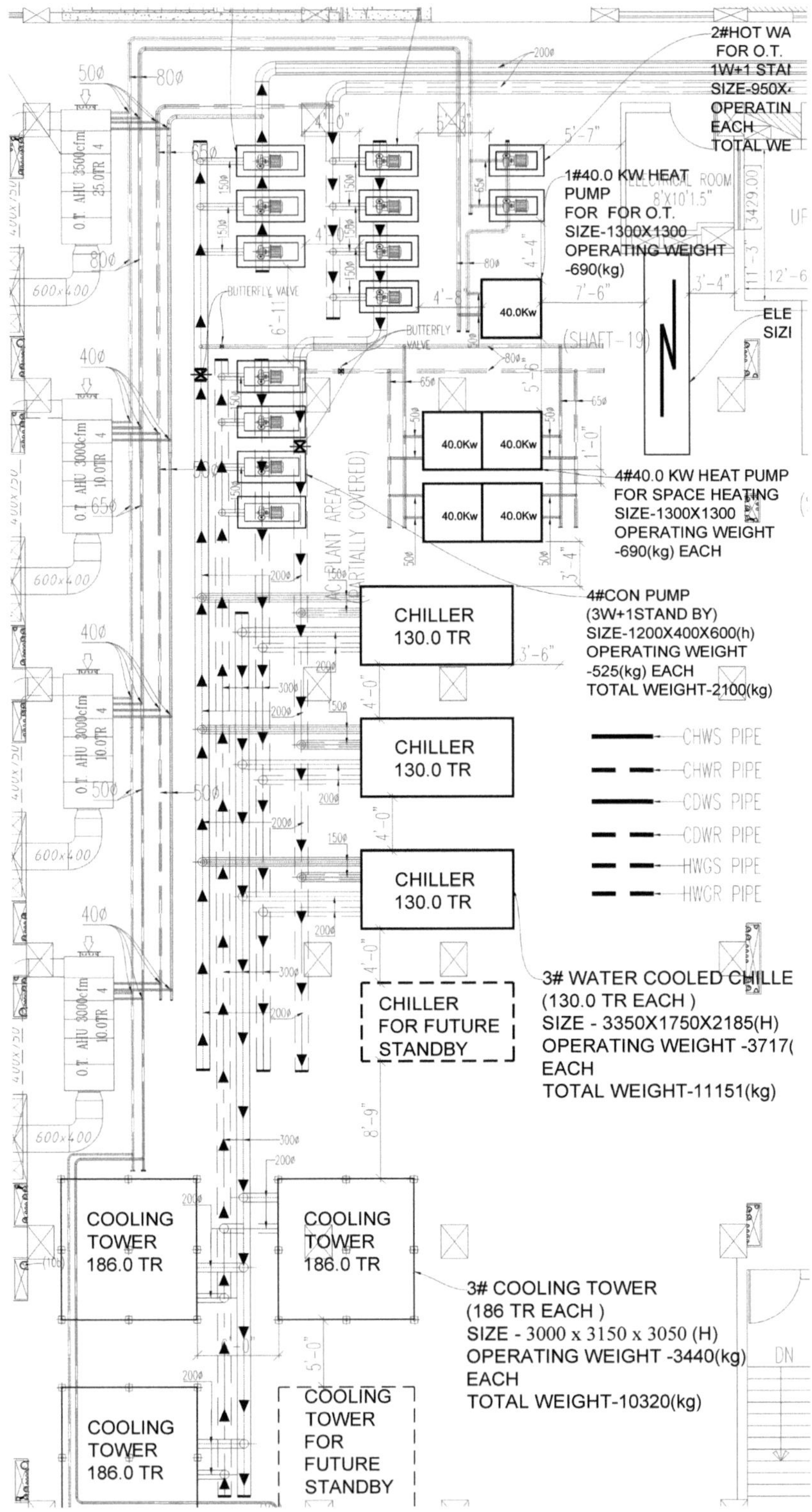

Fig. 38.1 Sample drawing of HVAC Chiller Plant

15. A space shall be provided for the electrical panel and main switches for supplying power to the system.

38.2.2 Cooling Towers

1. An open space shall be allotted either on the rooftop or in an open sky area for the installation of a pair of cooling towers.
2. The cooling towers shall be connected to the water pipelines for receiving and supplying water to the chillers. Also, a water pipeline shall be provided to make up the water in the cooling tower.
3. Power supply shall be provided for operating the cooling towers.

38.2.3 Air Handling System (Fig. 38.2)

1. The AHU shall be installed near the area where air has to be used.
2. For installing the AHUs, a separate room shall be provided, which shall have openings for installing the air ducts and an opening for taking the fresh air from the atmosphere.
3. Alternately, if the height of the floor permits and the ceiling of the floor has enough load-bearing capacity, ceiling suspended AHUs shall be installed, which are suspended from the ceiling with the help of screw rods and fasteners.
4. In case of Fan Coil Units, these are suspended from the ceiling at any convenient place in the room, preferably at the entrance of the room.
5. Required electrical power supply points shall be provided to the AHU/FCU.

38.3 DX (Direct Expansion) Chilling

In this system, instead of chilled water, the refrigerant (gas) circulates in the pipelines. In these types of HVAC central plants, the air which shall be used for spaces is chilled directly by the refrigerant present in the cooling coil of the AHU; thus the cooling efficiency of these chillers is higher.

DX type of central conditioning systems have three main compartments:

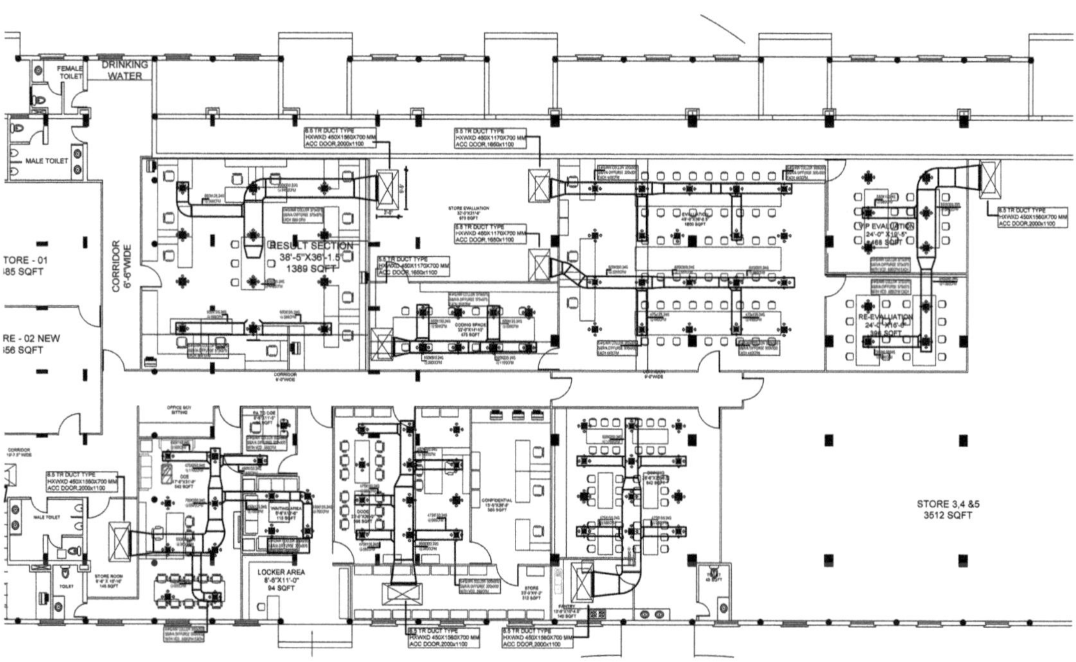

Fig. 38.2 Sample drawing of HVAC Ducting andAHU's

38.3.1 The Plant Room

The plant room contains equipment like refrigeration system (gas), condensers, and compressors (open type compressor or semi-hermetically sealed compressor).

The cooling of the semi-hermetically sealed compressors is done by the air blown by the fan, while water is used to cool the open-type compressors.

Condenser is a structure having shells and tubes, and is water cooled. Inside a condenser, the refrigerant gas flows along the tube side, and water flows along the shell side. With this process, the refrigerant is cooled faster. The cooling tower kept at the top of the plant room is used for cooling the condenser and the compressor. If required, a cooling tower can also be kept at other convenient location instead of the top of the plant.

38.3.2 Air Handling Unit Room

After leaving the condenser, the refrigerant enters the thermostatic expansion valve and ultimately the AHU, kept at a different place. The AHU is a box-like structure consisting of an evaporator or so-called 'cooling coil', air filters and a large blower.

After entering the AHU, the refrigerant enters the cooling coil, where it cools the air, which in turn is thrown into the room. To increase the efficiency of heat transfer from refrigerant to air, the coil is covered with fins.

Two types of ducts are usually connected to the AHU; one for return air and other for transporting the cool air to the rooms. The blower of the AHU absorbs the return air, which then passes through the filters and then over the cooling coil. Thereafter, the blower blows the air in the ducts of the room to pass the chilled air in the rooms.

38.3.3 Air-Conditioned Room

The ducts from the AHU open in the room. The ducts are terminated and connected to grills or diffusers, which in supply chilled air to the room. Once the air enters the room, it absorbs the heat, gets heated, and enters the return air grill located on the opposite side of the room, which is then transported to the AHU. This air is re-circulated by the AHU.

38.3.4 Benefits of DX Air-Conditioning Systems

1. DX systems has a flexibility for installation. This system can either be installed inside or outside the building.
2. The system has a great flexibility for expansion in order to increase the capacity or add a new building to the system.
3. These systems, once installed, do not require much maintenance, hence reduce the repair costs.
4. Occupies less space as compared to any other cooling systems.
5. Saves energy and reduces electricity bill.
6. This system has a provision to reduce or stop the flow of refrigerant to any desired indoor unit with the help of DX valve. Hence, individual room can be controlled.

38.3.5 Disadvantages of DX system

1. This system can be used only for small buildings, or otherwise if the rooms are located on a single floor. It is not practically feasible to lay the refrigerant piping for a large distance.
2. Another disadvantage is that if the piping is long, more amount of refrigerant will be needed, which in turn will make the system expensive.
3. More the length of the piping, more are the chances of leakage of the refrigerant.
4. The AHU and the refrigerant piping shall be close by, failing which the pressure of the refrigerant will drop, resulting in less cooling.

38.4 Split Air-Conditioning

This is basically a wall-hung system wherein the compressor and indoor unit are separate from each other but connected through refrigerant copper pipes. The outdoor units consist of compressor, and the indoor unit consists of blower fan and the refrigerant coil. One of the main advantages of this kind of air-conditioning is that it allows to control the temperature in each room individually.

These systems are generally preferred for a small area or a particular room.

38.5 HVAC—Room Side Design

The key design elements of various spaces in the hospital are as follows:

38.5.1 Operating Rooms

The ORs shall have the following for the comfort of doctors, staff, and patients and to reduce the chances of growth and transmission of microorganisms:

Temperature	Humidity	Ventilation system
18–22 °C	20–60% RH	20ACH SA/4 ACH OA

1. Each OR shall be provided with a dedicated AHU. The design and size of the AHU shall depend on the size of the OR.
2. To allow variable speed to cater to HEPA filter loading, AHU of OR shall be provided with VFDs.
3. AHU shall supply constant volume of airflow. However, if continued positive room pressure is to be provided in the OR, variable systems shall be used.
4. Air shall be introduced from the ceiling and exhausted through the exhaust diffusers provided on all the four corners of the OR.
5. HEPA filters shall be provided in the plenum of the OR, and the airflow shall be dissipated through laminar airflow diffusers fixed in the plenum.
6. Laminar airflow must be designed in such a fashion that clean air moves over the OT table and within the operating field at a maximum face velocity to sweep away particles in its path.
7. As an additional measure, Ultraviolet Germicidal Irradiation shall be provided to reduce infection risks.
8. While designing the HVAC system, low-temperature requirements of ORs, particularly cardiac and orthopaedic, shall be considered. This can be achieved using a low-temperature chilled water circuit.
9. Temperature and humidity sensors shall be provided in the rooms for system control. It will be better if such sensors are provided in the return air duct.
10. OR's AHUs shall be designed at the air velocity of 2 m/s at the coil to reduce the temperature of the air leaving the AHU.
11. Chilled water pipes coming to the AHU shall be designed at higher velocities and be in the range of 1.8–2 m/s.

38.5.2 Intensive Care Units

HVAC for different ICUs shall have:

Temperature	Humidity	Ventilation System
18–24 °C	30–60% RH	6ACH SA/2 ACH OA

1. For these areas of the ICU, AHUs shall be used instead of FCU.
2. For infective ICUs, the air exhaust shall be 100%.
3. The exhaust air of one ICU shall not be mixed with the return air of other ICU, i.e. the supply AHU and the return of each ICU shall be separate.

38.5.3 Patient Rooms

HVAC of Patient Rooms shall have:

Temperature	Humidity	Ventilation system
21–24 °C	60% RH	6ACH SA/2 ACH OA

1. For Single rooms, FCU shall be used instead of AHU.
2. A thermostat linked to the BMS system shall be provided in each patient room.

38.5.4 Isolation Rooms

Isolation rooms are classified as:

1. Negative Pressure Isolation Room—Generally used as Airborne Infection Isolation Rooms.
2. Negative Pressure Isolation Room with dirty and clean utility—Generally used as Quarantine Isolation Room.
3. Positive Pressure Isolation Room—Generally used as Protective Environment Isolation Rooms.
4. Standard Neutral Isolation Room—Generally used as Contact Isolation Room.

Negative Isolation Room

Temperature	Humidity	Ventilation System
21–24 °C	60% RH	12ACH SA/2 ACH OA

1. The room generally consists of a patient area, toilet and anteroom.
2. Inflow of the air shall be less than the outflow of the air.
3. Close monitoring and control of airflow direction are required.
4. Negative pressure shall be maintained through the communicating air valve even if the unit is unoccupied.
5. Differential pressure monitor along with alarm points connected to BMS shall be provided.
6. Seal the room if the air leakage is below 0.5 ft^2 (465 cm^2).
7. Exhaust air grill shall be placed above the patient's head end or otherwise at a low level near the head end of the patient.
8. Air shall be exhausted through HEPA filter, directly in the atmosphere with designed high plume dilution fans and released at 10 feet above roof level.
9. Recirculation of air is not recommended in negative isolation rooms.

Negative Isolation Room with Clean and Dirty Utility

1. All the requirements as of Negative Pressure shall be adhered too.
2. In addition, the room shall have a dirty utility. Air of the dirty utility shall be exhausted outside, as is being done for bedroom, anteroom, and toilet.

Positive Isolation Room

Temperature	Humidity	Ventilation system
21–24 °C	60% RH	12ACH SA/2 ACH OA

- These rooms are mainly for immuno-compromised patients such as those with organ transplant, BMT, leukaemia, burn, late-stage HIV etc.
- Inflow of the air shall be more than the outflow of the air.
- Inflow of the air shall be through HEPA filters.
- The flow shall be from the diffusers and in a laminar flow.
- Supply diffusers shall be installed in the ceiling above the patient bed, and exhaust shall be on the opposite side of the room, at a lower level.
- Differential pressure monitor along with alarm points connected to BMS shall be provided.
- Seal the room if the air leakage is below 0.5 ft^2 (465 cm^2).

Standard Neutral Isolation Room

1. This is basically a simple air-conditioned room in a separate zone of the hospital.
2. These isolation rooms are for patients having a non-airborne communicable disease and is used only for physical isolation of the patient.

38.5.5 Recovery (Post-Anaesthesia Care Unit)

Following shall be the requirements of HVAC for these spaces:

Temperature	Humidity	Ventilation system
21–24 °C	30–60% RH	6ACH SA/2 ACH OA

1. Return air grills shall be provided at a low level in the room to capture the exhaled anaesthetic gasses.

38.5.6 Emergency

Following shall be the requirements of HVAC of Emergency area:

Decontamination Room

Temperature	Humidity	Ventilation system
21–24 °C	60% RH	12ACH SA/2 ACH OA

1. The room shall be negatively pressurized.
2. 100% air shall be exhausted with separate exhaust ducting.

Examination/Treatment Room

Temperature	Humidity	Ventilation system
21–24 °C	60% RH	6ACH SA/2 ACH OA

Resuscitation Room

Temperature	Humidity	Ventilation system
21–24 °C	20–60% RH	15ACH SA/3 ACH OA

Triage

Temperature	Humidity	Ventilation system
21–24 °C	60% RH	12ACH SA/2 ACH OA

1. The room shall be negatively pressurized.
2. 100% air shall be exhausted with dedicated exhaust ducting.

Emergency Department Public Waiting Area

Temperature	Humidity	Ventilation system
21–24 °C	60% RH	6ACH SA/2 ACH OA

38.5.7 Burn Units

Following shall be the requirements of HVAC for Burn Units:

Temperature	Humidity	Ventilation system
21–32 °C	40% RH	6ACH SA/2 ACH OA

1. The room shall be positively pressurized.
2. Inflow of the air shall be more than the outflow of the air.
3. Inflow of the air shall be through HEPA filters.
4. The flow shall be from the diffusers and in a laminar flow.
5. Each patient room shall be linked with the BMS system and thermostat.
6. For controlling the humidity level, each patient room shall be provided with a dedicated humidifier and a humidistat.
7. Each patient room shall have provisions to raise the temperature to 32 °C if required.

38.5.8 Procedure Rooms

Following requirements shall be addressed for HVAC systems of the Procedure Room:

Temperature	Humidity	Ventilation system
21–24 °C	20–60% RH	15ACH SA/3 ACH OA

1. Room shall be positively pressurized.
2. Inflow of the air shall be more than the outflow of the air.
3. Inflow of the air shall be through HEPA filters.
4. The flow shall be from the diffusers and in a laminar flow.

38.5.9 Endoscopy Rooms

Following requirements shall be addressed for HVAC of the Endoscopy Room:

Gastrointestinal Endoscopy Procedure Room

Temperature	Humidity	Ventilation System
21–23 °C	20–60% RH	6ACH SA/2 ACH OA

1. Room shall be positively pressurized.

Endoscopy/Bronchoscopy

Temperature	Humidity	Ventilation system
20–23 °C	20–60% RH	12ACH SA/2 ACH OA

1. Room shall be negatively pressurized.
2. Inflow of the air shall be less than the outflow of the air.
3. Inflow of the air shall be through HEPA filters.
4. Hundred per cent air shall be exhausted outside through ducts.
5. The flow shall be from the diffusers and in a laminar flow.

Endoscopy ERCP Procedure Room

Temperature	Humidity	Ventilation system
20–23 °C	20–60% RH	15ACH SA/3 ACH OA

1. Room shall be positively pressurized.
2. Inflow of the air shall be more than the outflow of the air.
3. Inflow of the air shall be through HEPA filters.
4. The flow shall be from the diffusers and in a laminar flow.

38.5.10 Imaging Rooms

Following requirements must be taken care of while designing the HVAC system of Imaging Rooms, i.e. X-Ray, CT, Ultrasound, MRI, PET CT Scan, PET MRI, Mammography, DSA etc.

Temperature	Humidity	Ventilation system
18–21 °C	60% RH	6ACH SA/2 ACH OA

1. For Imaging rooms, separate AHUs are not necessary. Depending on the requirement and the area to be cooled, one or more AHUs can be designed.
2. For the specialized imaging rooms like Cath Lab, EP room, Fluoroscopy Room etc. it is recommended that the design standards of HVAC shall be the same as of an OR, because these rooms generally require more fresh air compared to other imaging rooms.
3. As machines in the imaging department produce a lot of heat, data about heat load dissipation shall be obtained from the original manufacturer of the machines before designing the HVAC for these areas.
4. Diagnostic rooms like PET and SPET CT Scan generally require 6 ACH SA/2 ACH OA of air. The air in these rooms shall be exhausted via the general exhaust system.
5. PET CT, PET MRI, SPECT, Gamma Camera, Hot lab and Radiopharmacy rooms shall be provided with BSC II hoods with a dedicated exhaust hood with filters for isotopes and general exhaust.
6. LINAC rooms require 6ACH SA/2 ACH OA air. The humidity of these rooms shall be less than 50%.

38.5.11 Central Laboratories

HVAC of central laboratories like Pathology, Biochemistry and Microbiology shall have:

Temperature	Humidity	Ventilation system
21–24 °C	60% RH	6ACH SA/2 ACH OA

- General exhaust shall be provided in all the laboratories to exhaust 100% air from the work areas.
- The exhaust of the Fume hoods and Bio-Safety cabinets shall be outside the building, through high plume dilution fans after proper filtration.
- Labs containing Fume Hoods or BSC cabinets shall have laminar flow diffusers.
- Ventilation system of the sterilization room of the laboratory shall be at 10 ACH SA/2 ACH OA.

38.5.12 Pharmacy

HVAC of Pharmacy shall have:

Temperature	Humidity	Ventilation system
21–24 °C	60% RH	6ACH SA/2 ACH OA

1. It shall be positively pressurized. Variable systems can be used in the pharmacy.
2. Clean room for hazardous drugs shall have BSC cabinets. The exhaust of BSC shall be filtered with carbon filters and HEPA filter before discharging.

38.5.13 Mortuary and Autopsy

HVAC of mortuary and autopsy rooms shall have:

Temperature	Humidity	Ventilation system
20–24 °C	60% RH	12ACH SA/2 ACH OA

1. Uni-directional diffusers shall be used to supply air.
2. Exhaust grilles shall be provided at both lower and upper levels.
3. Total air shall be exhausted outside through separate ductwork after required filtration.
4. For autopsy rooms (if provided), direct exhaust shall be connected with the autopsy table. Exhaust air shall be filtered through the HEPA filters. The exhaust air shall also be treated with UV lights, and carbon filter for odour and shall be discharged outside with a high velocity.
5. For Body Holding Refrigerator room, the heat loss dissipation shall be taken into account before designing the HVAC system.
6. Pressure display monitor connected to the BMS shall be provided for active monitoring of pressure.

38.5.14 Central Sterile Supply Department (CSSD)

HVAC requirements for CSSD shall be as follows:

Dirty Area

Temperature	Humidity	Ventilation system
16–23 °C	60% RH	6ACH SA/2 ACH OA

1. This zone shall have 100% dedicated exhaust and negative pressure.

Clean Area

Temperature	Humidity	Ventilation system
20–23 °C	60% RH	4ACH SA/2 ACH OA

Sterile Store

Temperature	Humidity	Ventilation system
20–24 °C	60% RH	4ACH SA/2 ACH OA

1. Supply air shall be through HEPA Filters.
2. Exhaust ductwork shall be made out of stainless steel.
3. Washers, disinfectors and sterilizers shall have a direct exhaust system.
4. ETO sterilization room shall be provided with 100% dedicated exhaust outside.

38.5.15 Server Room

Following shall be the requirements of HVAC for Server Room:

Temperature	Humidity	Ventilation system
19–22 °C	30–60% RH	12ACH SA/2 ACH OA

1. Heat load of the servers and other equipment in the room shall be considered while designing the HVAC.
2. Precision AC units or closely controlled AC units shall be used for Server Room, which shall provide both humidity control and cooling.
3. Server Rooms shall be provided with floor raised from the actual floor. This can be done by providing perforated floor tiles capable of bearing the rack load, and air-conditioning shall be done through these perforations.
4. Fan coils shall not be used in server rooms.

Note: The Temperature, Humidity and Ventilation System shown above for different departments are the standards laid down by various designers. However, the same may differ with the Temperature, Humidity and Ventilation system shown at various places in the book in respective chapters. The reason is that as per the practical experiences of the authors, these suggestions are appropriate. It is left to the actual designer that the standards may be revised depending on the requirement of a particular project.

38.6 Effects of COVID-19 on the Design of Air-Conditioning

It is also important to understand that in the past, the world has dealt with various types of infections caused by fungus, bacteria, parasites, and viruses, and today it is under a huge pressure to tackle the Novel Coronavirus. Tomorrow it might have to deal and fight with some biological infections, and there can also be some nuclear hazards that can be dangerous for the human race.

It is also true that day by day, the air quality of our planet will worsen and will be full of unrequired particles. And it will become a necessity to filter such particles for the healthy survival of human beings.

Therefore, it becomes necessary to design the HVAC system that is more flexible and sustainable to accommodate the addition and modification according to the need of the hour.

Following issues require special consideration in hospitals post-COVID-19:

1. Greater flexibility and movability should be taken care of while designing the HVAC.
2. Designs that can maximize infection control through filtration and induction of fresh air.
3. If possible, lobbies of hospitals can be left without air-conditioning, but shall be semi-open and well-ventilated. However, this may not always be true for extremely hot and/or cold localities.
4. It is a well-known fact that there is a high possibility of virus and bacteria being spread through recirculation of air, and if the supply and return of air are common in a large space, the chances of such spread would further increase.
5. *Use of fresh air*
   It is important to consider the air quality while designing the HVAC. Designs will have to ensure that based on the air quality, the filtration of the air to be thrown inside is proper and free from any type of foreign particles/pathogens/virus/bacteria/fungus.
6. *Filtration of fresh air*
   For filtration of air, filters have to be installed at the entry point of the fresh air. Many types of filters are available in the market which can filter the particles up to a defined depth and size. Sand and Dust Filters, Pre-Filters, Micro V filters, HEPA filters, ULVA filters etc. are widely used. But going a few years ahead, we can foresee that as the air quality worsens and induction of Biological and Nuclear particles in the air takes place, we may require additional filters to filter out these particles. Therefore, the provision of such filters has to be kept in mind while designing the HVAC.
7. *Treated Fresh Air Units (TFA)* is also known as Fresh Air-Handling Units (FAHU). TFAs are used when the requirement of fresh air is much higher, and that of recirculation is less, or when AHUs need to be fed to fulfil their fresh air requirements. For example if the ambient temperature (the outside air) is 36–40 degrees Celsius and after treatment, the temperature is brought down to 22–24 degrees Celsius, so that it does not increase the air-conditioning load. We recommend using Two-stage TFA to provide complete solution for the Quality of Indoor Environmental and Energy Saving. This single modular unit shall control features like cooling, heating, high-efficiency filtration humidification, mixing, sound attenuation etc. Two-stage TFAs can also provide the facility of heat recovery between incoming ambient air and building exhaust air without any cross-contamination.

8. *Ultraviolet Filtration*
   It is recommended that the fresh air to be inducted goes through the Ultraviolet filtration before being thrown inside. A UV-C lamp can be installed just at the end of the row of filters so that the air becomes free from any leftover pathogens before entering the hospital. But UV systems are not something that should be installed out in the open, as they can be harmful to human beings, and therefore they should be hidden safely in the ductwork.
9. *Automation of the filtration*
   It is recommended that this system of filtration shall be automatic and processor-controlled. Sensors can be installed at the entry point of the air to assess the quality of air and accordingly move the required and unrequired filters in their places to clear the duct for a free flow of air.
   i. An automatic system shall be in place to assess the quantity of fresh air and air exchanges required in the space. This requirement can also be pre-assessed while designing, which can be later modified by adjusting the openings of the dampers.
10. *Return and Exhaust of the air*
    Another important factor of HVAC is the treatment and use of the air which exists in the space. This air is either to be reused or otherwise exhausted. It depends on the zone and purpose for which the space is being used. If it is a sensitive and infected area, it is recommended to exhaust the entire air (but it depends on the design if some portion of it can be reused after proper filtration and treatment), and for other spaces, the air can be reused after filtration and treatment.
11. *Reuse of the return air*
    If the air has to be reused, it has to be collected through the return ducts and passed through various filters (as mentioned above) and even treated using UV-C before entering the AHU of the Fan Coil and being pushed into space. One important factor is that each area shall have a separate return air system with defined portioned space. Under no circumstances, the return air of one space should be mixed or combined with other, failing which might lead to cross-infection in the hospital.
12. *The exhaust of the air*
    In sensitive areas where infectious/contagious patients are kept, it is advised to exhaust the air completely and replace it with fresh air. In such spaces, return air is often not ducted to avoid cross-infection and is thrown out with a specified exhaust system. While COVID-19 is spread by droplets and does not flow around in the air for a long time, the next virus may not be so. Under such circumstances, the air-conditioning systems can easily spread it rapidly across the whole hospital if not handled with caution.
13. *HVAC for Intensive Care Units*
    For intensive care areas, the designs shall ensure proper zoning and exhaust system to take out air. Another precaution to be taken is that the exhausted air shall be thrown out in the atmosphere after proper treatment/filtration, so that microbes do not let open and pose danger to others outside the building. It is believed that if in a particular ICU the patients of only one particular disease are kept, the return air can be reused up to some extent after proper treatment by filtration and UV sterilization. But if there are patients of different diseases, it is recommended that total air should be exhausted (it depends on the design; if some portion of it can be reused after proper treatment; however, this is considered risky).
14. *HVAC for Isolation Units*
    Isolation units are generally designed for creating a negative pressure in the unit, which means less throw of the air and more exhaust of the air. The concept is that any pathogen/virus/bacteria should not remain in that space and be sucked out of the space. Negatively pressurized rooms help to prevent the spread of infectious diseases through the air. In such units, the air is pushed in the unit which has already been treated through fil-

ters and sterilized with UV. It is recommended that the air which has been exhausted from such units should also be treated and passed through the filters and sterilized with UV before being thrown to the outside atmosphere. This can be done by installing filters and UV lamps in the exhaust duct of such units.

15. *Conversion to Isolation*

    If the need be, hospital can also try to convert an additional wing (either the whole ICU or a few beds) of the ICU to a negative-pressure isolation ward to provide more space for accommodating additional infected patients.

    i. If the whole ICU is being converted, then it has to be negatively pressurized, for which special centrifugal fans can be installed while designing, which becomes operational when required. Apart from the ICU, this can be true for other areas as well like Emergency Rooms, Pre-and post-OP units etc.
    ii. If particular beds are to be converted, it can always be done with the help of collapsible shutters around the beds or fixing temporary acrylic partitions. For HVAC, Micro air-conditioning can be installed. In such technology, micro angle adjustable outlets are installed to induce the air inside, separately for each bed, above the patient, and a separate exhaust is given (with separate duct) for each bed. When this exhaust becomes operational, the common return duct is bypassed with the help of diffusers fixed in the exhaust duct.

16. *Humidity control*

    Properly controlled air humidification in hospitals provides a great comfort to the patients and staff, apart from efficient working of equipment, by reducing the dry air. Also, humidity is regulated to protect patients from nosocomial infections, bacterial attacks and prevent the spread of other infections. Higher air humidity can also reduce the airborne transmission of various type of viruses.

    i. One of the biggest concerns with equipment and humidity is the formation of electrostatic discharge (ESD). Although it is a general phenomenon, but it is more important in hospitals because it might be the reason for the life or death of a patient if the equipment malfunctions or fails due to uncontrolled humidity.

Further Reading

The importance of HVAC systems in hospitals [Internet]. Keyter. 2020 [cited 2021 Jul 12]. Available from: https://www.keyter.com/la-importancia-de-los-sistemas-hvac-en-los-hospitales/

New ASHRAE reference guides hospital HVAC design - Environmental Services [Internet]. Healthcare Facilities Today. [cited 2021 Jul 12]. Available from: https://www.healthcarefacilitiestoday.com/posts/New-ASHRAE-reference-guides-hospital-HVAC-design%2D%2D2389

Reijula J, Holopainen R, Kähkönen E, Reijula K, Tommelein I. Intelligent HVAC systems in hospitals. Intell Build Int. 2013 Feb 17;5:101–19.

Editor. HVAC System Design for Multi-Specialty Hospital I Cooling India Monthly Business Magazine on the HVACR Business I Green HVAC industry I Heating, Ventilation, Air conditioning and Refrigeration News Magazine Updates, Articles, Publications on HVACR Business Industry I HVACR Business Magazine [Internet]. [cited 2021 Jul 12]. Available from: https://www.coolingindia.in/hvac-system-design-for-multi-specialty-hospital/

HVAC design requirements for medical spaces [Internet]. [cited 2021 Jul 12]. Available from: https://www.hfmmagazine.com/articles/1755-hvac-design-requirements-for-medical-spaces

Ocana G. HVAC Design Manual for Hospitals and Clinics Second Edition. [cited 2021 Jul 12]; Available from: https://www.academia.edu/14124488/HVAC_Design_Manual_for_Hospitals_and_Clinics_Second_Edition

HVAC Design Manual for Hospitals and Clinics [Internet]. [cited 2021 Jul 12]. Available from: https://www.ashrae.org/technical-resources/bookstore/hvac-design-manual-for-hospitals-and-clinics

Saran S, Gurjar M, Baronia A, Sivapurapu V, Ghosh PS, Raju GM, et al. Heating, ventilation and air conditioning (HVAC) in intensive care unit. Crit Care. 2020 May 6;24:194.

Lenzer B, Rupprecht M, Hoffmann C, Hoffmann P, Liebers U. Health effects of heating, ventilation and air conditioning on hospital patients: a scoping review. BMC Public Health. 2020 Aug 26;20(1):1287.

Engineered Systems | For facility, consulting & mechanical engineers [Internet]. [cited 2021 Jul 12]. Available from: https://www.esmagazine.com/

5 Hospital HVAC Design Strategies for the Post-COVID-19 World [Internet]. Facilitiesnet. [cited 2021 Jul 12]. Available from: https://www.facilitiesnet.com/healthcarefacilities/article/5-Hospital-HVAC-Design-Strategies-for-the-Post-COVID-19-World%2D%2D19123

39 Electrical Services

In any hospital project, it is very important to assess the requirement of power for operating the equipment, providing general use electrical outlets, operating air-conditioning plants, lighting, etc. Apart from this, it is also important to identify the areas that may require special power considerations like MRI, PET CT, LINAC etc.

There can be different sources of power supply for hospitals such as:

39.1 Primary Power Supply (PPS)

It is the power supplied by the local power distribution company. This is considered to be the most reliable source of power. To get this power, based on the calculated power load for the hospital and after taking into account the redundancy, an application is made to the power distribution company for allocating the power load. Thereafter, the power load is sanctioned and the connection to the grid of distribution company is released. The power can either be released from the Low Tension (LT) line or High Tension (HT) line.

39.2 Secondary Power Supply (SPS)

It is the power generated and supplied from the in house on site power source such as Diesel Generator Set.

39.3 Tertiary Power Supply (TPS)

It is the power supplied immediately, which is automatically switched on to provide additional power source to the equipment where loss of power supply can lead to disastrous consequences. This power is usually supplied with the help of Uninterruptible Power Supplies (UPS) system.

39.4 Electrical Load Calculation

Before applying for the power connection, the requirement of the power load shall be calculated. This load is calculated considering the power requirement of the equipment, air-conditioning plant, lifts, and the lighting of the hospital. Apart from the power load connections, these figures of load will also help to design the electrical equipment like transformers, circuit breakers, and bus-bars.

The total connected load of the hospital shall be calculated in KVA. Based on this, the

A. Garg, A. Dewan, *Manual of Hospital Planning and Designing*,
https://doi.org/10.1007/978-981-16-8456-2_39

maximum demand is worked out with an overall diversity factor of 80% and power factor 0.8 (lagging). To meet this electrical load and assuming 80% transformer loading and 97% efficiency of transformers, a sub-station shall be designed.

Due to the advancements in the healthcare technology, there is an ever-increasing demand for more refined electrical power for hospitals and this trend will continue in the future. Considering the advancements, a small spare capacity shall be considered and added to calculate the total power requirement.

39.5 HT Distribution System

Power supply shall be received from the concerned Electricity Supply Board/Company either through the LT line or the HT line. If it is an HT line, it shall be 11 KV single circuit feeder two-pole structure and shall be terminated at the metering panel room located at the entrance of the hospital premises. The 11 KV supply from the metering room shall be terminated at the main HT VCB panel located at the sub-station area. Further, the HT power supply shall be connected to the transformers through 11 KV XLPE (E) cable which is laid underground or trenched.

The sub-station comprises of one number 11 KV indoor type 630 Amp VCB (may vary as per the load calculation) as incoming cum outgoing, and one oil-cooled OLTC type transformer, the capacity of which shall depend on the load calculated for the hospital.

39.6 LT Power Distribution

The power supply received from the transformer or the supply cable from the Diesel Generators is further connected to hospital's main LT cum synchronization panel through bus duct or LT Armoured XLPE, aluminium cable. Capacitor Panels shall be connected directly to the main LT panel cum DG panel to improve the Power Factor from 0.8 to 0.95 lagging. Hence, this main panel controls both the supplies, i.e. Primary Supply and Secondary supply from the source like DG set.

This main LT panel cum DG panel shall feed the supply to different panels like:

1. HVAC Panel
2. Imaging Department Panel
3. Central Laboratory Panel
4. Operating Theatre Panel
5. Cathlab Panel
6. LINAC Panel
7. Different Floor Panels
8. Plumbing Panel
9. Firefighting Panel
10. Utility panel
11. External lighting panel
12. Lift panel

The connections from the main panel to these panels are done through LT Armoured XLPE, aluminium cables or Rising Main Bus-bar.

The power supply from individual floor panels, located on each floor of each section, shall be terminated at the LDB/PDB installed at different locations of the floor. The LDB/PDB shall be separate for lighting and power application. It shall have incoming MCB cum ELCB and also outgoing MCBs. The rating of the MCBs shall be designed according to the load factor on a particular MCB.

From the MCBs, the power is distributed at various locations and to the electrical outlets through the underground LT copper cable. If required, cable trays can be used instead of going underground. Cable trays usually travel above the false ceiling, and the route shall be through the corridors. Avoid laying cable trays in the rooms.

39.7 Redundancy Due to Power Failure

There are a number of reasons in any electrical system by which the power supply may be disrupted at some point of time. Therefore a contingency plan needs to be in place by making provision for redundancy in power source to mitigate the impact of power failure.

The redundancy level shall be in accordance with the type and level of hospital and the number of lifesaving machines installed in the hospital. While creating a contingency plan, special attention has to be paid to the area. There may be some areas like OPD where power failure may not leave any detrimental effect related to patient's safety as compared to the power failure in an ICU where it can have disastrous consequences. While designing the power system in the hospital, the designer shall address the risks that may be involved because of power failure. Therefore, the designer shall design an optimum solution that can minimize the risk to the patient's safety and ensure the efficient operation of the hospital facility.

Keeping in mind the consequence of power failure which may affect the working of units or equipment in the critical areas like ICU, Emergency, OR, Diagnostic etc. a more robust power infrastructure shall be planned, which shall incorporate additional provisions of secondary and/or tertiary power supplies.

39.8 Emergency Power Generation System

Radiator cooled Silent Diesel Generating sets shall be provided as a secondary source of power to meet the power backup for all services (considering 100% power backup). To make the DG power supply more flexible and economical, it is proposed to install two or more numbers of DG sets. The rating of the DG sets shall be decided and calculated based on the peak load and normal non-peak load of the power required.

The DG sets shall be located near the substation, compatible with Programmable Logic Control (PLC) system panel. These DG sets shall provide power automatically in the absence of primary electricity supply or when the supply voltage drops below the pre-set value. The number of DG sets running at any particular moment of time shall depend upon the load requirement through PLC. If all DG sets are synchronized together, the PLC can automatically control the running of DG Sets. All the DG sets shall have the facility of auto start and auto shut down.

The DG sets shall be installed on a raised foundation, which shall be strong enough to tolerate the load and vibrations of the DG set. The DG set is fixed to the foundation with the help of fasteners, and anti-vibration pads shall be installed.

An independent exhaust pipe from each DG set shall be connected to the chimney of 30-metre height from the ground to let the smoke out in the atmosphere. Silencer shall be provided with each DG set. The ambient noise level from DG set shall not be more than 72 dB(A) during operation from one-metre distance. Maximum stack height of the DG set shall be as per the norms.

One of the main components of DG set is the batteries used for cranking the engine. Therefore, special consideration shall be given to the choice of starting batteries, and either VRLA or Ni-Cd type shall be used; however, the use of Ni-Cd batteries is highly recommended.

Facility for onsite storage of diesel for generator sets shall be provided. The quantity of the diesel to be stored shall depend on the estimated running hours of the DG set. However, to be on the safer side, it is recommended that hospitals shall provide storage capacity of diesel equivalent to a minimum of 2 days of fuel consumption at 80% average loading on the DG sets.

As far as the air-conditioning plant is concerned, it is not necessary to provide 100% power supply backup. However, few spaces like OR, ICU and emergency shall be provided with the backup. If the hospital has a single air-conditioning plant for the entire building, it will become necessary to provide backup to the entire plant. Therefore, the designer can plan to have one separate air-conditioning plant for each critical area like OR, ICU, and emergency, so that the power backup can be provided to the plant dedicated solely for these areas. However, DG set shall have enough capacity to serve at least that part of the HVAC system, including the central chilled and heating plant, that can fulfil the requirements of cooling and heating of the critical areas like ICU and OT.

Separate and dedicated main DB rooms shall be provided for critical care facilities like OR, emergency, and ICU, to segregate primary and secondary main DBs from other spaces.

39.9 Uninterrupted Power Supply System (UPS)

UPS system is an important source of uninterrupted power supply in the hospital. It shall be used to provide power supply to all emergency lighting. Most importantly, the UPS system is provided in the critical units and for sophisticated machines like MRI, CT and LINAC.

As far as critical care units like ICU, NICU, emergency etc. are concerned, each unit shall have a dedicated UPS system connected to the concerned unit. Few light points (it is not necessary to include all) and approximately half of the electrical outlets shall be connected through the UPS circuit. These outlets shall be used for connecting life-saving machines like monitors, invasive and non-invasive ventilators, etc. It is recommended that in ICUs, a three-phase on-line UPS shall be provided. The rating of the UPS shall be designed as per the requirement. On an average, for a 10 bed ICU, the rating of the UPS shall be about 5–10 KVA.

Each OR shall have a dedicated UPS system. The plenum and peripheral lights shall be connected through the UPS circuit. All the electrical outlets and sockets shall also be connected to the UPS, so that power could be supplied to the machines and equipment in the OR in case of failure of primary power. Also, there is a short time lag between the failure of primary power and time to switch on the secondary power. In this time, UPS plays an important role in power supply. It is recommended that in ORs, a three-phase on-line UPS shall be provided. The rating of the UPS shall be designed as per the requirement. Generally, the rating of the UPS for each OR shall not be less than 10 KVA.

Apart from this, a UPS shall also be provided for the hospital server and to the working nodes at different locations of the hospital. For server, one dedicated UPS shall be provided, and for working nodes, a small off-line UPS shall be installed. Otherwise, a dedicated UPS supply line is laid down in the building to provided power backup to all IT equipment like Computers, CCTV, Wi-Fi routers, Fire Panel, alarms etc. The rating of the UPS shall be designed as per the requirement.

For Major sensitive medical equipment like MRI, CT, PET CT, PET MRI, Cath Lab, Gamma Camera, LINAC, Brachytherapy etc. separate machine dedicated UPS system shall be provided. The UPS for these machines shall be able to take the entire load of the machine while it is operational. This UPS can save the machine from getting damaged due to sudden power failure. It is normal, that due to sudden power failure, the software of these machines corrupts. Also, this UPS helps to avoid hampering the ongoing procedure at the time of power failure.

For emergency lighting in the hospital building, single UPS or floor UPS can be used. The rating of the UPS shall be designed based on the load requirement.

Preferably, at least a battery backup of 20–30 min shall be provided with each UPS. Sealed maintenance free type of batteries shall be used for storage.

It is recommended that the static, double conversion type of UPS units, which is either monolithic or modular, shall be used.

For better performance, VRLA type batteries shall be connected in a dual string arrangement. By providing multiple string battery connection, it is easy to maintain the batteries while the UPS is in working condition as all the cables need not be disconnected, and a part of battery bank keeps giving back up to the UPS.

Since, life of the batteries largely depends on the room temperature, it shall be maintained between 18 and 22 °C in the UPS rooms. Alarm systems shall also be provided in the UPS room in case the temperature is above the normal range.

UPS units shall be provided with external bypass panel so that in case of total failure of UPS, power can be bypassed to maintain continuous supply.

All UPS units can be kept at a common place in the hospital. However, UPS connected to special medical equipment like MRI, CT, LINAC etc. shall be placed near the respective machine.

39.10 Switching Arrangement

Switching arrangement shall be designed in a manner that allows isolation to be achieved in any particular space for fault protection.

ACBs shall be used in the LT panel for switching incoming circuits. Similarly, for switching outgoing circuits up to 630 Amps, MCCB shall be used. Above 630 Amps, ACBs shall be used. Inside the main DBs and sub-DBs, MCCBs shall be provided. Final DBs shall have MCBs and RCCBs. Besides this, care shall be taken to prevent voltage drop which shall not exceed 5 volts in the cables.

39.11 Emergency Lighting

Ten per cent of common/parking area lights shall be designated as emergency lights for the period between main supply shut down and start of the DG set, in order to avoid complete blackout and shall be individually connected to UPS/inverter for uninterrupted illumination.

39.12 Earthing System

Earthing shall be provided to all the HT/LT distribution system. This can be achieved through local maintenance-free earth station and bonding the cables/equipment. Earthing shall also be provided for all the light and power points. This shall be done with the help of insulated copper earthing wire, which shall run throughout the length of circuits and shall terminate at boxes or electrical fixtures and shall be bonded to main earth.

Separate chemical earthing shall be done for the entire UPS system units, EPABX, server, lift, and low voltage system using copper electrodes.

Most importantly, equipotential bonding shall be provided for all the hospital equipment. This shall be achieved by connecting the metal bodies of the said equipment to the Earth Bonding Bar (EBB), which in turn shall be connected to the chemical earthing.

Critical units such as ORs shall be provided with a dedicated EBB which shall be located near the OR. For other areas, EBB shall be provided in the respective sub-electrical rooms, where the final DBs are installed. Major machines like MRI, CT, LINAC, chillers etc. shall have supplementary earthing and bonding with a dedicated EBB.

All electrical panels and sub-panels shall also be bonded and earthed with a separate EBB.

39.13 System of Wiring and Cabling

The system of wiring means laying of the PVC insulated copper conducted FRLS cables and wires in MS/PVC conduits in the entire hospital building. The size of copper conductor wires to be laid down shall be a minimum of 1.5 mm^2 for light points and 2.5/4 mm^2 for power points. Colour coding shall be followed for the entire wiring system in the hospital building and it shall be Red, Yellow, and Blue for the three phases, Black for neutral, and Green for earthing.

Besides colour coding, ferruling shall also be done on each cable with number coding for identification of the circuits for maintenance.

The wiring for points of light and power shall be done from the final DBs. Localized switching/dimmer shall be provided for each area for convenience and operations.

Power supply cables connected to the life safety equipment like fire pumps, fire fighting lifts, and smoke evacuation systems shall be fire proof and shall be connected to a separate power supply source (other than the main power supply source to the hospital).

Wires and cables to be used in hospitals shall have LS0H insulation. Armoured cables, which are used for outdoor installations or buried underground, shall have PVC outer sheath.

Separate cable trunking and conduits shall be used for Isolated Power Supply (IPS) final circuits.

39.14 Switches/Sockets and Boxes

White/coloured rocker switches 6/16 Amp shall be used for primary power supply sockets. Faceplate to be used can be made out of either plastic or metal. For aesthetic purpose, plastic/metal faceplates shall be of same colour as of the switch/socket. For DG set power supply, the colour of the sockets and switches can be changed like red colour which helps in easy identification of the switches. Similarly, for UPS power supply sockets/switches blue colour can be used.

If the switches/sockets are being provided in the bed head panel or the hanging pendent, wherein gas outlets are also provided, ensure that there is a proper partition between the switch/socket and medical gas outlets, so that there are no chances of sparking a fire.

39.15 Lightning Protection

The entire hospital premises shall be protected from sky lightning by providing suitable lightning arrestors connected to copper tape/cable. Suitable protected zone shall be formed through the mast and connected to earthing stations through cable/copper tape.

Special consideration shall be given to protect electronic devices and medical equipment in the hospital from damages due to lighting strike. Therefore, it is advised to provide Surge Protection Devices (SPDs) for sub-main electrical branch circuits serving critical medical equipment.

39.16 Power Quality

Sophisticated medical equipments are highly sensitive to power quality, and any electrical disturbances may cause equipment's failure, leading to fatal consequences. For any equipment, the power shall be in a pure sine wave form with no surges. The following precautions shall be taken:

1. For main equipment like CT, MRI, X-Ray, LINAC etc. power supply feeders shall be directly supplied from the main DB and not from the sub-distribution panels shared with others.
2. In case the supply from MDB is not possible, power can be supplied from the sub-main distribution board (SMDB), provided a dedicated appropriately sized SMDB is installed in the MDB room to serve a group of such equipment.
3. Surge protection devices shall be provided in the panels and also in the UPSs' to get a pure sine wave. The chances of damage to electronic boards of medical equipment can be reduced to a great extent, if the supplied power is with the pure sine waves.
4. To install harmonic filters, provision of breakers shall be made in the main DB's, and such spare breakers, designated for these filters, shall be clearly labelled as 'For Harmonic Filter Only'. Though it is not practically possible to accurately estimate the rating of harmonic filters in advance, power system harmonics of order 3rd, 5th, 7th, 9th, 11th and 15th order can create significant problems of over current and overheating of cables, bus-bars and transformers.
5. Harmonics shall be finally measured once majority of the medical equipment, mechanical, and electrical appliances are operational.

39.17 Power Factor Correction

Capacitor banks including reactor shall be provided in the main capacitor panels at the central power station for controlling the power factor as well as the harmonics. As per regulations, all bulk users are required to maintain a power factor of 0.9 and above, failing which stringent penalties are imposed by the power distribution companies.

39.18 Street Lighting System

LED lamps with suitable fixture mounted on 7 m high GI poles shall be used for street lighting, to maintain average lighting level of 18 lux with illumination density of 1.5 cd/m^2. The street lights shall be timer controlled for switching ON/OFF as per schedule.

39.19 Lighting Management System

39.19.1 Occupancy Sensor

Based on person's presence in an area, lights would automatically switch on/off. The sensor would have a time delay before the lights are switched off.

39.20 Illumination Levels

Following shall be the illumination level for general lighting of the hospital premises:

Room/Function	Illuminance in (Lux)	Colour rendering index (%)
Emergency unit		
Admissions/reception	300	80
Triage	500	90
Treatment area	500	80
Procedure room	500	90
Minor operation	500	90
Resuscitation room	500	80
Plaster room	500	80
Stores	300	80
Operation theatres		
Operating room	1000	90
Operating table	125,000	90
Scrub	500	80
Recovery–stage 1	500	90
Clean utility and dirty utility	100 to 150	80
Intensive care units		
Intensive care unit	100	80
High dependency unit	100	80
Simple observation / examination	300	80
Night light	10	80
Examination room	1000	90
Delivery suite		
Delivery room	500	80
NICU	100	80
Special care baby unit	1000	80
Circulation space	100	80
Formula room	300	80
Inpatient unit		
Patient bed	300	80
Treatment room	1000 (local)	90
Circulation space	100	80
Nursing station	300	80
Corridors	200	80
Laboratory		
Laboratories	500	80
Blood bank	300	80
Cold rooms	200	80
Radiology		
Angiography	500	80
CT/MRI scanning rooms	300	80
X-ray	300	80
Ultrasound	300	80
Screening-fluoroscopy	300	80
Mammography	500	80
Radiotherapy	100	80
Isotope store	300	80
Central sterile supply unit		
Decontamination and loading	500	80
Sterilization	300	80
Sterile store	150	80
Packing zone	500	80
Other treatment areas		
Dialysis	500	80
ECG	300	80
Endoscopy procedure room	300	80
Pharmacy	500	80
Laundry		
Linen store (linen department)	100	80
Packing and dispatching	300	80
Ironing and pressing	300	80
Mending room	500	80
Laundry	300	80
Outpatient unit		
Consultation and examination room	300	80
Treatment and procedure room	500	80
Allied health		
Gymnasium	300	80
Physiotherapy	200	80
Rehabilitation	200	80
Common and circulation areas		

(continued)

Room/Function	Illuminance in (Lux)	Colour rendering index (%)
Entrance lobby	200	80
Lift lobby	200	80
Lift car	150	80
Reception area	300	80
Corridors (general)	200	80
Lounge	150	80
Storage (general)	200	80
Toilets	200	80
Prayer rooms	100	80
Library	300	80
Changing room, lockers	150	80
General office	300	80
Loading bay	100	80
Shop/kiosk	300	80
Seminar room	300	80
Clean utility and dirty utility	150	80

Further Reading

says BAD. Tips for designing a hospital electrical system [Internet]. ETKHO Hospital Engineering. 2020 [cited 2021 Jul 12]. Available from: https://www.etkho.com/en/tips-for-designing-a-hospital-electrical-system/

Reiling J, Hughes RG, Murphy MR. The Impact of Facility Design on Patient Safety. In: Hughes RG, editor. Patient Safety and Quality: An Evidence-Based Handbook for Nurses [Internet]. Rockville (MD): Agency for Healthcare Research and Quality (US); 2008 [cited 2021 Jul 12]. (Advances in Patient Safety). Available from: http://www.ncbi.nlm.nih.gov/books/NBK2633/

the Electrical Distribution Systems for Hospitals [Internet]. [cited 2021 Jul 12]. Available from: http://www.electrical-knowhow.com/2012/02/electrical-distribution-systems-for.html

Farooq A, Alhalabi W. Smart Electrical Design of Medical Center to Vary Field Parameters: Sensor Network in Improving Health Care. J Eng Appl Sci. 2019 Feb 15;14.

Saving money in hospital electrical distribution systems [Internet]. Healthcare Facilities Today. [cited 2021 Jul 12]. Available from: https://www.healthcarefacilitiestoday.com/posts/Saving-money-in-hospital-electrical-distribution-systems%2D%2D2607

Owen S. NFPA 99 and the NEC: The Basis for a Healthy Electrical System [Internet]. EC&M. 2004 [cited 2021 Jul 12]. Available from: https://www.ecmweb.com/content/article/20891697/nfpa-99-and-the-nec-the-basis-for-a-healthy-electrical-system

Group TM. Hospital-Grade Standards for Power Cords and Other Power System Components for Global Markets [Internet]. [cited 2021 Jul 12]. Available from: https://www.medicaldesignbriefs.com/component/content/article/mdb/features/technology-leaders/21330

Hospital mechanical and electrical systems [Internet]. [cited 2021 Jul 12]. Available from: https://www.hfmmagazine.com/articles/1542-hospital-mechanical-and-electrical-systems

General rules of electrical installation design - Electrical Installation Guide [Internet]. [cited 2021 Jul 12]. Available from: https://www.electrical-installation.org/enwiki/General_rules_of_electrical_installation_design

Emergency and Standby Power Systems for Buildings [Internet]. Archtoolbox.com. [cited 2021 Jul 12]. Available from: https://www.archtoolbox.com/materials-systems/electrical/emergency-power-systems-for-buildings.html

Portal E-EE. Electrical Design Manual For New Hospitals [Internet]. EEP - Electrical Engineering Portal. [cited 2021 Jul 12]. Available from: https://electrical-engineering-portal.com/download-center/books-and-guides/electrical-engineering/electrical-design-manual-for-new-hospitals

Portal E-EE. Electrical design of healthcare facilities (essential system requirements) | EEP [Internet]. EEP - Electrical Engineering Portal. 2019 [cited 2021 Jul 12]. Available from: https://electrical-engineering-portal.com/electrical-design-healthcare-facilities

40 ELV, ICT and IBMS Services

ICT, Information and Communication Technologies, the system focuses on the services relating to processing information (data, voice, video) and connecting devices.

ELV, Extra Low Voltage, systems focuses on the services like connectivity, security, safety and automation.

Both the systems play an important role in the operation of the hospital. The LAN infrastructure in a hospital shall provide IP connectivity for various services in hospital, which may actually be located at some other spaces in the building, but it requires connectivity with the main source through the same physical network for sharing the data or command. The applications can be CCTV, data, public address, voice, video, nurse call, queuing systems, HIS, PACS etc.

40.1 Data System

All data cables shall be terminated at floor patch panel and then data shall be transmitted to the server through a backbone fibre optic cable.

40.2 Nurse Call System

It is the utility provided in the patient room to establish a communication between the nurse and the patient when the latter requires the services of the former. The following issues shall be considered while designing the nurse call system:

40.2.1 Desktop Console

The function of this unit is to a receive call and alarm from different locations of patients and staff. The unit is programmed in such a manner that if the patient activates the call from the bed, the console receives the call and displays the unique ID (may be room number or bed number) on the panel screen fixed on the console. Simultaneously, the alarm starts beeping. The nurse immediately comes to know caller's location. If the unit has bi-direction speech facility with the patient, the nurse can talk to the patient. The system shall be designed in a manner that the nurse shall not be able end the call from her end and has to go the patient bed for resetting and ending the call. This unit shall be placed at the nursing station and shall be in direct eye contact with the nurses.

40.2.2 Room Lights

These are colour coded lights installed at the main entrance of the area/room, above or beside each main door where the nurse call device is placed. This light is to assist the nurse to reach

A. Garg, A. Dewan, *Manual of Hospital Planning and Designing*,
https://doi.org/10.1007/978-981-16-8456-2_40

the patient who has activated the call. The light switches on when the call is activated and once the call is attended and the reset button is pressed, the light is switched off.

40.2.3 Patient Call with Handset

This is a device called Patient Hand Set which comprise of various buttons like staff assistance and emergency call buttons, microphone, speaker etc. to activate the call. This device has a jack for plugging the patient handset. This jack is plugged into the socket of the nurse call system. The socket is located at the head end of the patient, either on the wall or in the bed head panel. This device is provided at all locations where the patients are admitted and not continuously attended by a nurse.

The call button shall help the patients to communicate with the staff and to alert a nurse for any assistance, which in turn increases a sense of security in the patient.

40.2.4 Patient Call—in Toilets

These units are used to initiate an alarm call in emergency situation from inside the toilet. These units are usually fixed at a low height and within easy reach of the patient. These units shall have minimum buttons so that the patient is not in a confused state of mind while initiating the call. These units shall be waterproof and shall be able to be installed even at wet locations.

40.2.5 Staff Assist Call

This device is for the staff who is present at the patient location and requires additional help from other staff members, may be other nurses or doctors. The system has pre-configured locations, as to where the call will reach as soon as the call is activated. Once the call is activated, the alarm beeps at the other integrated place and a visual ID (from where the call is active) is displayed.

40.2.6 Emergency Call

This button is for the staff to raise alarm in case of an emergency to alert other staff members for help. Once the emergency call is activated, the system generates an audible alarm at the concerned staff station or designated mobile devices along with an alphanumeric display to indicate the location from where the call is initiated.

40.2.7 Wireless Handset

Nowadays, the patient unit is provided with a wireless handset to activate the call. This handset is connected using Bluetooth or infrared connection and functions similarly to that of a wired handset.

40.2.8 Wireless Console

Mobile wireless nurse call consoles work on Bluetooth or Wi-Fi technology. It allows the nurse to be aware of the call from a patient, other than the patient she is attending, or if the nurse is not present at the nursing station where the console is located.

40.2.9 Audio-Video Nurse Call System

This device is largely under development, which shall have an audio-video communication facility. Under this technology, the nurse console will have a small video screen, microphone, and a speaker. Similarly, at the head end of the patient, a small camera shall be mounted, and the handset shall have a small video screen along with a microphone and speaker. As soon as the patient activates the call, the audio and video are activated and the nurse can see the patient and talk to him/her. Further, the mobile of the patient can be connected to the nurse console through a dedicated IP.

40.3 Electronic Security and Video Surveillance System

40.3.1 Closed Circuit Television System (CCTV)

Being large, complex institutions, hospitals poses a great concern of ensuring the security of men and material in the premises. Hospitals generally have the presence of a lot of people, and some of them may be under mental stress. Therefore, there are all chances of self-harming or suicide. Moreover, there are high chances of theft of costly equipment and leakage of the medical data from the hospitals. Thus, to handle such issues, hospitals need to have extensive and effective CCTV solutions. The system is required to record all activities happening in the building, particularly the high potential areas like entrance lobbies, cash counters, OPD lobbies, ICU complex, emergency units, mortuary, kitchen, or any other cluttered and crowded spaces. If needed, this recording can be used for tracking an event.

The Closed Circuit Television System (CCTV system) facilitates an online display of video images on screen, records the same on real-time basis, and makes it available for tracking in the future if required.

The following issues need to be addressed while designing and planning the CCTV system and access control systems for hospitals:

1. Before deciding the location of the CCTV camera, patient's privacy shall be considered by the designer. Cameras shall never be installed in such areas where the privacy of the patient may be compromised, for example toilets, procedure rooms, OR, delivery suites etc.
2. The CCTV's and access control system shall be provided at all the important, crowded and sensitive locations of the hospital.
3. Coverage of CCTV shall be provided at the following locations but shall not be limited to:

Main Entrances of the hospital	Cash counters
Entrance Lobbies	NICU
Emergency and Triage Room	Nurse stations
Common Corridors	Staff rooms
Billing and Registration Counters	Body storage areas
Waiting Lobbies	Fire exit stairs
Staircases	Main entrances of public toilet
All exits of the hospital	Hot Labs
All receptions	MEP plant rooms
Pharmacy, medication dispensing areas	Air-conditioning Plant
Entrance door of medication rooms	Lift lobbies
Inside the medication rooms	Inside lifts
Inside the laboratories	Central Sterile Supply Unit
Blood Bank	Parking Lots and Garages

4. IP megapixel cameras shall be installed at the locations as mentioned above. Cameras shall also be installed in corridors, perimeters for perimeter protection, and each important area like server rooms, UPS room, hub room etc. Fixed cameras shall be used for primary surveillance of any area, but for areas like main entrance hall, additional secondary surveillance shall be provided with the help of PTZ cameras.
5. CCTV system cameras shall be connected to the DVR and PC for recording network video live images. These recordings shall be saved to the hard disk of the PC. The HDD shall have a capacity to record live footage for a period of at least two month. Back up the recordings shall be taken at regular intervals, on an external hard disk and HDD shall be made free for further recordings.
6. The entire system, including DVR, cameras and PC shall have a power backup through UPS. CCTV cameras shall be appropriately powered for continued functioning. The power supplied to these cameras shall be backed up by providing UPS power backup.

7. Due to operational and security authority requirements, separate and dedicated IT network shall be provided for IP CCTV network and access control.

40.4 Access Control System

A network shall be created within the campus for various systems to be deployed with the Integrated Security Management System (ISMS).

In hospital, at times, patients or family members of patients may become aggressive or even violent due to the anxiety and trauma the patient is undergoing. Further, the cases of quarantined patients need to be handled quickly and efficiently to prevent the spread of infection. Hospitals are also concerned about patient safety, as adverse issues can lead to patients being abducted, harmed, missing or committing suicide.

Furthermore, in hospitals, there is high risk of theft and abuse, particularly the expensive equipment distributed throughout the premises and pharmaceutical drugs. Therefore, a strong, comprehensive access control system shall be provided to improve the overall security, avoid hospital losses, and increase patient and staff safety.

These days different types of access control systems are available with different features and designs. Out of all these, there are a few which are suitable for hospital setup and can be used for restricting access to sensitive areas of the hospital like ICU's, OR, record room, isolation areas etc. which may prevent the spread of disease. The restricting access can also help in tracking and preventing the theft of medical equipment and drugs and can also protect both staff and patients.

40.4.1 No-Touch Access

Touch points are the points of access control system, which need to be necessarily touched in order to get through. These can be the door handles, push bar, keypad etc. In a hospital, these touch points can create a hazardous source of spreading infection. Hence, it is advised to reduce physical touch points and adopt touch-free devices like door readers, which reads and authenticates credential from a distance and then opens automatically.

The following sections describe the architecture and functional requirements of an integrated security alarm management system. The command and control system shall be the heart of the system, with all the system components reporting to it, and shall be modular and must have a highly scalable architecture.

1. Access control system shall consist of proximity readers for entry to common doors, which will eliminate the risk of un-authorized entry in the building premises. Main entry doors to the building through staircase and lift lobbies are ideal for implementing this system. The exit from these doors shall be planned through a card reader.
2. Biometric face readers shall be used at important locations, i.e. server rooms, control room and highly secured documentation area.
3. Access control system shall be integrated with IP CCTV and fire alarm system.
4. RFID cards/tags and reader-based access control system shall be used.
5. Fingerprint biometric readers, which requires touching a figure to scan the fingerprints, shall not be used in the hospital.
6. 'Infant Protection System' shall be used in the hospital in NICU and paediatric wards. This system shall have trackable tags, which shall be employed on the forearm of the infant and mother. This system shall be interfaced with access control system to disallow the access in case of any breach of security.
7. Discrete Panic Alarms shall be provided at all important locations like emergency triage area, cash counters, reception, ICU etc.

Electronic access control shall be provided at the following locations:

Radiotherapy LINAC Bunkers	Intensive Care Units
Server room or data centres	Entrances to staff only areas
CT Scan/MRI Room	Clean Storage of CSSD
Pharmacy	Dirty utility
Cash counters	All entries and exits to outside
Medical records	Entrances to back offices, insurance offices
Isolation rooms	Staff only corridors
Neonatal Units	

1. Entry doors locked with electronic access control system shall be accessible only for people with valid access cards. Access to these areas shall only be allowed by a designated door operator. Some of these areas are:
   (a) Doors between the control room and the patient treatment room of the radio therapy department.
   (b) Windows in the hot lab between the drug preparation and drug administration room.
   (c) Doors between the control room and the patient imaging room of the CT Scan or MRI.
   (d) Outside entry door and patient room in Isolation area/units.
   (e) Doors between dirty and sterile area of CSSD.
   (f) Window between the OR and dirty utility room attached to the OR.

40.5 Telecommunication System

In hospitals, either a combined audio/video intercom system or an audio intercom system shall be provided for a fast and easy two-way communication. IP-based solutions shall be preferred for better operational flexibility.

Telephone and data points shall be connected through four pair CAT 6 cables from the patch panel located on each floor. All the floor patch panels in turn shall be connected to the main patch panel installed in the LV rooms. Hook-up wire or patch cords shall be used for patching between incoming and outgoing patch panels.

Following issues shall be considered while designing the telecommunication system:

1. There shall be a central intercom EPABX system installed at a particular location in the hospital.
2. The telephone cable of the CAT 5 or 6 cable shall be laid down in the entire hospital building.
3. Each location shall be allotted a unique intercom number and connected to a cable/wire.

Telecommunication also includes the concept of the telemedicine and telemonitoring wherein home or remote healthcare facilities are provided by allowing real-time monitoring of off-site patients, visualize the investigation reports, providing general prescription etc. The efficiency and timely delivery of the results can only be achieved with telecommunication if an effective communication system is established between the patients, equipment, and healthcare personnel.

Until recently, Radio frequency (RF) was the most preferred technology to provide an effective communication channel for connecting the patients, equipment, and healthcare personnel. However, RF possesses issues relating to security, privacy, safety, interference generation, tolerance, spectrum congestion etc. Due to these shortcomings, wireless technology is being adopted now a days.

Then came in the Visible Light Communications (VLC) technology. VLC uses the lighting infrastructure of solid-state light sources like white LEDs for light-based wireless connectivity. VLC is an effective technology, particularly for hospital applications to provide services like telecommunication and remote health monitoring.

Further, a hybrid optical-radio network is considered to be the perfect connectivity infrastructure for hospitals. This hybrid network works with the combination of both radio and optical platforms to provide a high performance, highly secure, flexible, private, and safe communication network.

40.6 Patient Entertainment and Information Systems

Patients in the hospital shall be provided with an entertainment facility in their room. The patient entertainment and infotainment systems shall have the provision to view mainstream TV channels, videos, videos on patient awareness and education, health awareness shows, hospital informatics, diet menus, movies and shows on demand etc. based on the facility available in the hospital. The main points to be considered while designing this system are as follows:

1. A smart TV shall be located on the wall just in front of the patient in the patient room.
2. The height of the TV shall be such that the patient in head-up position can easily view it. Generally, the bottom of the TV shall be about 1524 mm from the floor.
3. An operating remote shall be provided at the bed of the patient.
4. The television shall be connected to the IPTV network. Also, it shall have the facility for multiple television channels by connecting it through satellite dish.
5. Use of mobile phones shall be allowed in the hospital. However, in critical areas like ICUs, the use of mobile phones shall be restricted.

40.7 Queue Management System

Areas where the patient/visitors have to wait for their turn like registration, billing, cash counter, OPD, investigations, pharmacy etc. shall have a queue management system in place.

1. Token system can be implemented wherein each person will be provided with a token mentioning a serial number for their turn. To facilitate this, token dispensing machines shall be provided at suitable locations under the supervision of a staff member.
2. Waiting area display: Suitably sized LED panel screens shall be provided in the lobbies, which shall display the token number and the counter or room number where the person has to report as their turn arrives. These screens shall be integrated with the IPTV systems of the hospital.
3. The calling station from where the call for token is raised shall be software controlled, and that could be operated from workstation of computer system, rather than using conventional hardware with keypad.

40.8 Public Address System

Communication plays an important role in providing better healthcare services and save lives in a hospital. Staff must be able to reach the required medical professionals at all times. Also, the staff must be able to make general and emergency announcements hospital-wide and know that the correct people are hearing it. This is where the hospital communication systems like intercom and public address (PA) system are of importance.

As technology has improved, so have communication systems. More and more communication systems are going IP by replacing old wired systems. This not only gives hospitals more flexibility but also provides better sound quality and more integration with other systems, like video surveillance, access control, and nurse call systems.

Apart from announcements in case of emergencies, public address system can be used in hospitals for broadcasting prayers, playing background music, announcements etc. in waiting areas and corridors.

1. *System Description*

   The public address system shall be designed in such a manner that the voice reaches all desired areas in the hospital. The quality of sound also matters, and the voice shall be clearly audible with no disturbances and echo.
2. *Zoning*

   Public-address system shall be zoned in the hospital building to suit the operational requirements of the hospital.

3. PA equipment shall include microphones for announcement, processing circuits, sound amplifiers, pre-mixers, ambient noise reductions, speakers, cabling and all other required equipment.
4. Microphones shall be highly sensitive, with minimum noise distortion and low sensitivity to feedback. They shall be connectable to the zone selection consoles, each with its own selectable priority, from which each operator shall send announcements to specific audio zones.
5. *Distribution Equipment*

   The distribution equipment shall primarily comprise line attenuators with line transformers and rotary/digital controls for selecting the output power of a line speaker.
6. *Speakers*

   The speakers shall be of various design, depending on the requirement of the area allocated/usage. If there is no false ceiling, the speakers can be column type and fixed on the wall of corridors at a specific distance. Wherever false ceiling exists, the speakers shall be of concealed mounting type with a wide bandwidth.
7. *Central Announcement Cell*

   The hospital shall have a central announcement cell which shall be manned round the clock. This cell shall have a microphone, amplifier and zone controller.

40.9 Integrated Building Management Systems (IBMS)

It is the pinnacle of automation controls that helps in the effective and efficient usage of various electro-mechanical systems in a building. With more emphasis on optimized energy controls and green building norms being the new focus area, IBMS helps in achieving the stringent norms by proper monitoring and control of the systems used like HVAC, electrical, DG, sprinklers, hydrant and security systems for optimized energy usage.

Building Automation System helps in conserving energy by planning and executing various energy conservation control schemes, which in turn helps in reducing manpower requirement for operating and maintaining the building services without compromising on the quality of services.

IBMS also acts as a strong Management Information System (MIS) by keeping the management informed about the critical operation of various equipment connected to IBMS and make available data required for analysing the working and further possibilities of conserving the energy.

The system shall be based on Micro Processor Control System, using various Energy Management Programmes to save energy with the latest techniques of controlling the environment. BAS shall be capable of performing the following main functions:

1. *HVAC System*

   In a hospital setup, HVAC system consumes maximum energy. If IBMS is used for HVAC, it can provide the opportunity to save lot of energy.
2. *Precision AC System*

   The IBMS can monitor and control the actual on/off status of the precision AC and display it on the BMS screen.
3. *Diesel Generator Set*

   The IBMS can monitor the status of alarm like low lubricant oil pressure low, fuel level low etc. for DG set. The status can also be displayed on the DG screen of the IBMS system.
4. *UPS System*

   Through IBMS, the UPS can be monitored via serial interface, and user can view the input, output, and interface parameters.
5. *Water Management*

   IBMS can control the water levels in the tanks through the automatic level sensors and can automatically switch on/off the water supply motors.
6. *Lift Monitoring*

   Through IBMS, the lifts can be easily controlled. It can control functions like floor position, alarm, and maintenance modes.
7. *Firefighting System*

   IBMS can easily monitor the pressure status in the hydrant and sprinkler line of the fire-

fighting system. If the pressure goes down in the line, it can automatically switch on/off the fire pumps to recover the pressure.
8. If the IBMS is connected and integrated with the fire control panel, it can monitor the status of the firefighting system.

Further Reading

Almotaeryi R, Khan F, Bouridane A, Jiang R. SMART CCTV SURVEILLANCE SYSTEM FOR HOSPITALS. 2017 Jan 1;Volume 72:.213-225.

Smart Building Technology | Optergy Best-in-Class BMS & EMS Solutions [Internet]. Optergy. [cited 2021 Jul 14]. Available from: http://optergy.com/smart-building-technology/

Public Address and Intercom System Design Guidelines | Clock | Telephone [Internet]. Scribd. [cited 2021 Jul 14]. Available from: https://www.scribd.com/doc/295754458/Public-Address-and-Intercom-System-Design-Guidelines

Miller ET, Deets C, Miller RV. Nurse call systems: impact on nursing performance. J Nurs Care Qual. 1997 Feb;11(3):36–43.

Nurse call system upgrades [Internet]. [cited 2021 Jul 14]. Available from: https://www.hfmmagazine.com/articles/1664-nurse-call-system-upgrades

Editor. Integrated BMS for Healthcare Building | Cooling India Monthly Business Magazine on the HVACR Business | Green HVAC industry | Heating, Ventilation, Air conditioning and Refrigeration News Magazine Updates, Articles, Publications on HVACR Business Industry | HVACR Business Magazine [Internet]. [cited 2021 Jul 14]. Available from: https://www.coolingindia.in/integrated-bms-for-healthcare-building/

Dašić P, Dašić J, Crvenković B. Improving patient safety in hospitals through usage of cloud supported video surveillance. Maced J Med Sci. 2017 Apr 15;5:101–6.

How to Create the Perfect Public Service Announcement [Internet]. GovTech. 2021 [cited 2021 Jul 14]. Available from: https://www.govtech.com/education/news/how-to-create-the-perfect-public-service-announcement.html

How good public address and intercom systems help save lives in hospitals - asmag.com Rankings [Internet]. [cited 2021 Jul 14]. Available from: https://www.asmag.com/rankings/m/content.aspx?id=30879

Hospital Building management system (BMS) [Internet]. Med & Tech. [cited 2021 Jul 14]. Available from: http://hospital-tech.com/solutions/hospital-building-management-system-bms/

Emergency Public Address System Requirements & Maintenance [Internet]. Jensen Hughes. [cited 2021 Jul 14]. Available from: https://www.jensenhughes.com/insights/public-address-systems-what-you-need-to-know

Aswin S, Narayanamurthy G, Jeyender S, Prasanna R, Kumar SP. Design development and implementation of wireless nurse call station. 2011 Annu IEEE India Conf INDICON. 2011 Dec 1;

CCTV in healthcare - The MDU [Internet]. [cited 2021 Jul 14]. Available from: https://www.themdu.com/guidance-and-advice/guides/cctv-in-healthcare

Building Management System (BMS) Research Papers - Academia.edu [Internet]. [cited 2021 Jul 14]. Available from: https://www.academia.edu/Documents/in/Building_Management_System_BMS_

Building management systems and integrated building management [Internet]. i-SCOOP. [cited 2021 Jul 14]. Available from: https://www.i-scoop.eu/building-management-building-management-systems-bms/

Building Management System - an overview | ScienceDirect Topics [Internet]. [cited 2021 Jul 14]. Available from: https://www.sciencedirect.com/topics/engineering/building-management-system

Zapatán RA, Armijos EE, Serpa-Andrade L, Pinos E. Analysis of a Nurse Call System Implementation using a Wireless Sensors Network. In: Torres I, Bustamante J, Sierra DA, editors. VII Latin American Congress on Biomedical Engineering CLAIB 2016, Bucaramanga, Santander, Colombia, October 26th -28th, 2016. Singapore: Springer; 2017. p. 638–41. (IFMBE Proceedings).

Advances in nurse call systems help to put patients in control [Internet]. [cited 2021 Jul 14]. Available from: https://www.hfmmagazine.com/articles/2790-advances-in-nurse-call-systems-help-put-patients-in-control

Rai M, Husain AA, Maity T, Yadav RK. Advance Intelligent Video Surveillance System (AIVSS): A Future Aspect [Internet]. Intelligent Video Surveillance. IntechOpen; 2018 [cited 2021 Jul 14]. Available from: https://www.intechopen.com/books/intelligent-video-surveillance/advance-intelligent-video-surveillance-system-aivss-a-future-aspect

41 Information Technology and Computerization

The IT or computer network has to be efficiently created in the hospital. This is necessary because the software required for operating the hospital, generally called HIS (Hospital Information System), is used at all the locations and departments of the hospital.

As the software is loaded in the central servers of the hospital, all the working places have to be connected to the servers to complete the network.

The following issues shall be considered while designing the network system and providing the IT hardware.

1. The main server shall be provided in the hospital and shall be located in a separate server room. This room shall be away from the patient area and the entry shall be restricted to this room. The flooring of the room shall be raised with a stage type floor free from the bottom. All the wires and cables shall be laid down under the floor. The temperature and humidity of the server room shall be provided as per the requirements of the manufacturers of the server.
2. Server cabinets shall be provided in the room, and the servers shall be placed in these cabinets.
3. As a precautionary measure, a second server shall also be provided, which shall be a mirror server to the main server, and the data of the main server shall be copied on the mirror server in real time.
4. Furthermore, another set of off-site backup servers can be provided either in another room of the hospital or other building or location. As the data is very crucial for hospitals, nobody wants to encounter the risks of losing data due to any breakdown, fire or flooding etc. in the main server.
5. All the servers shall be provided with a separate UPS power backup of the required rating.
6. An arrangement shall be made for additional backup of the data on the external devices like HDD, DVDs etc.
7. A separate room shall be provided to store these backup dives in or near the server room. For this, a separate air-conditioned room shall be provided. The room shall have a fireproof cabinet to store such devices.
8. The connectivity shall be done with the help of CAT 6 cables or optical fibre cables. From the main server the optical fibre cables shall be laid down and shall terminate at each floor of the hospital building. This cable shall be connected to the floor switch boxes. From the switch boxes, the cables shall be laid down till the user point and shall terminate at the connector jack RJ 45. The required work station shall be connected to this jack and ultimately it will be connected to the main server of the hospital.
9. The technology and design shall be based on set standards and only IEEE or IETF certi-

A. Garg, A. Dewan, *Manual of Hospital Planning and Designing*,
https://doi.org/10.1007/978-981-16-8456-2_41

fied protocols shall be used. The system shall be operative with the systems of other vendors also, hence the same standards such as HL7 and DICOM shall be used.
10. The IT network shall be capable of supporting multiple virtual IP addresses and shall allow multicast routed domains having a complete traffic separation.
11. The solution shall be provided with adequate security options to protect the network from hacking and exposure of IP. The security of IT shall be the main concern while designing the system.
12. Bandwidth requirements shall be carefully designed considering the network and data storage requirements.
13. Requirements of the Bandwidth and data storage shall be worked out based on the software and number of working nodes to be used in the hospital. Some software like PACS may require higher bandwidth, while software like Laboratory modules may require very less bandwidth.
14. Data storage capacity shall be planned in such a fashion that the space equivalent to data of minimum of 6 years' operation of the hospital can be stored.
15. If WIFI access is provided to the public in the hospital, Captive Portals shall be used to implement the system.

41.1 Health Information System (HIS)

A *Hospital Information System* (*HIS*) is a comprehensive and integrated information system for managing the hospital activities like Finance and accounts, in-patient treatment admission and discharge, Investigation departments like radiology and pathology, operation theatre, nursing care, outpatient management, procurements, asset management, materials management, pharmacy management, blood bank and payroll management. Most important is the reporting systems and analysis of the data to provide information to the management about actual performances and for framing policies and decision making, based on this analysis, for further improvement in the hospital.

Hospital information system is also known as *Hospital Management System* (*HMS*).

HMS is a common source of recording and retrieving information about a patient's health history kept at a secure place electronically and used or recovered as and when required. These systems help to enhance the ability and dependability of health care workers to provide care by keeping the track of the patient's history, diseases, medication, surgeries, visits, and health information that may be needed when required. Patient's diagnostic investigation like pathology and even visual images such as X-ray, will be available electronically to the health care professionals as and when required.

41.2 Modules of Hospital Information Software

The HIS is basically a bundle of softwares put together in one software and integrated to each other. Each such software, called 'Module', relates to the working of one activity. The HIS normally has the following modules:

41.2.1 Information Desk Module

This module is to provide answer to all types of enquiries relating to the hospital and also relating to the patients who are registered or admitted in the hospital like:

1. Patient's enquiry
2. Appointment's enquiry
3. Appointment for Investigation enquiry
4. Consultant's/Doctors enquiry
5. In-patient's enquiry
6. Tariff information
7. Estimates of treatment
8. Package's information
9. Investigations enquiry
10. Visitor pass management etc.

41.2.2 Patient Registration Module

Each patient who visits the first time to the hospital shall be registered before he/she goes in for consultation. Under this module, the registration staff fills up the patients' personal, medical, family, and demographic details during registration. These details are filled up in the system. Thereafter a unique ID is generated for each patient. This ID is used to maintain the patient's medical history and diagnosis and also facilitate the tracking of records. This module also helps generate the token numbers for doctor's consultation, print the patients' case sheets with barcode and photograph for easy tracking. Also the bills for registration charges and doctor's consultation can be raised through the module only. This module also contains information about the rosters of physicians and doctors and checks the availability of those physicians and doctors at any particular time and makes it easy for booking an appointment.

41.2.3 Outpatient Management Module

The Outpatient Department module helps in booking the consultations with the date and time of such consultation. It also facilitates the registration of the appointment along with the prescription and the receipt of the consultation fee deposited. This module also maintains a list of appointments for each day along with the time of consultation. Also, the booking of appointments is possible for investigating departments like laboratory and radiology. From this module, only the SMS and alerts can be sent to patients, informing them about their scheduled appointments. This module mainly deals with recording of the patients' medical treatment details along with the diagnosis and the investigation reports. The module is interfaced with other modules such as Registration, Laboratory test reports and Radiology reports to acquire the data from those modules.

1. Schedules for available doctors with date and time.
2. Appointment schedule.
3. Generating Token for consultation.
4. Recording Patient Basic parameters.
5. Diagnosis.
6. Result of the Lab orders.
7. Results of the Radiology reports.
8. Prescription of Medication.
9. Cross referral if required.
10. Details of the Procedures to be carried out.
11. Reports based on activities of user, patient and doctor.
12. Reports on OPD billing, revenue received and number of patient registered at the counters.

41.2.4 In-Patient Management Module

The In-Patient Department module mainly deals with the indoor activities of the patients and helps to monitor the activities and complete details of treatment for the entire duration of the indoor patients, i.e. from admission to discharge. It has a facility to count the beds occupied, class-wise bed allocation and also allot the bed to the patient after searching for a vacant bed. The IPD staff can view patient occupancy status of rooms/wards, which in turn can help the staff to make quick decisions about cleaning the vacant rooms and also the patient placement—from admission, inter ward transfer and discharge.

It also sends requests for interdepartmental consultations and maintains the record of the same. It also provides the link between newborns' medical records with maternal data records. The role of this module begins as soon as the patient is registered at the registration counter and a bed is allotted in the ward.

1. Admission of the patient
2. Bed allotment
3. Inter-departmental consultation requests
4. Records of Interdepartmental consultations

5. Inter-ward or Intra-ward transfers
6. Raising and recording the requisition of medicines and consumables from the central pharmacy
7. Raising and recording investigations and viewing report
8. Maintain the patient's sheet of charges to be billed to patients
9. Preparing RFID wristband for patient tracking
10. Reports of the counts, revenue, discount etc.
11. Dashboard for patient access

41.2.5 Admission, Transfer, Discharge (ADT) Module

This module takes care of admission, interdepartmental or inter-ward transfers and discharge of patients. It helps in searching the availability of beds and manages the allotment of bed, ward, or room to the patient based on the availability or costing. It also takes care of the discharge processes and ensures that the discharge summary is generated at the time of discharge of the patient.

1. Collection of data of admitted patients and the beds occupied.
2. Recording the notes of doctors relating to further treatment.
3. Recording nursing notes for reference of the doctor.
4. Detailed evaluation of the patient's vitals and condition.
5. Recording the special incidents happening during treatment.
6. Management of billing process.
7. Management of payments to be received from the insurance companies or third parties.
8. Bed allotment, ward allocation and inter-ward or inter-departmental transfers.
9. E-prescription of the medications during treatment.
10. Final billing and settlements at the time of discharge.

41.2.6 Consulting Appointment Management Module

With this module, advance appointments for consultation can be booked for follow-up patients as well as new patients. It facilitates to reschedule or cancel any appointment if required. At times some of the patients may land in the hospital only for laboratory/radiological investigations, for them also an appointment can be booked with this module. Apart from this, the registrations for these patients can also be carried out along with the bills for the services that have to be generated.

41.2.7 Bed Management Module

This module is to maintain the records of bed occupancy status at any point of time. It also helps to estimate the approximate waiting time for patients, which in turn reduces the bed turnover time. By reducing the bed turnover ratio, optimization of revenues can be done effectively.

41.2.8 Ward Management Module

This module provides a solution to the nursing staff engaged in wards, ICU's and other patient care units of the hospital. The module helps in nursing and clinical procedures, in-patient service, laboratory and blood bank and pharmacy order.

1. Patient health status monitoring.
2. Status of the patients' vital parameters.
3. Material requisition such as medicines and consumable for patient.
4. Nurses and assistants Roster management.

41.2.9 Nursing Management Module

This module facilitates nursing or other ward staff to manage their ward. This is of great use particularly for the critical units like ICUs and

OT and helps in effectively managing the respective ward. The module can keep records and tracks for all the services rendered to the patient in ward.

1. Information about the upcoming patient's arrival, status of the present patients etc.
2. Recording the vitals charts for monitoring the patient's vitals.
3. Investigations, tests and procedure to be performed and generating the request to the concerned department.
4. Ordering, receiving and recording the medicines given to the patient.
5. Booking theatre for surgeries.
6. Recording and preparing patient for surgery.
7. Recording admissions, discharge and interdepartmental/inter-ward transfers to update the bed census.
8. Communicating with support departments like security, housekeeping, maintenance etc.
9. Recording notes of the procedure performed.
10. Maintain Medication chart.
11. Maintain IN-take and Out-put Chart.
12. Prepare Temperature Chart.
13. Recording other events happening with the patient during treatment.
14. Recording any adverse reaction or adverse incidence to the patient.

41.2.10 Operating Room Module

This module helps to keep track of the surgeries performed in the hospital in respect to recording of the pre-surgery and post-surgery details. The Operation Theatre Management module helps to manage and pre-book OR's for surgeries and to manage the surgery team. It allows the OR staff to prepare for a surgery well in advance by preparing the surgical equipment and instrument required and record the same in the module. It helps coordinate with the blood bank in case blood is required, coordinate with laundry and housekeeping staff for their services. It also maintains a record of the drugs, and consumables used in the OR during the surgery and generates bill post-surgery. The module also maintains the records of the pre-operative and post-operative conditions of the patient.

1. Scheduling the surgeries by managing OR bookings
2. Preparing Pre-operative checklists
3. Maintaining the Anaesthesia record
4. Maintaining the Surgery record like procedure/surgery performed, time taken for surgery, surgeons and assistants details, complication during surgery if any etc.
5. Taking electronic multilingual consent forms
6. Recording and management of inventory and stock OR
7. Sterilization schedules, checks and audits etc.

41.2.11 Laboratory Module

The Laboratory module manages record and maintains the details of various investigations conducted for both OPD and IPD patients. Facility to email the results of these investigations directly to the patients and also sharing with the treating physician/surgeon for quick reference. It also allows the laboratory staff to manage their workflows smoothly. This module can also receive online orders of investigations from treating doctors.

1. Raise requisition for the tests, based on sample type and test wise
2. Feeding the master data with normal values
3. Create a template of reports
4. Investigation packages using different investigations
5. Raising the bill for investigation and issuing receipt
6. Sample collection processing
7. Interfacing with laboratory equipment for online data capture
8. Fetching results directly from the analyzer
9. Verification and authorization of the report
10. Re-processing the sample if required
11. Printing of the Report
12. Inventory management of the Laboratory equipment, reagents and kits

41.2.12 Blood Bank Module

This module is related to activities of the blood bank and facilitates registration of the donor, physical examination of donor, blood grouping, bleeding, blood screening, component preparation, blood requisition and cross-matching. Also helps to maintain records as per the requirement of the statutory controlling authorities of the country.

1. Donor registration
2. Donor Health Check-up records
3. Donation cancellation
4. Bag Labels Printers
5. Generate Bag and donor number
6. Blood grouping and its validation
7. Serology test of donated blood, entry and validation
8. TT tests of the blood, entry and validation
9. Separation of the blood component and its record
10. Crossmatch with the patient blood
11. Discard blood and blood components and their records
12. Blood and blood component requisition and issue
13. Apheresis records
14. Blood Bank Inventory records

41.2.13 Radiology Module

This module facilitates the management of the operations of the radiology department. This module supports the requisition, reporting of the investigations along with the records of the same. The module is also linked to the PACS for storing the images of the scan and X-rays.

1. Billing for the ordered radiological investigations.
2. Receiving requisition raised from the department for investigations.
3. Create masters for reporting.
4. Reporting the results of investigation.
5. Results authorization.
6. Re-investigation if required.
7. Report Printing.
8. Access previous images based on tests and UHID number.
9. Speech-to-text typing for radiologist to prepare report.

41.2.14 Picture Archiving and Communication System (PACS) Module

PACS is an imaging software of medical images that provides the facility of storage of radiological images based on the DICOM format. PACS is capable of handling images generated from various imaging equipment like X-Rays, CT Scan, MRI, PET Scan, Cath Lab, DSA, Ultrasound etc.

Multi-Site Connectivity available

1. Multi-Modality Connectivity
2. Online delivery of the images to others systems connected to the PACS server
3. Image processing tools
4. Option of 3D imaging
5. Image printing on Film/Paper
6. Linking and labelling of the Image
7. Multi-monitor support for medical-grade displays
8. Option for writing the images on CD/DVD with Autorun DICOM Viewer
9. Comparison of different patient images in single window
10. Tele-radiology module
11. Customizable and Secure user access
12. Expandability to connect different kind of medical imaging equipment

41.2.15 Casualty and Emergency Management System

The module deals with the working of an emergency department. The role of this module begins as soon as the patient arrives in the emergency and till the patient is either discharged or transferred to other departments or indoor areas in the hospital for further treatment.

1. Capturing data on patient's condition on the arrival of the patient.
2. Sending alerts to the corresponding departments, with the data on patient condition for planning and management of the patient.
3. Recording and booking the Medico-Legal Cases, preparing Police Information, Injury Report etc.
4. Consulting details.
5. Clinical follow-up scheduling.
6. Raising bills for emergency services and the receipt of the same.

41.2.16 Pharmacy Information System

The Pharmacy module is designed to manage the inventory of medicines, injectables, drugs, other medical consumables and implants or devices used in the hospital.

1. Provides a comprehensive list of available drugs
2. Suggests alternatives for drugs that are not available
3. Interfacing with drug databases
4. Raise purchase orders to vendors for ordering supplies
5. Generates alerts when stocks reach below a pre-defined level
6. Inventory analysis as per ABC, VED classification
7. Auto-generated alerts of stock when reaches minimum stock level
8. Alerts of Expiry of near expiry medicines
9. Generating reports for opening and closing stock balance
10. Printing drug sale bills
11. Maintaining stock of the drugs
12. Barcode/RFID for the items

41.2.17 Order Management System Module

Deals with raising the requests and orders for other services and includes;

1. Medicines, Drugs and consumables order to pharmacy
2. Laboratory investigation order
3. Radiology investigation Order
4. Diet order
5. Blood order to Blood Bank
6. Invasive/non-invasive Procedure order
7. Order to nurse for ward services

41.2.18 The Birth/Death Registration Module

Module facilitates registration of births and deaths, issues birth and death memos, sending reports to the concerned Govt. department for registering births/deaths, printing the birth/death memos, management of birth and death registers and generating statistical reports of births and deaths.

1. Registering birth data of new-born
2. Recording the exact date and time of birth
3. Registration of Death
4. Recording the exact date and time of death
5. Generate ID number after registering birth
6. Printing of birth/death certificates/memos
7. Providing statistical information of births/deaths
8. Porting Information on Govt. Portals

41.2.19 Electronic Medical Records Module

This module is dedicated to manage and store patient records, treatment records, diagnosis reports, investigation inventory, reports and billing electronically for easy tracking and quick retrieval.

Complete information of the patient about their medical history can be retrieved, and contact with the patient can be maintained by sending them alerts or messages about their appointment schedules, follow-up visits, self-care instructions and so on.

This module helps a lot in improving patient care since it is the main source of information about patient in terms of patient's history, demographic details, observation, complaint history, diagnosis, treatment provided, surgery/procedure observation, diagnosis, investigations done with reports, treatment provided, surgery/procedure performed and other therapeutic conclusions, it becomes easy for communication between hospital and patient and follow-up.

1. Medical record structure based on UHID
2. Scan hard copies of the reports and save in patient record
3. Checking and completing the patient record based on the checklist provided by the module
4. ICD codification based on diagnosis
5. Access controlled workflow
6. Indexing the record/data parameters like area, sex, problem, doctor, clinical department, diagnosis, lab parameter value, surgery/procedure, MLC, allergies, discharge type, summary etc.

41.2.20 Billing and Finance Module

The Billing module is for managing the billing of the patient towards the services provided in the hospital during the course of treatment.

1. Generate and issue bills for services availed by the patient in OPD and IPD.
2. Collect advance payments from the patient.
3. Collect payments at the time of final settlement of the bills and issue receipts of the same.
4. Issue refunds if any against the advance payments.
5. Creating daily estimated billing till date for collecting further advances from the patient.
6. Generate MIS reports of collection from OPD and IPD billing, cash flow analysis, calculation of the doctors share, summary of discounts offered, department-wise or service-wise billing done, and also aging reports that give useful insights into the hospital's financials.
7. Helps the staff to manage cash inflow and outflow, accounts receivables and payable, issue and process purchase orders, Bank reconciliation, daily cash day book, preparing hospital budgets and comparing the actuals with the budgets etc.

41.2.21 Insurance and Medi-Claim Module

This module deals with cashless patients and also the patients of empaneled organizations. The module helps for evaluation of the eligibility of a patient to get admissions for cashless treatment, for reimbursement in case of TPA or empanelled institutions, and process the settlement of bills online with the payee.

41.2.22 Human Resources Module

The Human Resources (HR) module manages all the issues related to hospital manpower like doctors, nurses, consultants, house-keeping staff, technicians and non-medical staff. It facilitates services like daily attendance, salary and incentives, leave records, resource engagement and scheduling. It also generates payslips for employee and payroll reports. It also includes preparing duty rosters and assessing staffing needs, recruiting, training and awareness towards various regulations and policies of the hospital and defining shift rotation.

1. Interfacing with the biometrics machine for daily attendance
2. Leave entitlements, records of the leave availed and leave sanctioned
3. Salary calculation taking into effect the provisions of PF, TDS, staff advances and loans etc.
4. Pre-defined Duty roster and comparison of actual duties with the roster
5. Bonus and incentive calculation
6. Overtime records and management
7. Outsource employee details, records and management

41.2.23 Materials Management System (Stock, Purchasing and Fixed Asset Module)

The module deals with the purchasing, stocking and issue of assets, medical equipment and consumables used in the hospital.

1. Raising indent for purchase
2. Inviting quotations from vendors
3. Preparing Comparative statements
4. Preparing Purchase Orders
5. Receiving material and gate entry
6. Store entry and preparing GRN
7. Quality and quantity verification
8. ABC analysis of material stored
9. Dead Inventory checking
10. Issue of material
11. Bill passing
12. Department-wise stock of equipment, material and consumables
13. MIS of purchases, stock and issued material

41.2.24 Dietary Module/Catering Module

This module is for a dietician to prescribe the suitable diet for the patient, based on the medical conditions of the patient or as instructed by the treating physician.

1. Create the list of food items to be supplied from the hospital kitchen
2. Calculate the calorie count and nutritional information of the food items
3. Sending information to the kitchen about various types of diets to be prepared and the number of such diets, like normal diet, diabetic diet, semi-solid diet and liquid diet etc.
4. Creation of daily menu of meals that has to be served in breakfast, lunch and dinner
5. Prescribing the recipes of food items along with the steps for preparation of recipes

41.2.25 Statistics and Reporting Module (MIS)

This is the most important module and tool for the management of the hospital to retrieve information about the hospital through various reports generated from HMS. These reports and analysis help the management to frame policies, revise policies and take the decisions at the right times. It also helps in measuring and monitoring the performance of different departments of the hospital. Various types of data can be retrieved as per the requirement and as per the analysis required.

1. Various types of dashboards used by the management.
2. Clinical dashboards.
3. Dash Boards for Top management.
4. Collection of department-wise patients served, services provided, total revenue collected, individual service-wise revenue received etc.
5. Customization of various reports as per the need of the management.
6. Ability to export the data and reports in other formats like Excel, Word and PDF.
7. Comparison of actual working with the Quality indicators as described by the accreditation institutes.

41.2.26 Hospital Analytics

The Hospital Analytics module helps to provide useful information and analysis of the data collected in the hospital. From the medical investigations, diagnosis, diseases and prescribed medications, clinicians can make informed decisions about patient care. These analyses also help doctors to make changes for improving the quality of health care services being provided in the hospital.

41.2.27 Interface Module

This module is to interface various electronic digitalized equipment and external software which are generally used in the hospital. These may include laboratory equipment such as biochemistry analyzers, monitoring equipment, digital camera, digital X-Ray Machines, Ultrasound Machines, CT Scanners, MRI, PET scan machines, LINAC, other radiology equipment using PACS technology and other such medical equipment and interfacing these with accounts module for Accounts and Finance management.

Further Reading

What is Hospital Management System | About Hospital Management Info [Internet]. Avanttec. 2019 [cited 2021 Jul 14]. Available from: http://www.avanttec.net/hospital-management-system/

Alotaibi YK, Federico F. The impact of health information technology on patient safety. Saudi Med J. 2017 Dec;38(12):1173–80.

The 'Must-Have' Modules of A Hospital Management System [Internet]. SD Global. 2017 [cited 2021 Jul 14]. Available from: https://www.sdglobaltech.com/blog/the-must-have-modules-of-a-hospital-management-system

Farzandipour M, Meidani Z, Nabovati E, Sadeqi Jabali M, Dehghan Banadaki R. Technical requirements framework of hospital information systems: design and evaluation. BMC Med Inform Decis Mak. 2020 Apr 3;20(1):61.

Thakare V, Khire G. Role of Emerging Technology for Building Smart Hospital Information System. Procedia Econ Finance. 2014 Jan 1;11:583–8.

System NA of E (US) and I of M (US) C on E and the HC, Reid PP, Compton WD, Grossman JH, Fanjiang G. Information and Communications Systems: The Backbone of the Health Care Delivery System [Internet]. Building a Better Delivery System: A New Engineering/Health Care Partnership. National Academies Press (US); 2005 [cited 2021 Jul 14]. Available from: https://www.ncbi.nlm.nih.gov/books/NBK22862/

Mehdipour Y, Zerehkafi H. Hospital Information System (HIS):At a Glance. Asian J Comput Sci Inf Technol. 2013 Aug 1;01:2321–5658.

Information Systems in Health Care [Internet]. Health Care Service Delivery. 2014 [cited 2021 Jul 14]. Available from: https://drdollah.com/hospital-information-system-his/

Hospital management system, HMS Software Development | KnowIT HMS [Internet]. [cited 2021 Jul 14]. Available from: https://www.rechnerinfo.com/knowit-hms.html

Hospital Management Software Development: Modules, Features, and Main Benefits [Internet]. [cited 2021 Jul 14]. Available from: https://steelkiwi.com/blog/hospital-management-software-development/

Aijing L, Jin Y. Design of the Hospital Integrated Information Management System Based on Cloud Platform. West Indian Med J. 2015 Dec;64(5):521–6.

Jay S, Anderson J. Computerized hospital information systems: their future role in medicine. J R Soc Med. 1982 Jun 1;75:303–5.

A detailed view of Hospital Management System (HMS) [Internet]. [cited 2021 Jul 14]. Available from: https://mocdoc.in/blog/a-detailed-view-of-hospital-management-system-hms

42 Water Supply and Drainage System

Water is life. The supply of water and a proper drainage system is necessary for the survival of the human beings. Particularly in case of hospitals, where it is the question of treating the ill and critical patients, the water supply and drainage system has to be excellent, and the importance of clean hygienic, good quality of water and drainage is critical. The quality of water supplied and the drainage system leaves a great impact on the issues like infection control, life of the medical equipment, staff, patients hygiene etc.

In the hospitals, many systems and operations are fully or partially dependent upon clean and treated water supplied for patients and staff. Also, the performance of some of the medical equipment depends on the quality of water being supplied to the said medical equipment. Similarly, the drainage and treatment of the wastewater are equally important.

The reliability of the water supply system is also important. Thus, it has to be ensured that uninterrupted water supply is available at all times in the building. On the other side, it has to be ensured that the volume of the water shall not be more than required and water stagnation in the tanks shall be avoided.

42.1 Water Supply System

42.1.1 Source of Water Supply

The following can be sources of water for hospitals:

1. Supply from the Water Network Supplier by connecting to their distribution network (may be Govt. Supply or others)
2. Bore Hole
3. Underground Water Wells
4. Connection for Portable Water Trucks

The following issues shall be considered related to the water source;

1. Generally, the TDS/PPM of the raw water varies from 80 PPM to 2000 PPM. However, it may vary depending on the water source. Hence the water needs to be treated so that the TDS/PPM reaches the level of 0–150 PPM.
2. Hospitals shall arrange for at least two sources of water so that a backup is available in case one source of water fails to supply water. Apart from this, one more source of water supply shall be arranged as an Emergency backup for water supply.

A. Garg, A. Dewan, *Manual of Hospital Planning and Designing*,
https://doi.org/10.1007/978-981-16-8456-2_42

3. The water supplied to the hospital shall be protected, so that the hospital is free from water-induced infections.
4. Before designing, the designer must calculate the maximum foreseeable water consumption daily along with the average as well as peak flow requirement of water and pressure required from the source of water.
5. While designing the water supply system, the designer shall take into consideration the expansion of the hospital that may occur in the future. On an average at least 25% spare water capacity to the system shall be considered as a buffer for future expansion.
6. For the water to be supplied, the temperature shall not be more than 40 °C. If so, the bacterial growth such as pseudonymous legionella shall grow in the water and it becomes risky. Many of the dangerous bacterias thrive in such an environment. The designer shall ensure that the water temperature shall be between 15 and 20 °C.

42.2 Water Storage

Hospital shall have storage of water equivalent to 3 days consumption. The main storage tank shall be made of concrete or Glass-reinforced plastic (GRP) tanks. Water storage calculation shall be based on the peak demand vis-à-vis the quantity of water available from the main external water source.

42.3 Water Storage Tank Locations

1. The location of the tanks shall be at Roof level and at floor level also. The main storage of the water can be done in the underground tanks. From there the water shall be pumped to the roof tanks for further supply. The rooftop tanks shall have a capacity to store water equal to 6 h consumption. But the system shall be provided to continuously fill up the tanks on a real-time basis.
2. To ensure the proper pressure of water supply on all the floors, one shall not fully depend on the approach of a gravity-driven roof water tank, but booster pumps shall be connected to emergency power.
3. The tanks shall be watertight so that the water inside the tank is not contaminated. Also, all around and beneath the tank sufficient space shall be provided for inspection and maintenance of the tank.
4. Each tank shall have
   (a) A drain valve just at the bottom of the tank. The drain pipe invert shall be located at the extreme bottom of the tank to fully drain the tank.
   (b) An overflow pipe connected to the tank. Overflow pipe shall be directly connected to the drainage.
   (c) Internal and External access ladders.
   (d) An air vent pipe along with an air inlet properly covered with corrosion resistant mesh.

42.4 Systems of Water Treatment

In hospitals, the treatment of water is essential for controlling the microbiological growth in water. Hence the arrangement shall be provided for treatment of the water depending on the purpose for which it has to be used.

For controlling the microbiological growth in the water, methods shall be provided to control the temperature, chemical components of the water. The methods that can be used are the following:

42.4.1 Pasteurization

Pasteurization or hot water flushing of the system is a method that is used in some of the hospitals. In this method, the water is heated by raising the temperature water to 70–75 °C. Then this water is used for flushing the entire supply system for at least 5 min, including the pipelines and the sanitary fittings. Of course, this method is a bit costly as a lot of energy will be required to heat the water. Also, if this method is adopted, the entire water supply system, including sanitary fitting, shall have to be shut down for those 5 min, which can be difficult for medium to large hospitals, but smaller hospitals can use this technique.

42.4.2 Chemical Treatment

For chemical treatment, Chlorine Dioxide is used. As Chlorine dioxide is an oxidizing biocide that reacts with the organic substances in the water, it oxidizes the entire growth in the pipelines and the sanitary fittings of the system.

42.4.3 Chlorine Water Treatment

Under this method, Chloramine is used for water treatment, as chloramine provides antibacterial activity with low levels of chlorine. As compared to free chlorine, which is rapidly lost, chloramines remain for much longer time hence more effective. But care has to be taken not to use this water for some of the procedures like dialysis unit, as it can cause haemolysis to the patient.

42.4.4 Water Softener Plants

This method is used where the contents of Magnesium and Calcium are higher in the water, as it can lead to deposition of scales in the pipelines and the sanitary fittings. This method is used for water being supplied to Steam Boilers, Laundry, Hot Water Systems, Cooling Towers and toilets of the hospital.

42.4.5 Silver–Copper Ionization

Copper–Silver Ionization is used for organisms that exist in contaminated water. In this method, the Copper–Silver ions are released into the water by passing electric current in water through the copper–silver plate.

42.4.6 Reverse Osmosis Treatment

This is the most commonly used treatment process in hospitals. This is a technology that removes maximum contaminants in the water by passing it through a semipermeable membrane under pressure. This water can be used in critical units like ICU's, Dialysis NICU etc. and can also be used for drinking. RO filtration has various methods of filtration like pre-filter, sand filters, charcoal filters, reverse osmosis and Ultraviolet filtration.

42.4.7 Ultraviolet Treatment

Ultraviolet (UV) is used to deactivate or kill the bacteria in water. This is achieved with the help of UV light, which disrupts the natural makeup of bacteria. For proper treatment, Ultraviolet light with optimum wavelength close to 254 nm shall be used for the destruction of biological matters.

42.4.8 Ozone Water Treatment

For Ozone treatment, an unstable gas made up of 3 oxygen atoms is used, which lasts for a few milliseconds. Ozone Water Treatment has proved to be a good disinfection method as it reduces the concentration of iron and manganese elements in the water. Under this technique, an ozone concentration is created by passing dry and clean water through a high voltage electric discharge. When the raw water is passed through the venturi throat, it creates a vacuum and pulls the ozone gas into the water for treatment of water.

42.4.9 Distilled Water

It is made from condensed steam after it is cooled and liquefied.

42.5 Drinking Water

For drinking water taps and fountains, some hospitals provide a separate water supply line. The following issues shall be addressed for drinking water;

1. The quality of drinking water, even after Chemical treatment, shall be safe for human consumption.
2. To prevent the temperatures of drinking water from exceeding 20 °C and stagnation of the water, the water shall be supplied from a central water storage tank that is made for drinking water only.
3. If a central drinking water system is not available, then the provision shall be made for bottled drinking water through water coolers.

42.6 Water Booster Pumps

In hospitals, high flow of water is essential for hygienic hand wash and cleaning. Therefore, the hospital shall have a system for constant and high flow water pressure to ensure hygienic and clean infection-free environment. Hence the following shall be provided;

1. The pressure at fixtures of cold water supply shall be appropriate.
2. The flow velocity of the cold water piping shall be appropriate.
3. A booster pump shall be provided to ensure that an adequate pressure of water is available throughout the hospital.
4. Multi-stage booster pumps shall be used instead of single-stage pumps.
5. An emergency power supply shall be provided to the booster pumps.

42.7 Hot Water System

In hospital, hot water is needed at a number of places like Hand Wash Basins, Scrub Sinks, CSSD, Kitchen, Patient's bathrooms, Maintenance Areas and Instrument washing area. The following issues shall be kept in mind while designing the hot water facility;

There are different types of hot water systems that are generally provided in the hospitals as follows:

42.7.1 Electrical Hot Water Generation

Under this system, a hot water generator is provided to heat the water. This is a cylindrical tank made out of stainless steel and is insulated to avoid any thermal losses. At the bottom of the tank, high-rated heating elements are provided, which heat up the water in the tank. These elements are controlled by the thermostat, which monitors the temperature of the water. Once the water temperature falls below the set temperature, the elements are switched on and switched off when the water reaches the preset temperature.

42.7.2 Hot Water Generation from Boiler/Steam by Burning Fuel

In this technique, a steamer or a boiler is provided for heating up the water. Below the water tank, fire place is provided for burning the fuel. As the fuel burns, water gets heated. The fuel that can be used is Gas, Wood, Coal or waste oil etc.

42.7.3 Solar Hot Water Generation

In this system, solar cells having conductive copper pipe capillary lines are installed on the rooftop where solar cells are exposed to sun rays. The water flows in these copper tubes within the solar cells and gets heated. This water is then stored in an insulated water tank, from where it is supplied to desired places. The biggest disadvantage of this system is that when the sun rays are poor or on any rainy day when sun rays are not available, water cannot be heated. Hence solar water systems shall be backed up by providing a standby system for heating water.

42.7.4 Stand-Alone Hot Water Geysers

In small hospitals, where it is not feasible to install a central hot water system, individual stand-alone geysers are used to supply hot water. These geysers are installed at different locations and the inlet pipeline and outlet pipeline have to be laid down. At the location of the geysers, the required power switch/socket shall be provided.

1. In hospitals, the design shall be such that it provides a backup plan of heating the water by adopting any of the techniques mentioned above. Generally, the technique of electrical heating element is considered to be the best backup as compared to any other techniques.
2. The temperature of the hot water must be kept at between 60 and 65 °C to prevent any growth of microorganism in the water.
3. The water serving supplied to the hot water plant shall be properly treated with Ultraviolet rays before connecting to the hot water system.
4. The pipeline to supply hot water shall be insulated with a moulded insulation and shall be flame-proof with a jacket suitable for temperature control.

42.8 Sanitary Fittings

As compared to any other commercial building, the sanitary fittings of the hospitals are different. The goal is to have an environment that is free from any infection and shall be safe and hygienic. The following issues shall be considered while designing the sanitary fittings;

1. In hospitals, the design shall provide leverage for future maintenance of the sanitary system and shall be durable.
2. Isolation valves shall be provided at the main entrance of sanitary fixtures in toilets.
3. In hospitals sensor taps should be preferred for hand wash basins.
4. Spray-type mixer taps shall not be provided in the hospitals.
5. As some of the mixing taps are provided with the flow restrictors at the point of discharge. As these restrictors can be a source of bacterial growth, and also hampers the free flow of water, the flow restrictors or aerators shall not be used in the taps and the mixers.
6. Adjustable spray options shall not be provided in the shower heads as this can lead to water stagnation issues.

42.9 Irrigation Water Supply

Dedicated irrigation water tanks shall be used to supply water for irrigation and shall not be mixed up with any other water supply line. The irrigation can be either for internal landscape areas or the external landscape areas.

42.10 WC Flushing Systems

The treated water can be used in some areas of hospital like Non-Loitering Irrigation Areas and WC Flushing Systems etc. The water discharged from Showers, Wash Basins, Floor drains and RO rejection water can be used for flushing systems.

42.11 Steam System

There are various locations in the hospital where the steam is required like laundry, food and beverages, laboratories, sterile store, CSSD etc. As the usage of different units is different, the quality of steam to be supplied to a unit will depend on the application for which it will be used, e.g. the areas like laundry or food and beverages may have ordinary plant steam, the CSSD and critical areas shall be provided with clean steam and the sensitive areas like laboratories or pharmaceutical preparation may require pure and filtered steam. The following are the important points that shall be considered while designing the steam system;

1. *Source of Steam System*

   Generally, in hospitals, there are two sources from where the steam can be generated. These are Central Steam Boiler System or Local or Central Electrical Steam Generator

2. *Plant Steam*
   Plant steam is normal steam prepared with the normal water, but some chemical may be added for controlling pH level of the steam.
3. *Clean Steam*
   Clean steam is generated by the RO or DM water supplied to the steam generator.
4. *Steam System Pipeline*
   Piping must be made out of stainless steel as it is hard and non-reactive metal and can resist corrosion as well. The pipeline shall be insulated properly to maintain the temperature in the pipeline. If the temperature of the steam falls down, it may be converted back to liquid.
5. *Central Steam Generation Vs. Local Steam Generation*
   There is an option to the hospital whether to have a Central plant for steam generation or the localized plants at different locations. While setting up a central plant is more economical, it is not that efficient. Secondly, if the stem consumption is too low, the operational cost of the central plant will be high. The next factor is the distance between the generation site and the user site. If the distance is more, more shall be the cost of laying the pipeline and maintaining the pipeline. Another advantage with localized plants is that in case any one of the plants fails, the other systems are working and providing backup. However, some hospitals prefer to operate using a combination of both the systems.

42.12 Water Drainage System

Hospitals shall have an effective drainage system. This is still more important, because the quality of effluent generated in the hospital is generally ineffective as compared to the effluent generated in any other building. Also the quantity of the effluent generated shall be considered while designing the system.

The following issues shall be addressed while designing the drainage system of the hospital;

1. Considering the location of the hospital, the nearby network of drainage, main holes and connection points shall be assessed.
2. The level differences between hospital drain and the drainage network shall be assessed.
3. Assess the type of effluent that may be discharged from the hospital like chemical, radiation and grease etc.
4. For the external drainage network, the connection points shall be as per municipality requirements.

42.13 Drainage Strategy

1. The drainage system shall be gravity driven for general effluent. Whereas Pressure drainage system is for draining effluent from the areas like basement via sump and pump connection.
2. Odours coming out from the drainage system due to broken or dried floor traps shall be prevented.
3. The drainage gradient shall be sufficient to discharge waste into main sewer lines.
4. As far as possible, the drainage discharge from the sanitary fixtures shall be direct to the drain line instead of the floor trap or any other fixture.

42.14 Types of Drainage Systems

Various types of drainage systems of hospital shall be kept separate from each other. This is necessary to control the infection and also for optimizing the drainage system.

The following are the drainage systems:

42.14.1 Wastewater Drainage

This is the general drainage from sources like Wash Basins, Sinks, Showers, Scrub Sinks, Bathrooms and Floor Drains. This type of drainage normally does not contain any human waste or discharge of contaminated water.

42.14.2 Soil Water Drainage

This type of drainage contains human waste and is created from WC's, Urinals and Dirty Linen washrooms etc.

42.14.3 Storm Water Drainage

This is a drainage from water collected due to rain, or sprinkler water etc.

42.14.4 Chemical Drainage

This is a drainage from the laboratories where the effluent needs to be neutralized before discharging it to the main system.

42.14.5 Radiation Drainage

Is drainage generated from the areas like hot labs, settlement toilets etc.

42.15 Methods of Drainage

42.15.1 Vent Pipes

To avoid the foul smell of the effluent coming out of the drainage, all the drainage systems shall be provided with the vent pipes in the drainage system to vent out the odour in the atmosphere.

42.15.2 Floor Drains

Floor drain and clean out drains shall be through the trap to prevent odours. As the floor drains usually dries out due to evaporation, there is a need to make arrangements that the trap is refilled with water if it dries. It can be done by providing the primer valve connected to the water supply to timely refill the trap.

42.15.3 Soil Water Drainage

Soil drainage is usually the discharge from Toilets (WC's), urinals and dirty utilities. This can be drained using the S-Trap or P-Trap discharge systems. However, the use of a P-trap system is recommended as it is easier to maintain.

The WC drainage connection must be at least 150 mm in diameter, if the numbers are more the size of the drainage shall be increased.

Bends of 90° shall be avoided as these can be the points of blockage.

42.15.4 Rainwater Drainage System

For Rainwater, the roof of the hospital shall be designed in such a fashion that the rainwater is collected through horizontal pipes from the roof and transferred to the vertical pipes provided for this purpose. These vertical pipes shall in turn be connected to either the holding tanks or to the soak pits used to increase the underground water level.

42.15.5 Infectious Contaminated Drainage

In hospitals, usually there are drainages that may consist of bio hazardous material with suspended living organisms which may create a risk of infection. These types of drainage can be from the areas like isolation rooms etc. For these types of effluents, the holding tank, called 'Kill Tank', shall be connected to all the concerned areas from where the bio hazardous material is discharged. This kill tank is injected with a chemical to attack the hazardous organisms before finally draining the effluent.

42.15.6 Radiation Drainage

Radiation tank shall be provided at a location where it is harmless for radiation exposure. If the Local municipality does not allow for radiation drainage in the external drainage network before being diluted, a holding tank shall be provided.

42.15.7 Kitchen Grease Drainage

The drainage system of the kitchen shall be provided with the grease interceptor before discharging the effluent to the external drainage network.

Once the drainage system is complete and is connected to the main holes of the buildings, the drain water has to be treated before it is finally drained in the main sewerage network provided by the municipality or to be discharged in the soak pits.

For water treatment, please refer to the chapter of '*BIO-MEDICAL WASTE MANAGEMENT*' (Chap. 46) in this book.

Further Reading

Galowin LS. Water supply and drainage in buildings.:252.

Balwani KS, Nagarnaik DPB. Water and Waste Water Management of a Hospital- A Review. 2015;6(4):4.

Altin A, Altin S. Sustainable Water and Wastewater Management in Hospitals. Turk J Occup Environ Med Saf. 2017 Jul 14;2:1–7.

Paleologos EK, O'Kelly BC, Tang C-S, Cornell K, Rodríguez-Chueca J, Abuel-Naga H, et al. Post Covid-19 water and waste water management to protect public health and geoenvironment. Environ Geotech. 2021 May 1;8(3):193–207.

Hospital plumbing systems [Internet]. [cited 2021 Jul 14]. Available from: https://www.hfmmagazine.com/articles/2260-hospital-plumbing-systems

Emergency Water Supply Planning Guide for Hospitals and Healthcare Facilities | Water, Sanitation, & Hygiene-related Emergencies & and Outbreaks | Healthy Water | CDC [Internet]. 2020 [cited 2021 Jul 14]. Available from: https://www.cdc.gov/healthywater/emergency/ewsp.html

Council NR. Drinking Water Distribution Systems: Assessing and Reducing Risks [Internet]. 2006 [cited 2021 Jul 14]. Available from: https://www.nap.edu/catalog/11728/drinking-water-distribution-systems-assessing-and-reducing-risks

Vertical Transportation System 43

In any multi-storey hospital, everyone is greatly dependent on the vertical lifts for providing an efficient vertical transport system amongst different floors and it is essential for movement of patients, medical equipment, support services, staff and visitors.

Lifts are essential to provide firefighting and evacuation facilities in case of fire or accident. In most of the countries, lifts are subjected to prescribed statutory regulations of the country. Hence the lifts shall meet the statutory regulations as prescribed by the concerned municipality.

43.1 Lift Categories

Usually the lifts are a box type square or rectangular structure called car. This car moves inside the lift shaft and the doors are provided at each floor. Another option can be the slope elevators or the stair elevators. Both these elevators takes lot of space, hence generally not provided in the hospitals. However, if ramp has to be provided in the hospital, the designer can think of providing slope elevator. The lifts in hospital buildings can be categorized and provided based on the function as below:

43.1.1 General Passenger Lifts

These lifts are used for the general passengers like staff, doctors and visitors, including the patients on wheelchairs. Main issues relating to passenger lifts are:

1. The clear internal minimum dimension of the lift car shall
   a. Width—2000 mm
   b. Depth—1700 mm
   c. Loading Capacity—1250 kg
   d. Door Opening—1100 mm
   e. Internal Height—2100 mm
2. It is advisable to provide a separate lift intended for housekeeping services.
3. As far as practically possible, the passenger lifts shall be separate from the Bed, Service and Goods lifts and shall have separate lifts lobbies.

43.1.2 Bed Lifts

1. These lifts are used to carry patients on patient beds or stretchers along with the necessary support equipment and staff.
2. The clear internal minimum dimension of the lift car shall
   a. Car Width—1800 mm
   b. Depth—2700 mm
   c. Loading Capacity—2500 kg
   d. Door Opening—1400 mm
   e. Internal Height—2500 mm

A. Garg, A. Dewan, *Manual of Hospital Planning and Designing*,
https://doi.org/10.1007/978-981-16-8456-2_43

43.1.3 Service/Goods Lift

1. These lifts are to be used for movement of the items such as furniture, equipment, equipment maintenance supplies, building materials and hospital waste etc. This lift shall also be used to carry the food trolley and the linen trolley.
2. The clear internal minimum dimension of the lift car shall
   a. Car Width—1600 mm
   b. Depth—2200 mm
   c. Loading Capacity—2500 kg.
   d. Door Opening—1200 mm
   e. Internal Height—2500 mm
3. For smaller hospitals, say up to 50 beds, smaller sized goods lift can be provided.
4. However, in hospitals where heavier equipment is anticipated to be transported, larger service/goods lift with wider door openings shall be provided.

43.2 Design Considerations

Some of the issues that shall be kept in mind while designing the lifts are as below:

1. The operational speed of the lift shall be designed in such a fashion so as to optimize the operation, efficiency and comfort.
2. Due to vibration, lifts shall be located away from sensitive areas, particularly away from MRI due to magnetic distortion.
3. As far as possible, the design and size of the Bed Lifts and Service Lifts shall be identical, so that the flexibility is available, and when the need arises, both can be interchanged with each other. Hence, with this arrangement, the backup shall also be available.
4. The Service Lifts shall be categorized for different types of use, e.g Dirty Lifts and Clean Lift, and these shall not be exchanged with each other.
5. Dirty Lifts shall be used for transporting Dirty Linen, Dirty ICU goods, Waste bins/bags, diseased patients, Infected Patients, empty food trolleys and other similar goods.
6. Clean Lifts shall be used for transporting items from the central stores, medication, clean food trolley, clean ICU goods, and staff and may be patient beds when required.

43.3 Engineering Guidelines

In hospital building the size, capacity, operational speed and drive system shall be chosen effectively. Some of the main criteria that shall be considered are as follows:

(a) Expected number of patients to use lifts
(b) Expected number of staff members to use lifts
(c) Operation and visiting hours of the hospital
(d) Zoning of the hospital building
(e) Number of lift wells provided in the building
(f) Floor location of the critical units in the hospital
(g) Location of the service departments
(h) Location of the support departments like kitchen and laundry
(i) Evacuation system in Emergency
(j) Location of the Emergency department
(k) Daily visitors in the hospital
(l) Number of attendants allowed with each patient

1. The selection of an appropriate speed depends on the height of the building. In earlier days the fast speed lifts were not preferred in hospitals. But due to change in technologies, nowadays jerk less lifts are available, hence the speed of the lift shall be immaterial while choosing the lift. However, as per standards, the height of the building shall also be considered while deciding the speed. More the height of the building faster shall be the speed of the lift.
2. The average interval time of 30 s to 50 s from door opening to door closing shall be generally acceptable for hospitals.
3. Door openings of the lifts can either be Centre opening doors or the Side opening doors. Centre opening doors are better as

compared to side opening doors. Hence the lifts being used by patients and clinical staff shall have centre opening doors. Side opening lifts shall be used for goods lifts or service lifts. For general passengers and visitors, either of the two lifts can be chosen.

4. The Machine Room Less (MRL) lifts shall be preferred as in these lifts, the machine room on the top floor is not required.
5. Emergency lighting shall be provided in lifts with at least 1hr battery backup.
6. The hall buttons shall be provided on each floor to call the lifts. Similarly, all the floors shall have the lift indicator to know the position of the lift car.
7. Lift shafts, including walls and ceiling, shall be properly sealed and painted to reduce the risk for the transmission of infection across the floors as the lift well penetrates all floors of a hospital.
8. Lift car doors shall have Infrared Curtain Door Sensor protection device for contact-free detection of the obstruction to avoid the risk of accident due to door collisions.
9. The lifts shall be provided with an intercom line so that in case of emergency, the passengers may contact the emergency service department.
10. The lift shall also be provided with a hooter, so that the passenger can press the hooter button in case of emergency.
11. There shall be provision of CCTV cameras in the lifts to record live images inside the lift car.
12. The ARD (Automatic Rescue Device) shall be provided in the lifts so that in case the lift stops due to power failure, the ARD device shall bring the lift to the nearest lower floor, and the doors open automatically to rescue the passengers.
13. Bed lifts shall be provided with a feature of priority lift car call option for patients in critical care.
14. As far as possible the lifts shall be provided with the power backup either by UPS or other alternate power source.
15. Power supply to lifts shall be directly from the MDB provided near the machine room of the lifts.
16. Handrails shall be provided in the cars on at least two long sides of the car for patient safety.
17. The flooring of the car shall not be slippery and shall be easily cleanable.
18. Fire-rated doors shall be preferred in for the lifts.
19. The lift shall have a provision of Overload device to warn when the lift is overloaded.
20. The lift shall have provision of Emergency Firemen's service.
21. The lift shall also have a provision of automatic Belt Inspection device.

Further Reading

Vertical Transportation - Lift System Design I WSP [Internet]. [cited 2021 Jul 14]. Available from: https://www.wsp.com/en-GB/services/vertical-transportation

Al-Sharif L. The Design of Elevator Systems in High Rise Buildings, Part 1. Lift Rep. 2017 Oct 1;43:46–62.

Shrestha A. Safety Considerations for the Design of Modern Elevator Systems. Honors Theses [Internet]. 2019 Jan 1; Available from: https://egrove.olemiss.edu/hon_thesis/1195

Health C for D and R. Patient Lifts. FDA [Internet]. 2019 Apr 26 [cited 2021 Jul 14]; Available from: https://www.fda.gov/medical-devices/general-hospital-devices-and-supplies/patient-lifts

Going up: Hospital lift technologies [Internet]. [cited 2021 Jul 14]. Available from: https://buildingbetterhealthcare.com/news/article_page/Going_up_Hospital_lift_technologies/102242

Elevator I vertical transport [Internet]. Encyclopedia Britannica. [cited 2021 Jul 14]. Available from: https://www.britannica.com/technology/elevator-vertical-transport

Shirley E. Circulation analysis and lift placing in hospitals. Comput-Aided Des. 1974 Oct 1;6(4):206–10.

An Architect's Guide To: Elevators and Escalators - Architizer Journal [Internet]. Journal. 2018 [cited 2021 Jul 14]. Available from: https://architizer.com/blog/product-guides/product-guide/elevators-escalators/

44 Pneumatic Tube Systems (PTS)

Pneumatic Tube Systems (PTS) is basically an internal logistics and transport system and is used for transporting small articles or documents within the hospital building. In this system, the item and documents are placed in a container or carrier (a capsule-like structure) and transported from one point to another through a tube network that is air pressurized.

The PTS is an air pressurized operated system having the air pressure pump attached to the control station. This system is used as a transport system of documents, material and medicines. This is the best, accurate and quickest mode of transport for documents, specimens, material and medicines.

In a hospital setup, at all the important receiving and sending locations, the terminals of PTS are provided. These are also called stations. The station has an outlet and a control unit. Some of these locations can be ICUs, Emergency, Operating Room, Indoor wards, Pharmacy, Laboratory, Blood Bank, Billing Counter etc.

It is very simple and easy to operate. The user has to just put the item or document in the carrier, close it and put it in the PTS station. Press the predefined station number, and the capsule starts moving to that station, and the item shall be delivered to that place in seconds (Fig. 44.1).

The PTS can either be a single-zone-system to be used only in one zone of the hospital. Otherwise, for multiple zones, the multi-zone-system can be used.

44.1 Pneumatic Tube System Components

The PTS system comprises components that, when combined, make a complete system. The following are the system components:

44.1.1 Blower and Air Reverse Valve

The role of the blower is to generate pressurized air that moves the PTS carriers in the piped network provided throughout the hospital under pressure or vacuum suction. The blower shall be installed in the plant room of PTS system. Along with the blowers, the system control unit and inter-zone/linear coupler are also installed in the plant room.

44.1.2 Carrier

Carrier is a reusable plastic container that holds and carries the contents through a pneumatic tube system to the desired places. The contents can be such as medicines/drugs, consumables, laboratory specimens, blood or blood products, documents etc. The carriers are available in different sizes to serve the requirements of the hospital. The type of carriers can be:

1. Standard carriers: Used for transportation of items like medicines, small instruments and solid particles.

A. Garg, A. Dewan, *Manual of Hospital Planning and Designing*,
https://doi.org/10.1007/978-981-16-8456-2_44

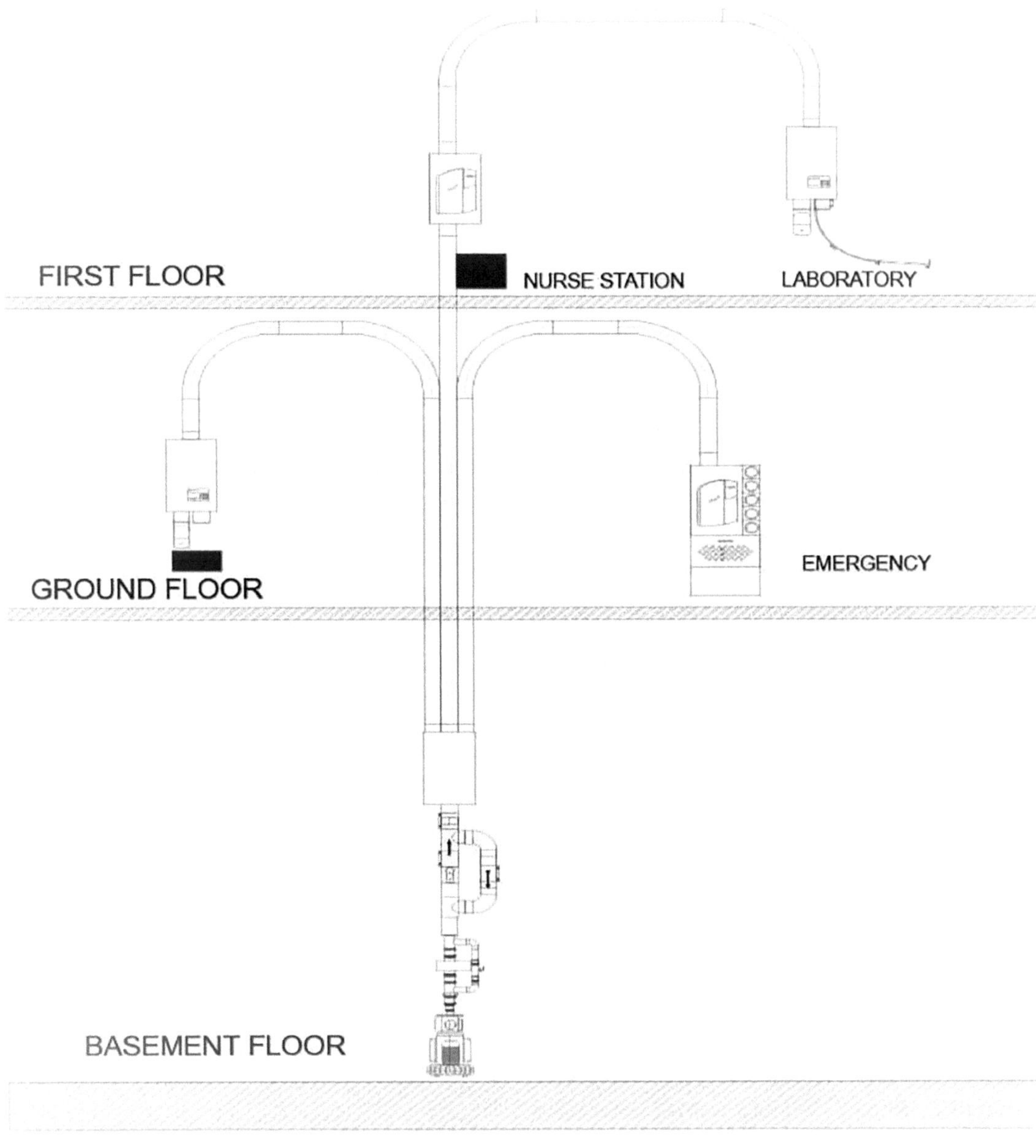

Fig. 44.1 Sample layout of multi-floor PTS system

2. Leak-proof carriers: Used for the transporting liquids or samples like blood samples which are very sensitive.
3. Special carriers: These are specially designed carriers such as lead lined or cooled carriers. These carriers are for specific use and are rarely used.

44.1.3 Control Centre

This is software that controls the movement of the carriers between the stations and users. This software is also capable of locating the live position of the carrier with the help of a user interface.

44.1.4 Database

A details of the carrier movements along with the date and time along with the station details are stored as a repository in the system for each of the PTS systems.

44.1.5 Inter-Zone Connection

This is a section of tubing network and is used to connect one zone with another zone.

44.1.6 Station

The station is a place used for sending and receiving the carrier of PTS system. Station is a user interface unit and includes an interactive touch screen, along with a dialling system and RFID scanner used to send or receive the carriers. The station has a platform where the carrier is placed for sending the material. Apart from this, the station is also provided with a receiving basket where the carrier is received.

44.1.7 Diverter

It is a device that switches the route of the carrier and is used within a tube network at branching points to allow the carrier to divert from one path to another.

44.1.8 Tubing

Tubing or piping is used for creating the network of PTS. This tube is used to carry the carrier. Generally, the size of the tubing is 110 mm or 160 mm. Tubes of different varieties are available, like PVC tubes which can be Grey and transparent, or GI and SS tubes. Based on the environmental conditions of the site, the tube is chosen. If required or if the hospital has a bulk load to be transported, the pipe greater than 160 mm can be used.

44.1.9 Zone

Zone is a set of stations which are connected directly to each other by tubing connections. E.g. a particular floor of the hospital can be one zone, and the next floor can be another zone. Further, the Zones can also be connected to other zones. A single zone can accommodate about 10 stations, whereas a Blower Group Zone can accommodate about 60 stations.

44.1.10 Slow Speed Device

Where any sensitive goods like laboratory samples and blood samples are required to be transported at a reduced speed, this device is used.

Further Reading

TranspoNet Pneumatic Tube System for Hospitals - Swisslog Healthcare [Internet]. KUKA AG. [cited 2021 Jul 14]. Available from: https://www.swisslog-healthcare.com/en-cn/products/transport-automation/transponet-pneumatic-tube-system

Maasz S. Specimen Transport Systems- Design Issues in Creating Efficient Pneumatic Tube Transport Networks. JALA J Assoc Lab Autom. 2000 Feb 1;5(1):68–71.

Isken M, Littig S. Simulation Analysis of Pneumatic Tube Systems. J Med Syst. 2002 Mar 1;26:9–19.

PDF guidelines - IOP Conference Series: Materials Science and Engineering - IOPscience [Internet]. [cited 2021 Jul 14]. Available from: https://iopscience.iop.org/journal/1757-899X/page/PDF%20guidelines

Dr. Arun. Mavaji. Innovative Methods To Improve Hospital Efficiency- Study Of Pneumatic Transport Systems (Pts) In Healthcare. IOSR J Bus Manag. 2013;9(6):10–5.

How pneumatic tube transport works [Internet]. Explain that Stuff. 2010 [cited 2021 Jul 14]. Available from: http://www.explainthatstuff.com/pneumatic-tube-transport.html

Abhinandu K, Kumar KVSP, Srikanth T, Prashanth BN. Design and Development of Pneumatic Drug Delivery System. IOP Conf Ser Mater Sci Eng. 2019 Dec;577:012128.

Design issues Pneumatic Tube Systems in a hospital [Internet]. [cited 2021 Jul 14]. Available from: https://www.telecomtubesystems.com/Design-issues-for-Pneumatic-Tube-Systems-in-Hospitals

Koroglu M, Erkurt MA, Kuku I, Kaya E, Berber I, Nizam I, et al. Assessing Safety of Pneumatic Tube System (PTS) for Patients with Very Low Hematologic Parameters. Med Sci Monit Int Med J Exp Clin Res. 2016 Apr 20;22:1329–33.

45 Signage System

Wayfinding or so-called the Signage System is a concept that is used to orient and navigate people through the space in a hospital setup. In hospitals, the purpose of wayfinding systems is to direct and guide patients, visitors and staff from entry points and car parks to reach their destinations and back again.

A well-designed wayfinding system can guide the patient, visitors, staff to their destination without any inconvenience or adding to the confusion, stress and worry that they are already suffering from. Whereas inefficient or poor wayfinding systems may cause stress, frustration, disorientation and helplessness.

An ineffective wayfinding system also leads to people becoming lost and wastes the time of staff, patient and visitor in just enquiring the locations.

Effective wayfinding systems make it easy for people to use the spaces and areas inside the hospital building.

45.1 Categories Using Wayfinding

The following categories generally use the wayfinding systems.

45.1.1 Patients and Visitors

Patients are the most common users of the wayfinding systems in a hospital. As the patients and visitors are generally unaware about the locations and passages of the hospital setup, the wayfinding systems help a lot in providing the information to these patients and visitors. Visitors may also include representatives of units providing commercial service, people arriving in the hospital for deliveries of stores, supplies and spaces, medical representatives, equipment suppliers, consumable suppliers, Govt. Officers like police officers and fire brigade officers, other health and welfare workers and other official representatives of various services.

45.1.2 Staff

As such the way finding system is of not much use for the staff, as being regular users of the system, most of them become familiar with the locations of the hospital setup over a period of time. The wayfinding can help the staff in making people aware of the spaces and locations, who are lost or in need of assistance.

45.1.3 Users with Special Needs

Wayfinding is also important for people with sensory, physical, language and intellectual disabilities. For such types of users, the universal signage system shall be used to help them find the way.

A. Garg, A. Dewan, *Manual of Hospital Planning and Designing*,
https://doi.org/10.1007/978-981-16-8456-2_45

45.1.4 Sensory Impairment

Blind people or the people with low vision and people with hearing impairment usually find it difficult to find the way and reach their location. Those with limited vision have to rely strongly on colour recognition, highlighted and clearly readable signboards and audible clues etc. Similarly, people with hearing impairment rely more on written messages, signboards, lip-reading and hand commands to communicate.

45.1.5 Language and Illiteracy

Due to illiteracy, the wayfinding systems shall have a provision for standardized symbols and pictographs along with alphabetical signage that can support the people to find the way who are functionally illiterate.

45.2 Principles for Designing Wayfinding System

While designing the wayfinding system, the following principles shall be followed:

1. Create a unique identity, say room number or hall number, for each location of the hospital.
2. Different zones of the regions shall be created like Diagnostic zone, Intensive Care Zone, OPD zone etc. Each zone shall be differentiated either by colour scheme of the different visual characters.
3. Use of floor or wall strips to show the route and the display what is ahead of this place shall be considered.
4. Provide the sign boards right from the entry point or from reception onwards so that the user can follow the wayfinding from that point onwards.
5. The sign boards shall be clearly visible, and the fonts shall be kept in such a size that it is easily visible from a distance.
6. The colour scheme of the signboards shall be in contrast colour. E.g. if the background colour of the sign board is dark blue, the text shall be in white colour, so that it is easily visible.
7. The indoor sign boards shall be well lit with background light to make it more readable, even in the night or low light.
8. The placement of the sign boards shall be such that it comes in eye contact while the user is moving in the building. E.g. the sign boards can be placed at the front wall at the end of the corridor, in landing of the staircase and hanging sign boards in the corridors etc.
9. The routes and the paths shall be well structured and shall be clear and as short as possible.
10. Sign boards for the handicapped users shall be clearly written in text as well as symbols.
11. The use of landmarks shall be promoted to provide orientation and memorable points to orientate the user.
12. The fire exit plans shall be provided as per the norms of the country. Fire exit sign boards shall be specifically well lit with a power backup available.
13. The hospital route plan or the site plans can be printed on the hospital brochure to make the user aware of the routes of the locations well in advance before landing in the hospital building.
14. At the main reception, display charts shall be provided displaying the details of the departments with room number and location, the list of indoor plans with room number and location, the list of doctors with their room numbers, days and timings. Apart from this, the floor plan indicating the zones, regions, and the follow through colour strip coding shall be provided.
15. Right from the first point like parking lot, the sign boards shall be provided depicting the main entrance route, emergency route or the OPD route etc.
16. The entry and exit gate of the hospital building shall also be provided with clear and readable sign boards and shall be well lit to be used at night.
17. In hospitals where there are multiple entrances and exits points, the sign boards

shall be provided at all such major entrances and exits.

18. The emergency department shall have large size sign boards, so that it is visible right from the entry point of the hospital.
19. The sign boards depicting the room number and the purpose of the room shall be provided at the entrance door of all such rooms or halls. Also a name plate shall be provided at the entrance door of the room or hall to show the name and designation of the person occupying the room/hall.
20. The serving counters like the reception counter, cash counter, help desk or the nursing counter etc., shall be clearly marked and numbered.
21. Where ever required, the directional arrows shall be provided on the sign boards.
22. Vehicular sign boards shall be displayed on the side of the roads to provide indications to the drivers and display signs such as zebra crossing, one-way entry, speed limit and stop signs etc. shall be provided.
23. Proper sign boards shall be provided in the parking lots depicting the parking position and reserved parking locations for VIP, Staff etc.
24. Do not place the sign boards too high, making it difficult to read. The maximum top-end height shall not be more than 1600 mm above the floor level. Generally, sign boards should be located within the 1200 mm–1800 mm band.
25. A directory shall be organized as per the user needs and not by bureaucratic hierarchy of the hospital. E.g. the directory of the doctors shall be placed above in the list and not the CEO or directors of the hospital. As the patients are more concerned with the doctors and not with the executives of the hospital.
26. Letterforms should be clearly readable, and the fonts shall be chosen which are legible. The capital height ratio of the typeface shall be approximately 3:4. Use of capital letters shall be preferred for signage.
27. Size of the letters shall be such that it is legible from a distance. The standard size of 25 mm letters is generally legible from 15 m away. If the sign board is viewed from angle, angular distortion occurs. If the font is distorted by a 45-degree angle, the legibility will decrease by 75%. Also poor lighting may further reduce the legibility. Therefore, the letter height of 45–50 mm shall be used to make it readable from a distance of 15 m.
28. Along with the text, icons or symbols that represent the department, facility, object or service shall be used for the users who are not literate. Through the combination of colour, text, symbols and icons, more information can be delivered in a small space.
29. Messages can be aligned left, centred or right. Out of these left-aligned text is considered to be the most effective alignment. However, the justified alignment from both sides is recommended to be used.
30. Keep terminology that is simple and understandable by the user. E.g. for the department of ENT, the terminology 'Otorhinolaryngology' is not understandable by the user, hence the terminology 'ENT' shall be used.
31. Signs boards shall be bi-lingual, one of them shall be English and other the Local language which is easily understandable by the user. The layout shall display both languages one above the other.
32. In all the lift lobbies and the staircases, the building levels shall be clearly displayed on each and every floor of the building. Hence the marking shall not create confusion about the floors. Therefore, the ground floor shall be termed as 'Ground Floor' and not the first floor. Similarly, the Service floor shall be termed as 'Service Floor' and not 'SF' as this may give the appeal of the second floor or the fifth floor because sometimes it looks like 5.
33. The size of the sign boards shall be carefully planned, so that it is visible to the user from a required distance. Too large sign boards shall also be avoided, as they look shabby and are a waste of funds.
34. The size proportions of sign boards shall also be planned well so that it does not look disproportionate.
35. Signs should be located keeping sufficient distance and spacing from each other.

36. Notice sign boards shall be placed at the desired places where the notices have to be displayed. The notices can be such as ‘not a thorough passage’, ‘No Smoking’, ‘Silence area’, ‘Restricted area’ etc.
37. General Information sign boards are used for users who need to know what can and cannot be done in the hospital complex. These sign boards shall depict the activities which are prohibited in the hospital premises. The examples can be No smoking, Walking on the grass prohibited, No loud talking, No horn, No spitting, Photography prohibited, Using mobile phones prohibited etc.

45.3 Types of Sign Boards

Sign boards can be of different types like:

45.3.1 Classified by Function

Based on the information that the user requires, the wayfinding sign boards, installed in the interior or exterior of the building, can be classified based on the type of information provided by the signboard. Some are like:

1. *Orientation*
   These sign boards give an overview of the building or site and the locations. These sign boards also provide other relevant information such as Waiting areas, IPD areas, visitors lounge and cafeteria etc. These sign boards may also be provided with maps, directories, floor plans etc.
2. *Directional*
   These types of sign boards are used to provide the defined route, path, or direction needed to guide the users to their destinations. Along with the messages, clear directional arrows shall also be provided.
3. *Identification*
   These sign boards depict the identity, name or function of specified rooms/halls, departments, floors, buildings or locations etc. These sign boards include name and number of building, floor/level, department and room.
4. *Statutory*
   These are the sign boards that are necessary to be installed as required by regulation and statute and are mandatory to do so. These sign boards can be like fire evacuation plans, fire exit, radiation area warnings, electrical danger sign boards etc.
5. *Traffic and Parking*
   All the sign boards which help to control traffic or assist the drivers fall under this category. These can be like No entry, One-Way only, Pedestal Crossings, No Horn, No left/right turn, speed limit etc.

45.3.2 Signs Classified by Physical Characteristics

This classification is based on the mounting methods with which the sign boards are displayed like:

1. *Self-Supporting*
   The sign boards which are self-sustained, free hanging, mounted on a pole, fixed on the plinth, or self-weight bearing signboards are called self-supported signboards.
2. *Wall Mounted*
   Are those sign boards which are fixed on the walls.
3. *Ceiling Suspended*
   Sign boards that are hung or fixed from the ceiling.

45.3.3 Other Factors of Classification of Sign Boards

There are some other factors based on which the sign boards can be classified. Some of them are:

1. *Single Sided*
   Single side sign boards are generally those sign boards that display the information on one side only and are generally fixed on the walls or the counters.
2. *Double Sided*
   Double-sided sign boards display the information on both the sides of the sign board

and are generally used as ceiling suspended sign boards.

3. *Illuminated Sign Boards*

   These are the sign boards that are illuminated with the internal self-illumination from the background, externally illuminated with the bollard or spotlights. All these sign boards require lighting by some means may it be the natural or artificial light.

4. *Dynamic or Static*

   The static sign board displays the same information and until replaced physically. Dynamic signs are used where the information changes often. E.g. information regarding patient room allocations, token numbers of waiting patients and information of the hospital facilities etc.

Further Reading

Devlin AS. Wayfinding in healthcare facilities: contributions from environmental psychology. Behav Sci Basel Switz. 2014 Oct 31;4(4):423–36.

Guenther R, Vittori G, Atwood C. Values-Driven Design and Construction: Enriching Community Benefits through Green Hospitals. :40.

Hospital & Healthcare Signage: Improving Patient Satisfaction [Internet]. DGI Communications. 2018 [cited 2021 Jul 14]. Available from: https://www.dgi-communications.com/hospital-signage/

admin. Healthcare Wayfinding and the 6 Rules for Effective Systems [Internet]. ID Signsystems Architectural Signage, Design & Lighting. 2015 [cited 2021 Jul 14]. Available from: https://idsignsystems.com/six-rules-of-healthcare-wayfinding/

Rodrigues R, Coelho R, Tavares JMRS. Healthcare Signage Design: A Review on Recommendations for Effective Signing Systems. HERD. 2019 Jul;12(3):45–65.

Lee S-C, Kim Y-J, Kim T-H, Yun S-J, Lee NK, Kim W-J. Impact of obesity in patients with urolithiasis and its prognostic usefulness in stone recurrence. J Urol. 2008 Feb;179(2):570–4.

Potter JS. Best Practices for Wayfinding in a Hospital Setting. :60.

Murphy P, Projects SS. 3 Innovative Wayfinding Solutions for Expanding Healthcare Facilities [Internet]. GNU Group. 2019 [cited 2021 Jul 14]. Available from: https://www.gnugroup.com/resources-innovative-wayfinding-solutions-for-expanding-healthcare-facilities/

46 Biomedical Waste Management

Biomedical Waste Management is governed by the legislation of individual country or state, which issues their own set of rules and regulations to manage such waste.

In India, the Directorate General of Health Services, Ministry of Health and Family Welfare, has issued such rules known as 'Biomedical Waste Management Rules, 2016'.

As it is not possible to define and discuss the rules and regulations of all countries, we have tried to highlight the 'Biomedical Waste Management Rules, 2016' issued in India for understanding this chapter.

The content of this chapter is the synopsis of the Biomedical Waste Management Rules, 2016 and shall not be considered as Plagiarism.

Biomedical waste, also known as 'Hospital waste', is the waste that may contain infectious (or potentially infectious) materials. It can also include waste originating from the laboratory. However, it differs from normal trash, kitchen waste or general waste. It also differs from other hazardous waste, such as chemical, radioactive, universal or industrial waste.

Biomedical waste can be in any form or shape; solid, semi-solid or liquid. Some examples of such infectious waste include discarded laboratory specimens, blood, body parts, amputated limbs, other animal or human tissues, removed bandages and materials used for dressing, used surgical gloves or any other medical consumables, catheters and other devices used for penetrating the skin. Also, discarded sharps objects like needles, lancets or blades, are considered to be a biomedical waste, as there are all the possibilities of them being contaminated with body fluids or blood.

46.1 Classification of Hospital Waste

It is the primary responsibility of the hospital to manage the biomedical waste generated within the hospital, which includes collection, segregation, storage, transportation, pre-treatment and disposal of such waste.

The waste generated from the hospitals is classified as:

- Biomedical Waste
- General Waste
- Other Wastes

46.1.1 Biomedical Waste

It is the waste generated from a hospital that can adversely affect the health of a person or environment, if not disposed of properly. These wastes are generated during diagnosis, treatment and other interventions. This is approximately 15% to 20% of the total hospital waste.

A. Garg, A. Dewan, *Manual of Hospital Planning and Designing*,
https://doi.org/10.1007/978-981-16-8456-2_46

Biomedical Waste is disposed in colour coded bags, where each colour defines the type of waste to be put into it as follows:

(a) **Yellow Category** is for human or animal anatomical waste, soiled waste, expired or discarded medicines, chemical waste, discarded linen, mattresses and beddings, routine mask and gown and clinical laboratory waste.
(b) **Red Category** is for disposable items such as tubes, bottles, intravenous tubes and sets, catheters, urine bags, syringes without needles, vacutainers and gloves.
(c) **White Category** is for needles, scalpels, blades or any other contaminated sharp object that may cause puncture and cuts.
(d) **Blue Category** is for broken, discarded and contaminated glass including medicine vials and ampoules.

Such wastes shall be handled and disposed of as per the rules and regulations of the respected country and/or state.

46.1.2 General Waste

Any waste, except biomedical waste, is considered general waste and may consist of paper, cardboard boxes, newspaper, food containers, plastic bottles, packaging materials, Aluminium cans, organic/biodegradable waste like left over food, construction and demolition waste etc.

Such wastes shall be handled and disposed of as per the rules and regulations of the respective country and/or state.

46.1.3 Other Wastes

It consists of electronic wastes, batteries, chemicals, radioactive waste etc. These may/may not be harmful to humans or environment.

Such wastes shall be handled and disposed of as per the rules and regulations of the respective country and/or state.

46.2 Steps Involved in Biomedical Waste Management

Biomedical waste management involves five steps:

(a) Segregation
(b) Collection
(c) Pre-treatment
(d) Transportation
(e) Storage

46.3 Biomedical Waste Segregation

1. Segregation shall be done at the point from where the waste is generated.
2. Posters depicting the segregation process shall be displayed at the point of segregation.
3. Colour coded bins, bags and containers shall be provided at the point of segregation.
4. Staff shall be provided with personal protective equipment.

46.4 Biomedical Waste Collection

46.4.1 Time of Collection

1. General waste shall not be collected along with biomedical waste.
2. Biomedical waste shall be collected from each ward, daily at a fixed time interval.
3. Best time to collect general waste is immediately after the visiting hours.
4. Collection time shall correspond to the time of waste generation. For example, OR waste shall be collected immediately after the completion of surgeries in a day so that the waste is not kept at the generation place for a longer time.

46.4.2 Packing of Biomedical Waste and Labelling

1. Biomedical waste bags shall not be filled more than three quarters.
2. Bags shall be tied with a cable tie and never stapled.
3. For replacement, empty bags shall be available at the collection point.
4. Biohazard symbol shall be printed on colour coded waste bags.
5. Details like collection date, waste type and quantity shall be labelled on the filled bags.
6. The bags shall have a bar coded stickers to allow tracking till final disposal.

46.4.3 Interim Storage

1. For interim storage of biomedical waste, dirty utilities shall be used and the waste shall not be stored in wards or departments.
2. Similarly, it shall not be stored in the patient care area, clinical area, procedures areas and OR.
3. If dirty utilities are not available, waste shall be stored away in a low traffic area.

46.5 Transportation of Biomedical Waste in Hospital

46.5.1 Transportation Trolleys

Transportation of such waste shall be done using closed trolleys or containers.

46.5.2 Route of Transportation

A route having fewer patients and visitors shall be chosen to transport such waste.

46.5.3 Central Waste Collection Room for Biomedical Waste

1. Hospital shall have a central waste collection room, located on the hospital premises.
2. The waste shall remain there until it is finally disposed.
3. This room shall be at a distance from public spaces and shall be restricted.
4. The space shall have the capacity to store waste generated for at least 2 days.
5. This room shall have an RCC roof with the facility to be locked. It shall also be guarded round the clock.
6. The room shall be provided with a ramp to transport trolleys.
7. Flooring shall be made out of tiles or other glazed material, and shall have a slope to wash the room.
8. Exhaust fans shall be provided for ventilation.
9. Fire extinguisher, smoke detector and sprinkler system shall be installed to prevent fire.
10. Tap water shall be supplied to wash the room and containers.
11. Signboards and logo of Biomedical Waste Hazard shall be fixed.

46.6 Record Keeping

1. Hospital shall maintain the records of the location of waste generation point, quantity of the waste generated, details of waste transported and date and time of disposal.
2. Quantity of waste generated shall be recorded category wise in the Biomedical Waste Register/logbook.
3. A weighing machine shall be provided in the central waste collection centre.
4. Records shall be prepared as an annual report and submitted to authorities.
5. Records of training provided to the people handling and segregating biomedical waste shall also be maintained.
6. Annual health check-up and immunization records of all the employees shall be maintained.
7. Records and minutes of Biomedical Waste Management committee meeting shall be maintained.
8. Records of any accident that may have occurred shall be maintained along with details of corrective and/or preventive actions taken.

9. Records of the operation of biomedical treatment equipment installed (if any), testing of effluent generated from hospital, and recyclable waste like plastic or glass, shall also be maintained.
10. Hospital needs to retain all these records for at least 5 years.

46.7 Updating Information on the Website

Hospital shall develop its own webpage/website for displaying all information relating to biomedical waste. This information shall be provided in the format prescribed by the rules and regulations of the country/state.

46.8 Management of General Waste

1. General solid waste generated from the hospital shall be segregated and collected in separate bins and shall be filled in bags that are non-chlorinated, and the same shall not be mixed with biomedical waste.
2. General waste is generally of two types: dry waste and biodegradable waste, and both shall be segregated separately. Green bins shall be used for biodegradable waste and blue for dry waste.
3. Waste collected in bins shall be disposed as per the rules.
4. Items like sanitary pads and diapers shall preferably be wrapped in pouches before disposal.
5. Horticulture and garden wastes shall be disposed as per the rules.
6. General waste shall not be thrown or burnt in open public spaces and shall not be put in drain or water bodies.

46.9 Management of Other Wastes

46.9.1 Used Batteries

These shall be disposed only by handing it over to authorized dealers, recyclers or any other authorized agency.

46.9.2 Management of Radioactive Wastes

These shall be re-exported to the manufacturer. For this, the hospital shall enter into an agreement with the manufacturer.

46.9.3 Management of E-Wastes

E-waste shall be handed over to authorized E-Waste Recyclers/Dismantlers or any other approved agency for disposal.

46.10 Effluent Treatment Plant (ETP/STP)

Waste water generated from the hospital has to be treated properly before final disposal, failing which can result in serious adverse effects on the environment and cause infectious diseases in humans. Hence, an effluent treatment plant is a must for hospitals.

Generally, waste water contains chemicals and biological wastes such as microbial pathogens, harmful bacteria and viruses, radioactive isotopes, pharmaceuticals, hazardous chemicals and heavy metals. Hospital continuously generates waste water from various units like pathology, OR, emergency, hot lab, ICU, radiology, kitchen and laundry.

Effluent Treatment Plant (ETP/STP) is used for removing organic matter and suspended solids from water before it is reused in the hospital or discharged in the environment.

Following are the different stages involved in the working of ETP/STP:

46.10.1 Preliminary Stage

This stage is also known as 'pre-treatment stage' where bar screens are used to remove larger suspended solids like debris, paper, rags, metal, plastic and other items that are present in the raw waste water/sewage. It is necessary to remove such items, failing which may cause serious damage to ETP/STP plant. After this, a process known as sedimentation is carried out, where waste water enters a grit chamber, and the water flow is slowed to remove sand, grit and sandstones from the water.

46.10.2 Primary Stage

In this stage, physical and chemical methods are used to improve the quality of waste water. A process called skimming is performed after sedimentation, where lighter particles float at the surface of water and the same are skimmed. This removes 60–65% of the total suspended solids from the waste water. For this process also, a grit chamber is used where the sludge settled in this process is sent to a sludge digester for further processing.

46.10.3 Secondary Stage

In this stage, organic matter is removed by the process of biological treatment. Once the water enters the secondary clarifier, floatable matter is removed and heavier matter settles down at the bottom, which is known as 'active sludge'.

46.10.4 Tertiary Stage

This is the final stage and is known as disinfection stage. In this stage, all leftover residual suspended solids particles and other materials are removed.

This chapter discusses the highlights of Biomedical Waste Management. However, the actual management of such wastes solely depends on the set of Rules and Regulations as framed by the respective country or state.

Therefore, the designer and the hospital management are advised to go through such rules and regulations before planning and designing the facilities and infrastructure of Biomedical Waste Management.

Further Reading

Adu RO, Gyasi SF, Essumang DK, Otabil KB. Medical Waste-Sorting and Management Practices in Five Hospitals in Ghana. J Environ Public Health. 2020 Mar 4;2020:e2934296.

Ali S, Wang W, Nawaz Chaudhry M, Geng Y. Hospital waste management in developing countries: A mini review. Waste Manag Res. 2017 Jun 7;35.

Aljabre SHM. Hospital generated waste: a plan for its proper management. J Fam Community Med. 2002;9(2):61–5.

Farzadkia M, Akbari H, Gholami H, Darabi A. Management of Hospital Waste: A Case Study in Tehran, Iran. Health Scope [Internet]. 2018 May 31 [cited 2021 Jul 15];7(2). Available from: https://sites.kowsarpub.com/healthscope/articles/61412.html#abstract

Kalantary RR, Jamshidi A, Mofrad MMG, Jafari AJ, Heidari N, Fallahizadeh S, et al. Effect of COVID-19 pandemic on medical waste management: a case study. J Environ Health Sci Eng. 2021 Mar 18;19(1):831–6.

Khan BA, Cheng L, Khan AA, Ahmed H. Healthcare waste management in Asian developing countries: A mini review. Waste Manag Res. 2019 Sep 1;37(9):863–75.

Kumar. Bio-medical waste disposal in India: From paper to practice, what has been effected [Internet]. [cited 2021 Jul 15]. Available from: https://www.ijournalhs.org/article.asp?issn=2542-6214;year=2019;volume=12;issue=3;spage=202;epage=210;aulast=Kumar

Kwikiriza S, Stewart AG, Mutahunga B, Dobson AE, Wilkinson E. A Whole Systems Approach to Hospital

Waste Management in Rural Uganda. Front Public Health [Internet]. 2019 [cited 2021 Jul 15];0. Available from: https://www.frontiersin.org/articles/10.3389/fpubh.2019.00136/full

Letho Z, Yangdon T, Lhamo C, Limbu CB, Yoezer S, Jamtsho T, et al. Awareness and practice of medical waste management among healthcare providers in National Referral Hospital. PloS One. 2021;16(1):e0243817.

Peng J, Wu X, Wang R, Li C, Zhang Q, Wei D. Medical waste management practice during the 2019-2020 novel coronavirus pandemic: Experience in a general hospital. Am J Infect Control. 2020 Aug;48(8):918–21.

Rao D, Dhakshaini MR, Kurthukoti A, Doddawad VG. Biomedical Waste Management: A Study on Assessment of Knowledge, Attitude and Practices Among Health Care Professionals in a Tertiary Care Teaching Hospital. Biomed Pharmacol J. 2018 Sep 21;11(3):1737–43.

Wafula ST, Musiime J, Oporia F. Health care waste management among health workers and associated factors in primary health care facilities in Kampala City, Uganda: a cross-sectional study. BMC Public Health. 2019 Feb 18;19(1):203.

47 Fire Safety

Fire safety, protection, and detection norms governed by the legislation of individual country or state, which issues their own set of rules and regulations to manage fire safety, protection, and detection.

There are some set codes and standards as prescribed by National Fire Protection Association (NFPA) that are accepted internationally. Similarly, In India, the 'National Building Code of India 2016', has issued a set of such rules.

As it is not possible to define and discuss the rules and regulations of all countries, we have tried to highlight the 'National Building Code of India 2016' for understanding this chapter.

The content of this chapter is the synopsis of the 'National Building Code of India 2016' and shall not be considered as Plagiarism.

Considering the importance of fire safety and protection, the hospital building shall be designed to easily deal with such emergencies and avoid any untoward fire incidence.

Hospital building has a lot of patients, visitors, and staff. Some patients may be sick and bedridden, and their evacuation may become difficult in case of fire. Hence, the hospital building shall have all provisions to minimize the possibility of a fire emergency. Hospitals shall also have adequate provisions to detect fire as soon as it occurs and suppress it before spreading.

47.1 Planning for Fire Safety in Hospitals

While designing a hospital building, the following points related to fire detection and fighting shall be considered:

1. Compartmentalization of the hospital building shall be done.
2. Open spaces shall be provided as mentioned in the norms.
3. Fire resistant doors shall be provided.
4. Lift lobbies, lift wells and staircases shall be pressurized.
5. Vertical shafts shall be pressurized.
6. Refuge area shall be provided.
7. Smoke ventilation system shall be provided.
8. Fire dampers and fire hydrants shall be provided.
9. Automatic sprinkler system shall be in place.
10. Fire alarm system shall be provided.
11. Public address system shall be provided.
12. Automatic detection system including smoke/heat detectors shall be provided.
13. Manual call point shall be provided.
14. First aid shall be placed.
15. Firefighting appliances like extinguisher shall be provided.
16. Alternate power supply shall be provided.
17. Signage for easy evacuation shall be in place.

A. Garg, A. Dewan, *Manual of Hospital Planning and Designing*,
https://doi.org/10.1007/978-981-16-8456-2_47

47.2 Structural Elements for Fire Safety

The following structural elements shall be provided while designing a hospital building:

47.2.1 Compartmentalization

Building shall have proper compartments and barriers to each compartment as described in the rules and regulations of the country or state. While designing these compartments, the following points shall be taken care of:

1. If any bedridden patient area is more than 280 m^2, the provision shall be made to shift the patient along with the bed to other smokeless compartment.
2. If any section of the building is larger than 500 m^2, compartmentalization shall be done, which shall be fire resistance for at least 2 h.
3. The patient area on each floor shall have at least two smoke compartments.
4. If any floor is occupied by more than 50 people, it shall be divided into two smoke compartments.

47.2.2 Open Spaces

Open spaces shall be provided outside the building as described in the rules and regulations of the country or state. While designing these spaces, the following points shall be taken care of:

1. Open space shall be provided around the building for the free movement of emergency/fire vehicles.
2. Open spaces shall be kept motorable and free from obstructions at all times.
3. Passage shall be provided for emergency vehicles to enter hospital premises.
4. The width of the entrances, roads and turning radius shall be as described in the rules and regulations of the country or state.
5. Outside storage and other tanks shall be covered with slabs and shall be strong enough to take heavy vehicle load.
6. Open space left for this purpose shall not be used for any other purpose like parking etc.
7. Access roads shall be provided around the building and shall not be terminated with dead ends.

47.2.3 Basements

Basement shall be designed considering the issues related to fire as described in the rules and regulations of the country or state. While designing the basement, the following points shall be taken care of:

1. Basements shall be made out of concrete walls.
2. It shall have provision of automatic sprinkler and smoke evacuation system.
3. Dampers shall be provided for fresh air.
4. The basement ceiling height shall be as described in the rules and regulations of the country or state.
5. Access to the basement shall be through a separate staircase and/or ramp. The width of the staircase and ramp and the slope of the ramp shall be as described in the rules and regulations of the country or state.
6. Basement shall have at least two independent exits.
7. The staircases shall be protected with fire resistance doors.
8. There shall be no cutouts to the upper floors from the basement.

47.2.4 General Exit Requirements

Exits shall be designed as described in the rules and regulations of the country or state. While designing exits, the following points shall be taken care of:

1. Exits from the building can be provided via staircase or ramps, but lifts shall never be

used in case of fire. Exits shall land in an open space near/outside the building.
2. Width, height and number of exits shall be in accordance with the rules and regulations of the country or state.
3. Exit doors shall open in the direction of exit, and not inside, so that in case of hurry, the door can be pushed outside than pulling inside.
4. Exit doors shall open in an enclosed stairway.
5. Exit doors shall be openable without any key.
6. Fire-rated doors, assembly and hardware shall be certified and labelled by the manufacturer giving details about the type of door, serial/batch number of door, manufacture details like year/month, fire resistance rating etc.
7. Access-controlled doors or electro-magnetic doors, if provided, shall be fire rated as described in the rules and regulations of the country or state. Manual release device shall be provided with the access-controlled doors.
8. Such provisions shall be made that boom barriers, turnstiles, access-controlled exit doors, and other such exits open automatically in case of fire or smoke.
9. Walking surfaces of exit area shall comply with the rules and regulations of the country or state.
10. Number of exits access, width of corridors, aisles or ramps, capacity of exit access, and travel distance to an exit shall be in accordance with the rules and regulations of the country or state.
11. Obstruction due to objects like chairs, tables, cupboards or any other obstructions shall be avoided in the exit access.
12. The exit access shall be properly lit with floor light strips or fluorescent strips for easy identification of access.
13. Exit signages of adequate size shall be placed in the exit access and suspended on the ceiling. Evacuation plan shall be affixed on the wall of all important places in the building.
14. Exit access shall not pass through any room or hall.
15. The travel distance of exit shall be as described in the rules and regulations of the country or state.

47.2.5 Corridors and Passageways

1. The width and height of corridors and passageways shall be as described in the rules and regulations of the country or state.
2. The width of the exit corridor and passageways shall never be less than the width of the exit doorways.
3. Corridors shall be well ventilated and shall be free from any obstruction.
4. In cases where the door of rooms open in the corridors, such doors shall open inside the room and not in the corridors, to permit free flow of traffic in the corridor.

47.2.6 Staircases

The hospital building shall have staircases. The numbers of staircases required, width of the staircase, width of the staircase thread, height of the riser, number of risers per flight, and minimum headroom shall be as described in the rules and regulations of the country or state.

1. If internal staircases are provided, they shall be constructed with an external wall and shall be made out of non-combustible materials. These staircases shall not be built around the lift shaft.
2. Metal staircases shall be avoided as they get heated in case of fire.
3. Pipelines or ducts of chimney, HVAC, gas or electrical lines shall neither be allowed in the stairway nor shall they pass through the staircase.
4. On one side of the staircase, handrail shall be provided, the height of which shall be as described in the rules and regulations of the country or state.
5. Lifts shall not open in staircase.
6. All external stairs shall directly open on the ground, in an open area.
7. Avoid using spiral staircase.

47.2.7 Ramps

1. If ramps are provided in the hospital, the width of the ramp, width of the minimum headroom, and inclination of the ramp shall be as described in the rules and regulations of the country or state.
2. Flooring of the ramps shall be non-slippery.
3. Turnings of the ramps shall never have a slope.
4. Ramps shall have landings on both the ends, i.e. top and bottom.
5. Both sides of the ramp shall have handrails.

47.2.8 Electrical and Emergency Power

Emergency power shall be planned as described in the rules and regulations of the country or state. This helps to ensure efficient and reliable power supply to the critical fire and life safety system and equipment. While designing the hospital electrical plan, the following points shall be taken care of:

1. In hospitals, the provision of emergency lighting shall be provided either using a standby generator with automatic changeover facility or UPS.
2. Emergency power shall feed facilities like emergency lighting, escape route, way finding strips, exit sign boards, fire alarm system, public announcement system, smoke detection control panel, hydrant/sprinkler fire pumps, pressurization fans, dampers and actuators, fireman's lift, access-controlled electro-magnetic doors etc.
3. Emergency power shall be automatic and activated within 1 s of failure of normal power.
4. For emergency power system, non-flammable material shall be used.
5. The panel or DB feeding the fire and life safety equipment shall be located in a fire-safe zone.
6. Cables for fire detection and suppression system shall be laid down in a metal conduit and not in PVC conduit.

47.2.9 Air-Conditioning, Ventilation and Smoke Control

Air-conditioning and mechanical ventilation of the hospital shall be done as described in the rules and regulations of the country or state. While designing the hospital air-conditioning and ventilation system, the following points shall be taken care of:

1. While designing such systems, the danger of the fire spreading from these devices shall be minimum.
2. While designing such systems, care shall be taken to curb the spread of smoke to other floors and even suppress this smoke.
3. Separate air handling units (AHU) shall be provided for different floors, as far as possible. It is better if AHUs are for smaller compartments, as it can prevent the spread of smoke through AHUs.
4. Ducting of air-conditioning shall be separate for floor or compartment and shall not be interconnected with each other. Use of metal ducting is highly recommended instead of any other combustible material.
5. AHUs shall have proper filter to curtail smoke and minimize the spread of smoke. The filters shall also be non-combustible.
6. Opening around the ducts in the wall shall be properly sealed.

47.2.10 Fire Barrier

Proper fire barriers shall be provided, horizontally or vertically, as described in the rules and regulations of the country or state. All openings in the shaft shall be properly sealed to prevent the spread of fire and smoke to other floors.

47.2.11 Glazing

While designing glazing, the following points shall be taken care of:

1. If a glass façade is used for the elevation of a building, it shall completely be a tempered glass with non-combustible assembly.
2. Sprinklers shall be located near the glass façade and shall provide full coverage to the glass.
3. All gaps in the glass façade shall be properly sealed.
4. Sufficient number of fire openable panels shall be provided in the glass façade.

47.2.12 Surface Interior Finishes

Use of non-combustible walls and ceiling surface finish is recommended, and they shall be designed as per the guidelines described in the rules and regulations of the country or state.

47.2.13 Fire Command Centre (FCC)

FCC shall be provided on the ground floor, just at the entrance of the building, and shall have a direct access to the user. While designing the FCC, the following points shall be taken care of:

1. A control room shall be provided with the main fire alarm panel, along with a public address system.
2. All controls and monitoring of the fire detection system and the fire suppression system shall be taken care of from this control room. This shall also include fire alarm, pressurization systems and smoke management.
3. A CCTV monitoring station shall be provided in this room.
4. The control room shall have a detailed floor plan along with the location of doors and windows, escape route, refuge area, staircases, lifts, ramps etc. which shall be clearly marked in these floor plans.

47.3 Fire Detection and Alarm

Adequate provision shall be made for providing fire detection system in the building as described in the rules and regulations of the country or state. While designing the fire detection and alarm system, the following points shall be taken care of:

1. For fire detection, an intelligent, analogue or addressable fire detection and alarm system shall be provided in the building. It shall consist of smoke detectors, heat detectors, response indicators, manual call stations, hooters/strobes, fault isolators and control cabling. The system shall be connected to a microprocessor-based fire alarm control panel.
2. Fire detection and suppression systems shall be so planned, programmed and integrated, so that in case of fire, the control panel can activate all systems like alarms, hooters/strobes, public announcements, sprinklers, pressurization fans, opening of access doors, glowing of way finding lighting, the release of fire barriers, switching on the fire pumps, AHU filters, smoke evacuation fans and dampers. The control panel shall also monitor the fire water storage tanks and pumps, hydrant and sprinkler pressures etc.
3. The smoke detectors, heat detectors, alarms, hooters, manual call points and response indicators shall be installed as described in the rules and regulations of the country or state.
4. All cabling for installation of the detection system shall be done with conductor FRLS insulated wires in MS conduits.

47.4 Fire Extinguishers/Fixed Firefighting Installations

1. Based on the guidelines prescribed in the rules and regulations of the country or state, the hospital building shall be protected by providing fire extinguishers of all types: Powder, CO_2, ABC, Foam, wet risers with hose reels and nozzles, down-comer, automatic sprinkler installation, yard hydrants, high/medium velocity water spray, water mist spray systems, manual/automatic fire alarm system etc.
2. Extinguishers shall be wall mounted and accessible to all.

3. The specifications and number of extinguishers, wet riser, down-comer, automatic sprinkler, yard hydrants, high/medium velocity water spray, water mist spray systems and manual/automatic fire alarm system to be used shall depend on the guidelines as described in the rules and regulations of the country or state.

47.4.1 Static Water Storage Tanks

Water supply for firefighting devices like hydrant, sprinklers, downcomers and yard hydrants shall be provided from form an underground/terrace static storage tank with the capacity as described in the rules and regulations of the country or state.

47.4.2 Fire-Fighting Pump House

A fire pump house shall be provided for supplying water to the hydrant, sprinklers, and yard hydrant.

The pump house shall have two auto-start main pumps, two jockey pumps, and one diesel engine operated fire pump set connected to the emergency power supply.

47.4.3 Automatic Sprinkler Installation

It shall be installed as described in the rules and regulations of the country or state.

1. The distance between sprinklers shall be as described in the rules and regulations of the country or state.
2. The sprinkler system shall not be installed in the OR, ICU, record room, CT, MRI, PET or other such areas, where water spray can damage the medical equipment.

This chapter discusses the highlights of Fire Safety Management. However, the actual management of fire safety measurements solely depends on the set of Rules and Regulations as framed by the respective country or state.

Therefore, the designer and the hospital management are advised to go through such rules and regulations before planning and designing the facilities and infrastructure of Fire Detection, Suppression, and Safety Management.

Further Reading

Fire safety in healthcare environments [Internet]. [cited 2021 Jul 15]. Available from: https://buildingbetterhealthcare.com/news/article_page/Fire_safety_in_healthcare_environments/139696

Fire Safety Management [Internet]. Fire magazine | Safety magazine | Security magazine | Disaster relief equipment and services. 2016 [cited 2021 Jul 15]. Available from: https://firesafetysecurityindia.com/fire-safety-management/

Fire safety and protection in hospital [Internet]. Scholarly articles on hospital infrastructure, renovation, upgradation, refurbishment, setting up new hospital in India. [cited 2021 Jul 15]. Available from: http://www.hospitalinfrabiz.com/fire-safety-and-protection-in-hospital.html

Fire safety technologies advance on many fronts [Internet]. [cited 2021 Jul 15]. Available from: https://www.hfmmagazine.com/articles/3778-fire-safety-technologies-advance-on-many-fronts

Loria G, Choudhry N, Sharma K. Fire management in hospitals. Apollo Med. 2012 Mar 1;9(1):74–6.

Omidvari F, Jahangiri M, Mehryar R, Alimohammadlou M, Kamalinia M. Fire Risk Assessment in Healthcare Settings: Application of FMEA Combined with Multi-Criteria Decision Making Methods. Math Probl Eng. 2020 Oct 19;2020:e8913497.

Ravenstein HV, Ravenstein HV. Fire safety of hospitals a guide for designers. Fire Saf Hosp Guide Des [Internet]. [cited 2021 Jul 15]; Available from: https://www.academia.edu/41708228/Fire_safety_of_hospitals_a_guide_for_designers

Tabish SA. Fire Safety in Hospitals. 2010.

48 Green Hospitals

There is no existing global definition of green hospital, but it can be defined as a building that is planned and designed utilizing maximum natural resources in an efficient and environment-friendly manner, which can enhance patient care, reduce cross-infection, improve patient's well-being and provide an aid towards the curative process.

The main motive of hospitals is to provide the best medical treatment and care to the patient, adopt measures to prevent diseases and create awareness amongst the community for prevention of diseases. To achieve these objectives, hospitals have to use various resources like water, electricity, petroleum products, chemicals, food articles, construction material and gases. Out of all these, some are natural resources like water, food articles, energy, petroleum etc., whereas others are man-made resources.

The painful reality of the day is the deteriorating health of our environment, which has become an issue of grave national and international importance, as the environment has a direct effect on the health of human beings, animals and plantations. In fact, that in the latter half of the twentieth century, human beings have tinkered with the ecosystem of the planet where climatic changes, chemical pollution and contamination and unsustainable resources are the main factors affecting the ecosystem.

As hospitals use all these resources, they produce carbon footprint which adversely affects the environment. Today, the world is talking about global warming, and scientists, leaders and researchers are struggling to find the solution to curb pollution and improve environmental conditions.

Though, hospitals cannot provide quality services without exploiting natural resources, but if all these resources are deployed and utilized in simple, smart and sustainable manner, hospitals can reduce carbon footprint up to a great extent.

To find the solution for improving the environment, the concept of green building is being promoted throughout the world. Government of various countries is giving a higher rating to green buildings, and similarly green hospitals are rated higher than ordinary hospitals.

To promote green building, different countries have designated different agencies to frame policies, guidelines, controls, conduct pieces of training, provide ratings, certifications and accreditations to such buildings. In the United States, Canada, China and India, Leadership in Energy and Environment Design (LEED) has been granted this responsibility. In India, in addition to LEED, the Bureau of Energy Efficiency (BEE) and the Indian Green Building Council (IGBC) also work for promoting green buildings. Similarly, for the UK and Netherlands—Building Research Establishment Environmental Assessment Methods (BREEAM); Green Star for Australia, New Zealand and South Africa; Comprehensive Assessment System for Building

A. Garg, A. Dewan, *Manual of Hospital Planning and Designing*,
https://doi.org/10.1007/978-981-16-8456-2_48

Environmental Efficiency (CASBEE) for Japan; and Green Mark Scheme for (Singapore) performs the same duties.

Different countries have different policies, guidelines and set of rules and regulations to promote green buildings. For example, LEED has classified green buildings into four categories: LEED-certified, Silver, Gold and Platinum.

48.1 What Is Green Hospital?

A Green hospital increases patient care and adds to the treatment of patients, while utilizing natural resources in an efficient and environment-friendly manner. To achieve this objective, the hospital shall take initiative and promote the following:

1. Choose an environment-friendly site, for example a location that puts less pressure on the environment, and where clean air, water and soil are available, biodiversity is not disturbed, which enhances public health by protecting wetlands, agricultural land and open spaces.
2. Utilize sustainable and efficient designs.
3. Promote using green building materials and products.
4. Think green during the construction phase and maintain the greening process.
5. Promote recycling and reuse of materials, reduce waste and produce cleaner air.
6. Take measures to reduce CO_2 generation.
7. Use more sustainable building materials.
8. Avoid products made of mercury, latex, plastic and PVC.
9. Promote energy conservation.
10. Promote water conservation.
11. Procure environment-friendly tools and resources.
12. Provide maximum outside greenery by plantations.
13. Integrate pest management.
14. Provide provisions for proper waste disposal and transportation.
15. Use more green electronics.
16. Manage pharmaceuticals effectively.
17. Promote environment-friendly chemicals.
18. Increase fresh air ventilation.
19. Introduce active and passive measures to improve indoor air quality.
20. Use clean and green interior building materials.
21. Design more gardens and landscape.
22. Reduce sound.
23. Maximize use of daylight in the building.
24. Optimize artificial lighting requirement.

48.2 Benefits of Green Buildings Hospitals

Following are some examples of advantages of designing green hospitals:

1. Energy savings, which can extend up to 40–50% of the ordinary hospitals.
2. Water savings up to 20–30%.
3. Improved indoor ambience.
4. Improved productivity of healthcare workers.
5. Improved indoor air quality.
6. Appealing exteriors and interiors of the building.
7. Designs can enhance natural lighting by providing glazing facades, translucent skylights with soothing colours, transparent and operable openings to green courtyards etc.
8. More daylight and landscapes create a positive effect on the patient, reduce their stress levels and improve hospital's overall operational efficiency.
9. Patient recovery rate is faster.
10. High level of patient and attendant satisfaction.

48.3 Barriers to Create Green Hospitals

It is easy to say that the planners and designers should promote green hospitals, but there are a lot of barriers that restrict the design of an excellent green hospital. Some of them are as follows:

48.3.1 System Redundancy

As the hospital has to operate round the clock, it needs to create a backup of the facilities like energy and water. However, in reality, the creation of secondary and tertiary backup systems sometimes becomes difficult because of various restrictions.

48.3.2 Infection Control

Hospitals are one of the most infection-prone buildings; thus, the main motive of hospitals is to prevent infection by placing strict infection control protocols, which sometimes becomes a hurdle in creating green hospitals.

48.3.3 Regulatory Compliance

As different countries have a different set of codes, policies, by-laws and standards for designing and constructing hospital buildings, it sometimes imposes a barrier for creating a perfect green hospital.

48.3.4 Intense Energy and Water Consumption

Hospitals usually consume a large number of resources like energy and water, which can even be up to two times as compared to any other commercial buildings, which puts a barrier to creating a perfect green hospital.

48.3.5 Ventilation Rates

As hospitals are infection-prone buildings, they usually require more fresh air intake, and hence more exhaust of the indoor air, which requires higher ventilation.

48.3.6 Accreditation and Licensing Demands

In most countries, hospitals have to obtain licenses or accreditation from regulating authorities/agencies. The authorities/agencies have their own set of rules, policies and standards, which need to be fulfilled before licensing or accreditation. Such rules, policies and standards might prevent hospitals from creating a perfect green hospital.

48.3.7 Higher Volume of Hospital Waste

Hospitals generally produce a higher quantity of waste, out of which a vast majority can be hazardous. It is necessary to dispose of this waste as per the policies and guidelines prescribed by the regulating authorities, which becomes a hurdle for creating green hospitals.

48.3.8 Chemical Use

Usage of hazardous chemicals are generally unavoidable in hospitals as these may be necessary for cleaning, disinfecting, sterilizing instruments, disposables and cleaning equipment, treating certain diseases, and largely used in clinical laboratories for testing. Some of these chemicals can be extremely toxic and hazardous, which is another issue in designing green hospitals.

48.3.9 Frequent Upgradations and Renovations

Usually, hospital buildings demand upgrade and renovation because of various requirements like addition of new medical equipment, creation of isolation areas and redefining hospital zones. These renovations and upgrades defeat the purpose of green buildings.

48.4 Elements of a Green Hospital

During the planning and designing phase of a hospital building, the following elements shall be considered to create a green hospital:

1. Energy Conservation.
2. Alternative Means of Energy Generation.
3. Water Conservation.
4. Indoor Environmental Quality and HVAC Optimization.
5. Chemical Management.
6. Solid Waste Management.
7. Environmental Services.
8. Food Services.
9. Environmentally Preferable Purchasing.
10. Sustainable Construction Materials.
11. Pharmaceutical Minimization, Management, and Disposal.
12. Reducing Transportation Cost.
13. Greenery.

48.4.1 Energy Conservation

Hospitals are prone to more energy consumption as compared to other commercial buildings because they use energy for innumerable medical equipment and other appliances, water heating, air conditioning and ventilation units, water pumps, lighting, ventilation and various clinical processes. Apart from this, energy is also consumed for services like catering, laundry and instrument sterilization.

The following issues can be addressed for energy conservation in the green hospital:

1. Switching over to light-emitting diode (LED) light bulbs/lamps/fittings instead of compact fluorescent lights or conventional fluorescent tube light fittings.
2. Turning down thermostats of the HVAC system just by few degrees, depending on the temperature inside the room, to achieve an optimum temperature.
3. Replace conventional electrical fittings with energy-efficient fittings, for example replace ceiling fans with DC fans.
4. Create an awareness campaign to reduce energy use throughout the hospital building.
5. Promote turning off office equipment, medical equipment and computers when not in use.
6. Switching off the AHUs or split air-conditioning system when not required or if the rooms are vacant.
7. Provide maximum natural light during daylight hours in the rooms and corridors of the hospital.
8. Plug all leakages in the room for effective air conditioning.
9. Regular checks and maintenance of electric motors and compressors of electrical equipment including the HVAC system.
10. Use light sensors for detection of occupancy and automatically switch on/off lights in the passage, rooms, washrooms and other areas of the hospital.
11. Usage of occupancy sensors shall be promoted in areas like offices, storage rooms, toilets, nurse stations, clean/soiled utility rooms, workspaces and break rooms as these areas are occupied inconsistently.
12. Provide in-row cooling combined with enclosed racks in data centres or the server rooms.
13. Active heat reclaim systems can be installed to gain low- and medium-grade heat from the data centre to contribute to the heating base load, thus reducing fossil fuel consumption.
14. Use controllers to reduce the voltage of electrical supplies for external lighting of roadways and external car parks.
15. Vestibules can be created to allow automatic opening and closing of windows and doors between spaces with different temperatures.
16. Periodic checking and maintenance of the boilers shall be promoted.
17. Restricting the time for use of hot water.
18. Replace doors and windows made of conventional metal, with thermal-resistant sustainable materials.
19. Provide proper insulation to the HVAC ducts, chilled water pipeline, hot water supply lines and the surfaces of boilers.

20. Prefer thermal insulation of exterior walls, roof and flooring.
21. Replace common manual faucets with faucets controlled by a photocell.
22. Adopt heat recovery systems from the condensates with a heat exchanger. Heat recovery elements can capture heat that goes out the smokestack or is otherwise lost outside.
23. Introduce an Energy Management System (EMS) to review the current data on a hospital's energy usage.
24. Upgrade hospital's energy-consuming equipment with more energy-efficient equipment to reduce energy usage.
25. The building's envelope shall be created including structures such as foundation, roof, walls and windows that create a physical barrier between the outside elements and the conditioned facility.
26. Adopt cogeneration systems like combined heat and power (CHP) systems to convert the facility's waste heat into energy. This energy can then be used for heating and cooling.
27. Arrange for periodic energy audits to review the pattern of energy consumption in the hospital and how the procured energy is consumed. The aim is to detect inefficiencies in a building and comprehensive analysis.
28. Usage of variable-frequency drives (VFDs) shall be encouraged. VFDs help to save energy in pumps and fans run by alternating-current motors.
29. Consider using a heat-recovery chiller. In hospitals that require both chilled water for cooling and hot water for heating, a heat-recovery chiller can be used to capture and use heat that otherwise would be wasted in the environment.
30. Promote cold-rinse for cleaning and washing in kitchen and laundry as hot water rinse is not required for all washings and cleanings.
31. Consider planting shaded trees or shading devices on the exterior to eliminate direct sunlight from the building.
32. Try replacing the existing magnetic ballasts (some of which may contain PCBs) with electronic ballasts.
33. Super insulate the roof and wall (exposed to direct sunlight) to reduce heat transfer into the hospital and apply light colours that do not absorb much heat. This will help in utilizing less energy to cool rooms in summers and heat rooms in winters.

48.4.2 Alternative Means of Energy Generation

Usually, energy utilized in the hospital is procured from energy supply agencies which are usually produced outside and are wheeled to the hospital. Apart from this, the hospital may have its energy generation system through a diesel generation plant or smoke-belching standby power generation sets.

The energy produced in the thermal plants uses coal as raw material, which increases the carbon footprints. Similarly, atomic plants are harmful to the environment.

To avoid this, the following sources of renewable energy can be deployed:

1. Solar energy can be of three types, photovoltaic (PV), solar thermal or concentrated solar power.
   (a) Solar power refers to solar PV panels that convert energy from the sun into electric power. Advantages of solar PV include the predictability and free availability of the sun around the globe. Solar power can even be stored in Lithium-ion batteries, which can be used as and when required.
   (b) Solar thermal technology uses energy from the sun to heat water that is economically cheaper for heating water and buildings or augmenting conventional steam or hot water systems.
   (c) Concentrated solar power (CSP) uses light-focusing technologies and mirrors to concentrate the power of the sun, producing steam that generates electricity or powers other thermal applications.
2. Wind turbines use the natural flow of air to produce power. Moving air passes over blades that create a pressure drop, which spins a shaft

and induces an electrical current within a generator to create electricity. Wind power may have negative impacts on birds and bats, and it can create concerns about land use and landscape views if sited inappropriately.
3. Hydropower uses the water stored in dams and flowing in rivers to create electricity. Falling water rotates the blades of a turbine, which spins a generator and converts mechanical energy into electrical energy.
4. Geothermal technology, wherein the earth's energy is transferred into heat or electricity. There are two different geothermal technologies, geo-exchange and geothermal hydrothermal power.
5. Biomass energy source comes from organic plant material. Plants capture carbon dioxide in the atmosphere and biomass transfers energy through chemical decomposition such as anaerobic digestion and create biogas, which can be burned to generate power. Biomass fuels can be burned in boilers to produce steam to make electricity or heat hospitals.
6. Biogas is formed when organic material decomposes in an anaerobic environment versus decomposing aerobically (with oxygen). The main component of biogas is methane. Biogas can be used in its raw form as a heating fuel or for electricity production with a turbine or engine.
7. Renewable Natural Gas (RNG) can be injected into the natural gas pipeline and used for heating or base-load electricity production.

48.4.3 Water Conservation

Hospitals in the normal course consume large quantities of water. Globally, due to the climatic changes and glacier melt, water scarcity is increasing. With little effort or change in designs, hospitals can conserve water.

The following issues need to be addressed for the conservation of water:

1. Provide the system for rainwater harvesting by capturing the rainwater in the monsoon season. The rainwater of roof and grounds be collected in the water storage pits to be used later when required for irrigation etc. Otherwise, the rainwater can be poured back into the earth through rainwater soak pits.
2. The rainwater collected in the water storage pits can also be recycled and used for flushing, cleaning or irrigation.
3. The collected rainwater can also be used to operate cooling towers, which the hospital uses for their air conditioning system.
4. The use of low-flow water-efficient fixtures and technologies shall be promoted to be used in the urinals, toilets and showers to save millions of gallons of water every year.
5. Promote using sensing devices in sinks to turn off the water from devices when not needed.
6. The drained water from the hospital can be recycled by installing ETP and aerobic/oxygenated Sewage Treatment Plant (STP). Even otherwise the STP plants are essential in hospitals. This recycled water can be used for irrigation, cleaning activities, cooling towers etc.
7. Stress routinely checks plumbing and pipes to prevent leakages in the water supply line throughout the hospital building.
8. Prefer using drought-resistant plants for landscaping and plantation to minimize water requirements for irrigation. Also, use more mulch landscape plantings to help retain moisture around the root system.
9. Design landscaping to include rain gardens as these gardens use storm water runoff generated from roofs or hardscape/impervious surfaces.
10. For irrigation use Drip Irrigation and sprinkler irrigation system as it is a more efficient method of irrigation with less consumption of water.

48.4.4 Indoor Environmental Quality and HVAC Optimization

Heating, Ventilation and Air Conditioning (HVAC) is a system used in hospitals for cooling, heating and ventilation. HVAC is one of the systems which consumes major energy in the hospital. Further, the HVAC system in the hospital is operative round the clock throughout the year. If the HVAC system is designed properly, a lot of energy can be saved.

The following measures can be adopted to reduce energy costs of the HVAC system:

1. Preventive maintenance service shall be carried out periodically to make sure that the HVAC system runs efficiently.
2. HVAC equipment shall be calibrated at regular intervals.
3. Timely cleaning replacement of the air filters, canvas, valves, insulation and gaskets can reduce the energy in the long run.
4. Ensure the quality of water used in the HVAC chillers. It will increase the life of the chillers and also reduce energy costs.
5. Temperature Control thermostats shall be provided at the patient end wherein the patient can switch on/off the air-conditioning as and when required. This will help the patient to maintain temperature as per his/her choice. These thermostats can also help in energy conservation.
6. Variable Air Volume (VAV) systems shall be promoted. VAV saves energy when the airflow is at the box minimum flow. VAV boxes generally increase airflow with cooling demand, but designers traditionally set them to fixed cubic feet per minute in heating to ensure that supply air does not get too warm and stratify.
7. Usually, the hospital prefers the HVAC system which can cater to the needs of the future expansion of the spaces in the hospital. But if the airflow demand under the present scenario is less than the capacity of the HVAC plant, the airflow shall be reduced to save energy.
8. Optimization of the chillers is another measure. The chillers should be upgraded as and when necessary. The hospital shall prefer to install more upgraded chillers, which shall have the provision to get synchronized with the actual load of cooling on the chillers. For example, the screw chillers. Screw chillers automatically slow down as soon as the requirement of chilled water goes down and vice versa. These upgraded chillers can reduce energy costs to a great extent.
9. Install Building Automation System (BAS) to control the HVAC system. The BAS keeps systems running according to operating schedules, setpoints and fundamental sequences of operation. The programming coordinates the operation of thousands of components, including everything from boilers and chillers, air handlers and exhaust fans, dampers and valves. One disadvantage of the BAS is that it typically prioritizes the indoor environment (i.e. temperature, humidity or air changes per hour) over energy efficiency.
10. FDD is another software that helps the management to reduce energy costs. FDD uses analytics software to continuously collect performance data from the BAS and identify potential faults. Faults are identified by evaluating a set of algorithms that are applied based on the system configuration.
11. Operating rooms in the hospital have very strict requirements for environmental conditions such as air changes per hour, humidity, pressure and temperature, hence a major space for energy consumption. A handsome amount of energy savings can be achieved by reducing their energy consumption by switching off the HVAC system of OR when not in use.
12. The refrigerant devices containing Chlorofluorocarbons (CFC) shall be replaced with other devices which do not contain CFC as a refrigerant. Preference shall be given to buy equipment that uses refrigerants that contain less potent ozone-depleting substances (ODSs) and with reduced global warming potentials (GWPs).

48.4.5 Chemical Management

Chemicals are very much prevalent in hospitals. The chemicals are generally used in the hospital building for maintenance, infection control and also during the treatment of the patient. Out of all the chemicals used in the hospital, some chemicals or the components of the chemicals are considered to be harmful and toxic to human beings and/or the environment.

Chemicals and fuels used in or around the hospital should be used with caution to prevent contamination and reduce exposure to staff, patients, visitors and the surrounding community. Antibacterial/antimicrobial products and sterilization and disinfecting chemicals also are commonly used in the health sector.

The following issues shall be addressed to manage the chemicals effectively:

1. Never dispose of liquid waste that contains cleaning or disinfection chemicals and agents down the drains.
2. Necessarily frame the chemicals and materials policy and protocols to protect patient, worker and community health and the environment. The policy shall have a specific chemicals action plan with benchmarks and timelines.
3. Create Mercury-Free Hospital by substituting all mercury thermometers and blood pressure devices with safe, accurate and affordable alternatives.
4. Monitor and manage the use of chemicals like glutaraldehyde, halogenated fire retardants, solvents and disinfectants, soaps, chlorine, radioactive substances, PVC, DEHP, and BPA. If possible, replace them with other safer alternatives and substitutes.
5. Try using chemicals which undergone at least basic toxicity testing.
6. If very high chemicals like carcinogenic, mutagenic or toxic for reproduction are used, hospitals should make it a high priority to replace them with safer alternatives.
7. Use equipment that is more efficient and uses less hazardous chemicals.
8. All the chemicals shall be labelled properly to avoid and accident or spilling.
9. Where ever possible prefer using natural cleaning products instead of chemicals.
10. Carefully and safely apply the pesticides and other chemicals for plantation in the exterior or interior of the hospital building.
11. Arrange for a good, experienced and reputed waste disposal agency if the hospital does not have its own incinerators.
12. Strictly follow the national chemical management policy of the country to reduce the purchase and use of hazardous chemicals.
13. Careful storage of hazardous chemicals with limited access is necessary.
14. Proper training shall be given to the staff and users as to how to handle, store and apply the hazardous chemicals.
15. Correctly label and properly store all chemicals as per the manufacturer's recommendations.
16. Try to phase out the use of Ethylene Oxide and the high-level disinfectant (HDL) glutaraldehyde and other hazardous substances and replace them with safer alternatives. Alternatives to Ethylene Oxide can be low-temperature sterilization methods such as vaporized hydrogen peroxide, hydrogen peroxide gas plasma, liquid peracetic acid and ozone.

48.4.6 Solid Waste Management

Hospitals usually generate a lot of waste. The waste generated by the hospital can be biodegradable, recyclable or hazardous. Proper segregation, storage and safe and effective disposal of such waste are essential to achieve the concept of the green hospital. It has been seen that about 10% to 15% of the total waste generated is from hospitals.

Improper disposal of such waste, in open dumps areas or the rivers etc., attracts a lot of disease vectors, release unpleasant odours and may also lead to transmission of diseases like malaria, typhoid, cholera, HIV and Tuberculosis. The sharp instruments, if not handled and disposed of properly, may lead to infections like Hepatitis B and C through injuries from such sharps contaminated with human blood.

The hospital can reduce waste and emissions through composting, recycling, minimizing packaging, using reusable rather than disposable products, buying recycled products and minimizing waste transport.

Operating rooms of the hospitals in themselves produces waste of about 20–30 percent of total hospital waste. Out of this packaging material used to protect and maintain the sterility of supplies and equipment accounts for a large part of the waste. Increased use of disposable supplies and equipment further adds to this problem.

The following issues need to be addressed for an excellent waste management:

1. Strictly follow the norms, policies and guidelines of the country for handling and disposal of hazardous waste.
2. Reduce the construction waste is also beneficial in building green hospitals.
3. Promote using recycled and renewable materials along with more sustainable construction methods.
4. Try avoiding toxic materials such as mercury, plastic, PVC and unnecessary disposable products.
5. Set up a waste management committee and allocate a budget for waste management.
6. Hospitals shall have a policy of segregation of waste at the source itself and non-hazardous wastes shall be sent for recycling.
7. Implement a comprehensive waste management training program and awareness campaigns to control waste.
8. Train and vaccinate the waste handlers and promote using personal protective equipment while handling waste.
9. Disposal of the waste shall be done in an economical, safe and environmentally friendly manner.
10. Establish the policies and guidelines to achieve zero waste and align the operations and procedures of the hospital to achieve this goal.
11. Storage of the waste shall be in a secured and restricted space.
12. Biodegradable wastes such as papers, cardboard, vegetable and plant wastes, food items etc. shall be composted at a proper place as demarcated by the local authorities.
13. The infected plastics shall be landfilled after disinfection, rather than incinerating because the burning of plastic produces greenhouse gases and toxic pollutants such as dioxins and furans.
14. Reducing inhaled anaesthetic atmospheric waste by utilizing low fresh gas flows, avoiding high impact inhaled anaesthetics like Desflurane, Nitrous Oxide and considering intravenous and regional techniques.
15. Reduce intravenous pharmaceutical waste by preferring prefilled syringes, appropriately sized vials and disposing of unused medications and vials as per laid down policy and regulations.
16. Reduce anaesthesia equipment waste by opening equipment intended for immediate use, preferring using reusable or reprocessed equipment instead of disposables, and reprocessing or recycling suitable disposable items.

48.4.7 Environmental Services

A clean environment in and out of healthcare facilities is important to reduce and control infections, provide quality air and reduce pests etc.

A clean environment protects the healthcare workers, patients and visitors in the hospital from exposure to pollutants and chemicals that could irritate, trigger medical conditions or cause serious harm.

Some of the measures that can be taken for a better environment is as below:

1. Attention shall be paid to the components of cleaning agents, pest control chemicals and all other such materials used inside and outside the hospital. If any of these are toxic and harmful to the environment, they should be discouraged.
2. The concept of Integrated Pest Management (IPM) shall be adopted to reduce the use of harmful chemicals, target specific pests and

shall increase the use of safer alternatives and techniques and limit exposure of applicators, humans and other organisms.

3. Avoid using or minimize the use of products that are manufactured with carcinogens, mutagens and teratogens; aerosols; respiratory irritants; neurotoxins; endocrine modifiers; asthma-causing agents, and chemicals that aggravate existing respiratory conditions; benzene-based solvents, highly acidic or alkaline products; butoxyethanol, chlorinated organic solvents, paradichlorobenzene; anti-microbial agents in hand soaps; bioaccumulative and toxic chemicals (PBTs) and products requiring disposal as hazardous waste.
4. Minimize atomizing chemicals.
5. Reduce use of virgin paper in janitorial paper and prefer using disposable paper products, such as paper and hand wiping towels which contain recycled content.
6. Promote usage of microfiber-based cleaning equipment which cut chemical waste, increase performance and reduce labour.
7. Improve the air quality inside and outside the hospital as it is one of the most vital components of any green building. The environment is suffering from poor quality air due to rising pollution. This can be achieved if more and more indoor plants are provided, which produces oxygen and reduces indoor pollutants from the air and are the natural air purifiers.
8. As hospitals are exposed to many pathogens and bacteria, it becomes necessary to have a ventilation system and a well-designed cleanroom to continuously provide fresh and filtered air.
9. Protect and restore natural habitat and minimize the combined footprint of buildings, parking, roads and walks.
10. Avoid materials such as lead and cadmium-containing paint and coatings, as well as asbestos.
11. Create facilities for natural ventilation and if required the mechanical systems for increasing the ventilation.
12. Improve the lighting and acoustical settings to reduce stress and support health and productivity.
13. Providing courtyard spaces with native and adaptive plant free from allergic effects improve fresh air of the environment.
14. Ensuring those roof parapets and caps are properly sealed and do not allow the pests to enter the roof and grow.
15. The bird nests, honey traps are checked regularly and removed immediately as and when noticed.
16. Repair and plug and orifices, cracks and holes in the walls to keep pests out of them.
17. Inspect the grounds around buildings and fill burrows with gravel.
18. Keep vegetation at least 1000 mm away from the main building perimeter.
19. Use physical barriers to block entry of pets, animals inside the hospital premises.
20. Prohibit smoking in the hospital. If any smoking area is designated, make sure it is at least 50 feet from the hospital to reduce the impact of smoke on patients, healthcare workers staff and visitors and also to prevent interior surfaces from absorbing the smoke.
21. Ensure that the smoking area is downwind and away from main entrances/exits, windows, air conditioning units and air intakes.
22. Ensure that all windows are openable to take full advantage of prevailing breezes of air. However, despite the energy savings and reduced environmental impact, it may not always be practical to use natural ventilation at all times. In that case, the mechanical systems shall be given for ventilation.
23. Avoid foam being used in the furniture like chairs, sofa sets, beds etc. as it is likely treated with a variety of flame retardants. Prefer using furniture with mesh instead.

48.4.8 Food Services

Agriculture and food systems have a significant impact on the environment and human health. Diets habits with increased saturated fats, refined carbohydrates and processed foods are some of the factors that are increasing the burden of diseases amongst the community. This leads to more and more long-term therapies and treatments. The treatment and therapies increase the healthcare cost and also the healthcare sector's environmental footprint.

Hospitals can promote health by providing fresher, good tasting, nutritious food choices for patients, healthcare workers and visitors by supporting food production that is local, humane and protective of the environment and health.

Large inputs of pesticides and chemicals lead to the degradation of soil, water and other natural resources. The use of energy such as fire to burn left out roots in the farms releases pollution in the atmosphere and contributes a lot to climatic change.

The farm processes like planting, reaping, transportation, processing, packaging, shipping and the use of man-made inputs make the global farming system unsustainable. Similarly, livestock, contribute greenhouses gases to the atmosphere and pollute other resources as well.

To achieve an environmentally friendly food system, the hospital shall keep in mind the following few issues:

1. Strive to eliminate using disposable food containers and bottled water as plastic from food services and bottled water will likely end up in a landfill or incinerated. If still there is a need to use disposable products, use biodegradable/compostable food service wares.
2. Paper products such as napkins often used in food services consume natural resources and generate additional waste, hence the use shall be minimized. Instead of that paper products with recycled content offer a better, more sustainable option.
3. Food waste can be removed from the waste can be composted on-site, to other designated places and this compost can be reused in farms and add to the overall sustainability of the agriculture sector. Even commercial composters are available on the market that can turn discarded food into compost.
4. To make hospitals and the overall health sector more sustainable, it has to be ensured that the food products have been produced in an environmentally safe and sustainable manner and the changes must be made as to how food is prepared, provided and served.
5. Implement a sustainable food plan and policy and increase the procurement of locally and regionally produced foods.
6. Examine ways to reduce food waste by implementing innovations such as room service, meals on-demand and just-in-time food preparation.
7. Supporting the habit of donating food that remains at the end of daily operations to food banks, churches and other community groups rather than disposing of it.
8. If space permits, promote community and staff to start an organic garden onsite.
9. Declare the hospital as a 'fast food free zone' and as far as possible eliminate sugar-based soft drinks in hospital cafeterias and vending machines.
10. Encourage vendors to supply food that is produced without using synthetic pesticides and hormones or antibiotics given to animals. This will support farmers' health and welfare, as well as ecologically protective and restorative agriculture.
11. Promote, educate and bring awareness to the patients, healthcare workers, visitors and the community at large about nutritious, socially equitable and ecologically sustainable food practices and procedures.

48.4.9 Environmentally Preferable Purchasing

During the normal course of operation, the hospitals have to necessarily purchase a lot of products such as pharmaceuticals, chemicals, reagents, disposables, consumables, equipment, fixtures, food and cleaning and other general supplies. These items leave a significant impact on the hospital's carbon footprint.

If environmentally friendly products are purchased, it can have a significant impact to improve sustainability.

Hence, the products purchased with the environment in mind should be less toxic; minimally polluting; more energy-efficient; safer and healthier for patients, workers and the environment; contain higher recycled content; have less packaging and shall be fragrance-free.

For environmentally preferable purchasing, the following shall be taken care of:

1. As far as possible the products such as pharmaceuticals, chemicals, disposables, consumables or any other articles shall be purchased with minimal packing as the packaging and other materials add to the waste stream and contribute to environmental degradation.
2. As incinerating or disposing of mercury-containing items in landfills is not recommended, Introduce the policy to phase out the instruments and equipment containing mercury and replace it with other sustainable items.
3. Wherever and whenever possible insist on procurement practices and patronize local vendors who supply the third-party certified sustainable products and follow sustainable and ethical practices.
4. Insist the suppliers disclose chemical ingredients and safety testing data. Once satisfied, only after that product shall be purchased. Preference shall be given to the suppliers and products meeting these specifications and are environmentally preferable.

48.4.10 Sustainable Construction Materials

As the world is preferring and thinking of more sustainability, construction also is one part of such thought and effort. Sustainability is important for a better quality of life and environmental quality. To have thriving and healthy communities, the need is to have clean air, natural resources and a non-toxic environment.

Sustainable construction is creating a healthy environment that is designed and constructed based on ecological principles. Sustainable construction focuses on principles like protect nature, high quality, conserve, reuse, recycle/renew and create non-toxic effects on the environment.

Over the years due to evolvement, the construction techniques, resources and building practices have been improved and new methodologies and materials are being used in the construction. Even new methods, technologies and techniques have been evolved to make the construction more sustainable and promote energy conservation.

For sustainable construction the following issues shall be addressed;

A. Materials

To introduce sustainability in construction, the choice of construction has to be very careful. The hospital shall prefer purchasing new generation stronger, lighter and more sustainable building materials. The materials that add to protect the environment and reduce the carbon footprint of the buildings shall be preferred.

B. Methods

Apart from the material, the building methods also enhance renewable and sustainable efforts. Some of these methods are like

1. Cutting and reshaping the materials precisely to reduce wastage.
2. Using material that produces less wastage like wooden flakes that wood is planed to wood dust arising during cutting of the plyboard etc.
3. Using iron scaffolding instead of wooden scaffolding.
4. Constructing green buildings.
5. Adaptive reuse projects that transform old buildings.
6. Managing construction sites by properly managing the materials to improve the environment like treating water on-site, properly covering the construction materials, no smoking and recycling food containers.
7. Conserving Energy while construction.

48.4.11 Pharmaceutical Minimization, Management and Disposal

For a healthy environment the procurement, management and disposal of the pharmaceuticals in a prescribed appropriately, safely manner are necessarily required. As the leftover and expired pharmaceuticals shall not be disposed of by just dumping in the landfill, it has to be disposed of in a prescribed manner. Hence the following measures shall be adopted:

1. Prescribe small initial quantities of pharmaceuticals during new prescriptions.
2. Avoid providing samples of medications to patients, as these often end up in the waste stream, but prefer to the poor patients who find it difficult to purchase medicines.
3. Provide necessary training for safe and proper disposal of the leftover expired pharmaceuticals.
4. Develop training programmes for healthcare workers to optimize their medicine prescribing practices.
5. Introduce the concept of centralized procurement and distribution plans for pharmaceuticals. This shall help in controlling the purchased quantity, over procurement, expiry and will also streamline the distribution of the pharmaceuticals.
6. While procurement of the pharmaceuticals, enter into contracts with the suppliers to ensure the return of excess pharmaceuticals.

48.4.12 Reducing Transportation Cost

More the utilization of transport, more the pollution, resulting in leaving a powerful impact on health issues. The transport sector is considered to be a major source of greenhouse gas emissions, and thus an important focus of climate change mitigation.

The hospital can reduce its transportation emissions by effective following a few of the following measures:

1. Arranging or providing public transportation infrastructure near to the hospital.
2. Preferring usage of alternate fuel like CNG and electric vehicles.
3. Promoting the healthcare workers, patients and visitors to use bicycles, public transportation and carpools.
4. Prefer purchasing products from local suppliers or/and suppliers who use fuel-efficient transportation.
5. Promote telemedicine as it reduces travelling resulting in the reduction of air pollution.
6. Provide off-site small healthcare of the hospital at a different location, that is easily accessible to patients, staff and visitors, hence avoiding unnecessary travel.
7. Dispose of hospital waste near to the point of a generation hence avoiding unnecessary transportation of the waste.

48.4.13 Greenery

Greenery in and around nursing homes, hospitals and clinics is beneficial for the climate inside and outside the organization and has a positive effect on the patients' state of mind and ability to recover, as well as the general well-being of patients, staff and visitors.

Greenery inside and outside the hospital can reduce stress among patients and staff, purify air, reduce concentrations of CO_2 and volatile organic compounds, reduce heat in and around buildings in summer, reduce heat stress, reduce the need for air-conditioning, increase insulation capacity, make surroundings more attractive, moves the focus away from pain and stress, releases water vapour thus humidifying the air and lower city temperatures.

The below-mentioned measures can be adopted for increasing greenery inside and outside of the hospital:

1. Create courtyards and other gardens which can be used for relaxation, treatment, sunbath or other naturopathy procedures.
2. Create green roofs, facades and walls.

3. Provide indoor gardens in central areas, company restaurants, waiting rooms and some treatment areas.
4. Provide attractive landscaping of the hospital grounds, including green borders and trees.
5. Green roofs top or rooftop gardens reduce heating and cooling costs inside the hospital rooms.
6. Increase planted surfaces around the hospital and plant trees on nature strips to reduce the heat-island effect.
7. Provide larger green zones in and around the hospital, which can create a pleasant climate.
8. Promote indoor plants to improve the air quality inside buildings as indoor plants can remove pollutants, especially CO_2 and volatile organic compounds by improving humidification.
9. Try planting shaded trees in the car parking area to reduce the evaporation of fuel from fuel tanks, reduce visitors' heat stress and lower fuel consumption by reducing the use of air-conditioning in cars.
10. Planting dense vegetation on the boundary of the hospital can act as a barrier and can help to protect the hospital's property.
11. Design the rooms in a manner that outside greenery is visible from the patient's bed.
12. Create attractive green outdoor gardens for ambulatory patients to relax.
13. Ensure easy access to the indoor and outdoor green areas.

Further Reading

Greening the Operating Room [Internet]. [cited 2021 Jul 28]. Available from: https://www.asahq.org/about-asa/governance-and-committees/asa-committees/committee-on-equipment-and-facilities/environmental-sustainability/greening-the-operating-room

Healthcare [Internet]. Healthcare | Johnson Controls. [cited 2021 Jul 28]. Available from: https://www.johnsoncontrols.com:443/en_sg/solutions-by-industry/healthcare

Inc B. Sustainable Construction: Methods and Benefits | BigRentz [Internet]. 2020 [cited 2021 Jul 28]. Available from: https://www.bigrentz.com/blog/sustainable-construction

PatientEngagementHIT. Smart Hospitals Making the Future of Patient Experience a Reality [Internet]. PatientEngagementHIT. 2020 [cited 2021 Jul 28]. Available from: https://patientengagementhit.com/features/smart-hospitals-making-the-future-of-patient-experience-a-reality

SHT_GreenChecklist.pdf - Section III THE GREEN CHECKLIST AND DISCUSSION GUIDE Hospitals use the greatest proportion of energy during daily operations | Course Hero [Internet]. [cited 2021 Jul 28]. Available from: https://www.coursehero.com/file/45576348/SHT-GreenChecklistpdf/

Smart hospitals: the digital future of global health | Hospitals [Internet]. Healthcare Global. [cited 2021 Jul 28]. Available from: https://healthcareglobal.com/hospitals/smart-hospitals-digital-future-global-health

What is smart hospital? What are the characteristics of smart hospital? [Internet]. ResearchGate. [cited 2021 Jul 28]. Available from: https://www.researchgate.net/post/What_is_smart_hospital_What_are_the_characteristics_of_smart_hospital

Part VI

Equipment Planning

49 Equipment Planning

The term equipment may have different definitions in respect to different contexts but for hospital it is generally defined as 'the articles and implements required to perform specific activities'. If analyzed for a hospital, the equipment are the tools and methods which facilitates the care providers in performing the diagnostic investigation to diagnose the disease and help in treatment of the diagnosed disease. In a true sense, the equipment in the hospital refers to the medical and mechanical machines used for diagnosis and treatment but are different from the fixtures and fittings.

Equipment in hospital can be either Fixed Equipment or Loose and Mobile Equipment. Fixed equipment is generally the equipment that is fixed to the building and can be like MRI, CT Scan, X-ray, LINAC, Mammography or a large sterilizer etc. Loose equipment are items that are not fixed to the building and can be moved easily as and when required to any other place. These can be items like monitors, surgical instruments, ECG machines and Ultrasound.

As medical equipment is the most vital component in any hospital. Therefore, the planners of hospital need detailed planning and coordination, assess the clinical needs and the equipment requirements and then only move forward for procurement.

Efficient planning of the hospital equipment requires a clear understanding of the clinical need along with detailed knowledge about budgeting, architectural design and building process.

The ultimate objective of equipment planning is to ensure all products selected are suitable for the hospital functioning, within the allotted budget and are procured, delivered and commissioned within the stipulated time frame and in accordance with project requirements.

The equipment planner shall plan the requirements either for the medical only or both the medical and non-medical equipment. An assessment of major and minor equipment shall be made to evaluate the need for equipment in terms of functionality and cost. While assessing the requirement of the equipment the following factors shall be considered:

1. What is the need for equipment?
2. Financial cost of equipment.
3. Functionality of equipment.
4. Frequency of use of equipment.
5. Income likely to be generated by the equipment.
6. Useful life of the equipment.
7. Period of return of investment for equipment.
8. Expected technology changes of the equipment.
9. Determine equipment reuse and relocation options.

While planning, the planner shall understand equipment preferences, concerns and priorities after conducting interviews with the departmental heads. He/She shall also review the

A. Garg, A. Dewan, *Manual of Hospital Planning and Designing*,
https://doi.org/10.1007/978-981-16-8456-2_49

architectural drawing and details to ensure that all the elements of the building fulfil the requirement for an efficient functioning of the equipment.

49.1 Choosing the Desired Equipment

Once the list of equipment is finalized, the planner has to choose the desired equipment out of the lot available in the market.

In today's competitive market, there are a lot of manufacturers manufacturing the same equipment, and each manufacturer has different models of the same equipment. Different models may have different costs depending on the specifications, configuration, capacity, size, performance and facilities. It is the planner who has to decide as to what is needed and which model best suits the requirement.

49.1.1 Quality of the Equipment

While choosing the medical equipment, tools and devices, the issues related to the quality of these items shall not be compromised. One shall look for a vendor with a quality mindset, which focuses on patient safety, product quality and compliance.

All the healthcare facilities use a lot of medical equipment and devices, which are from simple equipment to a complex machine combined with different technologies. Whatsoever it may be, the quality of such devices and equipment shall be ensured and shall never be compromised even if the cost of such quality equipment is bit more. The main factors in favour of quality assurance are:

1. Non-quality products may have defects or disturbances in functioning and may expose patients to serious risks like injury, sickness and even death.
2. The non-standard equipment may not have been calibrated as per the standards, which may give wrong results and the physician may not be able to diagnose the ailment properly.
3. Non-standard devices may have defects or malfunctions that could lead to severe consequences.
4. Quality products are generally safe, and by that said, free from unacceptable risks for persons, property or environment.
5. Throughout the globe, the medical equipment and devices are subject to extensive rules and regulations and there are a number of different standards and regulation systems to follow. Hence, the medical equipment and devices shall ensure the standards of the regulating authorities like US Food and Drug Administration (FDA); (QSR) to ensure product performance and safety; Standard ISO 13485 complements the Medical Device Directive etc.
6. This is true that if the quality of the medical equipment and devices is as per the laid down standards, the life of the equipment shall be more as compared to non-standard equipment and devices.
7. The repair and maintenance cost of the quality equipment and devices will be less as compared to others.

49.2 Points to Be Considered While Purchasing the Medical Equipment

Finalizing the specification and configuration of equipment: Before finalizing the equipment the specification, configuration of the equipment has to be finalized and depending on these specifications the vendors shall be sorted out. While finalizing the specification and configuration of the equipment, the planner shall try to choose the equipment with the latest technology and specification. On the other hand, the financial feasibility of the latest technology shall also be considered before choosing the specifications. Why we insist on the latest technology is that, in today's world the technologies are changing rapidly and the present technology may be outdated in a few years. In such a case, the hospital will be left with no other options but to replace the equipment in a few years' time. However, a careful comparison shall be done between the increased costs of latest equipment versus the technology requirement of the hospital.

49.2.1 Warranty

Go for the maximum warranty period. The longer the warranty period, less the worries of the hospital authorities about maintenance of the equipment.

49.2.2 Maintenance Contracts

Many equipment manufacturers provide the Annual Maintenance Contract. The maintenance contract can be with or without space parts. The maintenance contract without spares is called as AMC and with spares called CMC (Comprehensive Maintenance Contract). It is advisable to choose the CMC instead of AMC as it eases for management of the hospital to be least worried about the cost of spares required to be replaced.

49.2.3 Availability of the Service Engineers and the Workshops

Before procurement, the planner has to ensure that the vendor has their own workshop and the team of engineers available near the hospital so that the breakdown call can be attended in the shortest time period. Further, the preventive maintenance schedule can be carried out regularly. Further, it shall also be ensured that the vendors maintains sufficient stock of the spare parts of the machine to enable repair of the machine immediately, without calling the spares parts from a distinct place, which may ultimately lead to time delay and may increase the dead time of the machine.

49.2.4 Period of Spare Part Availability

Before procurement, the planner has to ensure the period or years for which the vendors shall be able to provide the spare part of the equipment. This period shall not be less than 10 years.

49.2.5 Cost of Consumables

Some of the medical equipment, e.g. laboratory analyzers, generally require consumables for day to day working of the equipment. Before purchasing the equipment, the cost of such consumables shall also be checked and compared with the cost of other vendors. Some of the laboratory equipment are designed on the technology of Closed System (means the reagent of the same manufacturer can be used) others are Open System (any make of reagents can be used). It is better to choose open system instead of closed system, otherwise hospital shall have to depend only on the same supplier for reagents, and he/she may charge whatever amount he/she likes.

49.2.6 Life Expectancy of the Equipment

Before purchasing the equipment, the expected life of the equipment shall be ensured. Also, the assessment has to be done regarding the technology changes and improvement in the design or specifications of the equipment.

49.2.7 Plan for Space and Development

As far as the space for equipment is concerned, every room in a hospital, of whatever nature it may be like patient room, ICU, diagnostic lab, radiology or emergency, has its own unique demands. So, before assigning a space or a room, ensure that there are sufficient and efficient spaces to install the desired equipment.

49.2.8 Vendors Evaluation

Planner has to check the track record of the vendor with respect to the quality of the after-sale service provided by him/her, efficiency, availability of the spare parts, infrastructure for after-sale service etc.

49.2.9 Checking Regulations

As some of the equipment are bound by the regulations of the local building codes, accreditation agencies, controlling authorities, other norms and regulations of the federal and state legislature and industry standards that the equipment must conform to. Therefore, during the planning phase itself, all such norms and regulations shall be identified and followed while purchasing the equipment.

49.2.10 Inspection and Testing Before Transfer of Ownership

Before transferring the ownership and signing the final commissioning reports, the Biomedical Engineer shall inspect and test the equipment. Thereafter, the equipment shall be commissioned and dummy tests to be performed for testing the operation of the equipment. While testing the issues like electrical safety inspection and radiation safety shall also be taken care of before giving the final affirmation.

49.3 Equipment Used in the Hospital

In hospitals, there are a lot of different equipment which are required for the efficient working of the hospitals. Some of them are too small and less costly whereas others may be the big equipment which requires large spaces and are costly.

It is not possible to compile the list of all the medical equipment available in the market today, but we have tried to list out a few of them along with the purpose for which it is used.

List of Medical Equipment Generally Used in the Hospital

49.4 General Items Used in Intensive Care Units, Wards, Pre & Post-Operative Units, Post Labor Wards, Triages Area and OPD's Etc.

Department and name of the equipment	Usage and purpose
Air bed	Air bed is a mattress that prevents bedsores and also relieves pain from sore spots, pressure spots and pressure ulcers.
Analyzers blood gas/pH	This analyzer is used to determine pH levels, partial pressure of carbon dioxide and oxygen in the blood.
Bipap machine	This is also called non-invasive ventilator and is used to supply pressurized air in the airway of the patient. As the device helps open lungs with the air pressure, it is also called 'positive pressure ventilation'.
Blood warmer	At times the blood or fluids needs to be heated before transfusion to the patient. For this, the blood warmer is used. It is particularly used when a large volume of cold fluids are to be transfused.
Defibrillator	Defibrillator sends an electric pulse or shock to the heart which restores the normal heartbeat. Defibrillator is also used to prevent or correct arrhythmia. Defibrillators can also be useful in restoring the heart's beating, in case the heart suddenly stops. This device is also a life-saving device. In hospitals, it shall be kept ready all the time so that it can be used when suddenly required.
DVT pump	DVT pump is a pneumatic compression pump that is designed to prevent the patient from developing deep vein thrombosis (DVT). This pump delivers a set pressure resulting in increased blood flow in the venous system of the limbs, which prevents blood clotting.

Department and name of the equipment	Usage and purpose
ECG machine	ECG machine (electrocardiograph) is used to measure and record the electrical activity of the heart.
Echocardiograph	Echocardiograph is used to see the anatomy of the heart. For echocardiography, the technique of sound waves is used to produce live images of the heart. Echocardiography also allows to monitor the functioning of valves of the heart. With echocardiography, the information about blood clots in the heart chambers can also be obtained.
Electrolyte analyzers	Electrolyte analyzers measure electrolytes in serum, plasma and urine.
Hemoglubinometer	A hemoglobinometer is to measure haemoglobin blood concentration. It uses the spectrophotometric technique to measure the haemoglobin concentration in the blood.
High flow nasal cannula	Hi flow nasal cannula (HFNC) is a nasal cannula to provide very high oxygen flow rates. Apart from this the device actually takes oxygen that can be heated to 37 °C with a 100% RH and can deliver 0.21–1.00% FiO_2 at flow rates from 20 to 60 litres/min.
Humidifier	Humidifier is used to add moisture contents in the oxygen which in turn prevents dryness which may otherwise cause irritation in different parts of the body.
ICE lined refrigerator	Ice lined refrigerators are used to save vaccines and store blood bags with temperature range from +2 °C to +8 °C.
Infusion pumps	An infusion pump is to deliver fluids, such as medications and nutrients, to patient's body in preset and controlled amounts or volume.
Invasive ventilators	Invasive mechanical ventilator is a lifesaving device used after intervention for patients suffering from respiratory or breathing problems. The primary purpose of mechanical ventilation is to provide oxygen to the patient, remove CO_2, decrease the efforts involved in breathing and reversal of life-threatening conditions such as hypoxaemia, insufficient oxygenation of arterial blood, and acute progressive respiratory acidosis, or build-up of CO_2 in the blood.
Multi Para Monitor	This monitor is used to keep track of the vital of the patient. Generally, the fixed parameters are blood pressure, heart rate, respiratory rate, pulse oximetry and temperature. Multipara monitors help provide information on multiple parameters like ECG, blood pressure, respiration, oxygen saturation and temperature to understand the condition of patients and monitor vital signs. Apart from these fixed parameters other parameter modules can be attached to the device like $EtCO_2$.
Pulse oximeter	Pulse oximeter is a non-invasive equipment used to measure oxygen saturation level, or the oxygen levels in the blood.
Suction machine electrical	Suction machine is a tracheostomy care device used to remove any obstruction from a patients' airway. The machine uses the technique of suction to pull out mucus, saliva, blood, secretions or other fluids stuck up in the airway, hence clearing the airway for easy breathing.
Syringe pumps	To gradually administer specific amounts of fluids to the patient (which has been preset), the syringe pump is used. Syringe pumps push the fluid in the patient's body via syringe, to inject a predetermined volume of fluid or medication in a gradual manner.

49.5 Department of Cardiology and CTVS

Department and name of the equipment	Usage and purpose
ACT machine	Activated clotting time (ACT) is used to monitor anticoagulation effects, after administration of the intense amount of anticoagulation medicines like heparin. ACT machine is used to monitor ACT before, during and shortly after surgeries that may require higher doses of anticoagulation medicines, such as CTVS and interventional cardiology.
Ambulatory ABP monitor (ABP)/ELR	Ambulatory blood pressure (ABP) monitor is to monitor the blood pressure continuously at the specified intervals over 24 h and thus get an overall profile of blood pressure variation in a day.

Department and name of the equipment	Usage and purpose
Cath Lab	A Cath lab is basically imaging equipment used to see the conditions of the arteries and check how well blood is flowing to and from the surface of the heart. Cath lab helps to diagnose and treat blockages that may have occurred in the arteries. It is used to perform procedures like coronary and peripheral angioplasty, angiography, cardiac catheterization, artherectomy, stent implantation and thrombectomy.
Electro physiology Lab	Electrophysiology (EP) lab is used for electrophysiology studies (EPS). This is to monitor and map the electrical systems of the heart as well as treat heart rhythm problems (arrhythmias).
Holter monitoring system	Holter monitor is a portable device used to monitor the electrical activity of a cardiovascular system for at least 24 and up to 72 h.
Intra-aortic balloon pump	An intra-aortic balloon pump, or IABP, is to control the flow of blood through aorta. The device uses a balloon, which gets deflated when the heart pumps blood, to give way to the blood to flow out in the body. On the other side, the balloon gets inflated when the heart relaxes to retain more blood in the heart.
Pacemaker temporary	When the patient suffering from Brady dysrhythmia, and temporary treatment has to be provided, the temporary pacemaker is used. Such conditions may arise when either the permanent pacemaker is not necessary or is not immediately available.
TEE probe with ultrasound	TEE is basically an ultrasound probe that work on high-frequency sound waves to take detailed pictures of the heart and the arteries that lead to and from it, from the backside of the heart. The probe of the TEE passes to the backside of the oesophagus to capture images of heart structures and valves.
Tilt test table	A tilt table test is to adjust the body position from horizontal to vertical for simulating standing up. The test is used to access faulty brain signals that may be causing low blood pressure.
TMT	TMT is basically a treadmill used to make the patient run and put the heart under stress. During different phases of stress on the heart, the ECGs are taken to detect any abnormal heart rhythms (arrhythmias) and also to diagnose any coronary artery disease.

49.6 Department of Gastric Sciences

Department and name of the equipment	Usage and purpose
24 h pH impedance	Oesophageal 24-h pH/impedance reflux monitor is used to measure the amount of reflux (both acidic and non-acidic) in the oesophagus during 24-h period. This is also used to assess any symptoms that may be correlated with the reflux.
Breath analyzer	A breath analyzer is an instrument to estimate the alcohol contents in the blood (BAC) from a breath sample.
Capsule endoscope	A capsule endoscope is a small capsule-like device having a tiny wireless camera that is swallowed while performing the procedure. This capsule endoscope takes pictures as it passes through the stomach, large intestine and small intestine. These images are then transmitted to the recording device worn on a belt around the waist of a technician. These recorded images are ultimately processed in the central processing unit to get the report.
Cholangioscope/ Choledochoscope, flexible or rigid	Cholangioscope is an endoscope to visualize inside of the bile ducts. It is used to treat the removal of bile duct stones. When coupled with the visualization of the pancreas, it is called cholangiopancreatoscopy.
Colonoscope	The colonoscope is used to examine the colon, and another such device called proctosigmoidoscope is used to examine rectum and lower colon. These devices are passed through the anal orifice into the colon or the rectum as the case may be.
Duedenoscope	Duodenoscopes allow seeing the top of a patient's small intestine, or duodenum. It is mostly used for endoscopic retrograde cholangiopancreatography (ERCP).

Department and name of the equipment	Usage and purpose
Electro surgical cautery with argon	Argon plasma coagulation (APC) is for controlled electrocoagulation via high-frequency monopolar energy through a contactless method. It is used to monitor rates of initial haemostasis, causes of recurrent bleeding that may require urgent surgery.
Endoscopic Ultrasound (EUS)	Endoscopic ultrasound (EUS) consists of high-frequency sound waves endoscope and is used to assess gastrointestinal and lung diseases. The EUS produces a clear and detailed image of the lining and walls of the digestive tract and chest along with the nearby organs such as the pancreas, liver and lymph nodes.
Enteroscope	An enteroscope is a device used to look inside of the small bowel. It is basically an endoscopy procedure that may be used for diagnosis and treatment of different types of digestive conditions.
Manometry unit	The manometry system is used to evaluate the motor functions of the oesophagus. The system provides useful information for diagnosis of diseases like dysphagia, achalasia and hiatal hernia.
Upper gastro intestinal scope	An upper gastrointestinal (UGI) is used to examine the inside lining of oesophagus, stomach and the duodenum. The tip of the scope, having a light bulb and camera, is inserted from the mouth, gently moved down the throat into finally into the oesophagus, stomach and duodenum, where it takes the images under bright light conditions and transmits the images to the central processing unit for further processing of the images.
Upper GI endoscope PEDIA	An upper gastrointestinal (UGI) is the same as in adults but with the difference that being smaller in size is used for paediatric patients.
Video processor	The processor is used for processing and displayable the image signals received from the endoscopes.

49.7 Nephrology and Dialysis

Department and name of the equipment	Usage and purpose
Colorimeter	To measure the concentration of a known solute in a given solution with the help of the Beer-Lambert law, the Colorimeter is used.
Dialysis chairs	Dialysis chair is basically a recliner and is used during the procedure of dialysis. Earlier the patient beds were used for dialysis. As the patient has to lie down ideal for 3–4 h, it was difficult to pass time and was uneasy for the patient. With the chair, the positioning of the chair can be changed as per the convenience of the patient and he/she can also watch the TV etc.
Dialysis machines	A dialysis machine is used to filter out the metabolic waste products and remove excess water from the blood and for this the artificial kidney or so called dialyzer is used.
RO plant	Reverse osmosis (RO) is a device used to purify water using the technique of reverse osmosis. The permeable membrane fitted in the device is used to remove ions, unwanted molecules and larger particles from water.

49.8 Neurosurgery

Department and name of the equipment	Usage and purpose
Auditory system, evoked response	Auditory evoked potential (AEP) machine is used to examine and determine the functional integrity of the auditory system. AEP is a type of EEG signal emanated from the brain scalp by an acoustical stimulus, which reflects the auditory ability level of the patient.

Department and name of the equipment	Usage and purpose
Aversive conditioning device	An aversive conditioning device is used for the administration of an electrical shock or other noxious stimuli to a patient which helps in modification of undesirable behavioural characteristics.
Biofeedback device	To gain control over involuntary bodily functions such as blood flow, blood pressure and heart rate, the biofeedback is used which basically uses the mind-body technique that involves using visual or auditory feedback.
Electroconvulsive therapy device	Electroconvulsive (ECT) is a device used to treat seizures in the brain, which are electrically induced in patients to provide relief from mental disorders.
Hypothermia device for spinal-cord injury	Therapeutic hypothermia is used in various types of neurological injury such as stroke, traumatic brain injury and post-anoxic encephalopathy.
Interferential current therapy	Interferential current therapy is used to provide relief from the pain and accelerate the self-healing process. In this therapy, the high-frequency signals are penetrated by the IFC through the skin into deeper lying muscular tissues.
Intracranial pressure monitoring device	The intracranial pressure monitoring devise is used to monitor the intraventricular catheter inserted into the lateral ventricle through the brain.
Neurosurgical fragmentation and aspiration device	Cavitron ultrasonic surgical aspirator (CUSA) is to remove the tumour by fragmentation, irrigation and aspiration.
Ophthalmodynamometer	This device is used for the detection of hemodynamically significant carotid stenosis. In this technique, the reliability of two pressure-dependent methods, namely ophthalmodynamography and ophthalmodynamometry, is established to get the desired results.
Pinwheel	Pinwheel is used to measure the nerve reactions when the instrument is rolled against the skin. This device consists of 7″ stainless steel handle with a wheel of evenly spaced sharp pins called the spur. The device helps to test the extent of neurological damage, and to ensure nervous system communication after surgery.
Probe, lesion, radiofrequency	This device is used for the insertion of a probe transcutaneous into an orifice (foramen ovale) in the base of the skull under sedation.
Skin potential measurement device	This device is to acquire skin potential response (SPR) signals. SPR is a branch of electro dermal activity (EDA) and involves reading of nervous electric pulses that may arise when the sympathetic nervous system activates the sweat glands due to any external stressing stimulus.
Stimulator intracerebral/subcortical	Intracerebral/subcortical stimulator is implanted in the body and is used for pain relief by applying electrical current to subsurface areas of a patient's brain.
Stimulator nerve	A nerve stimulator sends low levels of electrical impulses directly into the nerves to give relief from the pain. Nerve stimulation is used most often for nonsurgical pain treatment.
Stimulator neuromuscular	Neuromuscular electrical stimulation sends electrical impulses to nerves. Due to these electrical impulses, the muscles contract.
Stimulator peripheral nerve	Peripheral nerve stimulation (PNS) is used to treat chronic pain. In this process, a small electrical device (a wire-like electrode) is placed next to one of the peripheral nerves by surgery, which in turn stimulates the nerves.
Stimulator spinal-cord	A spinal cord stimulator is a device that is implanted inside the body which then sends low levels of electrical impulses directly into the spinal cord to relieve pain.
Stimulator Vagus nerve	Vagus nerve stimulator sends regular, mild pulses of electrical energy to the brain via the Vagus nerve to prevent seizures to the patient.

49.9 Neurology

Department and name of the equipment	Usage and purpose
Electroencephalograph (EEG)	In electroencephalogram (EEG) small, metal discs (electrodes) are attached to the scalp and is used to detect electrical activity in the brain. The cells of the brain communicate via electrical impulses and are active during the procedure. This activity is recorded in the form of wave and is then analyzed.

Department and name of the equipment	Usage and purpose
EMG (electromyogram)/ NCV/EP machine	EMG is used to measure the muscle response to the nerve stimulation and evaluates electrical activity within selected muscle fibres. This test is used to differentiate between a muscle disorder and a nerve disorder. NCV is to measure the speed at which an electrical impulse travel along a nerve.
Nystagmograph	To measure, record or visually display the involuntary movements (nystagmus) of the eyeball, the nystagmograph is used.
Plethysmograph, ocular	Plethysmograph is used to measure changes in volume in different parts of the body. The test is to check for blood clots in the arms and legs and also to measure the capacity of lungs as to how much air the patient can hold in lungs.
Polysomnography (PSG)	Polysomnography, also known as a sleep study, is to diagnose sleep disorders. This test records the brain waves, oxygen level in blood, heart rate and breathing, as well as eye and leg movements during the study.
Transcranial magnetic stimulation (TMS)	Transcranial magnetic stimulation (TMS) uses magnetic fields to stimulate nerve cells in the brain to improve symptoms of depression and is a non-invasive procedure.
Video electroencephalography (VEEG)	A video EEG records what the patient is experiencing or doing on videotape while the EEG test records the brainwaves.
VNG	Videonystagmograph (VNG) is used to measure a type of involuntary eye movement called nystagmus.

49.10 Plastic Surgery

Department and name of the equipment	Usage and purpose
CO_2 fractional laser	Fractional CO_2 laser is for steady rejuvenation of the face, neck, chest and hands by stimulating natural collagen production in the skin. It can also be used for facelift or neck lift by laser resurfacing in combination with aesthetic facial surgery.
Cryosurgical unit and accessories	Microfine jets of cryogen are used in a variety of different conditions including skin tags, acne, dermatofibroma, wrinkles, viral warts, lesions as well as scar tissue, burns and keloids, keratosis, small skin cancers, abrasions, basal cell carcinomas, solar lentigo etc.
Diode laser	A diode laser is to target specific chromophores in the skin by using a light beam with a narrow spectrum.
Electric dermatome	Electric dermatome is a skin grafting instrument and is used for providing skin graft with capabilities of variable thickness and width.
Ervium Yag Laser	Erbium laser resurfacing is to remove surface-level and deep lines and wrinkles on the face, hands, neck or chest.
Hair growth laser	Laser hair growth system is to treat hair loss for both men and women as it stimulates hair follicles to grow thicker and dense hair.
Hyper boric oxygen therapy machine	Hyperbaric oxygen therapy is used to treat decompression sickness, bubbles of air in the blood vessels, serious infections, and wounds that may not heal due to diabetes or radiation injury.
KTP laser	A KTP laser is a solid-state laser that uses the technique of potassium titanyl phosphate (KTP) crystal. A beam of green visible spectrum is produced and directed through the KTP crystal.
ND Yag Laser Long Pulse	An Nd:YAG laser produces near-infrared wavelength, which penetrates deep into the skin and is easily absorbed by haemoglobin and melanin chromophores.
ND Yag Laser Q Switch	Q-switched mode Nd:YAG produces dual wavelengths, one of the infrared ranges (1064 nm) and the second beam of 532 nm wavelength. These waves are useful for superficial skin lesions. It is mainly used for melisma and tattoo removal as it produces a high-intensity beam in very short pulses.
Osteotome	An Osteotome is used for cutting or preparing bone and is just like a chisel but is bevelled on both the sides.

Department and name of the equipment	Usage and purpose
Pulse Diode Laser	Pulsed lasers emit light in the form of optical pulses. However, depending on the pulse duration, pulse repetition rate, pulse energy and wavelength required, different methods for pulse generation and different types of pulsed lasers are used.
RF Cautery	In radio frequency, high-frequency radio waves are passed through soft tissue to cut, coagulate or remove the said tissue.
Varicose laser	Varicose vein laser is used to reduce varicose veins with heat technology. The laser sends a thin beam of radiation in the form of light.

49.11 Pulmonology

Department and name of the equipment	Usage and purpose
Body box diffusion	Body plethysmograph is used for pulmonary function test which determines the quantity of air in the lungs after the patient takes in a deep breath. It also measures the amount of residual air left in the lungs once the patient exhales as much as he/she can.
Broncho fiberscope adult/ pediatric	This is an endoscope that passes through the trachea to inspect the interior of the tracheobronchial tree for endobronchial diagnosis and treatment. It is also used to take specimens for culture and biopsy and removal of foreign bodies from the tracheobronchial tree.
Diffusion for DLCO	DLCO is to predict abnormal gas exchange during exercise.
EBUS	Endobronchial ultrasound (EBUS) is an instrument which is used to diagnose lung cancer, infections and other diseases causing enlarged lymph nodes in the chest.
Endobronchial ultrasonography TBNA	EBUS TBNA is to see inside the lungs and carry out the procedure with the help of a special kind of thin and flexible bronchoscope.
FENO (fractional exhaled nitric oxide)	Fractional exhaled nitric oxide (FeNO) is measured in the human breath test because of airway inflammation.
PC based spirometry	Spirometry is used to assess how well the lungs are working by measuring the quantity of air the patient inhales, quantity of air exhaled and how quickly the patient can exhale. Spirometry is used for diagnosis of diseases like asthma, chronic obstructive pulmonary disease (COPD) and other conditions affecting breathing.
PFT system with diffusion, Ros Q MEP/ MIP	This is to measure maximal inspiratory pressure (MIP) and maximal expiratory pressure (MEP) for maximal strength of respiratory muscles.
Polysomnography (Sleep Lab)	Polysomnography, also known as a sleep study, is to diagnose sleep disorders. This test records the brain waves, oxygen level in blood, heart rate and breathing, as well as eye and leg movements during the study.
Rigid Bronchoscope	Rigid bronchoscopy is for accessing the patient's airway and also allows to pass the larger airway instruments and cameras for diagnosis and treatment of airway disease.
Video Broncho scope	A video bronchoscope uses a CCD camera located at the distal tip of the bronchoscope to sense, capture and transmit images to the processor for further analysis.
Video Thoracoscope set	Thorascope is used to evaluate and treat pleural effusions in patients suffering from pulmonary tuberculosis.

49.12 Radiation Oncology

Department and name of the equipment	Usage and purpose
Brachytherapy	Brachytherapy is used for planting radioactive substances inside the body of the patient. Brachytherapy is a type of radiation therapy used for treating cancer. Brachytherapy is also known as internal radiation.

Department and name of the equipment	Usage and purpose
Cyber Knife 6MV	Cyber Knife is a Stereotactic Radio Surgery (SRS) system. SRS is a combination of principles of stereotaxic, or three-dimensional target radiation. In this procedure, the radiation beams from multiple directions cross-fire the tumour precisely at the desired point. Due to the high degree of precision, it becomes possible to deliver higher doses of radiation to the targeted area with minimal damage to the normal tissues and structures surrounding the tumour.
Linac linear accelerators	A linear accelerator, or also known as LINAC, is a machine used to deliver external beam radiation to treat cancer patients. A linear particle accelerator is a type of particle accelerator that accelerates charged sub-atomic particles or ions to a high speed by subjecting them to a series of oscillating electric potentials along a linear beamline.

49.13 Urology

Department and name of the equipment	Usage and purpose
Automatic device for monitoring and detecting kidney damage	This device is to automatically monitor and detect kidney damage of the patients. The sentinel device in this machine continuously monitors the urine output and measures urine flow rate and volume in real time.
Columns, Immunoadsorption in Extracorporeal Systems	Extracorporeal Immunoadsorption (ECI), using protein A columns, is used for selectively removing circulating immune complexes (CIC) and immunoglobulin's (IgG) from patients in whom these substances are associated with their diseases.
Cystometric device, hydraulic	Cystometry is used to measure the amount of urine actually in the bladder Vis-a-Vis how full the bladder feels. It is used for diagnosis of the main muscles of the bladder wall (the detrusor) or urethra (the urethral sphincter).
Erectile dysfunction device	A vacuum constriction device (VCD) is a device used by a man with erectile dysfunction. This is an external pump with a band on it to get and maintain an erection of the penis. The VCD system consists of an acrylic cylinder with a pump and the constriction ring or band. The cylinder and pump are used to create a vacuum to help the penis become erect whereas the band helps to maintain the erection
ESW lithotripter	Extracorporeal shock wave lithotripsy (ESWL) is used to break the kidney stone into small pieces using shock waves. These tiny pieces can more easily travel through the urinary tract and pass out from the body. By precisely locating the stone with the help of X-rays or ultrasound, the shocks are delivered to the stone, where it breaks into tiny pieces.
Uroflometer	Uroflometer is a device to measure urine flow rates during micturition, including peak flow rate, average flow rate, voided volume and time of voiding.
Wearable, smartphone controlled device for treating premature ejaculation (PE)	The device once placed on the perineum area, deliver a mild form of electrical energy through four electrodes, which confuses the ejaculatory nerves before they go up to the brain.

49.14 Robotic Surgery

Department and name of the equipment	Usage and purpose
Surgical robot with master control, magnified 3D HD vision, slave control, foot pedals for electrosurgery, clutch for camera and instrument control, surgical manipulator; endowrist functionality etc.	Robotic systems are used for robotic surgery. In this technique, the patient is laid on the OT table, and the surgeon gives command from the joystick from control room and the arms of the robot, fitted with the desired surgical instruments, perform the surgery. Mainly it is used for urological surgeries. But also now being used for cardiac surgeries, GI surgeries and plastic surgeries.

49.15 Orthopaedic

Department and name of the equipment	Usage and purpose
Goniometer	A goniometer is used to measure an angle or permitted rotation of an object to a definite position. This art and science of measuring the joint ranges in each plane of the joint is called goniometry.
Plaster Cutter	Plaster cutting saw is used by technicians to remove plaster and fibreglass casts from the patient.
Sensory Evoked Potential (SEP)	A somatosensory evoked potential test (SEP) is the study related to relay of body sensations to the brain and how the brain receives those sensations. In this process, the stimulating electrode is placed on the arm or leg, which generates an electrical signal.

49.16 Dermatology

Department and name of the equipment	Usage and purpose
Cryotherapy unit	Cryotherapy, also known as 'cold therapy', is a technique where the body is exposed to extremely cold temperatures for several minutes. The patient is made to stand in an enclosed chamber with head outside the chamber from top and the body is exposed to cold temperature for therapy.
Derma Abrader	Dermabrasion is used to remove the outer layers of skin which are damaged. With this, the new layers of skin are exposed.
Derma Peel	Derma Peel helps to erase fine lines and wrinkles, reduce enlarged pores, help build collagen and elastin, which helps to tighten and firm the skin. It is also used for reduction or even eliminating hyperpigmentation and melisma. The device is also helpful to remove acne and acne scars.
Dermatoscopes	Dermatoscope is a device that uses visible light like LED bulbs and is used for examination of suspicious skin lesions.
Electro-Cautery machine	Electrosurgery Cautery is used to cut, coagulate, dissect, fulgurate, ablate and shrink tissues. During process, the high-frequency DC current at various voltages is passed through tissue where the heat is generated.
Fractional CO_2 laser	Fractional CO_2 laser is used to stimulate natural collagen production in the skin of the face, neck, chest and hands. This leads to steady rejuvenation for several months which lasts for several years. This device is also used along with aesthetic facial surgery for facelift or neck lift.
Iontophoresis unit	Iontophoresis is used to treat bursitis, tendonitis/tendinopathy and to manage scar tissue. The technique used is electrical stimulation which helps in administering medication into the body through skin.
Ultraviolet lamp	Ultraviolet lamp is used for treatment for certain skin diseases such as psoriasis, acne, eczema and vitiligo.
MIPL laser	Intense pulsed light (IPL) is used to perform various skin treatments like hair removal, photo rejuvenation such as skin pigmentation, sun damage and thread veins.
Puva Chamber	PUVA (psoralen and ultraviolet A) is an ultraviolet light therapy and is used for the treatment of skin diseases like Eczema, Psoriasis, Graft-versus-host disease, Vitiligo, Mycosis Fungoides, Large-Plaque Para psoriasis and Cutaneous T-Cell Lymphoma.
RF Cautery	Radio frequency is used to cut, coagulate or remove the soft tissue by passage of high-frequency radio waves through tissue.
Skin biopsy punches	Skin biopsy punch is used to obtain full-thickness skin specimens. The device consists of a circular blade or trephine attached to a pencil-like handle.
Skin ultrasound imaging systems	High-resolution ultrasonography (HRUS) is used for non-invasive assessment of skin nodules and cutaneous diseases.

Department and name of the equipment	Usage and purpose
Woods lamp	A Wood's lamp uses long-wave ultraviolet light and is used to diagnose diseases like tinea (a type of ringworm fungus). When viewed by Wood's light, the fungus glows to detect the fungal scalp or skin infection.

49.17 ENT

Department and name of the equipment	Usage and purpose
Audiometer	Audiometer is a machine used to evaluate hearing acuity. The patient is given headphone to wear which is connected to the machine.
Electroglottograph	The electroglottograph, or EGG, (Laryngograph) is used for the non-invasive measurement of the degree of contact between the vibrating vocal folds during voice production.
ENT EXM unit, endoscope, camera, chair	ENT examination unit consists of adjustable electric chair and the exam unit has the facility for endoscope and other diagnostic instruments like throat mirrors, nasal and ear speculum etc. this unit is used for initial examination and diagnoses of diseases of the head and neck, ear, nose and throat regions.
Esophagoscope (flexible or rigid)	An esophagoscope is used to figure out what is causing abnormal throat, stomach or intestinal symptoms. Take a tissue sample (biopsy) for diagnosis of cancer or other conditions, such as dysphagia or gastroesophageal reflux disease (GERD).
Filli Form Set, Eustachian	Eustachian Tube Catheter is a device consisting of a bougie of filiform catheter and is used for probing or dilating the Eustachian tube.
Impedance Audio Meter	The impedance audiometry is used for tympanometry to determine the status of the tympanic membrane and middle ear. It is also used to evaluate acoustic reflex pathways including cranial nerves and auditory brainstem.
Laser, ENT microsurgical carbon-dioxide	CO_2 lasers are used for less invasive and highly precise head and neck surgeries like removal of cancer tissues while protecting the healthy structures, nerves and tissues.
Nasopharyngoscope (flexible)	Flexible nasopharyngoscope is used for examination of the nose, throat and airway.
Otodyamics Otoport (DP + TE) (OAE)	Otoport DP clinical handheld OAE instrument is used for OAE examination and can easily be switched between analytical clinical modes and screening modes.
Otoscope	An otoscope also called auriscope is a device used to look inside the ears. With the help of the light bulb and lenses built in the device, it gives a view of the ear canal and tympanic membrane or eardrum.
Speech Trainer Software	Speech trainer 3D provides an animated 3D video and audio model for 24 consonants and 7 vowel sounds.
Strobo Laryngoscope (Endoskope)	In stroboscope connected to a strobe light is used to register the frequency of the voice. The stroboscope is applied to the skin of the neck overlying the larynx, which then flashes just slightly out of sync with the frequency. The video image of the vibration of the vocal fold is produced for analysis.
Temporal Bone Lab Station	In the temporal bone lab, residents work at four operative stations to learn the complex anatomy of the temporal bone and the ear at the base of the skull.

49.18 Gynaecology

Department and name of the equipment	Usage and purpose
Colposcope (and Colpomicroscope)	Colposcope is a device used to examine the vulva, vagina and cervix with the help of a magnifying lens and bright light. It depicts the abnormal epithelium to identify abnormal biopsy and to evaluate the cervix followed by pap smear.

49.19 Ophthalmology

Department and name of the equipment	Usage and purpose
Applanation Tonometer	Applanation tonometer is used to measure the intraocular pressure, or IOP, of the eye. IOP is determined by the amount of force that is needed to flatten or appellate, a consistent area of the cornea.
A-Scan	A-scan ultrasound biometry provides data on the length of the eye and is used to determine sight disorders. This machine is also used for calculating the power of IOL lenses before cataract surgery.
A-Scan with water immersion	This device allows the scans of the eye to be taken without compressing the cornea. Under this technique, a small immersion scleral shell is placed onto the eye between the lids, filled with BSS and immersing the probe into the fluid without contacting the cornea. The BSS acts as an ultrasonic coupling media allowing scans.
Auto Keratometer	A keratometer, also known as an ophthalmometer, is used to measure the curvature of the anterior surface of the cornea for assessing the extent and axis of astigmatism.
Auto Refractometer	Auto refractometer is used to measure the degree of refractive error in the eye and the suggested correction powers lenses to be used.
B-Scan with UBM	B-scan is a two-dimensional cross-sectional view of the eye as well as the orbit. B-scan helps to view accurately the other structures of eye-like lens, choroid, sclera, vitreous and retina. The machine is particularly helpful to diagnose retinal detachment.
C3R Machine	C3R is Corneal Collagen Cross-linking with Riboflavin. In the device, ultraviolet light is used to promote increased cross-linking between collagen fibres within the cornea.
Contrast Sensitivity Chart	A sine-wave grating test is a contrast sensitivity test. Patient looks at several parallels, fuzzy bars of dark and light. This test provides the details as to how eyes view contrast.
Exophthalmometer	An exophthalmometer is used to measure the degree of forward displacement of the eye in exophthalmos.
Femto Lasix	It combines femtosecond technology with high-precision lenticular extraction. This device can cut the cornea precisely without opening a large corneal area.
Fornixscope	A fornixscope is a device used to pull back and hold open the eyelid for proper examination of the conjunctiva.
Frame, Trial, and Trial Box—Ophthalmic	An eyeglass frame for holding trial lenses while a person is being fitted for glasses. Trial box is a set of glasses of different powers and the glasses are mounted in the steel rings. This is used for clinical examination used by optometrists and ophthalmologists to determine a patient's need for refractive correction.
Fundus Camera	A fundus camera is a low-power microscope with an attached camera.
Humpry Automated	Humpry is used in neuro-ophthalmic conditions, early detection of glaucoma and general screening. The device is also used to measure 24° temporally and 30° nasally at 54 points.
Indirect Opthalmoscope	The indirect ophthalmoscope is used to inspect the fundus or back of the eye. The device produces a stereoscopic image with magnification ranging from 2× to 5×.
Keratometer	A keratometer (ophthalmometer) is used to measure the curvature of the anterior surface of the cornea, for assessing the extent and axis of astigmatism.
Lensometer	A lensmeter or lensometer, also known as a focimeter or vertometer, is used to verify the power of the lenses of eyeglasses. It is also used to properly orient and mark uncut lenses and ensure correct mounting of lenses in spectacle frames.
NA Yag Laser (Long Pulse Yag Laser)	Nd: YAG laser is used to correct posterior capsular opacification.
O.C.T	OCT is used to generate an image of the retina to examine patients with glaucoma. The picture is made by precisely measuring the amount of dim red light that reflects off the retina.
Ocular Esthesiometer	An ocular esthesiometer is a device is to assess corneal sensitivity, by touching the cornea with a single-hair brush.
Ophthalmic Camera	Retinal cameras are used to take images of the retina to diagnose disease or progression of disease in the retina. These images can also be used to view the central and peripheral retina, optic disc and macula.

Department and name of the equipment	Usage and purpose
Ophthalmic Refraction Unit	Ophthalmic refraction chair unit is used for initial examination of the eye. The chair has a facility to mount slit-lamp, auto-refractometer, projector and near vision holder on the chair.
Ophthalmoscope	Ophthalmoscope allows seeing inside the fundus of the eye and other structures of the eye. It is used as a routine physical examination of the eye.
Orb's Scan	The Orbscan corneal topography system is used to evaluate the anterior and posterior corneal surface topography along with the thickness of the entire cornea.
Pachymeter (NCT)	Pachymeter is used to measure the thickness of cornea. A probe of the device is gently placed on the cornea to measure its thickness.
Radiation Beta Unit	Beta radiation is a valuable therapeutic adjunct in the management of lesions of the anterior segment of the eye.
Retinoscope	Retinoscope is used to observe the light that is reflected from the retina by illuminating the inside of the eye.
Slit-lamp	A slit lamp is a microscope with a bright light used for an eye examination. The device gives a closer look at the eye both from the front and inside the eye.
Synapthophare	This instrument is used to diagnose imbalance of eye muscles and treat them by orthoptic methods.
Tonometer, non-contact (Pachymeter)	A non-contact tonometer with the help of a small puff of air measures the pressure of the eye known as pneumotonometry.

49.20 Operating Rooms

Department and name of the equipment	Usage and purpose
Anesthesia Workstation	The device is used to administer anaesthesia to the patients before and during surgery. It is designed in such a fashion that can mix and control the flow of nitrous oxide and oxygen. This device also consists of the invasive ventilator and the gases are delivered with the help of this ventilator.
Arthroscope set with accessories for knee and shoulder	Arthroscope is a small endoscope-like instrument, about the size of a pencil and is used in the arthroscopic surgery. An arthroscope consists of camera, lighting bulb and lens, which allows a surgeon to view inside a joint. With the help of this device only small incisions are required to be made and the joint need not be fully opened.
Boyles Machine	Boyle's machine is a device to mix the medical gases along with the accurate concentration of anaesthetic vapor, and to deliver this to the patient continuously at a safe pressure and flow.
Camera HD	The HD camera is one part of the laparoscopic surgery and is used to record the high resolution, full-featured, colour and multi-format images. The camera is mounted on the distal end of the endoscope to provide an unobstructed view of the surgical site.
C-ARM	A C-arm is an X-ray-based imaging intensifier. The CCD camera/X-ray detector and the X-ray source is mounted on the C-shaped arm in the opposite direction to each other. C-arm is used for fluoroscopic intraoperative imaging during surgeries and procedures.
Cryogun	The patented Cryogun allows works in situ for the most accurate sample collection possible. When structural and biochemical integrity is a must, the patented Cryogun assures of the best frozen and/or vitrified samples.
ECT Machines	Medical device intended to treat catatonia or a severe major depressive episode with depressive or bipolar disorder and older who are treatment-resistant or who require a rapid treatment response.
EES Generator (Harmonic)	The harmonic scalpel is just like surgical cautery but more advanced and is used to cut and cauterize tissue simultaneously.
Elec. Surgical Cautery	Electrosurgical is used to cut, cauterize the tissue with a pencil-like probe attached to the machine. The pencil probe procedures, the tissue is heated by a high voltage DC current and is heated up.

Department and name of the equipment	Usage and purpose
Fetal Doppler	A Doppler foetal monitor is a hand-held ultrasound transducer used to detect the foetal heartbeat for prenatal care.
Head light	Head-light is a LED light fitted with microscopic lenses and is used for microsurgery or for routine examination also.
Heavy Duty OT Table	Heavy duty operating table is safe for bariatric patients.
Holmium/Thulium YAG Laser	Holmium:YAG laser is the preferred laser for lithotripsy and is used in urology. The holmium laser operates at 2120 nm and delivers energy through optical fibres with core diameters ranging from 200 to 1000 μm.
Hyperthermia system, extracorporeal	The aim of whole body hyperthermia is to raise the overall core body temperature up to 107–108 °F to kill malignant cells. This is often achieved through the use of hot water blankets or thermal chambers, which resemble large, human-sized incubators.
Insufflator	Insufflator is to blow CO_2 in the stomach while performing the laparoscopic surgery.
Laparoscopy set	Laparoscopes are a thin telescope fitted with a cold light source and a video camera on the distal end. These scopes pass inside the body and the image is captured by camera under brighter conditions and displayed on the screen. The laparoscopic instruments are passed inside the body through the laparoscope and the desired surgery is performed.
Laser scalpel	The light scalpel is a CO_2 laser that produces a concentrated beam of light. The highly focused CO_2 laser beam vaporizes and seals the blood vessels simultaneously very cleanly and precisely.
Light source with Fibreoptic cable	A fibre light source is to produce high intensity light and transmit it to the tip of the endoscope through the fibre optic cable. The light source is available with halogen bulbs or led bulbs.
Micro processor controlled electrosurgical unit	ESU is basically a surgical cautery for cutting and cauterization but is controlled by the fast microprocessor processing all operating parameters.
Mobile ultrasound system	Portable ultrasound is a small and light device and is basically used in the OR the patients' bedside for ultrasound. The machine operates with the battery power backup.
Modular operation theatre with pendants	Modular operating theatre is a theatre built-in with the modules having a provision of air filtration through Hepa filers and airflow in a laminar style. It consists of a modular wall, ceiling with slanted panels, plenum, control unit, PDR, Hepa filters with a provision of laminar flow to maintain the positive pressure in the OR. The OR has the facility of electrical points and medical gas outlets along with surgical or anaesthetic pendants.
Morcellator	A power morcellator is used to cut bigger chunks of tissue into smaller ones, usually during laparoscopic surgery.
Multi Para monitor with $ETCO_2$	The machine provides the facility to monitor CO_2 for intubated and non-intubated patients. It is mainly used in the ORs when the patient is on anaesthesia workstation. At the time, it is also used in the ICU for sick patients.
Operating microscope	Operating microscope is a device fitted with light and high-powered lenses for magnification. This device is used for surgeries like neurosurgery, vascular surgery or the eye surgery where magnification is required.
OT light	An OT light is a ceiling mounted LED light with adjustable high lumen light used for surgery. These lights are shadow less and no heat is generated. The light is used to aluminate the surgical field.
OT table	An operating table is a table where the patient is laid down for surgery. The table has a provision for multi-positional adjustments and provisions to attach the required attachments to ease the surgery. The table can be operated hydraulically, electrically or a combination of both.
Pneumatic tourniquet electric	Pneumatic tourniquet is to apply pressure on the arterial blood flow, through cuffs, in a limb to create a bloodless surgical field. The cuffs are inflatable and the machine consists of a pressure-regulated control unit.
Portable OT light	A portable OT light unit with battery backup and flexibility of clamping it to OT table.
Recording system	Recording system is used to record the live and still images in HD format from the endoscopes/laparoscopes during surgeries. These captured images can either be displayed on the screen or can be saved for later revival.

Department and name of the equipment	Usage and purpose
Scrub Station	Scrub sink is used by surgeons and other surgical staff for scrubbing before surgery. Scrub sinks are normally foot operated, sensor operated or hand operated.
Surgical Loupe	Surgical loupe is a head wearable device that enhances and magnifies the field of surgery.
Telescopes	The telescopes transmit light coaxially through each barrel, to provide converging light at the operative site. The telescopes eliminate the need for constant realignment of loupes and headlights.
Vaporizer	Vaporizer is a device used to vaporize substances for inhalation.
Vitreous aspiration and cutting	A vitreous aspiration is an ultrasound-based device and is used for removing the vitreous matter from the vitreous cavity or removing a crystalline lens from the eye.
Operative Room CTVS	
Cardiopulmonary Bypass Blood Pump (Heart Lung Machine)	Cardiopulmonary bypass blood pumping machine (CPB) or so-called heart lung machine, is used during surgeries where the heart needs to be stopped for surgery. The machine takes over the function of the heart and the lungs and maintains the circulation of blood and the oxygen content of the body.
Hypothermia device (blanket, plumbing and heat exchanger)	This device is used to control the temperature of the body of the patient. After the surgery when the heart starts beating again, the body temperature of the patient needs to be lowered for a short time.
Patient warming system	Patient warming system (PWS) uses a heated surgical table pad and optional over body blanket immediately upon transfer to the surgical table to provide heat to the patient before, during or after the surgical procedures.
Sternum saw	A sternum saw is a bone cutter used to cut the sternum bones for opening the patient's chest to perform surgery. The saw has a reciprocating type of blade and resembles a jigsaw in appearance.
Vacuum stabilizer system octopus	The octopus tissue stabilizer is used to immobilize the target site of the coronary artery while performing bypass cardiac surgery.
Operating Room ENT	
Drill & saw system	Bone Drills & saw System: Bone drill is an electrically/pneumatically operated device and is used to drill holes through the bones or cut the bones to fix implants during the orthopaedic and ENT surgeries.
ENT operating microscope	Microscopes for otolaryngology allow to carry out complex and minimally invasive ENT surgical procedures with a high level of precision to enable the best possible clinical outcomes.
Operating Room Eye	
Operating (Loupe), Ophthalmic	Surgical loupe is a head wearable device that enhances and magnifies the field of surgery. These loupes are used in oculoplastic procedures, strabismus cases and retinal cases.
Ophthalmic operating microscope	Operating microscope is a device fitted with light and high-powered lenses for magnification. This device is used for ophthalmic surgeries having small structures.
Ophthalmic laser (green)	This is basically an argon laser that emits blue-green wavelengths. These waves are absorbed by the cells under the retina by the red haemoglobin cells in blood.
Phacofragmentation unit	Phacofragmentation is used for the removal of eye lenses and is used during refractive and cataract surgery. With this device, the crystalline lens is manually deteriorated and is removed in the pieces through a 4–5 mm incision.
Operating Room Gynaecology	
Culdoscope	Culdoscope is a kind of endoscope that is introduced through the vagina into the cul-de-sac to visualize female pelvic organs.
Hysteroscope	Hysteroscope is a thin device for examination inside of the cervix and uterus and is inserted through vagina. Hysteroscope is also used to take a biopsy or remove polyps or fibroid tumours.
Operating Room Neuro surgery	
Neuro endoscopes	Neuroendoscope is an endoscope for minimally invasive surgery and is used to remove the tumour from the brain through small holes in the skull or through the mouth or nose. The biggest advantage of this endoscope is that it is possible to reach such regions of the brain which is otherwise difficult to reach by traditional surgery.

Department and name of the equipment	Usage and purpose
Neuro Surgical Operating Microscope & Spine drill	Like other operating microscopes, this microscope has a provision for higher magnification under illumination and provided a better and enlarged view of the field of surgery. The microscope also has a facility of recording by connecting the camera in the third eyepiece of the microscope.
O-arm navigation—Spine	The O-arm navigation is generally used for spine surgeries as it allows visualization in real time of the surgical site. Due to its mobility, lower doses of X-ray images and speedy image processing, it provides live 3D navigation during surgery.
Stereotactic frame	A stereotactic head frame is used to trace out the reference points for targeting for surgery. In the process, the frame is fixed at the patient's head using local anaesthesia to numb the scalp. Thereafter, the indicator box is then attached to the head frame, and the MRI or CT scan is done.
Operating Room Urology	
Cystourethroscope	Cystoscope, or cystourethroscope, is used to have an inside of the bladder and urethra in detail for diagnosis or surgery.
Flexible Fiber Urotero-Renoscope	The flexible Uretero-Renoscope is also a type of endoscope which is used to have better access and ability to perform surgery of the upper urinary tract. As it consists of high-resolution camera and light bulbs at the distal end, it provides clear, sharp imaging.
Lithotriptor	Extracorporeal shock wave lithotripter is used for treating stones in the kidney and ureter that do not require surgery. By lithotripter, high-energy shock waves are passed at the desired place to break stones into pieces as small as grains of sand which then passes from the body along with the urine.
Nephroscopes	Nephroscope is used for removal of small kidney stones and small tumours. In this procedure called PCNL, by a small cut the nephroscope is passed inside to remove stones up to about 1 cm.
Pediatric cystoscope	Pediatric cystoscope is slim in design. There are many types of cystoscopes of varying different straight or angled channels and with angled or straight ocular, both with 70° direction of view and 4.2 Fr channel.
Resectoscope	Resectoscope is used to remove tissue from the body. Due to its specific design, it is also used to cut, remove or destroy tissue and control bleeding.
Urethrotome	Urethrotome is used to treat urethral stricture under direct visualization endoscopically. This instrument has a knife blade that is deployed by the surgeon.
Operating Rooms Orthopaedic	
Bit, drill, micro motors, saw reamers etc.	These tools are used for different types of orthopaedic surgeries starting from simple surgeries like intramedullary nailing of long bone fractures to complex surgeries like total joint arthroplasty.
Navigator for hip replacement	Navigation helps to minimize errors during surgery. This device provides precise information on the implant positioning, accuracy of the bone cuts, ligament balancing and final alignment of the limb as it provides a real-time visual information about the surgical field.
Navigator for knee replacement	Knee navigation an infrared-based real-time tool used during surgery of total knee replacement. This device provides precise information on the implant positioning, accuracy of the bone cuts, ligament balancing and final alignment of the limb as it provides a real-time visual information about the knee site.

49.21 Dental

Department and name of the equipment	Usage and purpose
CBCT	Dental cone beam computed tomography (CT) is used for CT scan by dentists. This technology is used to produce three-dimensional (3-D) images of teeth, soft tissues, nerve pathways and bone in a single scan.

Department and name of the equipment	Usage and purpose
Electro surgical unit and accessories, dental	Dental electrosurgical unit is used for sculpture of living tissue without pressure, controlling bleeding and inducing heat in fluids.
OPG	An OPG (Orthopantomagram) is basically an X-ray machine that has a provision to scan the upper and lower jaw in a panoramic view. It shows a flattened two-dimensional view of a half-circle from ear to ear.
X-ray unit, intraoral	The intraoral X-ray unit is used for getting a precise positioning, straightforward imaging and good quality of images in high resolution.

49.22 In Vitro Fertilization Clinic

Department and name of the equipment	Usage and purpose
CODA extra inline filter	Coda filters are for use to filter VOCs and contaminants. Coda is used to improve the air quality in the incubator and in the laboratory, which helps a lot to improve embryo and cell development.
Heracell CO_2 incubator	CO_2 incubator provides optimal growth conditions to enhance cell growth. Heracell CO_2 incubators provide accurate, uniform and reliable culturing conditions. The fan-assisted convection provides samples with a uniform temperature CO_2 and humidity within the incubator.
Integrated vertical laminar flow with TFT monitor and FCG table	Integrated vertical laminar flow provides unidirectional airflow through HEPA filters over the entire surface of the work tables and effective air exchanges.
Inverted microscope with micromanipulator	Inverted microscope is used to imaging the live cell sinked at the bottom and onto the coverslip for adherence.
Recorder, pressure, intrauterine	Intrauterine pressure (IUP) transducers are electronic catheter–tipped and used to record intraluminal pressure changes by responding to increase and decrease in the diameter of uterine lumen. It also has one or two ultra-miniature pressure sensors at the distal end coupled by a cable to a computer.
Spermfuge	Spermfuge is a temperature regulated centrifuge. The instrument is used for regulating and maintaining the 'critical' inner chamber temperature before, after and during centrifugation.
Trinocular stereo zoom microscope	A trinocular microscope, apart from two eyepieces, has one extra eye tube for connecting a microscope camera. This is basically a binocular microscope with a moving prism assembly in which light is directed to the third eye tube.

49.23 NICU

Department and name of the equipment	Usage and purpose
Baby incubator	An incubator is a device that is capable of providing an ideal environment with required temperature, perfect amount of oxygen, humidity and light, which is an ideal condition for the infant to develop. Hence, this device is used for pre-term infants while their vital organs develop.
Infantometer	Infantometer is for measuring the size (length) of infants.
Neonatal CPAP (bubble)	Bubble CPAP is a non-invasive ventilation device used for newborns with infant respiratory distress syndrome (IRDS). This device provides positive airway pressure (CPAP) which is delivered for spontaneously breathing of newborn to maintain lung volumes during expiration.
Pediatric ventilator	The critically ill children who require total or partial assistance to maintain adequate breathing, this machine is used. This invasive ventilator provides temporary breathing support to the child.

Department and name of the equipment	Usage and purpose
Phototherapy upper and under surface	Phototherapy is a treatment with a special type of light with a specific wavelength for lowering bilirubin levels in neonatal.
Radiant warmer	Radiant warmer is a device to maintain the body temperature of the baby and limit the metabolic rate. The heat loss in some newborn babies is rapid; hence body warmers provide an artificial support to keep the body temperature constant.

49.24 Pain Clinic

Department and name of the equipment	Usage and purpose
Manujet III Transtracheal jet	The Manujet III is a kit that consists of injector and jet ventilation catheters. Jet ventilation catheters allow transtracheal access for oxygenation/ventilation with a manual jet (Manujet III) or an automatic high-frequency jet ventilator.
SpineJet discectomy unit	The SpineJet HydroSurgery system uses the power of water in surgery. In this machine, a controlled hair-thin supersonic stream of water is used which is capable of an effective cutting, ablation and collection.

49.25 Labor Room

Department and name of the equipment	Usage and purpose
Equipment for assisted delivery	These instruments/devices are used to assist in the delivery of a baby as an alternative to the ventouse (vacuum extraction). Obstetrical forceps are an instrument that can be used.
Labour table	Table used for the delivery of the babies.

49.26 Radiology

Department and name of the equipment	Usage and purpose
Camera Scintillation (Gamma)	Gamma camera catches gamma rays emitted by radiopharmaceutical material injected into the patient. This is then converted into visible light photons (scintillation).
Computed Tomography (CT)	CT is basically a computerized X-ray imaging machine wherein a narrow beam of X-rays is aimed at a patient and the gantry is rotated around the body at a high speed. These X-ray beams after passing through the body of the patient is captured by the detectors and sent to the processing unit for processing. In the processing unit, the cross-sectional images or slices of the body are generated. This is also called as the spiral CT.
Cyclotron/Radio Pharmacy	A cyclotron is a machine used to manufacture short-lived radioactive isotopes that can be used for medical imaging.
Densitometer, bone	Bone densitometry equipment is used to measure the mineral density of the bone. To perform the procedure, a small dose of ionizing radiation is used to produce pictures of organs like lower spine or hips in order to measure bone loss.
Digital Subtraction Angiography (DSA)	Digital subtraction angiography (DSA) is a fluoroscopic technique that is used to visualize the soft tissues and the blood vessels. As the machine is X-ray based, the radiopaque structures such as bones are also captured while performing the procedure. With the help of software in DSA machine, these radiopaque substances are eliminated ('subtracted') digitally from these captured images, thus providing an accurate depiction of the opacified soft tissues and blood vessels.

Department and name of the equipment	Usage and purpose
Laser Imager Camera	These are dry imaging devices or laser printers, to print the multi-format images of digital radiology on the emulation-coated X-ray films.
Leakage Tester	Leakage tester is used for checking the radiation escaping from within the source assembly except for the useful beam.
Magnetic Resonance Imaging (MRI) with Spectroscopy	Magnetic resonance imaging (MRI) is a magnetic and radiofrequency-based machine. The machine uses a high-power magnetic field and computer-generated controlled radiofrequency waves to create detailed images of the organs and tissues of the body. Magnetic fields align the protons of the cell in a unidirectional fashion. Then the radiofrequency waves are fired on the protons, due to which the protons oscillate. This oscillation is captured by the machine and image is produced.
Mammographic Machine	Mammography is used for X-ray imaging of the breasts.
MRI Fiber optic pulse oximeter	MRI pulse oximeter is used to monitor patient's pulse and blood oxygen saturation during MRI scans. As MRI is a magnetic device, a normal pulse oximeter cannot be used inside the MRI room.
Nuclear Computed Tomography (PET CT)	Positron emission tomography–computed tomography (PET-CT) is a combination of a positron emission tomography (PET) scanner and computed tomography (CT) scanner in the same gantry of the machine. Both these scanners capture sequential images in the same session, which when combined produces a single superimposed image. To perform the procedure, the nuclear medicine is administered to the patient and the scan is performed.
Nuclear Magnetic Resonance Imaging System (PET MRI)	A PET/MRI machine is a combination of a positron emission tomography (PET) scanner and MRI scanner in the same machine. Both these scanners capture sequential images in the same session, which when combined produces a single superimposed image. To perform the procedure, the nuclear medicine is administered to the patient and the scan is performed.
PACS	PACS is a picture archiving and communications system. This system electronically stores images and reports. This can also be used to transmit the images electronically through Wi-fi or the internet. Also, the images stored in the PACS can be retrieved at any time when required.
Pressure Die Injector	Pressure injectors is a device used to administer the contrast media to the patient, in a pre-calibrated fashion, for performing the procedure. The device consist of an injector head for placing the syringes filled with contrast material. It has a positron plungers which deliver the contrast from the syringes to the pressure tubing connected to the syringe, and the tubing, in turn, delivers contrast material in the vascular system of the patient.
Ultra Sound Machines	An ultrasound machine is used to take images of organs inside the body using the technique of high-frequency ultrasound waves. This machine sends out high-frequency sound waves, in the body, which reflect off body structures. A computer receives the reflected waves and considering the time lag of receiving the waves from different tissues of the body, creates a picture.
Vascular Doppler	A Doppler ultrasound is a pencil-like thin ultrasound probe to send ultrasound waves at the précised small points and is used to estimate the blood flow through blood vessels by receiving back the bounced high-frequency sound waves by the red blood cells in the vessels.
X-Ray Machine DR systems 800/500/300 MA with fluoroscopy	Digital radiography (DR) is the machine wherein the X-rays are directly received by the detectors. These X-ray photons are then directly converted into a digital image and are sent to the processing unit for further management of the image.

49.27 Biochemistry

Department and name of the equipment	Usage and purpose
Automated clinical chemistry systems	The automated bio-chemistry analyzer is used to quantitatively measure different chemicals and other characteristics of biological samples, with minimum human interference and assistance.

Department and name of the equipment	Usage and purpose
Automated urinalysis system	This is used to automatically analyze the urine.
Carbon-dioxide analyzer	Carbon dioxide analyzers are used to detect and quantify the amount of carbon dioxide in the sample.
Colorimeter, photometer, spectrophotometer	Colorimeter is to ascertain the concentration of a known solute. A spectrophotometer is a photometer to measure intensity as a function of colour, the wavelength of light.
Fully Auto. Immunoassay Analyzer	Immunoassay analyzers are used to test a variety of substances like antiarrhythmic, anticonvulsant, antibiotic and cardiac glycoside drug concentration determination; cardiac markers; endocrine hormone testing; allergy testing; infectious diseases and protein, viral or bacterial toxin determinations etc.
Microscope fluorescence/ UV	UV microscope is used for fluorescent microscopy. Technique wise, the UV light reflects the image of the sample stains to the fluorescence microscope to create and view the generated image.

49.28 Microbiology

Department and name of the equipment	Usage and purpose
Bact Alert System	BacT/Alert is used for growing microorganisms in an automated microbial detection system which is based on the colorimetric detection of CO_2.
Bio Safety Cabinet	This cabinet is used to protect the laboratory worker and the surrounding environment from harmful pathogens. The cabinet is provided with a system to exhaust the air through HEPA-filters. The cabinet is also provided with the ultraviolet lights for killing the harmful bacteria and viruses within the working space of the cabinet.
BOD Incubator	BOD incubator (bio-oxygen demand) for culture growth where a high degree of constant temperature accuracy is required to maintain temperature of the test tissue for culture growth, storage of bacterial cultures and incubation.
CD4 Counter	CD4 cell counter is used to count the CD4 cells (also known as CD4+ T cells) in the blood.
Deep Freezer	Deep freezer is used to store the reagents and kits used in the department under low temperatures.
Elisa Reader with Washer	ELISA plate reader uses the technology of absorbance, luminescence and fluorescence detection modes, including intensity, TRF and polarization to detect and process the biological and chemical data.
Immunofluorescent Microscope	Immunofluorescence microscope is used for tissue sections, cultured cells or individual cells that are fixed using various methods.
Laminar air flow	Laminar airflow is used to improve the quality of air of the workplace by providing unidirectional air at the same speed with no or minimal cross-over of air streams.
Refrigerated centrifuge	Refrigerated centrifuge works on the principle of sedimentation, by holding the sample tubes for rotation at a high speed around a fixed axis. Due to the centripetal force, the denser substances separate at the bottom of the centrifuge tube.
RT-PCR	Real-time polymerase chain reaction (real-time PCR) is used to detect and quantify the gene expression from DNA and RNA.
T.B. Culture Bact/Alert 3D	BacT alert 3D system is an automatic liquid culture machine to continuously monitor the mycobacterial growth and is used for mycobacterial culture from sputum samples.
Thermocycler	Thermocycler is used to amplify DNA and RNA samples by the polymerase chain reaction. The thermocycler, in discrete, pre-programmed steps raises and lowers the temperature of samples in a holding block, allowing for denaturation and reannealing of samples with various reagents.
Vitek	VITEK 2 is used to perform bacterial identification and antibiotic susceptibility testing.

49.29 Pathology

Department and name of the equipment	Usage and purpose
Automated Platelet Counter	Automated platelet counter is used to study distinction among platelets, small debris and erythrocytes.
Binocular Research Microscope	Binocular research microscope has flat-field achromatic objectives and high-performance eyepieces and the lenses, which are coated hard for anti reflection, anti-fungal and having reduced light.
Cell Counter, Normal And Abnormal	The cell counter is used to count different types of cells in the blood like WBC, RBC and platelet.
Cell-freezing apparatus and reagents	Cell freezing is used to successfully freeze cells and resuscitate them from liquid nitrogen storage.
Chromatography (GAS), clinical use	Gas chromatograph (GC) is used to analyze body fluids and tissue homogenates, for detecting chemical compounds that may serve as markers of infection.
Chromatography for bacterial identification	Gas chromatography-vacuum ultraviolet spectroscopy (GC-VUV) is used to determine fatty acid methyl esters (FAMEs) of bacteria, to identify and discriminate different environmental bacteria based on their fatty acid profile.
Chromatography, ion-exchange	Ion chromatography is for separating ions and polar molecules based on their affinity to the ion exchanger. It can work on almost all kinds of charged molecules including large proteins, small nucleotides and amino acids.
Chromatography, thin-layer, methadone	A thin-layer chromatography is used for simultaneous screening and confirmation of methadone and its primary metabolite in urine specimens.
Clinitek status analyzer	The Clinitek status analyzer is for urinalysis to read urine test strips and Clinitest hCG cassettes.
Coagulation, automated	Coagulation analyzer is used for the measurement of blood platelet levels. It is used to measure the coagulation pathway speed, as well as thrombolin and thromboplastin levels.
Counter, automated cell	Automated cell counters are used to automatically determine and count the number and types of cells present in the sample like blood or urine.
Cytocentrifuge/Cytospin	A cytocentrifuge, or cytospin, is a centrifuge used to concentrate on cells in liquid specimens onto a microscope slide to enable stain and examination.
Enzyme immunoassay	Immunoassay is used in which an enzyme bound to an antigen or antibody functions as a label is tested.
Fibrometer	FibroMeter is for blood testing for evaluation and management of liver fibrosis. This test was specifically for patients with chronic viral hepatitis.
Heamatology Analyser	A haematology analyzer is used to perform a complete blood count (CBC) or hemogram. It performs a quantitative and qualitative analysis of the formed elements of the blood: Red blood cells, white blood cells and platelets.
Mass spectrometer	Mass spectrometry is used to measure the mass-to-charge ratio (m/z) of one or more molecules in a sample. These measurements are used to calculate the exact molecular weight of the sample components.
Micrometers, microscope	Microscope micrometers are used for measuring or counting specimens. Eyepiece micrometres (reticles) are small glass discs with markings on them. The micrometre is mounted in one of the two eyepieces and superimposes an image of the markings over the image of the specimen.
Microscope inverted stage, tissue culture	In an inverted microscope, the light source of light and the condenser are placed on the top of the stage, pointing down toward the stage. The objectives are placed below the stage pointing upwards.
Microtome	A microtome is used to cut thin slices of the tissue to be examined. The cut tissues are made to float on the surface of water bath to eliminate wrinkles and distortion in the tissue. Thereafter, the tissues are taken on the slide for examination.
Platelet Aggregometer	A platelet aggregometer is used to check how well the platelets clump together to form blood clots.
Processor, tissue automated	Tissue processor is used for diffusion of various substances into and out of porous tissues.

Department and name of the equipment	Usage and purpose
Projection microscope	Projection microscope has an added feature to the microscope to project the microscopic image to a wall or projecting screen.
Radioimmunoassay	Radio immunoassay is used to check the specificity of an antigen–antibody reaction to detect and quantify target molecules in biological samples.
Rotary microtome	The rotary microtome is to reduce vibration during microtomy, in which stability is important during sectioning to prevent undulations in the paraffin sections.
Slide Stainer, immersion type	Automated slide strainers are devices that automatically stains the peripheral blood and other hematologic smears to facilitate laboratory microscope differential counts using Wright's stain.
Spectrophotometer digital	Digital spectrophotometer is for spectrophotometric analysis of any concentration.
Stereoscopic microscopes	Stereo microscopes is for 3D viewing of specimens visible to the naked eye. They are also known as low power or dissecting microscopes.

49.30 Blood Bank

Department and name of the equipment	Usage and purpose
Apherisis machine	An apheresis machine is used to separate the donors' blood into its various components like plasma, platelets, white blood cells and red blood cells.
Blood bag tube sealer	The blood tube sealer is to seal the tube of blood bag without causing haemolysis and leakage of blood.
Blood Bank refrigerator	The blood bank refrigerator provides a safe and convenient environment for storage of whole blood, blood components (e.g. blood cells and plasma) and reagents.
Blood collection monitor	A blood collection monitor is a device used to monitor the collection of blood during donation to protect over or under bleeding of the patient.
Blood donor couch (Mobile)	The blood donor couch is to provide a comfortable position to the donor during blood donation process. The blood donor chair has features for adjustment of height, arm and position.
Blood mixing and blood weighting device	A blood mixing device is used to mix blood or blood components by agitation.
Cryo Bath unit	Cryo baths is to control the temperature by microcontroller based PID controller up to an accuracy of 1 °C. to ensure uniform temperature, the bath unit is provided with a circulating pump.
Deep freezer –40 °C and –80 °C	Deep freezer is used for storage of blood components like plasma in the blood bank.
Dielectric sealer	Dielectric sealer is a device where radio frequency (RF) energy is used for joining thermoplastic films using wherein the molecules of the materials are excited to be joined from inside out, fusing the materials together.
Elisa reader with washer	ELISA plate reader uses the technology of absorbance, luminescence and fluorescence detection modes, including intensity, TRF and polarization to detect and process the biological and chemical data.
HB meter	A hemoglobinometer is to measure haemoglobin blood concentration. In this machine, the technique of spectrophotometric measurement is used for measuring the haemoglobin concentration.
ID centrifuge	ID centrifuge is an automatic balance controlled silent centrifuge machine with a capacity of up to 12 ID-cards.
Mechanical shaker	A shaker is used to mix, blend or agitate substances in a tube or flask by shaking them. A shaker contains an oscillating board that is used to place the flasks, beakers or test tubes.
Plasma extractor	Plasma extractor is used to extract plasma from the centrifuged bags of blood. This is done by applying pressure on the collected bag through spring loaded front panel.

Department and name of the equipment	Usage and purpose
Platelet agitator	Platelet agitator is to store platelet concentrates and provide continuous gentle horizontal motion to the packs at a fixed speed and temperature of 20–24 °C.
Platelet incubator	Platelet incubators provide accurate and stable storage conditions for platelets, small cell fragments.
Refrigerated centrifuge	Refrigerated centrifuge works on the principle of sedimentation, by holding the sample tubes for rotation at a high speed around a fixed axis. Due to the centripetal force, the denser substances separate at the bottom of the centrifuge tube.
Thawing Bath	Plasma thawing Bath is for rapid and uniform thawing of fresh frozen plasma (FFP) bags at 37 °C.
Water Bath serological	Serology water bath is used to incubate samples in water at a constant temperature over a long period of time.

49.31 CSSD

Department and name of the equipment	Usage and purpose
Cleaner, ultrasonic, medical instrument	Ultrasonic surgical instrument cleaner is used for cleaning the metallic or plastic surgical instruments, sharp instruments, endoscopic surgical instruments including suction tips and ET tubes.
Dry heat sterilizer	For the items that might be damaged by moist heat or that are impenetrable to moist heat, dry heat ovens are used to sterilize them.
Ethylene oxide gas sterilizer	Ethylene oxide sterilizers are used to sterilize heat- and moisture sensitive instruments, consumables like plastic or rubber items, that would be damaged by pure steam or liquid chemical. In this instrument, the ethylene oxide gas is used for sterilization.
Infectious waste burner (incinerator)	Incinerator is used to transform medical wastes into inorganic, incombustible matter which becomes non-infectious and leads to reduction of volume and weight of the waste.
Plasma sterilizer	Plasma sterilizer is a sterilizer using the technique called oxidation. The plasma when used produces a chemical reaction due to which all microorganisms are deactivated. The high heat turns the molecules of the hydrogen peroxide into free radicals, which are highly unstable.
Pressure sterilizers	An autoclave is a machine used for sterilization at elevated temperature and pressure.
Sterilizer (autoclave)	Autoclaves are also known as steam sterilizers, and this is a device that uses steam under pre-determined pressure to destroy harmful bacteria, viruses, fungi and spores on items that are placed inside the sterilizer.

Other Small Items, Consumables, Furniture Used in the Hospital

49.32 Misc. Small Instruments

B.P. Apparatus	Needle Holder
Baby Weighing Machine	Nebulizer heavy duty
Chetal Forceps	Otoscopes
Cidex Trays 222 × 82 × 41	Splints and tourniquets
Cidex Trays 400 × 70 × 50	Sponge holder
Ear Speculum	Syringe needle destroyer
Examination Lamps	Stethoscope adult
Formalin Chamber Medium	Stethoscope Paed.
Fumigator 5 Ltr.	Suction machine baby

Hammer small	Torch
Height scale	Tongue depressor
Humidifiers	Trauma packs and kits
Laryngoscopes	Weight machine adult
Mortuary cabinets (cooled)	X-ray view box double
Nasal forceps	X-ray view box single

49.33 Misc. Disposable Items

Bowls 10″	Feeding cup
Bowls 4″	Instrument tray 200 × 150 × 50
Dressing drum SS 9 × 11	Instrument tray 300 × 250 × 50
Dressing drum SS 9 × 14	Instrument tray 310 × 195 × 63
Dressing drum SS 9 × 9	Kidney tray 150 × 70
Dressing forceps jar	Kidney tray 250 × 100
Dust bins	

49.34 Linen

Bed sheets	OT linen
Blankets	Patient gown
Doctors dress	Patient kurta
Draw sheet	Patient lower
Linen sets	Pillow cover
Macintosh	Towels

49.35 Consumables

Caps	O.T consumables
Cleaning consumables	OPD consumables
CSSD consumables	Printing material
Emergency drugs	Sleepers
Gloves	Stationery
ICU's consumables	Ward consumables like cotton, bandage, gauze, betadine and Savlon
Masks	

49.36 Back Up Services

Ambulance	Hospital operating software
Autoclaves	Oxygen cylinders 'A' type
Bed partitions	Oxygen cylinders 'B' type
Cleaning equipment	Televisions
Computers with printers and UPS	Water coolers
Fridges	

49.37 Patient Furniture

Attendants stool	Dressing trollies
Attendants couch	I.V. stand
Bed screens	I.V. rod
Bed side locker deluxe	Instrument trolley
Bed side locker general	Mattress
Beds deluxe	Over bed table
Beds general	Patient stool
Beds ICU motorized	Pillows
Beds semi fowler motorized	Step stool (double)
Cribs	Stretcher trolley
Cylinder trollies	Wheel chairs

Further Reading

Bhawan P, Road CIG. MEDICAL EQUIPMENT MAINTENANCE POLICY (2012).:27.

Biomedical Equipment List [Internet]. MedShare. [cited 2021 Jul 15]. Available from: https://www.medshare.org/biomedical-equipment/

Glossary

°F Degrees Fahrenheit
3D 3 Dimensional
ABP Ambulatory Blood Pressure
AC Air Conditioning
ACH OA Air Changes per Hour—Outdoor Air
ACH SA Air Changes per Hour—Smart Air
ACT Activated Clotting Time
ADT Admission, Transfer, Discharge
AEP Auditory Evoked Potential
AHU Air Handling Unit
AMC Annual Maintenance Contract
Amp Amperes
APC Argon Plasma Coagulation
ARD Automatic Rescue Device
ATM Automated Teller Machine
AV Audio-Video
B.E.P Break Even Point
BAC Blood Alcohol Concentration
BOD Bio-Oxygen Demand
BP Blood Pressure
BSC Bio Safety Cabinet
BSL Bio Safety Lab
Cat Category
Cath Lab Coronary Catheterization Laboratory
CAV Constant Air Volume
CCTV Closed Circuit Television System
CD Compact Disk
cd/m^2 Candela Per Square Metre
CEO Chief Executive Officer
CFM Cubic Feet per Minute
CIC Circulating Immune Complexes
CMC Comprehensive Maintenance Contract
CNS Central Nursing Station
CO_2 Carbon dioxide
COPD Chronic Obstructive Pulmonary Disease
CPAP Continuous Positive Airway Pressure
CR Computerised Radiography
CRRT Continuous Renal Replacement Therapy
CSSD Central Sterile Services Department
CT Computerised Tomography
CTG Cardiotocograph
CTVS Cardiothoracic and Vascular Surgery
CUSA Cavitron Ultrasonic Surgical Aspirator
D & C Dilation and Curettage
D.G Diesel Generator
D.S.C.R Debt Service Coverage Ratio
dBA Decibel
Derma Dermatology
DEXA Dual Energy X-ray Absorptiometry
dia Diameter
DICOM Digital Imaging and Communications
DLCO Diffusing capacity of the Lungs for Carbon Monoxide
DNA Deoxyribonucleic Acid
DOT Directly Observed Treatment
DPR Detailed Project Report
DR Digital Radiography
DSA Digital Subtraction Angiography
DSE Dobutamine Stress Echocardiography
DVD Digital Video Disc or Digital Versatile Disc
DVR Digital Video Recorder
DVT Deep Vein Thrombosis
DX Direct Expansion
e.g. For Example
EBB Earth Bonding Bar
EBUS Endobronchial Ultrasound
ECG Electrocardiograph
ECHS Ex-Servicemen Contributory Health Scheme
ECI Extracorporeal Immunoadsorption
ECM Electronically Commutated Motors

A. Garg, A. Dewan, *Manual of Hospital Planning and Designing*,
https://doi.org/10.1007/978-981-16-8456-2

ECT Electroconvulsive Therapy
ECT Electroconvulsive therapy
EDA Electro Dermal Activity
EEG Electroencephalogram
EGG Electroglottograph
ELISA Enzyme Linked Immunosorbent Assay
ELV Extra Low Voltage
EMG Electro Mayo Graph
EMO Emergency Medical Officer
EMR Electronic Medical Records
ENG Electronystagnogram
ENT Eat Nose Throat
EP Electrophysiology
EPABX Electronic Private Automatic Branch Exchange
Epm Unverricht–Lundborg disease
EPS Electrophysiology Studies
EPS Earnings Per Share
ERCP Endoscopic Retrograde Cholangiopancreatography
ESI Employees' State Insurance
ESU Electrosurgical Unit
ESW Extracorporeal Sock Wave
ESWL Extracorporeal Shock Wave Lithotripsy
ETO Ethylene Oxide
ETP Effluent Treatment Plant
EUS Endoscopic Ultrasound
FAME Fatty Acid Methyl Ester
FAR Floor Area Ratio
FCC Fire Command Centre
FCU Fan Coil Units
FeNO Fractional Exhaled Nitric Oxide
FFP Fresh Frozen Plasma
FPI Fins Per Inch
FPM Feet Per Minute
FRLS Fire Retard Low Smoke
FRP Fibre Reinforced Plastic
FSI Floor Space Index
ft. Feet
G.I Galvanized Iron
G.I. Gastro Intestinal
Gastro Gastroenterology
GC Gas Chromatograph
GC-VUV Gas Chromatography-Vacuum Ultraviolet Spectroscopy
GERD Gastroesophageal Reflux Disease
GRN Goods Received Note
Gynae Gynaecology
H.R Human Resources
HDD Hard Disk Drive
HDMI High Definition Multimedia Interface
HDU High Dependency Unit
HEPA High-Efficiency Particulate Air
HFNC Hi Flow Nasal Cannula
HIS Health Information System
HIV Human Immunodeficiency Virus
HL7 Health Level Seven
HMS Hospital Management System
HOD Head Of Department
HP High Pressure
HRUS High-resolution Ultrasonography
HT High Tension
HVAC Heating Ventilation and Air Conditioning
I.A.B.P. Intra Aortic Balloon Pump
IBMS Integrated Building Management System
ICCU Intensive Cardiac Care Unit
ICD International Classification of Diseases
ICRA Investment Information and Credit Rating Agency
ICT Information and Communication Technologies
ICTC Integrated Counselling and Testing Centres
ICU Intensive Care Unit
ID Inner Diameter
ID Identity Document
IEEE Institute of Electrical and Electronics Engineers
IETF Internet Engineering Task Force
IgG Immunoglobulin's
IITV Image Intensifying Television
IOL Intraocular Lens
IOP Intraocular Pressure
IP Internet Protocol
IPD In Patient Department
IPL Intense Pulsed Light
IPS Isolated Power Supply
IPTV Internet Protocol television
IRDS Infant Respiratory Distress Syndrome
IRR Internal Rate of Return
ISMS Integrated Security Management System
IT Information Technology
IUP Intrauterine Pressure
IV Intra Venous
IVF In Vitro Fertilization
JCI Joint Commission International
kPa Kilopascal
KV Kilovolt
KVA Kilovolt Ampere
kW Kilowatt

L/min Litres Per Minute
LCD Liquid Crystal Display
LDB Lighting Distribution Board
LDR Labor, Delivery, and Resuscitation
LINAC Linear Accelerator
LIPA Line Probe Assay
LT Low Tension
Ltr. Litre
Lux Unit of Illumination
mA Mill ampere
MA Medical Air
MCB Miniature Circuit Breaker
MCCB Moulded Case Circuit Breaker
MDB Main Distribution Board
MEP Mechanical, Electrical and Plumbing
MEP Maximal Expiratory Pressure
MERV Minimum Efficiency Reporting Value
MGIT 960 Mycobacteria Growth Indicator Tube
MGPS Medical Gases Pipeline System
MHz Megahertz
MICU Medical Intensive Care Unit
MIP Maximal Inspiratory Pressure
MIS Management Information System
MLC Medico Legal Cases
mm Millimetre
MRD Medical Record Department
MRI Magnetic Resonance Imaging
MRL Machine Room Less
MS Mild Steel
N.P.B.T Net Profit Before Tax
N_2 Nitrogen
N_2o Nitrous oxide
NABH National Accreditation Board for Hospitals
NCV Nerve Conduction Velocity
NIBP Non-Invasive Blood Pressure
Ni-Cd Nickel–Cadmium
NICU Neo-natal Intensive Care Unit
O.T. Operation Theatre
O_2 Oxygen
OAE Otoacoustic Emissions
OBS Obstetrics
OCT Optical Coherence Tomography
OD Outer Diameter
OLTC On-load tap changer
Onco Oncology
OPD Out Patient Department
OPG Orthopantomagram
OR Operating Room
Ortho Orthopaedic
PA Personal Assistant
PA Public Address
PAC Pre Anaesthetic Check-up
PACS Picture Archiving and Communication System
PC Personal Computer
PCNL Percutaneous Nephrolithotomy
PDB Power Distribution Boards
PE Premature Ejaculation
Pedia Paediatrics
PERT Program Evaluation Review Technique
PET CT Nuclear Positron Emission Computed Tomography
PET MRI Nuclear Positron Emission Magnetic Resonance Imaging
PF Provident Fund
PFT Pulmonary Function Test
PICU Paediatric Intensive Care Unit
PLC Programmable Logic Control
PNS Peripheral Nerve Stimulation
POP Plaster Of Paris
PPE Personal Protective Equipment
PPM Parts Per Million
PPS Primary Power Supply
PRD Pressure Relief Damper
PSG Polysomnography
PTS Pneumatic Tube Systems
PTZ Pan Tilt Zoom
PUVA Psoralen and Ultraviolet A
PVC Polyvinyl Chloride
PVR Profit Volume Ratio
PWS Patient Warming System
RCC Reinforced Cement Concrete
RCCB Residual Current Circuit Breaker
RF Radio Frequency
RFID Radio Frequency Identification
RH Relative Humidity
RNA Ribonucleic Acid
RO Reverse Osmosis
ROI Return on investment
RONW Return On Net Worth
RR Respiration Rate
RT Radiation Therapy
RT-PCR Real-Time Polymerase Chain Reaction
S.S Stainless Steel
SEP Somatosensory Evoked Potential
SICU Surgical Intensive Care Unit
SMDB Sub-Main Distribution Board
SMS Short Message Service

SOP Standard Operating Procedures
SOW Scope of Work
SPD Surge Protection Devices
SPECT CT Single Photon Emission Computerized Tomography
SPO2 Unit of Measuring Oxygen Saturation
SPR Skin Potential Response
SPS Secondary Power Supply
Sq. Ft. Square Feet
Sq. Mtr Square Meter
SRS Stereotactic Radio Surgery
STP Sewerage Treatment Plant
T.B Tuberculosis
TBNA Transbronchial Needle Aspiration
TCFR Techno Commercial Feasibility Report
TDS Tax Deducted at Source
TDS Total Dissolved Solids
TEE Transesophageal Echocardiography
TMS Transcranial Magnetic Stimulation
TMT Treadmill Test
TPA Third Party Administrator
TPS Tertiary Power Supply
TSSU Theatre Sterile Supply Unit
TT Lab Transmissible Tests
TV Television
UGI Upper Gastrointestinal
UHID Unique Health Identification
UPS Uninterrupted Power Supply
UPVC Unplasticized Polyvinyl Chloride
USB Universal Serial Bus
UV Ultra Violet
VAV Variable Air Volume
VCB Vacuum Circuit Breaker
VCD Vacuum Constriction Device
VED Vital, Essential, Desirable
VEEG Video Electroencephalography
VFD Variable Frequency Device
VIE Vacuum Insulated Evaporator
VIP Very Important Person
VLC Visible Light Communications
VNG Videonystagmograph
VRLA Valve Regulated Sealed Lead Acid
WC Water Closet
WC Water Column
WDV Written Down Value
WTP Water Treatment Plant
XLPE Cross Linked Polyethylene